BOUNDLESS

UPGRADE YOUR BRAIN, OPTIMIZE YOUR BODY & DEFY AGING

BEN GREENFIELD

VICTORY BELT PUBLISHING INC.
Las Vegas

Cover design by Allan Santos
Interior design and illustrations by Charisse Reyes, Crizalie Olimpo, Allan Santos, and Elita San Juan
Printed in Canada
TC 0120

CONTENTS

INTRODUCTION

Boundless

Adjective: unlimited or immense

Synonyms: *limitless, unbounded, untold, bottomless, immeasurable, measureless, incalculable, inestimable, abundant, abounding, great, inexhaustible*

WELCOME TO YOUR
BLUEPRINT FOR
BECOMING BOUNDLESS.

The average person wanders through life with brain fog, bloating, gas, indigestion, constipation, crunching joints, insomnia, lost libido, fibroids, cysts, acne, and piles upon piles of a lifetime of accumulated excess fats releasing inflammatory molecules and squeezing the lifeblood out of their organs. And amid all this physical pain and fatigue, we're constantly searching for evasive meaning and elusive happiness. Look around you. We're a step away from being the useless, soft-drink-sipping blobs who float on hovering chairs through the hallways in the robot cartoon *Wall-E*.

This complete lack of realization of our full human potential begins when we're babies, as we can see in the host of health issues the up-and-coming generation is experiencing, including lack of proper muscle and brain growth, immune system weakness, low IQ, stunted growth, obesity, depression, attention deficit disorder, social anxiety, and other frustrating problems that parents, teachers, and society as a whole now accept as all too common.

But what if this didn't have to be?

What if our kids were tiny, optimized human machines?

After all, Mozart learned to play the piano at the age of four, composed his first piece at age five, and wrote his first symphony at age eight. Pablo Picasso, when he was just twelve, had an astonishing grasp of the fundamentals of art and was producing photo-realistic anatomical sketches. Gian Lorenzo Bernini was churning out intricate, lifelike stone sculptures at only eight years old. But these folks aren't special childhood prodigies, savants, or some kind of unique geniuses. These are normal human beings. Sadly, in our modern era, we've forgotten how to nurture and grow an amazing human mind, body, and spirit. Instead, we've settled for a generation of kids who wind up on PeopleOfWalmart.com—attached to leashes and chewing on Ritalin.

And what if we adults—you and I—could leap out of bed each morning and tackle the day with the extreme ferocity of an electrified tiger? What if our performance, fat loss, recovery, digestion, brain, sleep, hormones, and spirits were optimized and firing on all cylinders? What if we all walked around like superheroes with a body like Batman's, a mind like those of the heroes of the smart-drug movies *Limitless* and *Lucy*, and a spirit like an enlightened yogi's? What if you could speed-read, memorize cards, remember the names of everyone at the cocktail party, wear any jeans you want, step onto a beach with your chest out and abs in, age gracefully with zero Botox and liposuction required, and have an intense feeling of inner peace, love, joy, happiness, and spiritual satisfaction?

What if this ability to look, feel, and perform at the human body's full capacity wasn't the stuff of lore but was instead the status quo? Sure, there are UFC and NFL gladiators fighting for glory on television with optimized bodies, random monks and meditators wandering the planet with optimized spirits, and professional poker players, computer programmers, and race car drivers hunched over card games, keyboards, and steering wheels with optimized minds. But in a perfect world—a world that is fully attainable—you would have it all: total optimization of body, spirit, and mind.

You would be, in a word, *boundless*.

So what does being boundless actually look like and feel like?

Owning a boundless mind means you have balanced and complete levels of important neurotransmitters so that your nervous system can flawlessly communicate; your brain is free of inflammation and fog; you've developed potent stress-banishing and cortisol-decreasing strategies; your IQ is elevated, along with your working memory and executive function; you understand how to effectively use nootropics, smart drugs, and brain-enhancing foods, biohacks, gear, and tools; your sleep is pure, uninterrupted, and efficient; and, ultimately, you feel as though you actually have power and control over your thoughts, feelings, interactions, and communication.

Owning a boundless body means you know how to rapidly get lean and burn fat; you know how to build muscle in the safest, cleanest, and fastest way possible; you've fixed your gut, eliminated digestive issues, and maximized nutrient absorption; you know the ideal movements, exercises, tools, foods, supplements, and workouts for strength, power, speed, balance, mobility, and endurance; you've cracked the code on maximizing recovery and recovery speed; you possess an unstoppable immune system; and you have a potent arsenal of tools to increase your symmetry and beauty.

Owning a boundless spirit means that you can consciously control your thoughts and beliefs to positively affect your health; you have a thriving practice of gratitude, love, and joy; you understand how to use currently fringe methods such as sound healing and vibrational frequencies to enhance your physiology; you've optimized your social connections, friendships, and relationships; you've maximized tantra, love, and sexual satisfaction; you've optimized the hidden variables that can make or break your mind, body, and spirit, including air, light, electricity, and water; you've learned from residents of the world's Blue Zones and longevity hot spots how to optimize your life, happiness, and fulfillment; and your daily habits and routines have allowed you to create your perfect day.

This book is your blueprint to becoming boundless—to being able to defy the modern norm of staggering through life with low energy, brain fog, a sluggish body, and untapped potential and instead call upon every shred of energy you want whenever you need it, so that you can achieve the most adventurous, joyful, and fulfilling life possible.

WHO THIS BOOK IS FOR

Allow me to give you an example of the type of person who could use a guide for becoming boundless. Imagine a man named Kevin. Kevin is standing in front of his bathroom mirror: frowning, concentrating, and flexing all at the same time as he stares at and analyzes his thirty-two-year-old body. For the past five years, he's lived as a self-described health seeker and has even been accused of being a "woo-woo fitness geek," but it's certainly been an uphill, frustrating battle of perusing recommended books, scrolling through fitness blogs, and experimenting with low-carb, low-fat, low-gluten, low-dairy, low-lectin, and definitely low-taste diets. Yet his body still doesn't feel "right." At his desk job as a materials engineer, he scrunches the glasses up his nose and squints at the computer monitor when his afternoon brain fog sets in; he's never actually done that triathlon he keeps saying he'll eventually do; and his gut rumbles with mild, distracting bloating all through the day. Despite some success at hacking and upgrading his body and brain, he still feels empty, and he's considering signing up for his eighth ayahuasca retreat so that he can keep working on finding his purpose. He's also considering opting instead for a ten-day Vipassana meditation, which he just heard on a health podcast is a better way to discover how to live the adventurous, joyful, fulfilling life he craves and hasn't found yet.

Deep inside, Kevin wishes that he had some kind of a blueprint for the human machine that he could use to cut through all the confusion keeping him from getting what he wants—a blueprint he could understand without a doctorate in human science, but one also steeped in research and experience, with clear instructions that could finally allow him to look, feel, and perform the way he knows he can without wasting his time or using old-school, inefficient techniques.

That's the exact blueprint you're now holding in your hands: a complete prescription for becoming boundless. In this book, you're going to discover exactly how to connect with, nourish, feel, taste, and see what it is to be boundless for the remainder of your long and fulfilled life.

You can consider this book to be your step-by-step guide to optimizing your life force, achieving a plane of higher existence, and realizing the full potential of the human machine—including increasing your intelligence, decoding sleep and sleep cycles, maximizing symmetry and beauty, building muscle, burning fat, having mind-blowing sex, defying aging, achieving maximum longevity, and acquiring deep and lasting love and happiness.

You will learn the fine pursuit of becoming not just a good exerciser or a really fit person, but a completely optimized human being who is able to "crush it" in all aspects of life, from body to mind to spirit and beyond—a human being who, in the words of science fiction novelist Robert Heinlein, can "change a diaper, plan an invasion, butcher a hog, conn a ship, design a building, write a sonnet, balance accounts, build a wall, set a bone, comfort the dying, take orders, give orders, cooperate, act alone, solve equations, analyze a new problem, pitch manure, program a computer, cook a tasty meal, fight efficiently, die gallantly." In other words, all the push-ups and pull-ups and squats in the world don't matter unless you are able to live an adventurous, fulfilling, joyful, and limitless life with distinct purpose and meaning. To die having left your distinct mark on the world and having encountered everything our grand universe has to offer. I don't know about you, but I think that's a pretty cool way to experience life—and if, like me, you have been nagged by a restless feeling that there must be more to life than mere day-to-day existence, then this book is for you.

Upon diving into the first several chapters of this book, you will discover that you actually can look, feel, and perform the way you've always sensed that remarkable and complex human beings should be able to. You'll find that your willpower, cognition, decision-making, lack of procrastination, and focus can all be biologically enhanced without spending thousands of dollars on biohacks or an advanced mind-training vacation. With a new, sharpened mind, you'll go on to see how simple it is to look good naked while enhancing your body's power, speed, mobility, balance, and stamina. You'll crack the code on optimizing hormones, fixing digestion, determining the perfect diet for you, and never wasting a second in the gym again. Finally, you will receive the icing on the cake: the elusive and meaningful happiness the world's Blue Zones and longevity hot spots have discovered, along with exactly how to foster that same happy life for yourself by pursuing gratitude, love, relationships, purpose, and meaning. Upon turning the final page in this book, you will have transformed yourself, your body, and your brain into a living being capable of stepping out the door and into the sunshine to enjoy the ultimate joyful, adventurous, and fulfilling life.

ABOUT ME

But you may be wondering why you should listen to me: a messy-haired, biohacking, self-experimenting immersive journalist who lives his life off-grid in the backwoods of Washington State on a goats-and-chickens farm with my wife and twin boys.

Allow me to give you a bit of background.

I was raised in rural northern Idaho and homeschooled through twelfth grade. I was president of the chess club, a thirteen-year violin veteran, a fantasy fiction author, and a boy who spent most of his childhood years with his nose in a book or traipsing through the countryside with a handmade bow and spear.

I graduated high school at age fifteen and, after receiving an offer to play varsity tennis, began college at sixteen. For four years, I studied anatomy, physiology, biomechanics, pharmaceuticals, microbiology, biochemistry, and nutrition, eventually completing a rigorous series of strength and conditioning certifications and internships at Duke University and the NFL before graduating at age twenty as the top senior in my class at the University of Idaho—all while working as a bartender, personal trainer, lab assistant, nutritionist, spinning instructor, athletic trainer, and strength and conditioning coach. During this rigorous course of study, I competed as president of the triathlon club, middle for the volleyball team, hole set for the water polo team, and onstage as a muscle-bound bodybuilder at 215 pounds and 3 percent body fat, drenched in glitter and tanning cream with a hefty dose of red wine and dark chocolate to make my veins pop.

After completing my bachelor's degree in exercise science and getting married to a Montana farm girl, I was accepted at six medical schools. But I quickly became disillusioned with the failures of modern medicine and opted instead to attain a master's degree in exercise physiology and biomechanics, after which I leaped hard-core into the fitness world, partnering with physicians and opening a series of personal-training studios, gyms, and physiology and biomechanics labs across Idaho and Washington—eventually being voted America's top personal trainer in 2008.

In late 2008, I became the father of twin sons, sold all my studios and gyms, and pivoted into homeschooling my boys; writing, speaking, and consulting; launching one of the world's first fitness podcasts; becoming a *New York Times* bestselling author of thirteen books; and starting a blog that now reaches over two million rabid fans each month. During this time, while making a name for myself as a relentless self-experimenter and biohacker, I became a pro obstacle course racer, completed the coveted Spartan Delta (a collection of nine of the most brutal obstacle-course-racing events on the planet), trained with Navy SEALs, competed across the globe in open-water swims, mountain runs, and adventure races, won multiple USA bowhunting competitions, and appeared on the planet's toughest reality TV shows.

While building an empire in the fitness industry, I competed as one of the top-ranked amateur triathletes in the world, completing over 120 races spanning over 6,200 miles and 13 Ironman triathlons, winning gold medals for the USA in long course triathlon, and leading swim, bike, and run enthusiasts in guided adventures through Hawaii, Thailand, Japan, and beyond. In 2013 and 2014, I was named one of the world's one hundred most influential people in health and fitness and began to coach the world's top CEOs, chefs, biohackers, poker players, tennis players, motocross and endurance competitors, and professional athletes from the UFC, the NHL, the NBA, the NFL, and beyond—along with advising and investing in a multitude of companies in the health, fitness, and nutrition industry.

Along the way, I've had the privilege to travel the world to hunt down fringe superfoods and supplements, biohacks and blood tests, centenarians and scientists, and all manner of little-known but highly effective ways to optimize your life. Within the pages of this book, you'll find plenty of the wisdom and practical tips I've discovered from those experts, along with what I've learned in the trenches as I traveled the globe and subjected my body to the brutality of being bloodied, frozen, dehydrated, drained, and pushed to the absolute limits of human physical and mental performance.

Today, from my quiet home on ten acres in the forested wilderness of Washington, I grow all my own food, hunt all my own meat, and combine my experiences of intense time in the trenches with a dose of ancestral wisdom and modern science to operate as CEO of Kion, a mind-, body-, and spirit-optimization company that serves as my wheelhouse for creating new supplement formulations and health foods; inspiring media, articles, and books; and coaching and consulting for the world's health seekers, wellness geeks, biohackers, and hard-charging high achievers to help them live limitless lives with complete minds, bodies, and spirits; flawless brains and nervous systems; optimized performance, beauty, hormones, and beyond; and lasting health, happiness, and longevity.

I read a book every day, spend most of my mornings immersed in health and fitness research, still toe the starting line of ruthless endurance and strength competitions, and self-experiment with every biohack, fitness tool, and supplement on the face of the planet, figuring out via a process of immersion in research and self-experimentation what works, what doesn't, and what threatens to give you hair loss, insomnia, or explosive diarrhea.

So that's me. But although this book is richly enhanced with stories from my own immersive experiences and deep, meaningful conversations I've had with the world's leading experts on the topic of becoming boundless, it's not about me. It's about you.

HOW TO GET THE MOST OUT OF THIS BOOK

As you read, don't feel pressured to digest this entire book cover to cover. Instead, think of *Boundless* as a cookbook for any element of your mind, body, or spirit that you want to target with laser-like precision. Are you trying to heal an injury fast, recover from surgery, or simply banish your ever-expanding morning soreness? Flip to chapter 12. Are you sick of afternoon brain fog, curious about the emerging world of smart drugs, or want an extra edge for cognition? Read chapter 5. Do you want to combine the secrets of the ancients with modern biohacking science to live as long as possible with stellar health? Then chapter 19 is for you.

Sure, each chapter builds on the last in terms of developing your knowledge and understanding and allowing you to become an expert in all things related to what makes your brain tick, your body work, and your spirit happy, but please don't think you need to take on this entire book at once if that's not your desired approach. Yes, I've designed it so that professional athletes, coaches, physicians, medical researchers, physical therapists, personal trainers, nutritionists, and other health professionals can take their game to the next level with the information they discover. But I have also had non-experts in mind—like Kevin, our materials engineer yearning for something more—so that anyone can flip to any chapter and discover research-proven, reality-tested techniques to build muscle, burn fat, live longer, have mind-blowing sex, raise healthy and robust children, and much, much more.

When I first finished *Boundless*, it was a beast—over 1,200 pages long. Although I edited it down to the exact version you're now reading, I have painstakingly gone through the steps to ensure that every last piece of cut content and every relevant study, podcast, book, and much more are all online, with a special webpage devoted to each chapter. You'll find the necessary website URL at the end of each chapter. You can use these resource webpages to take an extremely deep dive into any topic you discover within the pages of *Boundless*.

Phew. That's it. You ready for this?

It's time to become boundless.

#beboundless

COFFEE, BOOZE & HORROR FLICKS

HOW TO REWIRE YOUR SKULL'S SUPERCOMPUTER

In 2013, on a brutally hot day at Ironman Canada, I officially bonked. The bonk hit me hard at mile 14 of the 26.2-mile marathon run course. Up until this point, through the entire 2.4-mile swim, 112-mile bike ride, and previous 13 miles of pounding the blistering pavement, things had been going quite well—as well as things can go when both nostrils are crusted with sweat and salt, piss is dripping down the insides of both legs and burning the spandex blisters on your skin, and your feet feel like dead fish mashed inside stiff running shoes.

If you are unfamiliar with the term *bonk*, allow me to explain.

A bonk happens when your entire body runs out of carbohydrates. Usually, the sugars stored in your muscles and liver, known as glycogen, can fuel about one and a half to two hours of exercise. When you shove carbohydrates down your gaping maw in the form of gels, sports drinks, energy bars, and, at this point in the race, just about anything else you can get your sweaty paws on, including cookies, Coke, and candy from Ironman aid stations, this time to exhaustion can be extended by several more torturous hours.

But eventually, the bonk occurs. When it finally strikes, your entire body and brain shut down, fast. Your tongue sags out of the corner of your mouth as if you were a drunken sailor. Your pelvic muscles lose their precious grip on your bowels. You forget third-grade math. Things get ugly. Since fat is not metabolized into ATP—your body's primary form of energy—as quickly as carbohydrates are, your pace slows to an embarrassing stroll-in-the-park speed, and a midrace nap by the side of the road becomes incredibly appealing.

But this bonk took me by surprise. See, I thought I had figured out a way to biohack the bonk. My bonk-proof strategy wasn't sexy back then, and nobody was talking much about it, but it's called *ketosis*. By forcing my body to adapt to an incredibly high-fat, low-carbohydrate diet in the months leading up to the race and then consuming primarily MCT oil, coconut oil, electrolytes, and low amounts of a slow-release form of carbohydrate during the race, I thought I could spare muscle glycogen and instead begin burning the tens of thousands of calories of stored body fat that even the leanest of endurance athletes possess. Sounds reasonable, right?

Not quite. Based on the fact that it took half a liter of sickeningly sweet Coke, two energy gels, and an entire plastic bottle of neon-green Gatorade to snap me out of my midrace stupor, the strategy was far from reasonable. Something went wrong.

So what happened?

It turns out I had neglected one critical variable. Five days after the race, I explained my Canadian conundrum to my friend Dr. Peter Attia, a physician and researcher who crushes twenty-four-hour bicycle rides and brutal CrossFit workouts in a completely fasted state.

"Oh, that's simple," he grunted. "You didn't bonk. You got central nervous system fatigue."

Central nervous system fatigue? I faintly remembered my exercise physiology professor describing this unique cause of burnout. It's a bonk-like feeling that occurs when something significant changes in the concentration of neurotransmitters, the brain's signaling chemicals. As the brain and body work harder and harder, muscle tissue is broken down, resulting in increased levels of a sleep-inducing amino acid called tryptophan. Tryptophan crosses the blood-brain barrier and, smack-dab in the middle of an adrenaline-pumping competition, causes you to crave a post-Thanksgiving-dinner siesta. Tryptophan is the precursor to the neurotransmitter serotonin, and increased levels of serotonin can cause lethargy, depress motor neuron excitability, alter nervous system and hormone functions, decrease the strength of muscular contractions, and even impair judgment.

In addition, during CNS fatigue, levels of excitatory neurotransmitters such as dopamine and acetylcholine plummet, which is why copious amounts of caffeine and, interestingly, amphetamines can help counteract it. I suspect this is why so many endurance athletes, beyond sucking down as much sugar as they can get their hands on, turn to heavily caffeinated fuels such as Red Bull, Coke, and even NoDoz tablets during a long race. (If you want a comprehensive resource on the central nervous system, check out the book *Endure* by Alex Hutchinson. It takes a deep dive into everything a human being can do to override mental and physical fatigue.)

But unhealthy boatloads of carbs and caffeine weren't Dr. Attia's solution. Instead, he presented one simple suggestion: "Amino acids. You just need to take a bunch of amino acids every hour during the race, and you'll need far fewer carbs and stimulants."

Dr. Attia went on to explain that amino acids are the building blocks of neurotransmitters. When your blood levels of amino acids are low—as might be the case when afternoon brain fog strikes, or you are struck with insomnia, or you can't stop thinking about food, or you feel like lying down for a nap during a workout—it is often because you are experiencing an epic bout of amino acid deficiency and neurotransmitter imbalance. So by mainlining amino acids during an Ironman triathlon, or a hard day at the office, or when you are craving a Snickers bar or a venti Starbucks coffee, you amplify your brain's resistance to fatigue.

So what's the solution that fixed the amino acids problem in every race I competed in from that point forward, and the same hack you can use when you need to balance your own neurotransmitters?

You are about to discover that solution in this chapter, as well as many other solutions to help you improve sleep and mood and banish CNS fatigue. You will learn how to balance your brain, how to test and fix your neurotransmitters, how to reboot your body's tolerance for caffeine, how to mitigate the damage from a night of drinking, and even why you should think twice before ever watching a horror flick again.

To begin your journey to becoming boundless, you must first reboot the communication between your nervous system and your body. If your brain can't talk to your body, then you've got an issue that drastically affects your emotions, intellect, motivation, drive, cravings, focus, and, ultimately, your ability to feel wholly human and tap into your own boundless life force.

NEUROTRANSMITTERS 101

Neurotransmitters, those busy bees buzzing around 24-7, are key in the communication between your body and brain. When your neurotransmitter levels and their signaling pathways are optimized, your nervous system can process information efficiently and communicate with your body during a board meeting, a workout, or sex. You can fall asleep and stay asleep, overcome anxiety, and resist the temptation of that extra pint of chocolate coconut milk ice cream in your freezer. You have the focus and concentration to pore over books and websites while absorbing the precious data you seek. You are, in effect, well on your way to becoming boundless.

But let's face it. Your brain ain't perfect.

Yep, that giant gooey mash-up of neuronal cells, white matter, gray matter, blood vessels, nerves, and squishy tissue sometimes goes south, and, as a result, most of us walk around with broken, inflamed, poorly functioning, and poorly trained brains. When you think about it, it's kinda sad that you have a supercomputer in your cranium that's currently firing like a set of cheapo, half-broken Christmas lights from the general store.

There are multiple ways this amazing machine can wind up functioning at subpar levels. But to understand how the brain can malfunction, you first need to understand how nerve cells communicate with each other.

How Neurons Work

Your brain communicates with the rest of your body by initiating a chain reaction that runs along a string of nerve cells, or neurons. Each neuron has dendrites at its head, where it receives messages, and axons at its end, from which it transmits messages. A neuron relays the message from its dendrites to its axons through an action potential, which is an electrical charge imbalance.

Neurons are not connected to one another physically. Between the presynaptic cell (the neuron sending the message) and the postsynaptic cell (the neuron receiving the message) exists a gap called a synaptic cleft. So how does the brain's message jump from one neuron to the next until it reaches the target gland or muscle?

The presynaptic cell releases neurotransmitters to initiate a new action potential down the postsynaptic cell. The pattern then restarts. What was the postsynaptic cell is now the presynaptic cell, which releases neurotransmitters for the next neuron, the new postsynaptic cell. This process of synaptic transmission repeats until the brain's message reaches its final destination.

Let's look at an example of synaptic transmission that involves the neurotransmitter serotonin. The presynaptic cell makes serotonin from the amino acid tryptophan and then packages that serotonin into vesicles located in end terminals on the presynaptic cell. When an action potential arrives from your brain, that signal passes down the presynaptic cell into the end terminals.

At this point, the serotonin-containing vesicles are released. They cross the synaptic cleft and then release the serotonin so it can bind to

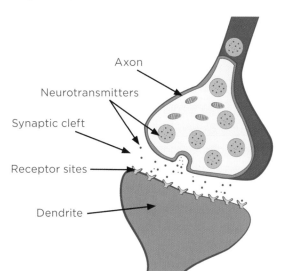

Axon

Neurotransmitters

Synaptic cleft

Receptor sites

Dendrite

receptors on the outside of the postsynaptic cell. If enough serotonin binds to the receptors, a threshold level is reached, the action potential is initiated in that cell, and the message moves on to the next cell. If you wanted to, say, contract your muscles to yank a barbell off the ground, the action potential would eventually reach the skeletal muscle fibers and cause that contraction.

So that the neuron doesn't remain in a constantly switched-on state, the remaining serotonin molecules in the synaptic cleft—the ones that didn't bind to a receptor—are destroyed by enzymes called monoamine oxidase (MAO) and catechol-O-methyltransferase (COMT). Some serotonin also gets returned to the presynaptic cell in a process called reuptake. All of this enables the neuron to switch off and prepares it to receive another signal.

But suppose you had a serotonin deficit, which would compromise the synaptic transmission of any signals dependent on serotonin. This could quickly lead to:

- Depression
- Food cravings
- Brain fog
- Reduced reasoning skills
- Anxiety
- Panic attacks
- Insomnia
- Eating disorders
- Migraines
- Distractibility

Of course, this sort of deficiency can also lead to your crumbling to the pavement during an Ironman. You have probably experienced at least one of these issues before, right? Fact is, millions of people walk around every day with some kind of neurotransmitter deficiency, excess, or suboptimal neuronal communication. The symptoms of a neurotransmitter problem depend on the kind of neurotransmitter involved.

The Most Common Neurotransmitters

In addition to serotonin, the most common neurotransmitters are dopamine, acetylcholine, and gamma-aminobutyric acid (GABA). We tend to associate neurotransmitters with their effects on the brain, but they also affect the body.

Dopamine is the primary motivating chemical; it can promote ambition, drive, and action by influencing the areas of the brain responsible for conscious movement.

Acetylcholine promotes focus, memory, and cognition and is necessary for motor neuron function and muscular movement.

GABA helps you relax and calm down. Without it, you become tense and anxious.

Serotonin also regulates gut motility (the movement of food through the GI tract) and is responsible for good bowel movements.

YOUR UNIQUE
NEUROTRANSMITTER DOMINANCE

In addition to neurotransmitter imbalances and deficits, you likely have some neurotransmitter dominance as well. Most of us naturally tend to have higher levels of a certain neurotransmitter, which causes us to exhibit behaviors associated with that particular neurotransmitter.

Neurotransmitter dominance isn't the same thing as neurotransmitter excess. While a neurotransmitter excess is most often caused by a dysfunction in neurotransmitter production or poor removal of a neurotransmitter from the synapse, a dominance is simply your distinct genetic predisposition to produce higher levels of a given neurotransmitter.

Each kind of neurotransmitter dominance has its strengths—such as better motivation, drive, emotional stability, or stress response—and its weaknesses—such as a tendency toward anxiety, burnout, or fatigue. If you're dominant in a particular neurotransmitter, there's no need to try to reduce your levels of that transmitter. Instead, use your understanding of that dominance to better determine your particular cognitive skills and which exercise and eating protocols could work best for you.

Here's my overview of neurotransmitter dominances, with my apologies if these read like astrological assessments. Trust me: they're far more accurate than astrology. You'll likely recognize yourself in one of the descriptions here, but if you'd like to confirm your dominance with a quiz, visit www.bravermantest.com.

Dopamine Dominance

If you are dopamine dominant, you are likely strong-willed, fast on your feet, and self-confident. You tend to be highly rational and more comfortable with hard facts and figures than with emotions and feelings. You take pride in achievement, strategic thinking, problem-solving, and inventing. You are overly alert, often hyperactive, and you may need less sleep than others. You likely get bored with frequent cardio, and you love explosive workouts and heavy weights.

When dopamine is in excess, you are tempted to engage in impulsive actions and push yourself too far beyond your limits. As a result, you are at constant risk of physically and mentally burning out. On the other hand, a dopamine deficiency can lead to fatigue, sluggishness, memory loss, or depression. You can boost your dopamine levels by using supplements that contain dopamine neurotransmitter precursors or naturally occurring levels of dopamine, such as amino acids, vitamin B complexes, *Rhodiola rosea* (rhodiola) and *Ginkgo biloba* (ginkgo); eating foods such as chicken, cottage cheese, eggs, pork, turkey, nuts, wheat germ, oats, milk, and yogurt; and aiming for a moderate intake of caffeine.

Acetylcholine Dominance

If you're acetylcholine dominant, you are tuned in to your senses, highly creative, and open to new ideas. You make the best of any situation, no matter how bad it may be. You can stick to the same workout program for a long time because you can sink your teeth into routines, but you are also flexible, creative, and spontaneous. You enjoy activities involving words, ideas, and communication—many artists and actors are acetylcholine dominant. You can handle high intensity and high volume, but your body needs more rest to recover. You are extremely social, charismatic, and charming, and you highly value relationships. You love adventure and travel and are constantly learning new skills and information.

In a state of acetylcholine excess, you may become paranoid, panicky, or anxious. An acetylcholine deficiency can result in poor memory recall, slow reactions to sensory stimuli, and a brain that generally feels slow. Acetylcholine-supporting compounds include choline, phosphatidylcholine, acetyl-L-carnitine, and many herbal nootropics (that is, natural compounds that improve cognitive functioning), such as ginkgo and ginseng.

I am quite notably inclined toward acetylcholine dominance. So what has worked best for me? Since acetylcholine is a neurotransmitter that is synthesized in the brain using choline, acetylcholine-dominant people burn through their choline stores faster than normal, so consuming more choline from the diet and from supplements is important. In addition to eating a diet high in healthy, choline-rich sources of fat, such as eggs, nuts, cold-pressed oils, and avocados, I have found it helpful to take 4 g or more of fish oil per day and the nootropic supplement Qualia, which contains a host of choline precursors and derivatives. This strategy can also be effective for serotonin or dopamine deficiencies and excess GABA.

GABA Dominance

GABA is an inhibitory neurotransmitter, so if you're GABA dominant, you often function quite well and stay calm in stressful or chaotic situations, operating in a state of level-headed confidence. You love organization and rigid schedules that eliminate uncertainty, and you're drawn to institutions and tradition. You tend to be emotionally stable and slow to anger. You thrive on creating peace, nurturing and caring for others, and creating stability in the relationships around you. You may have difficulty motivating yourself to exercise hard because you are too relaxed to crave the excitement that training and competing can provide. Instead, you likely enjoy laid-back outdoor activities and sports.

Excess GABA may amplify your tendency to nurture to the point that you ignore your own health and needs. A GABA deficiency can make you feel nervous, irritable, and anxious. Herbs and supplements that support GABA include melatonin, phenibut (at night), valerian root, and passionflower.

Serotonin Dominance

Serotonin reboots the brain while you sleep so that you can start fresh each morning. Delta brain waves, which are produced in abundance when you sleep, are amplified by serotonin and increase your ability to rest and regenerate. If you're serotonin dominant, you're highly responsive to sensory input and slightly impulsive, and you thrive on change and novelty—you like to try new foods, explore new hobbies, and travel to new places. You tend to be drawn to excitement, whether in movies, parties, or video games, and you prefer high-energy activities like gambling, mountain climbing, hunting, skydiving, and other extreme sports.

Excess serotonin can make you nervous and distracted and prone to emotional extremes. It can also induce desperation for interpersonal interactions. A serotonin deficiency—often brought on by too much excitement or insufficient sleep—can make you feel overtired and out of control. Serotonin-supporting compounds include fish oil, 5-HTP, magnesium, St. John's wort, and tryptophan.

TESTING YOUR NEUROTRANSMITTERS

A physician can determine your neurotransmitter levels by testing your blood, cerebrospinal fluid, or urine (the most common method). Typically, a testing panel will encompass some or all of the major neurotransmitters—in addition to serotonin, dopamine, acetylcholine, and GABA, these include glutamate, norepinephrine, and epinephrine (the last two are used to synthesize dopamine). Ostensibly, this information helps doctors treat a host of brain-related disorders, such as anxiety, depression, ADHD, memory loss, brain fog, mood swings, autism, and Alzheimer's.

Problem is, neurotransmitter tests don't actually measure neurotransmitter levels that are being released by vesicles within the nervous system and traveling between neurons in your brain. In fact, there is no established relationship between neurotransmitter levels in the brain and the levels in any other part of the body, including blood, cerebrospinal fluid, and urine—which are the usual suspects for testing neurotransmitter levels. The brain has a selective filter called the blood-brain barrier (BBB) that keeps out neurotransmitters, along with many other substances. And a significant amount of the neurotransmitters circulating in your body are produced outside of the brain—95 percent of your serotonin, for example, is produced in your gut. Some neurotransmitters are not even produced by you but rather by the bacteria that live inside you. Indeed, the bacteria that reside in your gut synthesize over thirty neurotransmitters!

Commercial lab neurotransmitter testing has also not held up under scrutiny. The physicians who use it often receive a referral commission, and in 2016, a company called NeuroScience, Inc. was fined over $6 million for violating testing requirements and was found to have intentionally manipulated test results. Not only that, but NeuroScience also recommended supplements based on the illegitimate results and then proceeded to sell those supplements! Plus, one study on the accuracy of neurotransmitter testing found plenty of evidence refuting its validity, demonstrating that these tests have no scientific foundation.

The circulating amount of any given neurotransmitter is also in constant flux. Each neurotransmitter has a different half-life, the time it takes for the total amount to fall by 50 percent. These half-lives can be as long as several minutes or as short as a fraction of a second. Everything you do, including thinking, impacts your neurotransmitter levels on a second-to-second basis, so neurotransmitter test results show only your levels at a particular moment in time. Perhaps this is why there are currently no scientifically established norms for ideal neurotransmitter levels.

However, there is one relatively new and more accurate method of assessing neurotransmitters: the DUTCH Complete panel. While in the past I've only relied on a panel like this for a urinary analysis of hormones, DUTCH is now able to provide valuable insight into specific markers associated with neurotransmitter breakdown, most notably homovanillate (HVA), a metabolite of dopamine metabolism, and vanilmandelate (VMA), a metabolite of norepinephrine and epinephrine metabolism. Low levels of HVA can be due to low levels of dopamine or poor conversion of dopamine to HVA, often caused by insufficient levels of methyl groups, magnesium, and NAD, which are needed to metabolize dopamine. This can be accompanied by addictions, cravings, and pleasure seeking (to boost levels) in addition to sleepiness, impulsivity, tremors, low motivation, fatigue, and low mood. Low levels of VMA in the urine may indicate low adrenal hormone output and often signal a copper or vitamin C insufficiency. This can be accompanied by addictions, cravings, fatigue, low blood pressure, low muscle tone, exercise intolerance, depression, and loss of alertness.

Aside from the DUTCH test, there are effective, symptom-based questionnaires that have been used for years to determine neurotransmitter imbalances. Dr. Datis Kharrazian, author of the book *Why Isn't My Brain Working?*, states, "There is no scientifically validated way to test neurotransmitter levels through lab testing. The best way is to assess your symptoms."

There are several free neurotransmitter quizzes and questionnaires online, including the following:

- Dr. Eric Braverman's Personality Type Assessment (www.bravermantest.com), which will help you find deficiencies in acetylcholine, dopamine, GABA, and serotonin levels. Dr. Braverman is the founder and president of the PATH Foundation, a nonprofit organization that researches brain health and healthy aging. The quiz is taken from the information in his bestselling book *The Edge Effect*.

- Dr. Mark Hyman's UltraMind Solution Companion Guide (drhyman.com/download-the-ultramind-solution-companion-guide), which is a set of quizzes to help you determine your levels of neurotransmitters, vitamin D, magnesium, fatty acids, zinc, inflammation, thyroid function, and more. It is adapted from his book *The UltraMind Solution*.

- Julia Ross's Mood Type Questionnaire (www.juliarosscures.com/mood-type-questionnaire), which helps you determine your serotonin, endorphin, norepinephrine, and GABA status. It can also help you determine how stable your blood sugar levels are.

Neurotransmitters and Your Gut

Neurotransmitters produced outside of your brain, such as those produced by the bacteria in your gut, cannot cross the BBB, though amino acid neurotransmitter precursors like tryptophan and B vitamins can. This may be a feature, not a bug: 95 percent of the body's serotonin is produced in the gut, and if all that serotonin were able to cross the BBB and accumulate in the brain, it could potentially cause similar effects to LSD. Basically, you'd be trippin' all the time.

But neurotransmitters in the rest of the body, such as those in the gut, can still affect the health and function of the brain. It appears this is most likely due to the fact that the vagus nerve serves as the primary communication nerve between the gut and the brain and can be both stimulated and inhibited by neurotransmitters, even if those neurotransmitters aren't crossing the BBB in any significant quantity. Some evidence suggests that supplemental forms of the neurotransmitter GABA might be able to cross the BBB and exert a calming effect. GABA can also exert its effects on the brain in a

bit more indirect way, specifically via an effect on the enteric nervous system in the gut. GABA, as an inhibitory neurotransmitter, inhibits the generation of the action potential of a neuron, which makes that neuron less likely to excite a nearby neuron.

When neurotransmitter activity in the gut or brain is disrupted, the neurotransmitters in the other area are also affected. For example, serotonin regulates healthy bowel movements by improving gut motility. IBS-D, which is a type of irritable bowel syndrome characterized by excessive gut motility and diarrhea, is modulated by serotonin levels in the gut. Research has shown that 46 percent of IBS patients exhibit depression, 34 percent exhibit generalized anxiety disorder, 31 percent exhibit panic disorder, and 26 percent exhibit somatization (medical symptoms not connected to any cause). So while neurotransmitter populations in the gut and brain are often separate and distinct, they can still dramatically affect each other.

9 WAYS TO FIX YOUR NEUROTRANSMITTERS

Once you've identified any deficiencies or excesses, the remainder of this chapter can help you implement supplemental, dietary, and lifestyle habits that will help bring your neurotransmitters back into balance—and if you're not experiencing any problems at the moment, they are generally supportive of neurotransmitter health.

1. Avoid Antidepressants

Prozac, Sarafem, Paxil, Zoloft, Celexa, Lexapro, Effexor, Cymbalta, Pristiq—the list of antidepressant drugs goes on, with hundreds of millions of prescriptions handed out and billions of dollars in sales each year.

Most antidepressants affect serotonin levels in one of two ways: by directly increasing the brain's level of serotonin or, more commonly, by blocking the reuptake of serotonin by nerve cells. Antidepressants that work this way are called selective serotonin reuptake inhibitors, or SSRIs. By preventing serotonin from being returned to neurons, SSRIs increase the brain's amount of available serotonin.

However, it's far from certain that SSRIs are safe or effective, especially with long-term use. Eventually, not only do you require increasing doses of SSRIs to have the same effect, but you also eliminate up to 60 percent of the serotonin receptors in your brain as they become downregulated due to long-term exposure to flooded levels of serotonin. The enzymes in the synaptic cleft that break down neurotransmitters also adapt to the higher levels of available serotonin by becoming more efficient and operating at higher activity levels, so serotonin is more rapidly broken down. Antidepressant use can also damage the serotonin receptors in your liver, kidneys, and colon and thus affect your delicate brain-gut connection (a crucial connection I'll explore in greater detail in chapter 13) and appetite regulation by lowering the sensitivity of these organs to signals from your nervous system.

A great deal of evidence suggests that antidepressants don't work well anyway. Meta-analyses of research have revealed that SSRIs have no clinically meaningful advantage over a placebo, and those studies that do show any clinically meaningful advantage over a placebo do not take into account that people taking the drugs also engage in supportive weekly visits with the physician overseeing the medication, which is a significant treatment in and of itself. There is also little evidence that antidepressants work better for more severe depressive conditions. The few studies that have shown antidepressants to have a small degree of superiority over placebos were poorly designed and, as a result, unreliable. Ultimately, antidepressants have not been shown to affect the long-term improvement of depression or suicide rates, and chronic exposure to SSRIs can make you feel apathetic and less engaged in your life.

Are there alternatives? You bet. Natural supplements such as acetyl-L-carnitine, probiotics, and even curcumin can all be highly effective antidepressant strategies with far lower risk than a pharmaceutical antidepressant. (An important note: If you're currently taking an antidepressant, don't stop taking it without talking to your doctor. Abruptly stopping an antidepressant can cause unpleasant withdrawal symptoms and other side effects, so make sure you work out a tapering schedule with your doctor.)

2. Limit Your Intake of Stimulants

My father was a gourmet coffee roaster. When I was as young as thirteen, I was sucking down espresso shots and gulping black coffee every day. By the time I was thirty, I was a bona fide addict. I was so tolerant of caffeine that I could never settle for anything less than a 20-ounce mug o' joe. At that point, I knew I had to do something to fix my excessive caffeine intake.

Sure, low doses of caffeine can improve mental performance and protect against Alzheimer's, so you don't need to avoid it entirely. But, like antidepressants, high doses of caffeine, ephedrine, ephedra, guarana, Ritalin, and other central nervous system stimulants can overwhelm the brain with excitatory neurotransmitters, creating resistance to neurotransmitters and long-term receptor damage. The more stimulants you take, the more you need to take to feel any benefit. As you increase your intake, you exacerbate this effect, and the cycle continues.

CAFFEINE

Caffeine is both water- and fat-soluble, which means it can easily cross your blood-brain barrier. When you frequently consume coffee, tea, soda, and other caffeine-containing drinks, you cause a gradual change in your brain's chemistry and physical characteristics, especially in the number of receptors for adenosine, a chemical that induces a state of tiredness and supports natural sleep rhythms.

The molecular structure of caffeine closely resembles that of adenosine, which means that caffeine can easily fit into your brain's adenosine receptors. With its receptors constantly plugged up by caffeine, adenosine can no longer bind to those receptors and make you tired. Your body's response is to create more and more adenosine receptors, so you need more and more caffeine to bind to those receptors and block the effects of adenosine. You need ever-increasing doses of caffeine just to function normally.

ADENOSINE

To kick a serious caffeine habit and reset your adenosine receptors, you have three options: First, you can avoid caffeine for seven to ten days, every four to eight weeks. Consider keeping a bag of decaf coffee or decaf tea in your freezer or pantry for this period so you can enjoy the wonderful aroma, taste, concentrated antioxidants, social benefits, bowel-moving glory, and many other health benefits of a hot morning beverage without exhausting your neurotransmitters. Second, you can drink one or two cups of coffee per day of a medium roast that is slightly lower in caffeine but contains a high amount of antioxidants. Third, you can consume 100 to 200 mg of L-theanine with every cup of coffee.

3. Avoid Toxins

Ten years ago, while passing through a mall or department store, I would think nothing of taking a big whiff of men's colognes and fragrances. These days, I suck in a giant freediver-esque breath prior to wandering through the personal care aisles at Macy's. I also open the window of my hotel room to pull in fresh air, avoid running on busy roads, and travel with my own soap, shampoo, and conditioner.

Colognes, perfumes, brake dust, smog, airborne heavy metals, and even Christmas tree–shaped car air fresheners contain toxins that can drastically affect neurotransmitter production as well as your sensitivity to those neurotransmitters. The results can include brain damage and brain fog. To avoid these effects, you can take the following measures.

Eat organic fruits and vegetables when possible and wash other vegetables in a water-and-vinegar solution.

 Use natural personal care products. Check labels and avoid parabens, dyes, and fragrances.

 Use natural household cleaners like lemon juice, vinegar, and baking soda.

 Fortify your home with air and water filters.

 Choose a holistic dentist for any dental work.

Once you begin to make these changes, you will find that when you do encounter an attack against your neurotransmitters, such as the wafting aromas in a department-store cologne section, you will be extremely sensitive and notice it almost immediately. Listening to your body in these situations is important. If it looks, tastes, or smells synthetic, avoid it. If you can't eat it without dying a horrible death, don't smear it on your teeth, hair, skin, or nails. (I'll talk in much more depth about avoiding toxins in chapter 20.)

Finding the Sweet Spot with Medium-Roast Coffee

The solution I've implemented in the past to not being overcaffeinated? Simple. For seven to ten days out of every month, I pull out a bag of Swiss Water Process (a low-chemical method for decaffeinating unroasted coffee beans), organic, decaffeinated coffee and make myself a piping-hot cup of decaf as a substitute for regular.

But if you prefer to pass on decaf, another option is to pay attention to the roasting process of your coffee. Roasting involves some pretty complicated science: it requires converting a substance that has three hundred volatile aromatic compounds into a substance with over one thousand volatile aromatic compounds. As you can imagine, this encompasses a lot more than simply tossing a metal bucket of coffee beans into a giant oven.

Why is the roasting process so important when it comes to your health and the purity of the coffee you drink? Even the highest-quality coffee beans contain a substance called acrylamide, which has been known to cause cancer in animals. Most roasters roast the hell out of the coffee bean to eradicate this substance, but

this dark-roast process often introduces other cancer-causing chemicals. For example, at high temperatures, roasting produces polycyclic aromatic hydrocarbons (PAHs) and results in the burned flavor that so many coffees are known for.

But if a smokeless roasting process is used (this is pretty rare, but a few folks still do it), it obliterates acrylamide without sacrificing the numerous antioxidants found in coffee or creating PAHs. In addition, and most important for the caffeine issue, it creates a coveted sweet spot of a dense amount of antioxidants and only a low-to-moderate amount of caffeine. Compare your coffee to a nice cut of beef: you wouldn't blast a filet mignon to well-done; you'd gently cook it to a tasty and tender medium-rare for the ultimate combination of taste and health.

In other words, with a medium roast and a smokeless roasting process, you can get all the benefits of coffee without all the issues of adrenal imbalances and the jitters. You can have your cup and sip it too, baby.

4. Avoid Sensory Overload

Fifteen years ago, I walked out of the horror flick *Saw*, hands trembling with adrenaline, and swore under my breath that I would never watch another scary movie at night. Since making that oath, my sleep has drastically improved, as have my daily focus and energy.

In the twenty-first century, most of us are bombarded with sensory information every day. We're exposed to all the following:

 Loud sounds, like honking cars and ringing phones

 Radio and EMF waves

 Violent entertainment like horror flicks

 Rapid visual and auditory effects in games and movies

 Fluorescent lighting

 The electronic flickering of monitors and screens

 Excessive working hours

All this sensory exposure overloads your central nervous system and can lead to severe neurotransmitter imbalances. Your brain has to calm itself down from these stimuli with higher levels of calming neurotransmitters like serotonin and GABA than it would normally require. You may be overloaded if you:

 Listen to loud music while exercising

 Spend much of your day staring at a computer monitor

 Are exposed to artificial fluorescent lighting all day

 Have a steady diet of fast-moving, exciting, or violent movies and video games, especially before bed

 Constantly play music in the background

To rebalance your neurotransmitter levels, you have to step back from the barrage of sensory input in your life and enjoy some silence and stillness. Turn down the midworkout heavy metal and pop music. Back away from the 3-D Blu-ray box set. Go for a leisurely walk through a nearby park, sit on the porch with a cup of chamomile tea or a glass of organic, biodynamic red wine, or engage in twenty minutes of quiet, mindful deep breathing and meditation. (See chapter 3 for effective breathing and meditation techniques.)

If you do find yourself accompanying a group of friends to the latest Halloween blockbuster, consider following it up with a dose of GABA-supporting compounds, such as passionflower extract, lemon extract, cannabidiol (CBD), or a phenibut supplement. Passionflower extract is known to promote healthy GABA activity and reduce anxiety; lemon extract and CBD have GABA-mediated antistress effects; and phenibut is the form of GABA that is capable of entering your brain through the blood-brain barrier.

5. Fix Your Gut

You have a second brain, and that second brain is not in your head. Think lower. Okay, fellas, not that low. Up a bit higher. Yes, the second brain is in your gut. The enteric nervous system (ENS) is a net of neurons that controls your gut and operates semi-independently from your brain. It uses more than thirty neurotransmitters, just like the brain, and up to 95 percent of your body's serotonin is actually produced in your gut. This makes sense when you consider that in the nine meters from your esophagus to your anus, there are more than 100 million neurons, more than in your spinal cord or your entire peripheral nervous system! Irritable bowel syndrome, which afflicts nearly every active individual now and then, arises partly from a serotonin imbalance in your gut. This is also why SSRI antidepressants, which change the balance of serotonin in your body as well as your brain, can lead to serious gut issues.

Neurotransmitters are produced in your gut lining and by the billions of bacteria in your gut. So if your gut lining is damaged or your gut flora is out of balance, then you are at serious risk for neurotransmitter deficiencies and imbalances. This may also be why probiotics and the consumption of a wide variety of fermented foods can be highly effective natural remedies for depression.

We'll explore the brain-gut connection in more detail in chapter 13, but a good first step in addressing neurotransmitter imbalances is a gut reboot: four to eight weeks of a squeaky-clean nutrition protocol—two of my favorites are the Autoimmune Paleo (AIP) diet and the low-FODMAP diet—combined with generous amounts of glutamine, colostrum, and bone broth or collagen.

6. Replace Your Building Blocks

Think back to my Ironman bonk and Dr. Attia's advice to use amino acids. Amino acids work so well to stave off central nervous system fatigue because they are the primary building blocks—along with vitamin B and minerals—of neurotransmitters.

First, examine your diet to ensure you are consuming adequate protein—a minimum of 0.55 g per pound of body weight per day. Some of the best high-quality amino acid sources are grass-fed beef, wild salmon, eggs from pastured chickens, raw organic dairy, almonds and almond butter, quinoa, and spirulina or chlorella. I have found that many people who struggle with sleep or

VITAMIN B_6	VITAMIN B_{12}	FOLATE	VITAMIN B SUPPLEMENTS
bell peppers	calf's liver	broccoli	full-spectrum blend with 5-methyltetrahydrofolate (5-MTHF)
turnip greens	snapper	beets	
spinach		lentils	
		calf's liver	
		asparagus	
		spinach	

Not all amino acids are created equal. Branched-chain amino acid supplements (BCAAs) contain only three of the nine essential amino acids (EAAs) that the body can't make itself: leucine, isoleucine, and valine. People take BCAAs hoping to stimulate muscle protein synthesis, fight fatigue, and increase focus during workouts. Unfortunately, these claims about the benefits of BCAAs are primarily based on 2006 studies done on rats. Since then, additional studies have shown that in humans, BCAAs have no effect on muscle growth and may cause a spike in blood glucose or insulin, along with an imbalance of the more important EAAs.

In contrast, supplements that contain the correct balance of all nine EAAs—which are more expensive than BCAAs but far more efficacious—have been shown to improve the retention of lean muscle, increase metabolic rate, and optimize brain and liver function, with no deleterious side effects and a very low calorie load.

Sure, you could simply eat a steak or suck down a whey protein shake to get all your EAAs, but the protein from food must first be digested and then broken down into amino acids, so food-derived amino acids not only come with far more calories than EAA capsules or powders but also take longer to be absorbed. It's also difficult to eat real food during, say, a workout or race. (Ever try to chew through a few hard-boiled eggs while weight training or gnaw on a chicken breast during a hot afternoon run?) My preferred brand of EAA supplements is Kion (GetKion.com).

motivation issues that are tied to neurotransmitter problems also benefit from 10 to 20 g each day of essential amino acid supplements, which combine the nine essential amino acids to supply all the necessary neurotransmitter precursors.

For the nervous system to synthesize and circulate the neurotransmitters formed by amino acids, you need to have an adequate intake of B-complex vitamins. Vitamins B_6, B_{12}, and folate (vitamin B_9) are especially important. Excellent food sources of vitamin B_6 include bell peppers, turnip greens, and spinach. Folate can be found in broccoli, beets, turnip and mustard greens, romaine lettuce, lentils, calf's liver, asparagus, parsley, and spinach. B_{12} sources include calf's liver and snapper. For vitamin B supplementation, look into full-spectrum vitamin B blends that use only the highly bioavailable form of vitamin B called 5-methyltetrahydrofolate (5-MTHF). (I recommend the Thorne Multivitamin Complex and the herbal smart drug Qualia, a nootropic with plenty more than B vitamins in it.)

If you are frequently sweating under high amounts of exercise or lifestyle stress, you should also consume a mineral-rich source of protein, such as a goat's milk–based protein powder, a daily dose of a liquid trace mineral supplement, and liberal amounts of a high-quality salt. The protein in goat's milk is higher in minerals than the protein in cow's milk, and combining Himalayan salt with Celtic sea salt or Colima salt provides a full spectrum of minerals.

7. Lube Your Nerves

Ever since I sat slack-jawed in the audience at a health symposium and listened to author Nora Gedgaudas explain that cholesterol levels lower than 200 are associated with lower IQ, I have gone out of my way to shun a phobia of dietary fats. Because a diet rich in healthy animal foods, like meat, dairy, and eggs, is associated with higher cholesterol levels, vegans and vegetarians are more likely to have lower cholesterol—and the side effects that come with it. Whenever I meet vegans or vegetarians who want to optimize their cognitive function, I warn them to be cautious with a strictly plant-based diet. In a wide body of research, vegetarians have been shown to

Creatine and Memory

Creatine is an important compound that's found mostly in meat, so it's notoriously missing from plant-based diets. David Benton, a psychology professor who specializes in diet and behavior, studied the memory of omnivores and vegetarians both before and after they consumed a placebo or creatine supplement. Before taking the pills, the omnivores and vegetarians had similar performance on a memory test. Then, each group was divided into two smaller groups, one taking a placebo, the other taking creatine.

A week later, all four groups took another memory test. The omnivores' results didn't change from the previous week, whether they took a placebo or creatine. The vegetarians who took the placebo also performed the same as the week before. But the vegetarians who took creatine not only improved from the week before but also outstripped all of the other groups in terms of cognitive performance.

Interestingly, this suggests that vegetarians could potentially have better memories than omnivores—most likely due to their high intake of antioxidant-rich plants and relatively low intake of overcooked or processed meat—but the same diet that gives them these advantages also gives them the disadvantage of a creatine deficit. It also suggests that creatine intake, either via supplementation, adequate meat (particularly beef) intake, or both, can address some of those deficits.

have elevated rates of depressive disorders, anxiety disorders, and other cognitive malfunctions. Though plant-based eaters are often unaware of the potential dark side of this diet, significant evidence suggests a link between going meatless or low-fat (a prevailing characteristic of a plant-based diet) and an elevated risk of severe mental disorders. Many vegetarians and vegans feel stellar on a plant-based diet for months or even years. But eventually, they experience nagging aches and pains due to amino acid deficiencies and cognitive decline due to fat and vitamin B_{12} deficiencies, which can cause dementia, depression, and other mental disorders.

When it comes to fats, another very good way to enhance the speed with which your brain communicates with the rest of your body is to care for the health of your nerves themselves. Your nerves are wrapped in insulating myelin sheaths, sleeves of fatty tissue that protect your nerve cells and assist with the transmission of messages between your brain and the rest of your body. A diet for a healthy nervous system should be rich in nutrients that support the formation of these sheaths. After all, it doesn't matter how many neurotransmitters you make if the action potentials they propagate can't be adequately transmitted because you have broken-down, degraded myelin sheaths. Omega-3 fatty acids, particularly docosahexaenoic acid (DHA), are important for the formation of myelin sheaths, so a neurotransmitter-supporting diet should include a high intake of omega-3s.

Flax seeds, walnuts, kale, collard greens, and winter squash contain high levels of omega-3 fatty acids, but the amount that is absorbed from them can be relatively low. Sources of more readily available omega-3 fatty acids include salmon, sardines, cloves, grass-fed beef, halibut, shrimp, cod, and tuna. In addition, anthropological evidence shows that, long before we discovered cashew cheese and tofu, animal flesh and organ meats could provide not only many of the omega-3s necessary to support myelin sheath health but also the calorie-dense foods necessary to fuel the energy-hungry human cerebellum. Many anthropologists believe that without the ability to use cooking to make raw meat more digestible, we would never have matured beyond the mental capacity of herbivores like gorillas. Today, stronger brains are still powered by many of the nutrients commonly found in animal proteins, including B vitamins, zinc, iron, and tryptophan, which is found almost exclusively in poultry.

That's not to say that a plant-based diet can't be neurotransmitter-friendly. Vegans and vegetarians can obtain myelin sheath–promoting nutrients and oils by consuming soaked, sprouted, and fermented seeds, nuts, legumes, and grains; vegan-friendly algae-based DHA supplements like chlorella, spirulina, and marine phytoplankton; and foods containing the monounsaturated fat oleic acid (which can comprise up to 30 percent of the myelin sheath!), such as olive oil, almonds, pecans, macadamia nuts, and avocados.

With each meal, include at least one source of oleic acid, such as olives, olive oil, or avocados, and at least one source of DHA, such as cold-water fish, fish oil, algae, or DHA-enriched eggs. My personal strategy is to keep a bottle of extremely high-quality extra-virgin olive oil on hand in the kitchen at all times and to travel with a fish oil high in DHA.

8. Repair Your Genes

I'll warn you: hardly anybody is talking about this strategy to hack your neurotransmitters. But when I interviewed Ben Lynch on my podcast about his mind-blowing book *Dirty Genes* and his genetic testing service, StrateGene, he explained to me that there's a list called the Super Seven, which is a list of so-called dirty genes—gene variants that directly affect not only neurotransmitters but also several other important metabolic functions. The Super Seven are:

- **MTHFR**, which supports methylation, a crucial process involved in more than two hundred of your body's vital functions
- **GST/GPX**, two gene variants responsible for regulating your body's energy levels as well as your glutathione levels, thus impacting your natural antioxidant responses
- **COMT**, which affects the metabolism of dopamine, norepinephrine, and epinephrine, thus regulating your mood, energy levels, and ability to calm down, sleep, and focus
- **DAO**, which affects your body's response to histamines from food and bacteria, thus affecting your vulnerability to food allergies and intolerances
- **MAOA**, which affects your relationship to dopamine, norepinephrine, and serotonin, thus governing your mood, energy, sugar cravings, and ability to sleep
- **NOS3**, which affects your circulation and nitric oxide levels and helps determine your cardiovascular health and vulnerability to heart attacks, circulatory issues, and stroke
- **PEMT**, which affects your cell walls, brain, and liver, impacting a range of health issues, such as gallstones, fatty liver disease, gut problems, and attention and focus deficits

You can test for these genes by taking an inexpensive salivary DNA test through a company such as 23andMe and then uploading the results to StrateGene for interpretation. Once you are armed with the knowledge of which dirty genes you possess, you can go about fixing them. For example, if you discover you possess the MTHFR gene pattern that directly affects methylation, you can supplement with 5-methyltetrahydrofolate while avoiding folate or folic acid, which are shoved into cheap multivitamins and used to fortify packaged foods.

9. Focus on Antioxidants

In his book *Nutrient Power: Heal Your Biochemistry and Heal Your Brain*, Bill Walsh describes the importance of antioxidants for stabilizing cognition and reducing overall brain inflammation. Multiple studies show the importance of one particular antioxidant, N-acetylcysteine (NAC), for reducing the neuronal damage and degeneration associated with excess levels of excitatory neurotransmitters like glutamate. NAC—best taken as a supplement—is now recognized as a crucial nutrient for treating neurological disorders such as schizophrenia and bipolar disorder. As an antioxidant, NAC neutralizes many free radicals before they cause damage in neural cells, and by inhibiting excess excitatory activity of glutamate receptors in the brain, it can also be very effective at treating addiction to everything from nicotine to cocaine to meth to gambling. It also works quite well for addiction because it affects dopamine reward pathways in the brain. Any

Mitigating the Effects of Alcohol

My StrateGene analysis revealed that because of my genes, alcohol has an extremely deleterious effect on my neurotransmitters. Turns out, this is primarily related to histamine intolerance. Alcohol and its metabolic breakdown product acetaldehyde can liberate histamine from its storage location in mast cells and depress histamine elimination by inhibiting DAO, resulting in elevated histamine levels throughout body tissues. So I asked Dr. Ben Lynch about his strategies for mitigating histamine intolerance and thereby reducing alcohol's negative effects.

He explained to me that histamines are bioactive, nitrogen-based compounds that play a part in immune responses and gut function. Histamine intolerance is associated with a combination of slower DAO, MTHFR, MAOA, MAOB, and NAT2 genes—a condition that Dr. Lynch refers to as "dirty." So my histamine levels are naturally elevated, and while this contributes positively to focus and attention, it also produces a potential risk for narcolepsy and adverse reactions to alcohol. If you drink alcohol, you may experience one or more of the following (typically a few occur simultaneously):

A red face

Flushing

Irritability

A runny nose

A bloody nose

Exacerbation of existing eczema

Exacerbation of existing psoriasis

Insomnia

Sweaty feet

Increased heart rate

Headaches or migraines

The following are dietary tactics you can implement to reduce these effects.

- **Limit your intake of high-histamine foods when you consume alcohol.** Cheese and aged meats are particularly high in histamines, and, ironically, they are often paired with wine.

- **Consume specific probiotics.** The DAO gene is partly responsible for breaking down histamines derived from food and bacteria. In the gut, DAO can often be overwhelmed in the presence of too many histamines and too much tyramine (an amino acid), both of which can be increased when consuming alcohol. One way to minimize this effect is to take probiotic supplements that contain bacterial strains involved in breaking down histamines.

addictive substance or behavior activates these pathways, which eventually creates a dopamine imbalance. Along with decreasing glutamate, NAC balances these reward pathways, which can reduce or eliminate cravings.

Two other antioxidants called luteolin and diosmin have been shown to reduce levels of beta-amyloid, which is strongly associated with Alzheimer's disease. Lemons are rich in diosmin, and luteolin is abundant in green peppers and tomatoes. Studies have also shown that flavonoids called anthocyanins—particularly those found in red berries—also play a key role in brain health and Alzheimer's prevention.

- **Take SAMe.** Like the DAO gene, the HNMT gene's job is to break down histamines in the blood. When your DAO gene is overwhelmed by the consumption of alcohol, your HNMT gene has to work harder to compensate. For HNMT to work, it needs a compound called S-adenosine-L-methionine, or SAMe, so taking a SAMe supplement can help. If taking SAMe makes you feel worse, you can instead consume nutrients that indirectly promote the breakdown of histamine, such as nettle leaves, quercetin, bitter orange fruit, and bromelain, or take enzymes such as DAO that break down histamine quite effectively.

- **Take PQQ.** If your genes are dirty, alcohol can lead to oxidative stress, which reduces your ability to process histamine. The molecule PQQ helps reduce oxidative stress far more effectively than vitamin E, vitamin C, or other common antioxidants. To get the benefits of PQQ, take one PQQ lozenge before drinking.

- **Take molybdenum and thiamine.** Sulfites are common in wines and contribute to irritability, insomnia, and headaches. They also bind to and prevent the absorption of vitamin B_1, which is necessary for energy and focus. Taking about 500 mcg of molybdenum helps reduce the effects of sulfites on your

mental performance and vitamin uptake. You should also consume about 50 mg of thiamine before drinking, as thiamine can prevent sulfites from binding to vitamin B_1.

In summary, my ideal booze stack—supplements I'd use anytime I'm planning to consume more than one drink—would include the following:

- Probiota HistaminX, a probiotic, to optimize the DAO gene. Consume two capsules before drinking.

- HomocysteX Plus to optimize the HNMT, MAOA, MAOB, and MTHFR genes. Consume one capsule before drinking.

- Molybdenum to optimize the SUOX gene. Consume one capsule before drinking.

- PQQ to optimize the MTR gene. Take one lozenge before drinking.

- Thiamine to optimize the PDH gene. Consume one capsule before drinking.

- SAMe to optimize the HNMT gene. One of my favorite such supplements is Histablock by Seeking Health. This one is optional if you are already taking HomocysteX Plus.

For any workout that lasts more than ninety minutes and any competition for which glycogen depletion and central nervous system fatigue are potential concerns, I recommend a blend of four ingredients to keep your energy high for hours on end, with very few blood sugar fluctuations or gut issues.

1. **Easy-to-digest carbohydrate.** Look for one that contains potato dextrin, dextrose, or highly branched cyclic dextrin. This will allow you to maintain liver and muscle glycogen stores without getting the blood sugar roller coaster or gut rot and fermentation caused by many common sports nutrition carbohydrates, such as fructose and maltodextrin. One product I like is GlycoFuse by Gaspari Nutrition. Because you'll be including the other substances listed below, I recommend far less of this carbohydrate than is normally recommended: about 100–150 calories per hour.

2. **Easy-to-digest protein.** Although many sports drinks now feature whey protein, I prefer a protein that is more easily digested and broken down for immediate assimilation. For this, you cannot beat essential amino acids, at an intake of 5–10 g per hour. I recommend a powdered version, such as Kion Aminos.

3. **Ketone or MCT source.** I recommend, if you can afford the relative expense, one serving of ketone salts or ketone esters per hour. In addition, or as a more budget-friendly alternative to ketones, you can consume 1 teaspoon to 1 tablespoon of MCT oil per hour, although there is a slightly increased risk of digestive distress with this strategy.

4. **Electrolyte source.** If you are mixing all of the above into one water bottle that you nurse for each hour you are competing, you should also include one serving (typically a single scoop) of electrolytes each hour. I prefer Thorne's Catalytes as a balanced blend of sodium, potassium, magnesium, chloride, small amounts of d-ribose, and more.

Simply mix all of the above in a blender or shaker bottle, then divide the drink among sports flasks or water bottles based on the number of hours. For instance, if you'll be competing for three hours, mix together the three-hour amounts of carbs, protein, ketones, and electrolytes and then divide it among three water bottles.

THE LAST WORD

So what happened after I struggled to the finish line of Ironman Canada, surviving on the fumes of Coke and sugar?

For the next race, I took Dr. Attia's advice and pulled out the big guns: amino acids. And voilà—that year at the Ironman World Championships in Kona, Hawaii, I crossed the finish line in a very respectable nine hours and fifty-nine minutes, with no central nervous system stimulants and one-quarter of the carbohydrates that white-lab-coat-wearing nutrition scientists normally recommend for endurance athletes. Since then, I have refined my fueling strategy and the nutrition tactics I recommend for endurance athletes to include other potent compounds such as dextrin and exogenous ketones (I'll talk more about these in chapter 14). I have also added 10 to 20 g of essential amino acids to my daily supplement protocol for neurotransmitter support, especially on days when I eat little protein.

Of course, you don't need to swim 2.4 miles, bicycle 112 miles, or run 26.2 miles in half a day to use these strategies. Not surprisingly, much of what you just learned can be used to enhance not only stamina and endurance but also power production and muscle contraction speed. These strategies can also help you increase focus, fall asleep faster, and banish brain fog.

In the next chapter, you are going to learn about another aspect of your brain that can break—the blood-brain barrier. But in the meantime, try implementing the neurotransmitter-supporting strategies from this chapter:

1. Use natural antidepressant alternatives.

2. Take a break from caffeine.

3. Remove toxins from your home.

4. Avoid sensory overload.

5. Reboot your gut with a squeaky-clean eating protocol.

6. Get adequate amino acids.

7. Eat fat.

8. Determine your neurotransmitter dominance.

ONE THING YOU CAN DO THIS WEEK

Today, take at least one step toward boosting the state of your neurotransmitters. Instead of drinking that afternoon cup of coffee, enjoy a cup of decaf or herbal tea or some sparkling mineral water with stevia. If you have already consumed a couple of cups of coffee and want to start undoing the potential damage, add fish or eggs to a meal, or add some chlorella or spirulina to a smoothie or shake.

> For citations for all the research studies mentioned in this chapter and a deeper dive into the topics of this chapter—including links to podcasts, blog posts, recommended tools and supplements, and much more—visit BoundlessBook.com/1.

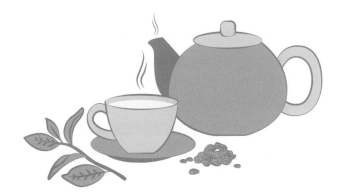

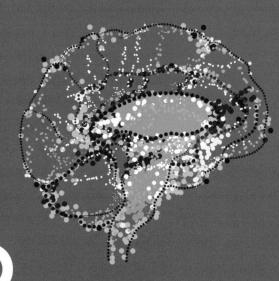

38 DEGREES BELOW ZERO

HOW TO FIX A LEAKY BRAIN

Silhouetted against the glow of the halogen floodlights in Spartan CEO Joe De Sena's big red barn in Pittsfield, Vermont, bundled up in a giant double-layered snowsuit, the emergency medical technician sighed and bent down for a closer look at my cold, hard, blue feet.

"Were you wearing double socks?"

I watched as he tugged at my ice-encrusted big toe. "Yeah, polypropylene liner with Smart-wool."

"Wiggling your toes a lot out there?"

I nodded.

"Can you feel this?"

He dug his fingernail into the underside of my toe. The pressure felt like a very distant pin-prick. "Barely."

He sat up. "Let's get your feet in a hot water basin for a few minutes and get you back out there."

I grimaced. He was referring to the 38-degrees-below-zero, snow- and ice-covered fields that lay just outside the barn and served as the playground and official location of the brutal Spartan Agoge. Formerly known as the Death Race, the Agoge is a punishing mash-up of obstacle course racing, brutal mental and physical challenges, and wilderness survival, an ultimate battle against the elements and the twisted, cruel minds of the race organizers. It is designed to build the perfect blend of grit, resilience, and perseverance to make you just as badass as Leonardo DiCaprio's character in the hard-core movie *The Revenant.* The Agoge was just one step in my quest to complete the coveted Spartan Delta, a calendar year of nine of the toughest obstacle-course races on the planet.

As the EMT placed my near-frostbitten feet into a hot water basin to thaw them out, I began to practice my four-count breathing. One year earlier, former Navy SEAL commander Mark Divine had taught me this invaluable box-breathing technique as I was getting bashed by the frigid Pacific Ocean for eight consecutive hours at the SEALFIT Kokoro Camp—an equally hellish crucible designed to simulate Navy SEAL Hell Week for those citizens who want to see what it feels like to be subjected to the extreme rigors used to sculpt a battle-worthy warrior and to be on the brink of hypothermia for seventy-two consecutive hours.

Four count in, four count hold, four count out, four count hold.

As pins and needles engulfed my feet, I continued to focus on my breathing, the same breathing I use when strolling through a chaotic airport, managing the lions jumping out from my email inbox, or sitting in a stressful traffic jam. My mind soon entered a state of pleasant and painless nirvana. Ten minutes later, I was trudging out into a tundra so cold that any exposed skin would be frostbitten within two minutes.

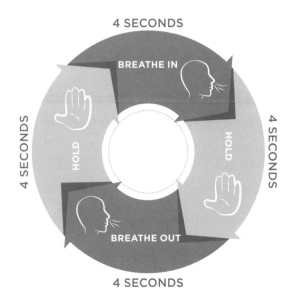

So what am I? Some kind of cold-obsessed masochist? Hardly. As a skinny-ass, relatively hairless author, extreme forays into icy landscapes and arctic plunges are not a regular or deeply desired habit of mine. But I highly value the power of cold exposure to heal and optimize the nervous system, particularly a critical part of the brain, the blood-brain barrier. In this chapter, you'll discover why I wander out for chilly winter morning walks in a T-shirt and shorts, why I begin and end each day with a refreshing cold shower, why I go out of my way to hop into a cold lake, river, ocean, or ice bath once a week, and why cryotherapy chambers are not just gimmicky ways to spend valuable cash on goose bumps.

BLOOD-BRAIN BARRIER 101

I first became interested in cold therapy when I learned about its benefits for one part of the human nervous system that is vital but often neglected: the blood-brain barrier (BBB). Fact is, when it comes to your mental function, supporting the BBB is one of the most important steps you can take, and maintaining it properly requires far more than mere cold therapy. To understand why the BBB is so critical, let's look first at what can happen when something goes wrong.

Chances are, you have heard of the gastrointestinal condition known as leaky gut. If you are a wellness enthusiast or you lurk on health forums, you may have already heard leaky gut described as "intestinal permeability." But the truth is that your gut is naturally and selectively permeable, allowing nutrients to pass into your bloodstream while keeping harmful toxins, large allergenic proteins, and pathogens out. When this process fails because your gut lining has been damaged by compounds such as herbicides, pesticides, excessive alcohol, sugar, and a variety of other assailants, your gut lining becomes more permeable than it should be, and you end up with a leaky gut. This can lead to indigestion, poor nutrient absorption, the development of food sensitivities, and systemic inflammation.

Similarly, when your BBB is punctured or damaged, you can end up with a leaky brain. No, a leaky brain has nothing to do with the zombie apocalypse or gray matter oozing out your ears.

The reality is much easier to digest and is based on the fact that your brain is very similar to your gut in at least one respect: it's protected by a membrane, the BBB, that's also selectively permeable.

Your brain requires compounds such as glucose, amino acids, fat-soluble nutrients, and ketones to function properly, so the BBB needs to allow them to pass through. For example, caffeine crosses the barrier quite easily and can be beneficial for brain health. At the same time, your brain also relies on the BBB to keep out harmful toxins, infectious pathogens, and rogue immune cells.

The BBB is formed by brain capillary endothelial cells, which are simple squamous (flat) cells that line the walls of blood and lymphatic vessels. The entire barrier includes three mechanisms that control the exchange of materials between your blood, brain, and cerebrospinal fluid and maintain the extracellular environment of the central nervous system:

- The cells that form the physical barrier between your blood and your brain

- Transporter molecules that mediate the flow of compounds between your brain and blood

- Enzymes in the endothelial cells of the brain and epithelial cells of the blood that metabolize neurotransmitters and toxins

Most of the research on the BBB in the past one hundred years has focused on formulating drugs to effectively reach the central nervous system by enabling them to cross the BBB. To understand the delicacy of this barrier, you have to understand that the endothelial lining of your blood vessels is only one cell thick—that's about one-tenth the thickness of a single strand of hair. Some of the largest vessels, such as arteries and veins, are also surrounded by thick walls of connective tissue and smooth muscle cells, but the vessel walls themselves are lined only by this thin sheet of cells.

Like every other cell in your body, endothelial cells can divide. The division of endothelial cells can actually help to quickly repair blood vessel walls. If left to themselves, they can live from a couple months (liver endothelium) to several years (brain endothelium). But when they are exposed to harmful compounds or stressors such as excessive inflammation, these cells can die prematurely and are forced to quickly divide in order to replicate in adequate quantity to repair the vessel wall. But when the vessel wall is exposed to a stressed state 24-7 without any breaks, the vessels that make up the BBB gradually weaken.

When the BBB is compromised, the brain is exposed to invaders such as toxins and bacteria. This can cause inflammation in the brain, and long-term, chronic inflammation in the brain can result in dementia, Alzheimer's, and other neurodegenerative diseases, as well as less-serious problems like brain fog, lack of focus, poor sleep, and food cravings.

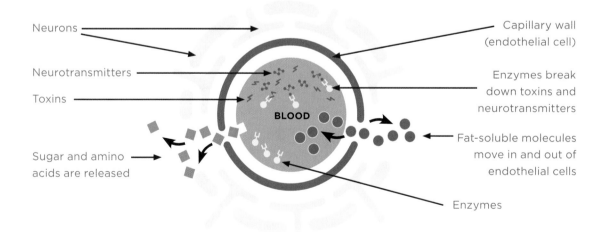

DO YOU HAVE A LEAKY BRAIN?

Getting tested for a leaky brain can be difficult. It often involves complicated and expensive protocols like electroencephalograms, spectrophotometry to track blue dyes that are injected into the brain, or tests of enzymes called matrix metalloproteinases. There is one decent blood panel from Cyrex Laboratories, called the blood-brain barrier permeability test, that looks for antibodies often associated with BBB issues brought on by traumatic brain injury or concussion, but you'll need a doctor to order that panel for you.

But you don't need to invest in these tests to determine if you're at risk for leaky brain. In fact, it is pretty simple to identify variables in your life that may be weakening your BBB. The following are the most common factors that can lead to a leaky brain.

Poor Sleep

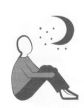

To properly regulate BBB function and integrity, it is crucial to get enough sleep. One group of researchers studied the effects of chronic sleep restriction on mice. Not only did it significantly diminish endothelial and inducible nitric oxide synthase, endothelin 1, and glucose transporter expression in brain microvessels of the BBB, but it also decreased the brain's uptake of 2-deoxyglucose, a sugar needed to maintain proper signaling between neurons. In other words, the mice's BBBs were less able to shuttle nutrients into the brain, and their brains were less able to properly send messages. This all coincided with increased permeability of the BBB.

Excessive Alcohol Intake

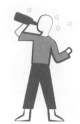

Research suggests that long-term alcohol abuse can lead to neuron degeneration, ranging from poor message signaling to full-on cell death, and can also cause damage that renders the BBB more permeable. Alcohol is primarily composed of ethanol, which enhances the activity of molecules called reactive oxygen species (ROS), which can damage brain cells. Chronic exposure to alcohol also increases the expression of CYPE1, an enzyme that converts ethanol into acetaldehyde, resulting in the formation of excess ROS in the process. Acetaldehyde is a close chemical cousin of formaldehyde (did someone say embalming fluid?) that's used in the manufacturing of adhesives and plastics. It's also a potent neurotoxin (thirty times more toxic than alcohol itself!) that can cross the BBB. When the BBB is punctured, ruptured, or loosened, heavy metals, toxins, molds, undigested proteins, and—you guessed it—excess acetaldehyde can cross the barrier and damage the brain.

Both ethanol and acetaldehyde can increase the permeability of the BBB. While a small glass of wine a day may not be a serious issue for your BBB, chronic, excessive alcohol intake will increase ethanol and acetaldehyde concentrations to dangerous levels.

High Blood Pressure

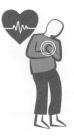

Research suggests that in rats, BBB dysfunction is related to the combined effects of elevated blood pressure and cerebral vasodilation, the widening of blood vessels in the brain. High blood pressure can be caused by anything from chronic stress and shallow chest breathing to poor diet and lack of sleep. Considering that one in every three adults in the US has high blood pressure, this factor should be taken very seriously.

Other Factors

While sleep deprivation, alcohol intake, and high blood pressure are the most common causes of a leaky BBB, there are also other well-researched factors, including the following:

- Systemic inflammation
- Stress, whether acute or chronic
- Bacterial infections
- Toxins like lipopolysaccharides, which are generated from high-fat, high-carbohydrate meals
- Mold exposure
- A leaky gut
- Liver damage
- Frequent blood glucose fluctuations
- Frequent sleep disturbances
- Anything that triggers oxidative stress in glial cells of the brain, such as high sugar intake
- Hypoxia (oxygen deficiency in the cells), especially from shallow, rapid mouth breathing rather than deep, slow nasal breathing
- In some people, high intake of glutamate and MSG. The glutamate that naturally occurs in many foods, such as milk, wheat, and vegetables, and the glutamate added to foods as MSG are exactly the same, which means that your body metabolizes them the same way. The problem arises if you have any of the following conditions, which can lead to excess inflammation that renders the BBB more permeable: histamine intolerance, glutamate sensitivity, gluten intolerance or celiac disease, Hashimoto's thyroiditis, type 1 diabetes, or autoimmune diseases that are linked to glutamate autoimmunity. In addition, if you're consuming very high amounts of glutamate (more than 20 g per day), it could be a problem, since excess glutamate in the brain can cause cell damage and cell death.

Many common health issues are associated with increased susceptibility to the factors listed above, including depression, head trauma, Lyme disease, obesity, and diabetes. These conditions lead to inflammation and oxidative stress and increase levels of MMP-9, a class of enzymes that are involved in the body's natural process of tissue repair and replacement. When inflammation is present, MMP-9 can break down various components of the BBB.

So, with all these threats to your brain and vascular system, how can you prevent leakage and seepage in your BBB?

12 WAYS TO FIX A LEAKY BRAIN

"Hi, I'm Ben Greenfield, and I'm naked."

Thus begins one of my most popular videos on YouTube. Over five million voyeuristic viewers have watched me strip off my clothes, take a deep breath, and step into an icy shower (and yes, it still surprises me how many people need a tutorial on taking a cold shower). I have religiously maintained this practice for the past three years, along with cold baths, cold river and lake swims, keeping my home temperature at goose-bump level, and even swimming in the nineteen-foot endless pool in the forest behind my house, which I filled with the chilliest water I could find.

I first became intrigued by cold exposure when, in 2013, I interviewed NASA materials engineer Ray Cronise on my podcast. Ray, who had just penned a fascinating article in *Wired* magazine, described to me during the podcast how he had just created what he called the Shiver System, a protocol to help people lose over 20 pounds of fat per month by taking a cold shower at the beginning and end of each day. Later, I discovered more about the effects of cold exposure when neurosurgeon Dr. Jack Kruse explained to me how he uses cold-water exposure with his patients to heal nerves and brain damage. Then, journalist James Nestor, author of the fascinating book *Deep*, informed me of the beneficial brain changes that occur in freedivers and humans in general when they immerse themselves in cold water.

I was convinced. Not only did I journey to Fort Lauderdale, Florida, to spend a full week learning to freedive and spearfish in deep, cold water, but I also began to experiment with chanting, meditation, deep breathing, and even fancy electronic vagus nerve stimulators, all to increase the integrity of the BBB.

There are plenty of measures you can take to prevent BBB permeability, repair holes that may already be there, and maintain the integrity of your endothelium. The following are twelve ways to fix a leaky brain.

1. Get More Sleep

Sleep loss is known to impair the immune system and increase levels of pro-inflammatory mediators. Sleep loss also increases sympathetic, "fight-or-flight" nervous system activity and causes endothelial dysfunction—which limits the ability of the cells that make up the BBB to divide and repair. The sleep study on mice mentioned earlier found that at the end of six days of sleep deprivation, the permeability of the BBB was restored to baseline after just twenty-four hours of recovery sleep. So to maintain the health of your BBB, you need to get a good amount of sleep each day, between seven and nine hours per twenty-four-hour period. A small dose of the sleep hormone melatonin—0.2 to 0.3 mg—half an hour before bed can help restore optimal BBB permeability and maintain its integrity, and the neurotransmitter-balancing strategies for serotonin and GABA in chapter 1 can also improve your sleep. (Chapter 7 will take a much deeper dive into sleep and sleep hacking.)

2. Limit Your Alcohol Intake

As you learned earlier, alcohol consumption is a major contributor to a leaky brain because of both the formation of ROS, which can damage the BBB, and the passing of compounds such as acetaldehyde across the BBB and into the brain. Sure, the low dose of ethanol from a glass of wine a day can migrate across the BBB and trigger the release of good endorphins and stimulate relaxing neurotransmitter receptors. But higher amounts of alcohol can result in damage from ethanol and acetaldehyde. So as much as possible, limit yourself to one glass of wine per day—preferably not of the giant fishbowl-size variety.

3. Control Blood Pressure

Both acute and chronic hypertension increase BBB permeability. Dark chocolate, magnesium, potassium, handgrip strength training, and even high-dose garlic can all help reduce blood pressure. If you're worried about your breath after consuming garlic, you don't have to mow through an entire bowl of elephant garlic to reap its benefits. Taking a supplement of allicin, the main bioactive component of garlic, is a far more efficient way to get the brain-boosting benefits of garlic, without acquiring vampire-killing breath. As far as handgrip devices go, you can take a Captains of Crush grip strengthener with you in the car or on an airplane or train. There is also a hand-grip smart device called Zona that has been clinically approved for treating blood pressure and guides you through a squeeze-and-relax regimen. Finally, do not restrict salt as a blood pressure–lowering strategy. A good mineral-rich salt is crucial for maintaining normal blood volume, blood pressure, and oxygen delivery to tissues. (For more on the myths behind salt consumption, I cannot recommend highly enough that you read Dr. James DiNicolantonio's book *The Salt Fix*.)

4. Be Cautious with High-Fat Diets

In one study, rodents that were given a diet that was 40 percent saturated fat experienced elevated BBB permeability. But if you happen to be a high-fat, low-carb diet enthusiast, there are ways to mitigate this effect. Adding aged garlic extract, alpha-lipoic acid (particularly R-ALA, its more biologically active form), niacin, or nicotinamide eliminated this elevation. Supplementing with bitter melon and vitamin D_3 has also been shown to be effective. Phytonutrient-rich plants and spices such as turmeric, *Astragalus propinquus* root (astragalus), and cruciferous veggies like broccoli, brussels sprouts, and cabbage produce a similar healing effect. Fiber-rich foods like sweet potatoes, kale, and beans are also helpful. If you follow a high-fat ketogenic diet, I recommend making it a clean, plant-rich one, like those advocated in Dr. Steven Gundry's *The Plant Paradox* and Dr. Terry Wahls's *The Wahls Protocol*. And be sure to consume plenty of dark, leafy greens like kale, spinach, and collard greens.

5. Drink Coffee and Tea

Caffeine is a known protector of BBB integrity, and a cup of coffee a day may even help inhibit BBB disruption, which could be one way that coffee helps to prevent Alzheimer's disease. Caffeine induces the production of cAMP, a molecule that facilitates intercellular communication and fortifies the tight junctions of the BBB. In addition, cAMP reduces inflammation in the brain. You can get a good, healthy dose of caffeine from an 8-ounce cup of coffee or green tea.

6. Take Supplements

Alpha-GPC, a type of choline that readily crosses the BBB, is known to improve endothelial dysfunction. Inositol from egg yolks or supplements also enhances BBB integrity. Berberine reduces BBB permeability and increases resistance to brain damage following head trauma. Vitamins B_{12}, B_6, and B_9 restore a damaged BBB to equilibrium. Research has shown that individuals who have had a stroke may have some success repairing their BBBs by using herbs and supplements such as astragalus, chlorogenic acid, ginseng, olive leaf extract, and rosmarinic acid. In addition, individuals who have had head injuries and suffer from a leaky brain have been shown to benefit from apigenin, butyrate, citicoline, and shilajit.

You can also use nutrients and supplements to help inhibit MMP-9, those enzymes that, in the presence of inflammation, can break down parts of the BBB—inhibitors of MMP-9 have been shown to restore BBB integrity. These inhibitors include curcumin, resveratrol, berberine, fish oil, ginger, broccoli, watercress, pomegranate extract, and many other natural anti-inflammatories found in fruits, vegetables, herbs, and spices.

7. Get More Magnesium

Adequate magnesium intake, between 300 and 400 mg a day, can attenuate BBB permeability—in a study, even people who were injected with an agent to induce leaky BBBs benefited from magnesium. You can get magnesium into your system by taking it orally, soaking in magnesium salts baths, or applying magnesium topically, as either a lotion or spray, on the back of your neck and head. Make sure to track how much magnesium you take in total, including all these applications. In amounts over 1,500 mg per day, magnesium can cause loose stools.

8. Stimulate Your Vagus Nerve

The vagus nerve is the largest nerve in your body and runs from your brain to your ears, tongue, lungs, and gut. It is the backbone of your parasympathetic system, and its health goes hand in hand with both emotional and gastric health. Multiple studies have shown that stimulating the vagus nerve strengthens the BBB. You can naturally stimulate the nerve with practices like massages, singing, chanting, meditation, deep breathing, and cold showers. A good vagus nerve stimulator device that delivers electrical impulses to the vagus nerve, such as the Fisher Wallace Stimulator, can also work quite well.

9. Avoid Frequent Snacking

Ghrelin, a hunger-stimulating hormone, can improve BBB integrity. Research has shown that ghrelin can reduce BBB breakdown after traumatic head injury. By avoiding frequent snacking and grazing, practicing intermittent fasting, and not eating until you're actually hungry, you can normalize your ghrelin levels.

10. Nourish Your Gut Bacteria

One study observed the effects of a transplant of gut bacteria from healthy mice with perfect BBB integrity to unhealthy mice with leaky brains. The researchers found that the transplant restored the integrity of the damaged barriers because of specific inflammation-modulating compounds released by bacteria that increase BBB integrity. Fortunately, you don't have to hunt down a willing donor to give you a healthy poop transplant. You can achieve similar BBB repair results by eating more prebiotic fiber, taking quality probiotics, and eating a wide variety of fermented foods on a regular basis.

11. Decrease Inflammation

According to Dr. Datis Kharrazian, a medical researcher specializing in chronic disease and nutrition, inflammatory cytokines—molecules that promote inflammation—that start in an inflamed gut can enter the bloodstream, make their way to the brain, and pass through even a healthy blood-brain barrier. Once in the brain, these cytokines can affect sensitive tissues, most notably the vagus nerve and autonomic nervous system, to the point that they cannot function properly. Both the vagus nerve and the autonomic nervous system play a major role in regulating the movement of food through the gut, so when they're not working properly, intestinal motility slows down. In a sort of vicious cycle, once intestinal motility slows down, the inflammatory cytokines in the intestines have even more time to make their way into the bloodstream and from there pass through the blood-brain barrier, creating a cycle of continuing inflammation and worsening intestinal function. Because poor vagal nerve tone can increase both cortisol and inflammatory cytokines, Dr. Kharrazian recommends stimulating the vagus nerve in order to reboot it, through singing, gargling, and gagging exercises, along with coffee enemas.

12. Cold Thermogenesis

With ten pale-blue fingers, I white-knuckled the steering wheel of my Toyota RAV4 and strained to remember how to turn on the engine. After staring blankly through the windshield at the parking lot for several minutes—teeth chattering and brain slowly coming back to life—I leaned to the right, fumbled for the keys that lay on the passenger seat, then cursed as my large intestine contracted and filled my soggy Speedo with a liquid bowel evacuation.

Ten minutes earlier, I had dragged my sorry ass out of the frigid Spokane River and stumbled like a drunk, waterlogged sea otter up across the pavement back to my Toyota. See, after studying the benefits of cold thermogenesis (which is the use of any type of cooling strategy to induce a metabolic effect) and practicing cold showers and ice baths for several weeks, I figured I would level up and try a real outdoor cold-water swim in the middle of March, when chunks of ice still floated down the river near my home. But rather than simply dipping in and out of the safe edges of the water, like a true hard-charging overachiever, I attempted to swim upstream for a good twenty minutes without a wet suit. Now in the car, as my body fought to restore its normal temperature after my foolhardy attempt at a health hack, I was paying the price.

Thing is, a long, frigid, lose-control-of-your-bowels ice-water swim is an unnecessary (and very much ill-advised) method of engaging in cold thermogenesis. With far simpler techniques, you can take full advantage of the many benefits of cold thermogenesis. By engaging in regular cold exposure such as cold soaks, cold showers, splashing cold water on your face, wearing body-cooling gear like the Cool Fat Burner vest, sitting in cryotherapy chambers, and even keeping your home a bit chilly, you can:

- restore BBB health by causing increased blood flow and nitric oxide delivery to your brain, which increases BBB integrity and suppresses BBB degeneration
- increase cell longevity
- support a robust immune system
- induce rapid fat loss in the absence of exercise
- lower your appetite and strengthen the appetite-regulating vagus nerve connection between the gut and brain
- cause internal temperature fluctuations that will send blood and nitric oxide to your brain (you will learn more about nitric oxide in chapter 3)

One simple option is to use Ray Cronise's Shiver System, a five-minute cold shower at the beginning and end of the day. It involves alternating from twenty seconds of cold water to ten seconds of warm water ten times through. If this sounds boring or monotonous to you, get a waterproof mp3 player or learn some rollicking shower songs.

Another option is a dip in the brand-new Morozko Forge, which is a prebuilt eight-foot-long ice bath that uses chlorine-free ozone treatment combined with an advanced water cooling system to maintain water temperatures as low as 32 degrees Fahrenheit—even in hot summer conditions of up to 110 degrees Fahrenheit.

Alternatively, for some DIY options, you can use my fellow biohacker Luke Storey's budget freezer hack or my friend and music producer Rick Rubin's slightly spendier luxury chiller system.

Interestingly, these types of strategies are all the more crucial for children. After all, babies aren't born with a BBB! If a leaky BBB makes an adult highly susceptible to toxins, chemicals, and other environmental and food-based pollutants, it really makes you rethink how you should optimally care for a newborn child, eh?

LUKE STOREY'S FREEZER HACK

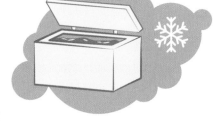

This $800 hack involves turning a chest freezer into an ice bath. It beats the hell out of spending $5,000 to $35,000 for a professional sports or spa version.

Step 1: Buy a 19.8-cubic-foot chest freezer. This is big enough for two average-size people to cram into at once, or for one person to sit comfortably in with legs extended. The minimum size for me to extend my legs fully is 17.5 cubic feet (I'm six foot two). You can always go to a store and jump in a few different freezers to find the one you want, but prepare to get some curious glances. I like a freezer like a Frigidaire because it comes with casters, which make it mobile—a helpful feature when it comes to emptying the water out. You might want to consider throwing in an extra $150 for an extended warranty, especially since you are not using the freezer for its intended purpose. That said, mine has been going strong for over a year with no issues.

Step 2: Using a garden hose with a chlorine filter attached, fill the freezer with water to about five to eight inches from the top. Next, plug the freezer in and turn it to the coldest temperature. Depending on the outside temperature, it can take from thirty-six to seventy-two hours for the water inside the freezer to become cold.

Step 3: Pour ½ cup of 35 percent food-grade hydrogen peroxide into the water. This will prevent or at least slow down the growth of bacteria. Use as often as needed, preferably each time you bathe. Do not use salt, which would promote rust.

Step 4: Once the water has reached the desired temperature (mine is 39 degrees Fahrenheit), plug the power cable of the freezer into a grounded twenty-four-hour plug-in mechanical timer so that the freezer turns on for approximately two to four hours per night. You will have to find the sweet spot where the water stays cold but doesn't freeze over. You can monitor your water temp to find the correct timer setting using a laser thermometer.

Step 5: Plug a breaker-safe grounding stake into any nearby ground and drop the opposite end's alligator clip into the tub. This will keep the water grounded, which confers additional health benefits. Bodies of water in nature are never ungrounded, and I find ice baths to be much more calming when they are grounded. To prevent electrical surges from lightning strikes, make sure you use a grounding cable with a breaker.

Step 6: Depending on how often you use the ice bath freezer, how sweaty you are, and how many users regularly get into the water, you will need to change the water in the tub once every one to two weeks. If you shower off sweat from workouts or saunas before getting into the bath, your water will last longer. You will know it is time to change it when it develops a swampy smell, which comes from bacteria. To change the water, pull out the drain plug on the bottom corner of the unit, empty all the water out, clean the tub, then refill it with filtered water.

Step 7: Always unplug the power from the unit when you are using it. It is unlikely that there is any danger in using the unit while it is plugged in, but when it comes to mixing water and electricity, it is better to be safe than sorry. Trust me, you do not want to create a "toaster in the bathtub" effect.

The following tips will help you maintain your freezer:

- If you see rust start to form on the seams inside the tub, empty the tub, dry it, and apply a clear silicone sealant to the affected seams to prevent future oxidation.
- Keep a doormat next to the tub and wipe your feet before entering.
- If you want a less ugly tub, consider building a wooden encasement around it. Alternatively, you could have the tub professionally painted at an auto body shop. Please note that if you do build an encasement, your water will likely freeze much faster, and this will affect the settings of your outlet timer.

RICK RUBIN'S CHILLER SYSTEM

In the backyard of his Kauai beach house, music producer Rick Rubin has a beautiful, highly effective ice bath system that's the Cadillac of cold thermogenesis setups. It's an ofuro (Japanese-style) hot tub attached to a hot tub cooling system and an ozonator, so the water stays clean without the use of chlorine or hydrogen peroxide. For this setup, you'll need the services of a professional contractor and a cool $6,000. You'll find everything at BoundlessBook.com/2.

MY OWN TECHNIQUE

After forgoing the painstaking process of swimming through ice chunks in the Spokane River, I took the admittedly elaborate and expensive step of hiring a crane to drop a nineteen-foot endless swimming pool in my backyard forest, then disabled the heater. In the cool, shady conditions of the Inland Northwest, the pool remains at a chilly 40 to 55 degrees Fahrenheit year-round.

THE LAST WORD

You don't want to associate the word *leaky* with any part of your body. After reading this chapter, you may be worried that you have somehow done irreparable damage to a delicate structure in your brain. But the good news is that your endothelial cells are designed to quickly regenerate and patch holes in your BBB. All you need to do is follow the tips in this chapter to give your body the environment that allows this repair to occur.

In the same way that a sound intestinal lining is necessary for optimized digestion and nutrient absorption, an intact and correctly functioning BBB is critical for precise cognitive performance. By combining all the strategies above with what you already discovered in chapter 1 about neurotransmitters and what you are about to discover in chapter 3 about breathing, you will be fully equipped to upgrade your brain health and cognition.

ONE THING YOU CAN DO THIS WEEK

The health of the vagus nerve, a raging appetite, and normalized blood pressure are all critical to a healthy BBB. Guess what addresses all three? Cold showers and cold water to the face. Each morning for the next week, try to take a two-to-five-minute cold shower or splash cold water in your face ten to twenty times.

> For citations for all the research studies mentioned in this chapter and a deeper dive into the topics of this chapter—including links to podcasts, blog posts, recommended tools and supplements, and much more—visit BoundlessBook.com/2.

BREATHWORK AND BEYOND

HOW TO BANISH STRESS AND KISS HIGH CORTISOL GOODBYE

Ron Penna, the founder of Quest Nutrition and a brilliant student of human physiology, flexed his python-like biceps and spoke a little faster. "But it turns out most of these so-called breathing experts are wrong and that carbon dioxide is a *good* thing."

I leaned forward at the dinner table, ignoring my sous vide rib-eye steak. I had always been taught, even in my master's-level nutrition and exercise science courses, that carbon dioxide (CO_2) was a metabolic waste product associated with lactic acid accumulation and poor breathing patterns, and that too much CO_2 in your blood resulted in nasty issues like metabolic acidosis and cell damage. Ultimately, I had been taught that the less CO_2 you have floating around in your bloodstream, the better.

Ron continued: "High levels of CO_2 in the body, if you can figure out how to get high oxygen levels at the same time, is actually one of the best ways to completely saturate your tissues with oxygen. As a matter of fact, the naked mole rat, an animal that lives an inordinately long amount of time, has rock-bottom levels of inflammation, and has never been known to develop cancer, lives in underground holes that allow it to maintain remarkably high levels of CO_2."

I was skeptical, but Ron went on to explain something called the Bohr effect: high levels of CO_2 cause the hemoglobin in red blood cells to dump their precious oxygen. Because this increases oxygen levels in the brain and muscles, it results in huge surges of energy and enhanced physical performance. He also described the fascinating practice of Buteyko breathing, a little-known form of breathwork that optimizes oxygenation, maximizes O_2 and CO_2 levels, and causes stress levels to plummet.

I had one more question for Ron. "So what's the best way to teach the body how to do this the right way?"

Ron's eyebrows shot up in surprise. "You mean you don't know? I would have thought you were doing this every night, Ben. It's mouth taping."

I nodded and gulped. It could be tough to convince my wife that I needed to tape my mouth at night during our normal snuggle-and-chat time, but I was willing to experiment with Ron's anticancer, cortisol-lowering, life-extending suggestions. Head spinning, I left dinner and immediately ordered the book *Normal Breathing: The Key to Vital Health,* by Artour Rakhimov, which changed my entire approach to breathwork—specifically, by altering my belief that you need to breathe deeply from the belly and exhale as much harmful CO_2 as possible and convincing me that, instead, shallow, infrequent nasal breathing could be a hidden key to longevity, decreased levels of the stress hormone cortisol, and reduced risk of cancer.

The power of breath to change emotions, chemicals, neurotransmitters, and hormones was not a new concept to me. Years before speaking with Ron, I first realized the importance of breath when I interviewed running coach and author Budd Coates, who taught me the rhythmic exercise breathing techniques I'll cover later in this chapter. When training with former Navy SEAL commander Mark Divine at his famous SEALFIT Kokoro crucible camp in California, I learned box breathing and holotropic breathwork, the latter of which got me the highest I have ever been sans psychedelics. Freediving instructor Ted Harty introduced me to static apnea tables for hypoxia (low oxygen) and CO_2 tolerance. World-famous holistic health coach Paul Chek taught me the best tricks for proper deep belly breathing. The Iceman, Wim Hof, taught me his body-charging breathwork tactics, and big-wave surfer Laird Hamilton showed me how to use my breathing to instantly enter the parasympathetic rest-and-digest state.

Quick Tips to Breathe Better

An easier-to-digest alternative to *Normal Breathing* is *The Power of Your Breath* by Anders Olsson. In Olsson's book, I found a host of breathing tips and science based on Buteyko breathing concepts, including these:

- Breathe in through whichever nostril correlates to the part of the brain you want to activate (keeping in mind that the left side of the brain is associated with the right side of the body, and vice versa). For example, if you have a more left-brain, analytical, logical task to accomplish, precede it with one to two minutes of inhaling only through your right nostril. If you need to accomplish a more right-brain, creative task, then inhale only through the left nostril. Breathing only through your left nostril is also an effective way to activate the parasympathetic nervous system before bed or a nap.

- To increase your CO_2 levels, you can mix 2 teaspoons of baking soda with a glass of water and drink it before, during, or after training. Alternatively, throughout the day, you can sip on a form of bottled water that is naturally high in sodium bicarbonate, such as San Pellegrino bottled water. I personally drink two to three big 32-ounce bottles of San Pellegrino per day.

- Use a device called the Relaxator to improve your breathing. I have been hanging this tiny breath-training device around my neck when I go on walks to train me how to retain oxygen and CO_2 simultaneously.

- Add one to two cups of baking soda to a bath and soak in it for twenty to thirty minutes to increase circulating CO_2 levels.

- Take three deep abdominal breaths prior to a meal to center your body and improve nutrient uptake.

In this chapter, you will learn everything I have been taught by these experts, the best-of-the-best breathing protocols. But first, you must understand something called the HPA axis, along with the reason your breath (which you can consider to be your life force, your invisible energy, your prana, and a primary source of boundless energy) is vitally important to your cortisol and CO_2 levels. Then you'll understand why breath is one of the most potent tools you can use to decrease stress, fix your nervous system, and even upgrade your genetics.

STRESS AND THE HPA AXIS

There is a thin beige kite string lying on the surface of my desk. Each day, when I arrive at my desk to write, I take that kite string and tie it around my waist. No, I am not obsessed with narcissistic waist measurements, nor do I have a kite fetish. Rather, the kite string trick is a method taught to me by Paul Chek, who discovered that everything from constipation and back pain to poor stress control is caused by squeezing one's abs in, a habit I developed to perfection during two years of competitive "abs in, chest out" bodybuilding. Paul also teaches that one of the best fixes for this habit—which he refers to as an inverted breathing pattern that locks up the abdominal wall, pulls the rib cage down, and puts extra tension on the chest and neck muscles, restricting the amount of oxygen your body receives—is to tie a string around your waist and focus on consciously expanding that string in and out with each belly breath. This is also a potent way to decrease stress because the pressure receptors in your chest can stimulate cortisol release during shallow chest breathing. Nifty trick, eh?

Don't get me wrong: stress can be good for you. Stress is why ripping muscle fibers apart with a barbell makes you stronger, why sucking wind and tasting lactic acid in your mouth during a run makes your heart healthier, why skipping a meal or fasting enhances longevity and blood sugar control, why eating bitter wild plants and tannic coffees and teas strengthens your immune system, why getting bombarded with sunlight radiation causes vitamin D synthesis, and why blasting through a hundred emails causes the growth of new neurons.

A heavy weight, a fast-moving treadmill, a morning without food, a mouth-puckering bite of raw kale, a bit of afternoon UVA and UVB rays, and even stress from a lion jumping out of your email inbox are all mild hormetic stressors. Hormesis is a biological reaction in which low doses of an agent that could be toxic or lethal at higher doses have a beneficial effect, such as improved health, stress tolerance, muscle growth, or longevity. Sure, exercise could kill you if you went to extremes, but in controlled doses, exercise can give you hormetic benefits, such as an increased ability to fight free radicals, manage heavy loads, or be more resilient to environmental stressors. Other examples of hormetic stressors include fasting, caloric restriction, exposure to heat or cold, low-level radiation, and even exposure to some bacteria and germs.

This concept of hormesis is why I do something mildly uncomfortable every day (like a cold shower, a sweat session in a sauna, or a hard-breathing workout) and something that scares the living hell out of me about once a quarter (like a hard obstacle course race, an off-road triathlon, or an open-mic-night performance).

But you run into problems when you expose yourself to too much of this type of stress. In many people, excessive exposure to hormetic stress from all those workouts, cold baths, sauna sessions, and more is often combined with:

- Physical stress from sleep deprivation
- Chemical stress from drugs, alcohol, caffeine, nicotine, cleaning chemicals, or pesticides

- Mental stress from anxiety or worry
- Emotional stress from anger, guilt, loneliness, sadness, or fear
- Nutritional stress from food allergies or nutritional deficiencies
- Spiritual stress from troubled relationships or financial or career pressures

When any of this stress—both the good and the bad—gets too high and too hard for too long, you can break your brain via a third system, which is the focus of this chapter. That system is the hypothalamic-adrenal-pituitary axis (HPA axis), and when it breaks, you end up with HPA axis dysfunction.

The HPA axis includes the hypothalamus (the part of your forebrain toward the front of your skull), the pituitary gland (just below the hypothalamus), and the adrenal glands (at the top of the kidneys). By producing a host of chemicals, such as corticotropin-releasing hormone (CRH), adrenocorticotropic hormone (ACTH), glucocorticoids, and cortisol, these three organs regulate functions such as stress response, mood, digestion, immune system function, libido, metabolism, and energy levels.

This entire axis operates on what are called feedback loops. A feedback loop occurs when the output of any system loops back to that system as an input. A positive feedback loop would increase a system's output, while a negative feedback loop would decrease a system's output.

Let's take a look at how a feedback loop would take place in the HPA axis—in this case, with regard to cortisol. You lift a heavy barbell at the gym, your body realizes it is stepping into a fight against that barbell, and cortisol is released to activate your sympathetic nervous system. At the same time, some of that cortisol sends one signal back to your hypothalamus to inhibit CRH production and another signal to your pituitary gland to inhibit ACTH production, which can decrease production of epinephrine and norepinephrine by the adrenal glands. The result of this negative feedback loop is that cortisol taps the brakes on your body's built-in stimulants, ensuring that you don't exhaust your energy stores by lifting barbells all day.

In healthy, low-stress individuals who are not, say, crushing a CrossFit WOD or destroying themselves at the gym each day, this HPA axis feedback loop works in harmony. But when cortisol and norepinephrine are overproduced, the HPA axis eventually becomes desensitized to the negative feedback telling it to calm down. This leads to chronic stress on the hypothalamus, pituitary

The HPA Axis Feedback Loop

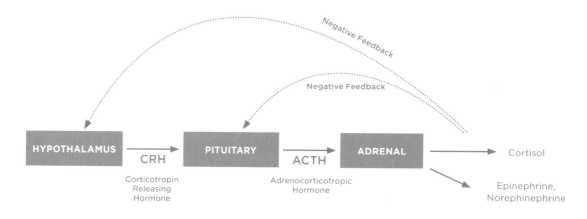

gland, and adrenal glands. Eventually, adrenal imbalances arise that cause hard-charging high achievers to wake up each morning tired, groggy, and unmotivated until they can get their paws on a piping-hot cup of liquid cortisol: coffee.

Interestingly, HPA axis dysfunction is associated with the neurotransmitter imbalances you learned about in chapter 1. For example, selective serotonin reuptake inhibitor antidepressants are very effective at treating panic issues. These drugs keep serotonin high, causing norepinephrine levels to fall, so you feel less of the effects of chronic stress. But this is a less-than-ideal way to treat stress since you simply need more and more antidepressants as time goes on and your body becomes desensitized to serotonin.

The Adrenal Fatigue Myth

I have made mistakes in the past. For example, I used to tell all my personal-training clients to eat six to ten small meals per day to keep the metabolism boosted, a myth I'll bust in chapter 8. I used to preach that having as much muscle as possible was a key to longevity, which is also not true, as I'll explain in chapter 9. And in my previous book, *Beyond Training*, I devoted an entire section to identifying and fixing "adrenal fatigue," which recent research has shown to be a bit more complicated than I first thought.

The term *adrenal fatigue* (AF) has been used by some medical experts to describe a condition supposedly caused by chronic stress, particularly exposure to stressful situations. It was first coined in 1998 by Dr. James Wilson to describe a group of symptoms that include body aches, fatigue, nervousness, sleep disturbances, and digestive issues, all of which were hypothesized to be the result of subpar adrenal gland function and are typically the reason a catch-all term such as AF is used as a diagnosis. When you experience stress, your immune system slows down and your adrenal glands release hormones like cortisol to regulate blood pressure and heart function. According to the AF theory, if you experience long-term chronic stress, your adrenal glands become incapable of continuously producing the amount of cortisol necessary to make you "feel good" or give you energy. At that point, supposedly, adrenal fatigue hits.

But the fact is that no endocrinology society has recognized AF. In fact, most endocrinologists claim there is no compelling evidence that the condition exists. There is an inherent fault with the theory of AF because the underlying biology is false: the adrenal glands are indeed capable of pumping out plenty of hormones like cortisol. To cope with increasing amounts of stress, the adrenal glands may also adapt and become larger. And even if cortisol levels are low, it doesn't necessarily mean that the adrenal glands aren't working. The hormone DHEA is also produced by the adrenal glands, and sometimes when cortisol levels are reduced, DHEA can be relatively high—so low cortisol levels do not necessarily point to subpar adrenal gland function.

There are a myriad of valid causes of symptoms attributed to AF, none of which arise from adrenal dysfunction. Sure, it is true that recommended treatments for alleged cases of AF have proven to be helpful. But the drugs prescribed for AF—which are typically corticosteroids—seem to promote a sense of well-being whether or not someone has been diagnosed with AF.

One of the other issues with AF is that diagnosing it usually requires examining a patient's cortisol levels. But there are any number of factors that could influence cortisol levels. In fact, you could probably name one common factor given everything you have learned thus far in the book: inflammation. Cortisol modulates inflammation, and there are many environmental factors aside from AF that could result in an acute or chronic inflammatory state.

How does inflammation lead to symptoms that could be misconstrued as AF? First, tiredness, a chief symptom of AF, is actually modulated by the hypothalamus. The hypothalamus is regulated in part by orexin neurons, and inflammation leads to the suppression of orexin neurons, resulting in an overall feeling of fatigue. One example of this effect is narcolepsy, which is thought to result from the loss of orexin: people with narcolepsy have a high level of general fatigue in addition to the excessive daytime sleepiness that also characterizes this disorder.

Inflammation also modulates tiredness through pro-inflammatory cytokines, small proteins that signal interactions and communications between cells. Pro-inflammatory cytokines in the brain have been observed to correlate with fatigue in many studies. One of the mechanisms by which this is thought to occur is the suppression of what is called the "circadian pacemaker output." Circadian rhythms, which govern sleep cycles, are controlled by a pacemaker in the su-prachiasmatic nucleus in the hypothalamus. Research suggests that inflammatory damage to the circadian pacemaker leaves a person feeling tired.

All of this is not to say that everyone who thinks they have AF is suffering from hypothalamic problems. Symptoms of alleged cases of AF could be the result of anything from sleep apnea to thyroid dysfunction. But let's say that you are indeed dealing with many of the symptoms of AF— whether due to inflammation, overtraining, or a combination of factors. What's the best fix?

First, many of the tactics covered in this chapter, from curcumin to cryotherapy, revolve around quelling inflammation to put you in a state that is more receptive to recovery. These tactics can help you minimize or resolve any symptoms stemming from inflammation.

There are also lifestyle changes you can make to reduce fatigue and other symptoms so often associated with AF. One of the first things to do is reduce sources of stress in your life. Stress can lead to the release of pro-inflammatory compounds like cytokines, blood cells, and platelets, which, in turn, lead to chronic low-level inflammation. Meditation is a simple method for reducing anxiety and stress, as are several of the breathing techniques in this chapter, especially box breathing. Getting adequate sleep is also critical for reducing fatigue. After all, your body can only fully repair itself if you get enough sleep. Visit chapter 7 and its guidelines for hacking your sleep schedule and circadian rhythms, even when you are on the road, and for properly timing your sleep.

Sun exposure helps to reduce fatigue-related symptoms as well. The infrared rays that the sun releases, particularly between 8 and 11 a.m. and 4 and 7 p.m., modulate several physiological processes related to stress and fatigue. Low-frequency PEMF therapy has also been shown to modulate and improve fatigue, which makes sense considering that the PEMFs given off by the earth are involved in regulating circadian rhythms. Blue-light-blocking glasses and blue-light-generating glasses can also help regulate your circadian rhythms.

As you can see, it's not just as simple as getting a diagnosis of AF and taking the giant plastic bag full of adrenal-support supplements that your old-school naturopathic doctor might hand you or the corticosteroids an allopathic physician might prescribe. Instead, you must change your lifestyle and your environment dramatically to manage these.

Finally, one other underlying cause of fatigue is mitochondrial dysfunction. When your mitochondria fail, ATP production drops, resulting in reduced energy levels, which affects everything from muscle contraction to hormone production. Your mitochondria often fail when the system responsible for producing ATP becomes excessively stressed. Here is how this might occur: In normal metabolism, ATP is converted into a compound called ADP and phosphate energy is released. ADP passes into the mitochondria, where ATP is then remade by a process called "oxidative phosphorylation." A person becomes fatigued when he or she requires energy faster than ATP can be produced. In this scenario, ATP is converted into ADP faster than it can be recycled, resulting in a buildup of ADP. Some of the ADP is converted into AMP-1 phosphate, but this cannot be recycled fast enough to keep up with ATP losses. The result is too much ADP and AMP-1 phosphate and not enough ATP. So any attempt to reduce fatigue and other related symptoms ought to include strategies for boosting your mitochondrial count and efficiency. Chapter 20 has more about how to reduce and fix mitochondrial dysfunction by addressing a host of invisible variables in your personal environment that can affect mitochondria. I also highly recommend the works of Dr. Sarah Myhill (drmyhill.co.uk) on mitochondria dysfunction, especially *Diagnosis and Treatment of Chronic Fatigue Syndrome and Myalgic Encephalitis*.

In addition, one important consideration for mitochondrial dysfunction is the concept of a "cell danger response," which is elucidated in a fascinating paper by researcher Dr. Robert Naviaux. In simple terms, your mitochondria can sense danger, such as a pathogen, toxin, or excessive sympathetic nervous system activity initiated by stress, and in response release ATP into the extracellular matrix. The ATP can bind to receptors on the outside of the cells and trigger an immune response, leading to cytokine cascades and massive inflammation. When mitochondria get stuck in this process because the pathogens are still there or danger is still perceived, chronic fatigue syndrome and mitochondrial dysfunction can result because you have very little ATP left for energy production (since it's all being dumped into the extracellular matrix, a network of molecules outside cells that give them structure and support). For people with chronic fatigue, some good functional medicine doctors are now using a medication called suramin (originally developed to treat African sleeping sickness) to block the extracellular ATP and calm the immune reaction. The reason this is important is that Dr. Naviaux believes that no amount of mitochondrial support will reverse the process of releasing ATP once it's begun, so you simply need to either eliminate the source of danger or switch off the "danger response" that has gotten caught in this loop.

HOW TO FIX YOUR HPA AXIS

So what can you do about HPA axis dysfunction? You can probably guess the single most important tactic I have ever discovered for dealing with the stress that causes HPA axis issues: breathing.

Research has demonstrated a link between stress and breath. In fact, scientists have figured out that you can relax your brain via deep, controlled breathing techniques and that you can speed up stress reactions and cortisol release via hyperventilation. This all has to do with your brain's respiratory pacemaker, which consists of a cluster of neurons in the brain stem that affect breathing, emotional states, and alertness.

Harvard researcher Herbert Benson coined the term "the relaxation response" in his 1975 book of the same name. He wrote that by using your breath, you can alter the basic activity of your cells and the expression of your genes. But more fast-acting than your breath's gene-altering effects is its ability to improve the body's reaction to stressful situations, reduce excessive stress hormones, and alter oxygen and carbon dioxide levels in the way Ron explained to me at dinner. Short, rapid breathing stimulates the fight-or-flight sympathetic nervous system, while slow, deep breathing stimulates the rest-and-digest parasympathetic nervous system.

As a hard-charging high achiever, I am infatuated with the power of breathwork. And in my quest to become a better breather, I have identified the best-of-the-best of the myriad of breathwork tactics, all of which you are about to discover.

THE BEST-OF-THE-BEST BREATHING TECHNIQUES

While there are a host of breathwork practices and tactics, I've personally discovered that those listed below are the most effective for me at managing stress, maintaining tissue oxygenation, enhancing sleep, increasing energy, and much more.

1. Buteyko Breathing

Years before I spoke with Ron Penna, Patrick McKeown, the author of the excellent book *Oxygen Advantage*, introduced me during a podcast interview to Buteyko breathing, a technique primarily used to reverse the host of health problems associated with improper breathing habits. The most common of these habits are overbreathing (excess oxygen consumption combined with excess carbon dioxide exhalation) and mouth breathing, which contribute to poor sleep and sleep apnea. Buteyko breathing—named after the Russian physician who developed the technique—is based on the fact that when you stop mouth breathing and learn to engage in slow, whisper-like nasal breathing, you can oxygenate your tissues and organs far more effectively.

As Ron described to me at dinner, the common belief among experts is that you must breathe deeply to remove excess CO_2. But you must still maintain ideal CO_2 levels in your lungs because lack of CO_2 constricts your blood vessels and may detrimentally affect your heart function, tissue oxygenation, and blood pH. Buteyko breathing keeps you from both excessive oxygen consumption and excessive CO_2 blow-off. In addition, Buteyko nasal breathing transports the gas nitric oxide (NO) more readily into your lungs because your nasal cavities produce and contain high levels of NO. Think of NO as Viagra for your entire body—it significantly dilates blood vessels and bronchial tubes, along with neutralizing germs and bacteria.

How can you learn to Buteyko breathe and reverse a mouth-breathing habit? The two best methods are the control-pause technique and nighttime mouth taping.

THE CONTROL-PAUSE TECHNIQUE (CP)

CP is a breath-hold after a normal exhalation of air until you experience the tiniest desire to breathe in. CP provides excellent feedback about your ability to efficiently raise your carbon dioxide levels and engage in nasal breathing.

To obtain an accurate measurement, rest for ten minutes before the exercise. Next, begin to breathe through your nose. After exhaling normally through your nose (not a full, deep exhalation), squeeze the tip of your nose with your fingers and look at a stopwatch. If you experience even the slightest inclination to breathe in or gasp air at six seconds, immediately let go. In this case, your CP is six seconds. If you have to take a big breath at the end of the breath-hold, then you held your breath for too long.

A good CP is thirty seconds, a very good CP is forty-five seconds, and Buteyko claimed that if someone had a CP of sixty seconds, then "he or she is insured against illness." A CP lower than thirty seconds indicates room for improvement, while a CP lower than

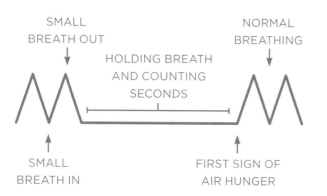

SMALL BREATH OUT

NORMAL BREATHING

HOLDING BREATH AND COUNTING SECONDS

SMALL BREATH IN

FIRST SIGN OF AIR HUNGER

fifteen seconds is indicative of symptoms such as respiratory issues, disordered sleep breathing, anxiety, and stress. My first CP was seventeen seconds, but via nasal breathing, mouth-taping, and many of the other tactics in this chapter, I am now up to forty-one seconds and still improving.

MOUTH TAPING

The concept of mouth taping is quite simple: you tape your mouth prior to sleep to force your body to learn nasal breathing. I personally mouth-taped for a month, after which I found that my body had simply become trained to breathe through my nose during the night. You will want to get 3M Micropore tape from Amazon or any medical supplies dealer, or a pre-cut mouth-shaped tape called Somnifix (which contains a hypoallergenic adhesive with fewer chemicals than 3M tape).

Apply a small amount of an edible oil such as olive or coconut oil to your lips and the edges of your mouth—this will make it easier to roll back the tape during the night if you need to speak or cough—then apply the tape your lips. Gently attempt to inhale through your mouth to make sure you didn't miss a spot. The next step is easy: fall asleep while breathing through your nose. You will find it relaxing and easy to learn. Amazingly, I found that I instantly adjusted to sleeping with the tape on, even when I was first learning the technique.

2. Box Breathing

Former Navy SEAL commander Mark Divine taught me this simple tactic for quieting the mind during periods of extreme stress, such as struggling to stay warm during an entire night of standing in the bone-chilling waves of the Pacific Ocean or sitting in a giant tub of ice for over fifteen minutes. I also use this tactic to resist the urge to flinch from syringes during procedures such as stem cell injections or blood draws. The deep, intentional breathing helps to regulate the autonomic nervous system and calm you down.

The technique is simple: close your mouth and slowly inhale through your nose for four seconds, hold your breath for four seconds, exhale through your mouth for four seconds, then hold the exhalation for another four seconds. Doing this a few times through will help you enter a relaxed state. Commander Divine has even developed an app, Box Breathing, that teaches you his own style of this technique, complete with audio cues and timers.

Box breathing is similar to another popular style of breathing called 4-7-8 breathing. For 4-7-8 breathing, begin by placing the tip of your tongue against the ridge of tissue behind your upper front teeth. Quietly inhale through the nose for four seconds, hold your breath for seven seconds, then exhale audibly through your mouth, making a whooshing sound, for eight seconds. Repeat this cycle at least three more times.

3. Kundalini Yoga Breathing

Of all the forms of yoga I have learned, Kundalini yoga is the most invigorating and the best at circulating oxygen throughout the body. In the Kundalini yoga tradition, a combination of movement and breathing techniques are used to ignite your Kundalini energy, which is coiled at the base of your spine. The first time that I performed a Kundalini session on the beaches of Kauai, I found myself in a trancelike state for hours afterward.

Kundalini yoga weaves several core breathing concepts into a single yoga routine.

BREATH OF FIRE

If you have ever watched a dog pant, you get the gist of Breath of Fire. This is one of the few forms of breathing I perform to invigorate the body and activate the sympathetic nervous system. To perform it, inhale and exhale as quickly as you can—preferably through your nose—while pressing your belly out on the inhalation and in on the exhalation. (This technique is considered to be activating for the sympathetic nervous system, so you may want to avoid it if you are in a stressed-out state.)

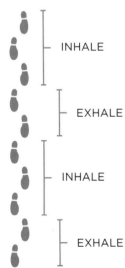

INHALE
through nose
EXHALE
through nose

INHALE ←
stomach out
EXHALE →
stomach in

SITALI BREATH

Also known as the "cooling breath," Sitali brings you into a centered, focused state of calmness. Close your eyes, curl your tongue, and inhale through your open mouth. Then close your mouth and exhale through your nose. I have found that simply performing six Sitali breaths when I am in stuck in traffic or overwhelmed by a stressful workday can be incredibly centering.

ALTERNATE-NOSTRIL BREATHING

In the Kundalini tradition, this form of breathing, traditionally known as Nadi Shodhana Pranayama, is a potent stress-reducing tactic. Begin by pressing your thumb on your right nostril and gently breathe out through your left nostril. Next, gently breathe in through the left nostril, and then press the left nostril closed with a different finger. Remove your thumb from the right nostril and breathe out through the right nostril. Next, breathe in through the right nostril, close it with your thumb, lift your finger from your left nostril, and then exhale from the left nostril.

4. Rhythmic Breathing

After reading the book *Running on Air* by Budd Coates, I began to use rhythmic breathing to get through long Ironman bike rides and runs. Then I realized that it could be used in just about every exercise situation. Whether you are lifting weights, running, or cycling, rhythmic breathing can be used to keep your body in a relaxed state no matter how hard you are moving. Learning to breathe rhythmically is difficult initially, but it becomes second nature within a few days of practice.

INHALE

EXHALE

INHALE

EXHALE

When you are running or cycling, you want to inhale more than you exhale. When you are lifting weights, you want the lengths of your inhales and exhales to be equal. No matter what you're doing, you never lose control of your breath or allow it to become nonrhythmic.

If you are running or cycling, take one active, deep nasal breath in for every three foot strikes or pedal strokes and one relaxed, more passive nasal breath out on the next two foot strikes or pedal strokes. As you increase your intensity and go faster, you can continue this breathing pattern while speeding up the breath frequency by taking one deep breath in for two foot strikes or pedal strokes and one deep breath out on the subsequent foot strike or pedal stroke.

If you are lifting weights, take in a deep nasal breath, exhale as you lift the weight, then take in another deep nasal breath as you return the weight to its starting position.

5. Decompression Breathing

Hunching all day at a keyboard, tilting our heads over our phones, commuting long hours, and slouching on the couch all promote poor posture and aggravate poor breathing patterns. This, in turn, causes unnecessary stress and strain on the joints, restricts organ function, and weakens force output. So if you can wake up in the morning and do something that fights the effects of gravity and restores your body to a decompressed state, so you can enhance circulation, breathe better, and stand taller all day long and have better digestion and no lower-back pain, why not try it?

Enter Dr. Eric Goodman. After watching Eric's TEDx Talk, "The Unexpected Physical Consequences of Technology," I interviewed him on my podcast about the decompressive breathing he teaches in his Foundation Training program, which trains your body to shift the burden of its weight to where it belongs: the large posterior chain muscle groups, specifically your shoulders, back, butt, and legs. Foundation Training was birthed by necessity when Dr. Goodman began suffering repetitive back problems in his midtwenties. He had blown out his L4 through his S1 vertebrae in his lower back and was told, at twenty-five years old, that he needed back surgery.

Instead, Dr. Goodman, who was in chiropractic school at the time, became a man obsessed. He used his knowledge of anatomy and his deep understanding of exercise to learn how to use breath and simple exercises to decompress the spine and restore nerve and lower-back function. Each movement incorporates the same basic decompressive breathing pattern, in which you inhale and expand your rib cage up and out to the sides of your chest. You then focus on keeping the rib cage expanded while you exhale, using your stomach muscles to expel the air from your lungs. I use this form of breathwork every day, typically during a quick break from computer work or while on a long road trip or flight.

6. Static Apnea Tables

Static apnea tables, which were introduced to me by freediving instructor Ted Harty, are sequences of timed breath-holds designed to accustom the body to an extreme lack of oxygen or excess CO_2. These can be quite useful for training inspiratory and expiratory muscles, increasing breath-hold time, and even as a mini-workout on an easy recovery day. The tables can be performed in water or on dry land (for instance, when you are on the couch at home or driving).

A CO_2 tolerance table is designed to accustom the body to high levels of carbon dioxide by reducing the duration of resting time between breath-holds. The following table, which requires about twenty-five minutes to complete, consists of eight cycles and is based on breath-holds of one and a half minutes:

1	Hold breath 1:30 min		5	Rest 1:30 min	Hold 1:30 min
2	Rest 2:15 min	Hold 1:30 min	6	Rest 1:15 min	Hold 1:30 min
3	Rest 2:00 min	Hold 1:30 min	7	Rest 1:00 min	Hold 1:30 min
4	Rest 1:45 min	Hold 1:30 min	8	Rest 1:00 min	Hold 1:30 min

In contrast, an O_2 tolerance table is designed to accustom the body to extremely low levels of oxygen by prolonging the duration of breath-holds between resting periods. The following table, which requires about thirty minutes to complete, consists of eight cycles:

1	Hold breath 1:00 min		5	Rest 2:00 min	Hold 2:00 min
2	Rest 2:00 min	Hold 1:15 min	6	Rest 2:00 min	Hold 2:15 min
3	Rest 2:00 min	Hold 1:30 min	7	Rest 2:00 min	Hold 2:30 min
4	Rest 2:00 min	Hold 1:45 min	8	Rest 2:00 min	Hold 2:30 min

Obviously, the math can get distracting when you are trying to focus on your breath, so I recommend using the Apnea app, which will walk you through tables for a variety of different breath-hold times with helpful audio cues or vibrations.

7. Breath-Hold Walks

Several afternoons each week, I duck out from writing and working in my home office and scramble up a steep hill through the forest to an old farm road that travels a mile out and a mile back. The road is dotted with telephone poles approximately one hundred yards apart. Every time I pass a telephone pole, I take one deep belly breath and hold it for as long as possible. Once I run out of oxygen, rather than gasping for air—which every muscle in my body desperately wants to do—I inhale only through my nose. After a brief, twenty-to-thirty-minute walk like this, I feel as if I have been in deep meditation for hours. These breath-hold walks are similar to apnea walks for freediving training and can be performed in a park or airport, on a treadmill, or anywhere you want to combine movement and breathwork.

Although it isn't based on breath per se, one other very interesting device I've discovered for these walks is a Counterpace. This combination heart rate strap and phone app plays a quiet metronome or timed music in sync with your heart rate, so that as you walk in time to the music, you match your step rate to your heart rate—for instance, a heart rate of 120 beats per minute and step rate of 120 steps per minute. By keeping your heart rate and step rate identical, you train your leg muscles to squeeze blood toward the heart exactly when it's relaxing and most able to receive it. Conversely, the heart contracts while the legs are relaxed, which delivers oxygen to the muscles while they are most receptive to blood flow. This favorable timing has been shown in research to lower central blood pressure and increase the speed at which blood flows to the brain. The concept is based on external counterpulsation therapy, in which a device squeezes the legs of patients with cardiovascular disease in time with their heartbeat.

8. Holotropic Breathwork

While Dr. Stanislav Grof was researching the effects of LSD, he became interested in altered states of consciousness and how they could help empower people to deal with trauma. He developed a method for achieving a psychedelic experience via breathwork alone and called it holotropic breathing, derived from the Greek holos, which means "whole," and trepein, which means "to move forward."

Dr. Grof explains that holotropic breathing works because your breath can help you "transcend the narrow boundaries of the body ego" and achieve a relaxed, spiritual high. The holotropic breathwork session I performed in San Diego got me higher than I have ever been without the use of psychedelic drugs, providing me with an intense out-of-body experience unlike anything I have ever encountered.

You can't do holotropic breathwork on your own or with some fancy phone app. Sessions are typically led by a certified holotropic breathwork facilitator, often in a two-to-three-hour group session. There is usually evocative, intense music that is rhythmic throughout the intense breathing portions and meditative towards the end as you enter a trancelike state. (You'll find guidelines and recommendations for finding a certified holotropic breathwork facilitator at www.holotropic. com/holotropic-breathwork/facilitator-listing.)

9. Basic Wim Hof Breathing

Wim Hof, a two-time podcast guest of mine, is a somewhat crazy and controversial but highly entertaining Danish yogi known for completing intense feats of physical endurance in extreme temperature conditions, often clad in little more than pasty white underwear. His Wim Hof Method is a series of breathing exercises that results in your ability to hold your breath for progressively longer periods of time. If you care to try it yourself, you can begin with his basic breathwork technique. It consists of thirty cycles of continuous breathwork, with no pauses between each inhalation and exhalation. Each exhalation should be relaxed—meaning you should not fully exhale but should instead leave some air in the lungs, so that you breathe in more oxygen than you breathe out.

At the end of thirty breath cycles, exhale and hold your breath for as long as possible with no air in your lungs. You will eventually get the urge to breathe. At that point, inhale and hold your breath for a final fifteen to thirty seconds, or for as long as you can. You can squeeze your forehead a little to get more blood flow to the brain. Repeat this process, starting with thirty breath cycles again, for two or three rounds. To complete the routine, take one more deep recovery breath to restore normal oxygen levels. Wim Hof also encourages doing bodyweight exercises such as squats or push-ups while holding your breath on an exhalation.

This breathwork technique dramatically stimulates hypoxia and even mimics hard training at high altitude. The effects of hypoxia are generated mostly through an ancestral mechanism to help the human body survive in low-oxygen environments. By holding your breath, you induce a positive stress response by turning on your "survival mode," just as when you expose yourself to sauna therapy or cold thermogenesis. The results include:

- An increase in red blood cells
- The production of growth factors that lead to the development of new blood vessels, even in people with heart disease
- The induction of nitric oxide synthase, which has a variety of positive effects on cell tissues and can even assist with vasodilation problems like erectile dysfunction
- The induction of tumor protein p53, the "guardian of the genome," which protects your cells' DNA and prevents cells from becoming cancerous

Finally, stem cells, which are incredibly important to your tissue survival and repair, as well as to your overall longevity, can only survive in a state of hypoxia. Stem cells are abundant in fetal circulation, where oxygen levels are low. The mother's womb is very hypoxic, with oxygen concentrations matching those at the top of Mount Everest! After birth, the stem cells survive in various locations called niches in the body, such as bone marrow.

Here is what's most interesting: research has shown that in rats, the number of active mesenchymal stem cells (MSC)—one of the most versatile and beneficial forms of stem cells—in the blood increases by as much as fifteen-fold during hypoxia! And when cultured in hypoxic environments of just 2 percent oxygen, instead of 20 percent oxygen, like normal air, stem cells keep their self-renewing abilities. This is likely because bone marrow stem cells and mesenchymal stem cells have low numbers of mitochondria and are more adapted to anaerobic environments than to oxygen-rich environments.

Just a few minutes of hypoxia per day may stimulate your stem cells to migrate from bone marrow to the rest of your body, where they can stimulate the repair and growth of new cells. This could benefit many degenerative disorders, including Parkinson's and Alzheimer's, and has been shown in rat models to stimulate neurogenesis in the brain by proliferating neural stem cells. Hypoxia can also help memory and cognitive function and even exert antidepressant effects.

A big thanks to my friend and breathwork expert Niraj Naik, the Renegade Pharmacist, for turning me on to this little-known fact about stem cells.

The Results

So has learning all these breathing skills paid off for me?

Absolutely. Not only can I breathe my way through intense, stressful, or painful parts of my life, but I can also use my breath to amplify my nervous system and focus for better performance, and I can freedive and spearfish for amazing, tasty seafood in just about any tropical locale on the face of the planet.

I have used quantifiable measurements such as heart rate variability and blood cortisol to analyze how proper breathing affects my nervous system and hormones. The results are astounding. So don't blow off breath: you can easily learn these tactics too. The ones I have described above—of the dozens and dozens of breathwork techniques that exist—are those that have moved the needle most for me. Should you want to learn even more about the breathing tactics I have discovered, visit BoundlessBook.com/3 for several of my podcast episodes and interviews with the world's top breathing experts.

THREE OTHER POTENT WAYS TO REDUCE STRESS

Of course, in addition to the breathwork techniques listed above, there are myriad other ways you can banish stress, kiss high cortisol goodbye, and fix HPA axis dysfunction. While breathwork is the fastest and best way to address stress, here are three other highly effective tactics.

1. Avoid Excessive Exercise

Overtraining, which can lead to chronically elevated cortisol levels, is the quickest path to HPA axis dysfunction and leads to many brain fog, mood, and irritability issues, especially in exercise enthusiasts and exceptionally active individuals.

Fact is, there are plenty of ways to move the body without crushing weights at the gym or pounding the pavement during a run. Even on rest days, you can engage in active recovery, which is far more effective than passive, unengaged recovery. Active recovery tactics include tai chi, qi-gong, yoga, heart rate variability training, hot-cold contrast therapy, cold thermogenesis, electro-stimulation, and heat shock training.

There is no rule that avoiding excessive exercise means you spend a day off from the gym lying on the couch with a big bag of vegetable chips. For example, a typical recovery day for me includes:

- Morning nasal breathing and a breath-hold walk in the sunshine

- Frequent movement breaks during office work to perform jumping jacks, bodyweight squats, push-ups, and mini-trampoline sessions

- Reading magazines or doing easy yoga in a dry or infrared sauna to move lymphatic fluid and to detox via sweat

- A few cold showers spread throughout the day, or a hot-cold contrast session of alternating sauna and cold pool immersion

- A full-body foam-rolling routine or deep tissue massage

You get the idea. Just because you are not performing an intense exercise session doesn't mean you can't improve your fitness or breathing, decrease stress, and satisfy that urge to do something other than lounge around.

2. Shut Down Inflammation

In mice, researchers have experimented with a protein called NF-kB, which is involved in inflammation in the hypothalamus. When NF-kB is switched off in mice, they live about 20 percent longer! On the other hand, chronically elevated levels of NF-kB not only accelerate aging but also decrease another protein called GnRH. When GnRH is turned down, fewer new brain cells are created, and aging is accelerated even more. As you can see, the effects of inflammation in the hypothalamus spread far beyond the HPA axis.

When I wake up with a fuzzy brain—which can happen after a late night out, too much alcohol, or a night of disrupted sleep—one of the first things I do is pop 1,000 mg of curcumin, the active component of the turmeric plant. Due to its potent anti-inflammatory effects, curcumin rapidly shuts down inflammation and mitigates the effect that a poor night of sleep has on the HPA axis (plenty more on that coming in chapter 7!).

3. Sleep

The only time your body fully repairs neurons is when you are asleep, specifically during the deep-sleep stages that occur, assuming you are going to sleep sometime between 9:30 and 11:30 p.m., as your body temperature decreases between 2 a.m. and 6 a.m. So if you are not getting quality sleep, then you are never going to fully recover and repair your HPA axis. In fact, because of the crucial role that sleep plays in the health of the nervous system, getting adequate sleep is the single most important strategy you could ever implement for fixing your brain and enhancing cognition. Even if you incorporate all of the other biohacks, nutrition tips, and strategies in the first three chapters of this book, you are never going to experience optimal brain and nervous system performance if you don't sleep properly. (I'll talk in detail about sleep hygiene and advanced sleep strategies in chapter 7.)

THE LAST WORD

Chronic stress can lead to HPA axis dysfunction and accompanying fatigue and brain fog. You can reduce stress and sharpen your focus just through conscious breathing techniques, like the eight I've described in this chapter:

- Buteyko breathing
- box breathing
- Kundalini yoga breathing
- rhythmic breathing
- decompression breathing
- breath-hold cycles from a static apnea table
- breath-hold walks
- holotropic breathwork

Avoiding excessive exercise, decreasing inflammation, and getting good sleep are also excellent stress-reducing tactics, and they're all interrelated and interdependent. As you implement each of these strategies, your HPA axis will work with wonderful efficiency. When you pair these techniques with the ones for fixing neurotransmitters and the blood-brain barrier described in chapters 1 and 2, you can venture forth into the next chapters of *Boundless* with a head that is fully primed and prepped for an upgrade.

ONE THING YOU CAN DO THIS WEEK

There are many forms of breathwork, but it is handy to know at least one energizing form and one relaxing form. So you have two tasks today: First, energize your body before a workout or during a bout of tiredness with one full minute of Wim Hof–style breathing (short, rapid, forced inhalations followed by short, rapid, unforced exhalations). Second, before bed or during a stressful time of the day, try to engage in one full minute of alternate-nostril breathing (breathing in through your right nostril with a finger covering your left nostril, exhaling through the left nostril with a finger covering the right nostril, then repeating with the opposite nostrils).

> For citations for all the research studies mentioned in this chapter and a deeper dive into the topics of this chapter—including links to podcasts, blog posts, recommended tools and supplements, and much more—visit BoundlessBook.com/3.

EAT YOURSELF SMART

HOW TO FUEL YOUR BRAIN

Apple chips. Coconut flakes. Roasted nuts. Standing in the "natural" section of the airport newsstand with nary a candy bar in sight, I felt proud, self-righteous, and überhealthy. I had not been lulled by the siren song of Cinnabon, nor had I fallen prey to the Starbucks bakery case or, heaven forbid, the $12 preservative-infused "healthy" snack pack on the airplane.

I grabbed a bag of organic, low-calorie, spirulina-infused popcorn and glanced at the ingredients label.

Popcorn. Spirulina. Organic agave syrup. *Canola oil.*

I gulped, set the bag back down, and walked away, shocked that the villain canola oil was still being shoveled into our gaping maws as we innocently perceived ourselves to be nourishing our bodies with so-called superfoods.

Why am I so adamantly opposed to something as seemingly inconsequential as a teaspoon of canola oil in a giant bag of spirulina popcorn? And why would I rather mow through an entire bag of pure white sugar than eat a few french fries, an apple fritter doughnut, or a big ole canola oil–soaked bag of trail mix from the gas station convenience store?

In this chapter, I'll explain why processed oils like canola oil are some of the worst foods for your brain and identify other all-too-common compounds that damage your neurons, as well as the best foods, nutrients, and diet-optimizing strategies for your brain.

BRAIN FOOD 101

You are what you eat. You have probably heard this phrase before, along with the slightly less well-known but equally important phrase "You are what what you eat ate." Yes, that's right: you'd better think twice about whether your steak was raised on grass or GMO corn, whether your chicken ate bugs or herbicide-laden grains, and whether your fish consumed worms or pieces of ground-up fish and fish farm meal. Nowhere is this more important than when it comes to fueling your brain.

I first understood the intense importance of this concept when I interviewed Dr. Cate Shanahan, the author of the book *Deep Nutrition*, who believes that a diet high in "crappy fat," like the vegetable oils and trans fats found in french fries, doughnuts, and most packaged foods, is far worse than a diet high in sugar. When she works with professional sports teams, she recommends that they switch to a diet based on bone broth, tubers, organic dairy, bone marrow, seeds, nuts, vegetables, grass-fed beef, and wild-caught fish. (Full disclosure: this is a controversial strategy she has caught some flak for, primarily because I think many professional athletes begin to consume adequate fats, which I do indeed endorse, but also shove carbohydrates and overall calorie consumption too low on the scale of importance.)

Why is this whole fat issue so important? You are fat. No, I don't mean that you are *fat*. But you are, at a fundamental level, made of fat.

Every living cell in your body has a membrane responsible for allowing compounds to move in and out of the cell so it can function properly. These membranes are primarily formed from the fats you consume. This means that how flexible and permeable these membranes are depends on the quantity and, more importantly, the quality of the fats you get from your diet.

If your diet is high in damaged fatty acids, like those found in corn, canola, safflower, or sunflower oil, or if your diet is high in trans fats, or if the fish oil you take is rancid and exposed to too much light and heat, or if your steak is a slab from a big ole corn-and-grains-fed cow, then those damaged fats get incorporated into the building blocks of your cell membranes—including those of your neurons.

Damaged, highly reactive fats are found in most brands of potato chips, french fries, fried packaged foods, and pretty much any other fatty food that has been (1) heated at too high a temperature for the fat to remain stable, or (2) exposed to too much pressure for the fat to retain its natural structure. A common example is olive oil that has been heated to above 400 degrees Fahrenheit and has been fried multiple times. Although a spicy, dense, flavonol-rich extra-virgin olive oil is great for you, olive oil that's been exposed to high heat is not, and you may be eating damaged olive oil at high-end restaurants without even knowing it. You can also encounter olive oil that has been cut with canola oil to save money (as I discovered in my interview with Dr. Shanahan, this happens even at five-star Napa Valley restaurants!). Your cells take these damaged fats, incorporate them into the membrane that wraps around the cell, and voilà! You have quite literally become what you ate: crappy, damaged fatty acids.

FAT/OIL	SMOKE POINT (UNREFINED/REFINED)	BEST USES
Avocado oil	520°F	• high-heat cooking • low-heat cooking • dressing • finishing
Butter, ghee	300/480°F	• high-heat cooking • baking
Coconut oil	350/450°F	• high-heat cooking • sautéing • baking
Duck fat	375°F	• high-heat cooking
Lard (pork, bacon fat)	375°F	• high-heat cooking
Macadamia nut oil	410°F	• low-heat cooking • dressing • finishing
Olive oil	320/465°F	• high-heat cooking • low-heat cooking • dressing • finishing
Peanut oil	230/450°F	• high-heat cooking
Rice bran oil	415°F	• low-heat cooking
Sesame oil	450°F	• dressing • finishing
Tallow (beef fat)	400°F	• high-heat cooking
Walnut oil	400°F	• dressing • finishing

No organ demonstrates this better than the brain. There are copious amounts of fat in neuronal membranes. These fats insulate your brain, protect it from shock, and help your nervous system maintain a healthy temperature. The transmission of electrical signals across neuron synapses also depends on fatty acids, as do neurotransmitter levels.

This is why I would rather mow through an entire bag of sugar than consume just about any fried food on the face of the planet: the sugars aren't going to serve as the building blocks of my body. Sure, sugar can spike my blood glucose, cause some vascular inflammation, produce gastric bloating, and create a surge of insulin. But at least I can do things to negate most of the damage and lower the sugar spike or burn the sugar away: drop and do some burpees, or go for a run, or eat some bitter melon extract, Ceylon cinnamon, or apple cider vinegar. You simply can't do that with bad fats: they get incorporated into your cell membranes whether you exercise or not, and there is no immediate way to undo the damage. So give me a choice between a stick of cotton candy and a bag of potato chips, and I'll eat the cotton candy, hands down.

Hidden Rancid Oils in Common Health Foods

You would be surprised at how many "healthy" or organic foods and so-called superfoods are jam-packed with rancid, damaged oils, just like the spirulina-infused popcorn I encountered in the airport. Don't be fooled by the fancy labels and certifications on the packaging: these oils have oozed into packaged foods far beyond the obvious threats like french fries, doughnuts, potato chips, and cookies. The following is a list of nineteen common "health" foods that may contain these rancid oils.

- Pasteurized dairy products, such as commercially produced milk, cheeses, butter, and, yes, even many organic yogurts
- Organic packaged pasta and rice meals (the "healthy" equivalents of Rice-A-Roni and similar foods)
- Many big-name trail mix blends, often marketed as high-protein, low-sugar trail snacks
- Many brands of organic nut spreads, such as almond butter, cashew butter, and peanut butter
- Store-bought bags of peanuts, almonds, cashews, and other nuts, including many of the nut mixes in the bulk food section of the grocery store
- Baking chocolate and semisweet chocolate, often marked as organic or non-GMO

- Many store-bought sauces, including those advertised as low-calorie
- Gluten-free or organic cereal bars, granola bars, and many protein bars
- Most salad dressings, even those from the organic or natural section of the grocery store
- Many non-GMO vegetable chips, sweet potato chips, and coconut chips
- Gluten-free and/or organic packaged pretzels, cookies, rice crackers, and multigrain crackers
- Fried eggs at many breakfast joints, or any eggs prepared with high heat
- Sautéed or stir-fried foods at most restaurants, including fish, vegetables, and leafy greens
- Many dairy-free ice creams, including those made with coconut, cashew, or almond milk
- Butter substitutes and spreadable fats like margarine
- Premade packaged popcorn, especially cheddar-flavored and caramel popcorn
- Both dairy and nondairy coffee creamers
- Most popular frozen meals marketed as healthy
- Gluten-free and/or organic frozen pizzas

The best defense? Check labels!

The role fats play in cell membranes is not the only reason to be careful with damaged fats. A consistent intake of these fats leads to chronic inflammation. Acute inflammation is part of the body's natural response to infection and tissue damage and is even important for muscle growth after exercise. But chronic inflammation can lead to many physiological problems, from obesity and muscle loss to atherosclerosis and arthritis. According to many nutritionists and scientific studies, sugar is the most inflammatory aspect of any diet. High sugar intake is indeed inflammatory, but it is not as terrible as consistent processed-oil consumption.

Processed oils like canola or vegetable oil are polyunsaturated fats, which are molecularly unstable and prone to cell-destroying oxidation. Oxidants are reactive molecules that are used to transfer electrons from one atom to another. They are naturally produced both inside your body and the environment, but in excess they can react with other cellular molecules in your body, such as proteins, DNA, and lipids, often contributing to disease and inflammation in the process. (This is why antioxidants are so important—they help prevent oxidation-related damage.)

So any brain-fueling strategy must begin with the elimination of every source of overheated, overpressured vegetable oils and polyunsaturated fats. Then you have to increase your consumption of healthy fats and cholesterols from natural, whole-food sources. Dr. Shanahan writes in *Deep Nutrition*, "A necessary outgrowth of the indictment of cholesterol is a rejection of the traditional, natural fats that have sustained humankind for thousands of generations. It's a little like the idea that Nestle successfully used in the 1940s to sell infant formula to my grandmother and many other women, claiming it was 'more perfect than breastmilk.' Those who mean to replace natural, traditional foods with modern-day food-like products in the name of health are championing the position that nature doesn't know best; a corporation does. This is an extraordinary claim requiring extraordinary evidence—a burden they have failed to meet."

Should You Eat at the Whole Foods Salad Bar?

If you are the average health enthusiast who doesn't mind paying $27 for a salad, you have undoubtedly spent time hunting and foraging at the hot bar and salad bar of a fancy, highfalutin grocery store like Whole Foods Market. Fact is, many of the prepared foods at these bars—from the marinated yams to the rotisserie chicken to the vegetarian Buffalo wings—are drenched in canola oil.

Should you be worried? It depends. Not all canola oil is created equal.

Whole Foods only uses non-GMO canola oil that's been expeller-pressed—a mechanical process that simply squeezes out the oil instead of using chemical solvents to extract it. So it is safe to say that compared to the average chemical-processed, GMO canola oil, the canola oil you find in the Whole Foods salad bar is relatively healthier.

But all canola oil is still refined, partially damaged, and high in erucic acid, a fatty acid associated with heart damage, high blood pressure, and blood clotting. It also contains trans fats. All of this can deleteriously affect cholesterol levels and cardiovascular health.

While the canola oil you consume at the salad bar of a health-food store is likely healthier than the canola oil you get in a basket of french fries and a burger, you are still filling your body with a less-than-ideal fat. I advise moderation, even with non-GMO, expeller-pressed canola oil.

Finally, to limit the potential damage that seed oils like canola, sunflower, and safflower oil can cause to your cell membranes, consider the advice of Dr. James DiNicolantonio, author of *Superfuel*, who says that supplementation with 20 g of glycine (preferably split into four servings of 5 g each) and 2 to 5 g of spirulina can significantly help mitigate the damage.

She goes on to explain that for centuries, fat has been an integral part of many ancestral diets. The ancestral Northern European diet, for instance, is high in fatty fish, red meat, and fermented, full-fat dairy products, which means that if your ancestors were Northern European, you have inherited a wealth of genes that rely heavily on fats. The same concept applies to a traditional Mediterranean diet. Sure, a Mediterranean diet includes ample carbohydrates like bread and pasta, but in coastal countries like Italy, a large part of the daily meal plan includes foods full of healthy fats, such as fish, nuts, full-fat milk and cheeses like pecorino or *mozzarella di bufala* (buffalo mozzarella), along with plenty of fasting and caloric restriction. Because your brain is composed of and uses so much fat (60 percent of your brain is fat!), a diet that is low-fat or fat-free, or that consists of inflammatory fats, can significantly damage your cognitive health.

There are several notable exceptions to this rule that will be addressed in chapter 14, including certain genetic populations who can get by on less fat. But for now, the important takeaways are that processed, damaged fats are bad for your brain and that healthy, natural fats are some of the best fuels for your brain.

9 FOODS THAT BREAK YOUR BRAIN

Damaged fats and vegetable oils are not the only foods that can break your brain. Here are nine additional foods to be cautious with if your goal is cognitive optimization.

1. Histamine- and Oxalate-Containing Foods

Histamines are compounds released by mast cells, a type of white blood cell that tends to proliferate as part of an immune response to stressors like cuts, scrapes, and allergens. Once released, histamines dilate blood vessels and increase blood flow to the stressed area (such as your nasal cavities during allergy season), resulting in inflammation.

Excessively high histamine levels can cause brain fog and headaches, especially in those sensitive to histamines. An inherited genetic condition called systemic mastocytosis, which can be aggravated by histamine-induced brain inflammation, is a mast cell disorder associated with psychiatric symptoms such as diminished attention and memory, anger, irritability, and depression. While low levels of histamines are necessary for brain function, motor activity, and healthy circadian rhythms, excessive levels cause parts of the brain to shut down in an inflammatory response, especially if you have mastocytosis. In addition, mast cell activation syndrome (MCAS) is an immunological condition in which mast cells inappropriately and excessively release chemical mediators that can also result in histamine sensitivities. MCAS can be brought on by a leaky gut, an infection, or even excess levels of chronic stress. To diagnose MCAS, a physician will often test for plasma histamine and diamine oxidase, but these are considered unreliable as they fluctuate significantly. Better tests will look at N-methylhistamine, prostaglandin D2, heparin, and tryptase, which can all indicate excess mast cell activity.

No discussion of mast cells and histamine would be complete without mentioning the work of Dr. Neil Nathan, whose excellent book *Toxic: Heal Your Body from Mold Toxicity, Lyme Disease, Multiple Chemical Sensitivities, and Chronic Environmental Illness* is a must-read for anyone who suspects they have a histamine sensitivity, excess mast cell activation, mold exposure, or Lyme disease. For stabilizing mast cells, Dr. Nathan's typical starting point is 500 mg of quercetin taken thirty minutes before each meal and at bedtime (for a total of 2,000 mg per day). This is because a mast cell stabilizer such as quercetin must be in the body before you eat or drink in order to work. In addition, Dr. Ben Lynch has developed a suite of histamine-blocking and histamine-digesting enzymes, including diamine oxidase (DAO), which is the main enzyme responsible for the degradation of ingested histamine. You'll find some of his formulas at BenGreenfieldFitness.com/seekinghealth.

One way to combat excess histamine in the brain, especially if you are sensitive to histamines, is to avoid foods that contain high levels of histamines. While many health-care practitioners feel this is unnecessary or ineffective, I personally know many folks who have eliminated headaches by simply eliminating certain foods, including the following:

- Fermented beverages, such as wine, beer, and kombucha. I personally limit myself to one such drink per day. (Yes, this means that if you drink a giant kombucha with lunch, you may want to consider forgoing your nightly glass of wine.)
- Fermented foods, such as sauerkraut, vinegar, soy sauce, kefir, and yogurt. I eat these foods but treat them more as condiments than as major components of my diet.
- Vinegar-soaked foods, such as pickles and olives
- Cured or smoked meats, such as bacon, salami, hot dogs, and smoked fish
- Soured foods, such as sour cream, sour milk, and buttermilk
- Dried fruit
- Aged cheeses
- Peanuts
- Leftovers, especially when they're more than a few days old. (This is a good reason not to eat at a restaurant on a Sunday or Monday, which are typically the two days of the week when a restaurant serves the least-fresh food.)

Don't get me wrong: I am not trying to completely rip the charcuterie platter out of your hands. But if you have brain fog and headaches, you should consider the fact that one person's superfood may be another person's villain, and reducing your intake of these foods could help. Instead, consume foods with lower amounts of histamines, such as the following:

- Freshly cooked meat, fish, and poultry (not smoked, cured, or preserved)
- Eggs
- Low-gluten grains, such as amaranth, buckwheat, millet, quinoa, sorghum, teff, and rice (brown, white, and wild)
- Fresh fruits, such as mangos, pears, watermelons, apples, kiwis, cantaloupes, and grapes
- Fresh vegetables (not canned or preserved)
- Extra-virgin olive oil and coconut oil
- Leafy herbs, such as parsley and cilantro
- Herbal teas

There is no single conclusive way that doctors can diagnose histamine intolerance, but the best currently available test for discovering sensitivities is the StrateGene analysis. If an allergist or immunologist suspects you may have a histamine intolerance, they will often begin by testing for food allergies and intolerances and place you on a diet that eliminates foods high in histamines to see if that relieves symptoms. Physicians can also request a blood test to check levels of DAO.

Although it tends to fly under the radar, many people are now discovering the benefits of limiting oxalates in their diet, which seems to provide relief from symptoms of inflammatory conditions, autoimmune issues, mineral deficiencies, and perhaps even autism. Many of the symptoms of oxalate sensitivity overlap with those of histamine sensitivity, and if the elimination of histamines does not relieve your issues, you may want to consider also limiting oxalate-rich foods, including beer, beets, chocolate, coffee, spinach, nuts, tea, and soy. In addition, if oxalic acid is elevated without an elevation in glyceric or glycolic acid, it is often because of a candida overgrowth or excessively high vitamin C intake. A urinary organic acids test (OAT) from Great Plains Laboratory that shows elevated glyceric, glycolic, and oxalic acids can give a clue that you are oxalate sensitive, have high oxalates, or both. Several genes that can be looked at on a 23andMe salivary genetic test, notably AGXT, GRPHR, and HOGA1, can indicate a tendency toward oxalate sensitivity or excess oxalates.

2. Glucose-Fluctuating Foods

Within your brain are cells called microglia and astrocytes. When these cells are frequently exposed to high amounts of sugar and blood glucose fluctuations, it can cause chronic neuroinflammation, neuronal loss, and progression in dementia and Alzheimer's disease. My friend Dr. Nora Gedgaudas refers to astrocyte-induced neuroinflammation as the neuronal equivalent of a bunch of tiny, rabid chihuahuas (your hyped-up astrocytes) sprinting around your brain while firing off machine guns. High blood glucose levels increase not only astrocyte-induced neuroinflammation but also the susceptibility of your neurons to injury. This means that a diet high in sugar and starch, which spike blood glucose levels, can be damaging to the brain. Excessive glucose fluctuation can also lead to hyperinsulinemia (elevated insulin levels), which, in turn, causes hypoglycemia (low blood sugar) and neuroglycopenia (a shortage of glucose in the brain, which affects neuronal function), all of which ultimately lead to brain damage.

The exact opposite effect is achieved by periods of intermittent fasting or adherence to a ketogenic diet or a low-carb, high-fat diet. (While the terms are often used interchangeably, a ketogenic diet is not necessarily synonymous with a low-carb, high-fat diet. The former creates a metabolic state in which fatty acids are broken down into ketones, which your body primarily uses for energy, and in addition to diet, this state can be achieved via the consumption of ketones, strict carbohydrate restriction, fasting, exercise, or a combination of all of the above. The latter simply involves eating a low amount of carbohydrates and a high amount of fat.) These strategies improve insulin signaling and reduce the side effects associated with roller-coaster blood sugar patterns. In fact, one study showed that after just six months on a ketogenic diet that restricted blood sugar fluctuations, one patient with congenital hyperinsulinism was free of epileptic seizures and showed marked recovery in psychological development. Mary Newport, author of the book *Alzheimer's Disease: What If There Was a Cure? The Story of Ketones*, improved her husband's Alzheimer's via coconut oil–derived ketones. The vast majority of people who have followed a diet like the one she prescribes have also reported surprising improvements in cognitive function. Finally, in his book *The End of Alzheimer's*, Dr. Dale Bredesen highly recommends a plant-based, mildly ketogenic diet that incorporates sugar restriction, ten to fifteen servings of vegetables per day, and at least twelve hours of intermittent fasting per twenty-four-hour cycle.

There are several kinds of diets that control carbohydrate intake, and the terminology can be confusing. What exactly is high-carb? What is low-carb? What is ketogenic? Here's the answer: Technically, a high-carbohydrate diet has more than 45 percent of calories coming from carbohydrates (the 2015 *Dietary Guidelines for Americans* recommends getting between 45 and

65 percent of your daily calories from carbs, and this is the way most Americans eat). A moderate-carbohydrate diet has 26 percent to 45 percent of calories from carbs. A low-carbohydrate diet, in contrast, needs to include less than 130 g of carbohydrates per day, which is less than 26 percent of a typical 2,000-calorie-per-day diet (although I personally consider hard-training athletes who eat 150 to 200 g of carbohydrates per day to easily be in low-carb mode). A very-low-carbohydrate diet or a ketogenic diet typically includes only 20 to 50 g per day of carbohydrates, or less than 10 percent of daily calories.

Of course, these percentages can vary widely, especially if you are a highly active individual or an athlete engaged in multiple workouts, practices, scrimmages, or competitions in any given week. Very active people often need to pay closer attention to ensuring they consume adequate carbohydrates to keep their liver and muscle glycogen stores topped up, and to maintain joints and other tissues that require glucose. Ideally, these individuals should consume carbohydrates before, during, or after physical activity, when they are far less likely to cause wild glucose fluctuations. (I prefer to eat carbohydrates toward the end of the day, when the post-carb serotonin release can assist with sleep.) Because of this, most of the athletes or highly active individuals I coach, including myself, engage in daily carbohydrate refeeds of 100 to 200 g, typically with the evening meal, every day except rest and recovery days.

Finally, while a diet that limits glucose fluctuation is important, don't get me wrong: your brain does indeed need some amount of glucose. As a matter of fact, every mammalian brain depends on glucose as its main source of energy, and tight regulation of glucose metabolism is critical for brain physiology. In adults, neurons demand more energy than any other kind of cell, requiring continuous delivery of glucose from blood. In humans, the brain accounts for about 2 percent of the body weight, but it consumes over 20 percent of glucose-derived energy, making it your body's main consumer of glucose. Problems with glucose metabolism in the brain underlie several diseases affecting the brain. For example, one of the earliest signs of Alzheimer's disease is a reduction in cerebral glucose metabolism, and both human studies and animal models suggest that disturbed glucose metabolism is associated with Alzheimer's progression.

So how many carbohydrates do you need to eat per day to give your brain enough glucose? While your brain consumes roughly 100 to 150 g of glucose every day, that doesn't necessarily mean that all this glucose needs come from dietary carbohydrates. During a process called gluconeogenesis, your liver can convert fatty acids and amino acids into glucose, which is then used by the brain. In addition, some amount of carbohydrate restriction can lead to the production of ketones, which serve as an alternative fuel source for the brain (and may possibly offer up to 60 percent of the energy the brain needs). But even with the contribution of ketones and gluconeogenesis, the brain still needs about 20 to 30 g per day of carbohydrates from dietary sources, which most people easily get unless they are on a severely carbohydrate-restricted diet, which I rarely recommend.

3. Artificially Sweetened Foods

In light of all the adverse effects of sugar, it might seem reasonable to turn to artificial sweeteners and sugar alternatives.

As reasonable as this may seem, many artificial sweeteners are known to be neurotoxic. In fact, in many animal studies, researchers have shown that artificial sweeteners can cause weight gain, brain tumors, and bladder cancer, and human studies have also linked them to cancer. There are five artificial sweeteners on the FDA's "generally recognized as safe" list of additives: saccharin, aspartame, sucralose, neotame, and acesulfame potassium. But just because they are thought to be safe doesn't mean they are optimum brain fuel. And it's disconcerting that the FDA establishes an "acceptable daily intake" of artificial sweeteners, similar to toxic substances like pesticides.

Take aspartame, for example. When aspartame is heated above 86 degrees Fahrenheit, as it is inside your body, the wood alcohol it contains converts to formaldehyde (embalming fluid). The formaldehyde then converts to formic acid and causes metabolic acidosis, a chemical imbalance in which your body produces or contains more acid than it can efficiently remove. In addition, one of aspartame's metabolic by-products is the amino acid phenylalanine. One in twenty thousand people is born with a genetic condition known as phenylketonuria. People with this condition cannot metabolize phenylalanine, which can accumulate and cause brain damage. (This is why diet sodas display the warning, "Phenylketonurics: Contains phenylalanine.") But even if you do not have phenylketonuria, phenylalanine can still cause DNA and protein damage in your brain.

Splenda isn't any better. Despite the claim that it is "made from sugar," Splenda, also known as sucralose, is not actually sugar. Like aspartame, it is a chlorinated artificial sweetener. In fact, Splenda is more chemically similar to the pesticide DDT than it is to sugar! While the FDA claims they reviewed over one hundred studies on the safety of consuming Splenda, what they don't reveal is that in animal studies, higher doses of Splenda are associated with decreased male fertility and brain lesions. In mice, consuming Splenda has also been shown to negatively impact the beneficial gut bacteria—bacteria like *Ruminococcaceae Ruminococcus*, *Streptococcaceae Streptococcus*, and *Lachnospiraceae Ruminococcus*—that regulate inflammation. Similarly, the artificial sweetener acesulfame potassium has been shown to negatively impact the gut microbiome in mice.

If you do opt for alternative sweeteners, the best options are stevia and monk fruit extract. Stevia is derived from plants in the *Stevia* genus, which contains more than two hundred species. Stevia has no negative effects on your brain and, unlike sugar, has little effect on blood glucose levels, making it a great option for preventing or managing diabetes. Monk fruit extract also has no negative effects on your brain and has little to no effect on your blood sugar, and it contains mogrosides, a group of potent antioxidants.

4. Condiments

As you may already know, most condiments (think soy sauce, mustard, and your average salad dressing) contain high amounts of salt. In fact, one tablespoon of soy sauce contains nearly 40 percent of your daily recommended sodium intake. Excess sodium can cause hypertension (high blood pressure), a condition that results in your blood vessels, including those in your brain, growing narrow and weak. Hypertension can lead to transient ischemic attack (a temporary disruption of blood to the brain), stroke, dementia, and mild cognitive impairment. Hypertension can also cause a myriad of other issues, including kidney failure, kidney artery aneurysm, retinopathy (damage to blood vessels in the eyes), sexual dysfunction, bone loss, coronary artery disease, enlarged left heart ventricle, heart failure, aneurysm, complications during pregnancy, aortic dissection (severe damage to the body's main artery), and obstructive sleep apnea.

Please don't interpret this to mean that salt is bad. Natural salt, such as mineral-rich Aztec or Celtic salt, is quite good for you and is necessary for healthy cellular activity. (I'm often asked "Why not Himalayan salt?" and the answer is simple: it tends to be higher in heavy metals and other contaminants.) In fact, the average adult male contains 92 g of sodium, half of which is found in extracellular fluid, making sodium crucial for normal cell function. But you run into problems with hypertension, nerve signaling, gastrointestinal irritation, and other issues when you consume high amounts of sodium chloride without also consuming other minerals. Unless you are consuming extremely high amounts of sodium chloride (over 4,000 mg per day), you probably don't need to reduce your sodium intake at all. What you need to do is increase your potassium and magnesium intake.

Sodium and potassium exist in your body in a delicate balance: while a high sodium intake can increase blood pressure, a high potassium intake can relax blood vessels and decrease blood pressure. Certain cultures, primarily Asiatic cultures, consume high amounts of sodium-rich foods like soy sauce and miso, but they don't suffer the negative effects of sodium chloride because they also consume other minerals, like potassium and magnesium, in foods such as seaweed. There is less conclusive evidence on the efficacy of magnesium compared to potassium in reducing blood pressure, but much of the evidence that does exist is positive and warrants further research. The ratio between dietary sodium and potassium should be about 1:1, so for every 100 mg of sodium you consume, match it with about 100 mg of potassium. You don't want to exceed a daily intake of 1,500 mg of magnesium, as higher doses can cause loose stool.

Even if you are consuming plenty of potassium and magnesium, you may want to consider the high amount of refined, processed vegetable oils in most mayonnaise and salad dressings, the neurotoxins chloropropanol and salsolinol in soy sauce, and the high-fructose corn syrup in barbecue sauce. Chronic exposure to these compounds leads to brain inflammation and, ultimately, cognitive decline. When it comes to condiments, check the labels and stick to the natural stuff, such as Primal Kitchen, Maranatha, Annie's Naturals, Trader Joe's, or your own homemade versions.

5. Trans Fats

Small amounts of trans fats, a form of unsaturated fatty acids, occur naturally in some meat and dairy products, such as beef, lamb, and butter. But most trans fats these days are industrially manufactured and are found in manufactured spreadable oils, where they form as a by-product of hydrogenation. Just about any spreadable oil found on grocery store shelves, such as margarine, frosting, or vegetable shortening, contains extremely volatile and highly oxidative trans fats—and most premade cakes, cookies, pie crusts, and crackers contain vegetable shortening, making them rich in trans fats. High blood levels of trans fat have been directly associated with poor cognitive function and low brain volume, along with heart disease, cancer, type 2 diabetes, low birth rate, obesity, immune dysfunction, impaired memory, and increased brain inflammation.

One study observed the effects of dietary trans fats on the word recall of 1,018 young men and women. The researchers discovered that the more trans fats an individual ate, the worse their word recall was. Trans fats also increase oxidative stress and promote endothelial dysfunction, which results in vascular damage that limits blood flow and the delivery of energy substrates to cells and tissues. Since memory is particularly sensitive to poor cellular energy delivery, trans fats can significantly reduce memory function.

6. Gluten

Gluten is a general term for the proteins found in wheat, including wheat berries, durum, emmer, semolina, spelt, farina, farro, and graham flour, as well as in rye, barley, and triticale (a cross between wheat and rye). Gluten acts as a glue to help foods maintain their shape, but because of its inherent stickiness and ability to create digestive difficulties, gluten has become the ultimate pariah among health enthusiasts and hippies. While they are less common than many people claim, gluten intolerances, cross-reactivities, and allergies can be legitimate problems and can even cause serious health complications, such as gut damage, autoimmune diseases, and neuroinflammation.

Even if you don't have an intolerance or allergy to gluten, or if it doesn't seem to cause perceivable gut issues, gluten can still damage your brain. Dr. David Perlmutter, a renowned neurologist, wrote the book *Grain Brain* to reveal how excess carbohydrates, especially gluten-containing grains, can cause a host of neurological problems. These problems range from dysregulation of the autonomic nervous system (the part of your nervous system responsible for automatic actions such as breathing and digestion), cerebellar ataxia (inflammation of or damage to the cerebellum, which causes loss of fine motor skills), hypotonia (low muscle tone), developmental delay, learning disorders, depression, migraines, and headaches. In fact, re-search has connected gluten sensitivities to neurological and psychiatric concerns like autism, schizophrenia, and hallucinations.

Fortunately, you can minimize the effect of gluten on your brain and the rest of your nervous system. For example, gluten can be broken down before eating via fermentation, which is why some of the only bread I eat is my wife Jessa's mouthwatering homemade sourdough. Through the process of slow fermentation, sourdough lactobacilli and fungal enzymes called proteases can eliminate gluten and, as a bonus, also reduce the bread's glycemic index—how quickly and how much it raises blood sugar. In contrast, ordinary yeast does not break down gluten and other harmful proteins like gliadin.

Sprouting is also another grain-preparation technique that may reduce the effects of gluten. There is a lot of debate over this technique, and there is no conclusive evidence to support it, but many alternative-diet and health experts recommend sprouting grains. The basic idea behind sprouting is that as a seed (such as a grain) germinates, it taps into and metabolizes stored carbo-hydrates to fuel its growth and may partially break down storage proteins such as gluten. Other sources claim that during the sprouting process, gluten gets broken down by the seedling as it taps into the energy contained within the seed's endosperm. Sprouting also releases vitamins, minerals, and other bioactive components that are unavailable for absorption in the unsprouted grain.

Ultimately, gluten-free foods can contain just as many chemicals, preservatives, and sugars as gluten-containing foods, and unless you have a condition such as celiac disease or you are fighting a leaky gut from years of poor eating, you don't need to avoid gluten entirely. Instead, eat gluten-containing grains only when they are prepared via ancestral processes such as fermentation and sprouting, think twice before snagging any old "healthy" goodie from the organic coffee shop, and support your ability to digest gluten by limiting your gut's exposure to chemicals such as pesticides and herbicides. You can also take supplements like Gluten Guardian or gluten polypep-tidases to help break down the gluten you do eat. That way, you can have your cake and eat it too, although you still shouldn't turn into a complete breadhead. (Read chapter 13 for more tips on managing gluten and getting a healthy gut.)

7. Foods High in Heavy Metals

Remember the Mad Hatter from Lewis Carroll's classic children's book *Alice's Adventures in Wonderland*? Like the saying "mad as a hatter," the character has its origin in the hat-making industry in England the 1800s, when a mercury solution was often used during the process of turning fur into felt. Hat-makers inhaled the fumes of this highly toxic metal and the mercury accumulated in their bodies, causing loss of coordination, slurred speech, loose teeth, memory loss, depression, irritability, and anxiety—a cluster of effects that came to be known as "mad hatter syndrome."

Mercury, found all too often in dental amalgams, fish, vaccines, and coal-burning power plants, isn't the only heavy metal that can cause neural issues like mad hatter syndrome. Aluminum, arsenic, lead, lithium, manganese, and thallium are also highly neurotoxic and have a host of deleterious cognitive effects. For example, lead inhibits the synthesis of heme, the nonprotein part of hemoglobin, the molecule that transports oxygen in your blood, and can affect brain function by interfering with neurotransmitters; methylmercury damages specific areas in the adult brain and especially developing nervous systems.

There are a plethora of ways to detox your body, such as ingesting charcoal or algae species like chlorella. But if you decide you are going to detox metals from your body and you don't go about it properly, you can suffer the same brain damage as those poor hatters. Why? Charcoal, chlorella, and other popular detox supplements are known as "weak binders." These binders act in much the same way that a magnet acts with metal shavings: they have a weak bond with the metals, and, as they pull the metals with them through your intestinal tract, some of those bonds can break, and the metal will then move back into your system, with the dangerous possibility of crossing the blood-brain barrier. In other words, rather than removing the toxins, these weak binders can end up allowing them to cross into deeper tissues, most notably the brain.

It is critical to use a true binding agent in a properly structured detox protocol to prevent toxins from recirculating after they have moved out of your cells. My friend Dr. Dan Pompa gave himself mad hatter syndrome by detoxing the wrong way but then went on to develop a unique detoxification protocol he calls True Cellular Detox. I interviewed Dr. Dan about the ins and outs of his protocol, and you can listen to my extremely detailed podcast with him on BoundlessBook.com/4, or visit chapter 13 for more details.

In the meantime, avoid frequent consumption of foods that are high in heavy metals, including these:

- Fish, especially larger fish or predatory fish such as king mackerel, bigeye tuna, sharks, and swordfish (mercury)
- Processed or powdered bone broth from nonorganic sources (lead)
- High amounts of brown rice (arsenic)
- Refined wheat flour (cadmium)
- Soft drinks from soda fountains (the machine may have cadmium in the pipes)
- Canned foods (lead)

If you want to test for heavy metals, you can get a Nutrient and Toxic Elements blood test from Genova Diagnostics, which will test for aluminum, arsenic, cadmium, lead, and mercury, as well as potassium, magnesium, calcium, zinc, copper, and selenium. Another good test is one from Doctor's Data called a urine provocation test, which involves "provoking" a release of metals with a chelating (binding) substance called DMSA, which pulls stored levels of toxic metals out of tissues and organs and makes it possible to detect them in urine. Another urine test is the Doctor's Data urine porphyrins test, since abnormal levels of urinary porphyrins are associated with high-level exposure to toxic chemicals or metals. Finally, the Great Plains Laboratory offers a hair test for metal toxicity and mineral deficiency. The problem with most tests is that they depend on your body's ability to excrete metals, and since most people with heavy-metal toxicity have compromised detoxification ability, testing can show low levels of metals even when someone is highly toxic. This is why most good functional-medicine practitioners use a variety of tests to get an accurate picture and may even prescribe a spectrographic test with a device called an OligoScan, an autonomic response test, or an energetic test. I recommend National Integrated Health Associates (NIHAdc.com) in Washington, DC; on their website you can find a list of integrative medical and naturopathic practitioners and dentists who can identify and treat heavy-metal toxicity, as well as similar toxic burdens. You can also visit HolisticDental.org for a list of certified holistic dentistry practitioners, although you'll need to ask if they specialize in removing metals from the mouth or metal detoxification in general.

8. Meals That Are High-Fat and High-Carb

Lipopolysaccharides (LPS) are toxic molecules found in the outer membrane of gram-negative bacteria. (You may recall from high school biology that the difference between gram-negative and gram-positive bacteria is that gram-positive bacteria lack this outer membrane. Gram-negative bacteria include *E. coli*, *Neisseria gonorrhoeae*, and other well-known pathogens.) LPS are classified as endotoxins—whereas exotoxins are released by bacteria, endotoxins are contained within the cell membrane until it is destroyed, at which point the endotoxin is released. In people, most endotoxins are produced by bacteria found in the gut.

Of all the small molecules floating around in human plasma, 25 percent to 33 percent are derived from gut bacteria, including LPS. When blood endotoxin levels get too high, they cause metabolic endotoxemia, a condition associated with cardiovascular disease, chronic inflammation, type 2 diabetes, lipid abnormalities, insulin resistance, nonalcoholic fatty liver disease, obesity, and stroke. Interestingly, one of the contributing factors to a higher risk of LPS-induced metabolic endotoxemia is a high-fat diet.

Wait a minute! Haven't I already claimed that fats are good for your nervous system? They are, but here is the deal: high-fat diets also have the *potential* to induce endotoxemia. Problems arise when you consume lots of fats alongside lots of carbohydrates—the classic potato chip, pork rind, cheesecake, baked goodie, follow-up-your-rib-eye-steak-with-a-chocolate-soufflé type diet. I have witnessed a fair share of healthy eaters complain of endotoxemia-like brain fog, then continue to chow down on dark chocolate peanut butter cups, roasted chicken glazed in brown sugar, and piles of avocados on rice crackers. And yes, this means that if one of your favorite meals (like mine) is a nice, fatty cut of rib-eye steak with sweet potato fries, you want to go easy on the fries, especially if your primary objective is cognitive enhancement.

How does endotoxemia happen? High-fat, high-carbohydrate meals are known to raise the levels of reactive oxygen species and inflammatory cytokines, leading to oxidative stress and inflammation. Consuming a high-fat, high-carbohydrate meal may also increase the permeability of your intestinal wall due to damage caused by the LPS. When your intestinal barrier permeability increases—a condition known as "leaky gut"— it allows bigger particles into your bloodstream, including LPS, pathogens, and allergenic proteins, all of which can exacerbate systemic inflammation. In addition, as you learned in chapter 2, a leaky gut is often associated with a leaky blood-brain barrier. So if you consume fats and carbohydrates together, it could potentially set off a chain reaction that results in brain damage or neuroinflammation. This means that any strategy to reduce your level of circulating endotoxins must include anti-inflammatory gut strategies (which are explored in detail in chapter 13) and a focus on reducing glucose fluctuation (as discussed above).

9. Moldy Foods

The word *mold* conjures images of decaying corpses, old hamburger meat in your refrigerator, or a nasty growth on your shower wall. Molds are collections of microorganisms that are decomposers of dead organic material such as leaves, wood, and plants. The tiny spores and hairlike bodies of individual mold colonies are too small for us to see without a microscope but constantly float about in the air around us. Some of the most harmful components of certain molds are mycotoxins, toxic substances that are capable of causing damage to the brain, along with disease and death, in both humans and animals.

The problems of mold in our homes have been well publicized. High amounts of indoor mold exposure can alter blood flow to the brain, affect autonomic nerve function and brain waves, and diminish concentration, attention, balance, and memory. It can impair the cognitive development of young children and cause hemorrhagic infarcts (areas of dead tissue caused by blocked veins) in the brain. A person who suffers from toxic mold exposure can go from being a highly efficient thinker able to analyze patterns and problems to experiencing complete brain fog, insomnia, anxiety, loss of appetite, and confusion and being misdiagnosed with depression or even bipolar disorder. Dr. Neil Nathan, author of the book *Toxic*, estimates that for 80 percent of his environmental toxin–sensitive patients, mold toxicity is the primary trigger for their symptoms (the remaining 20 percent are triggered by Lyme disease).

You can have tests such as an ERMI (environmental relative moldiness index) performed by a licensed contractor to determine if your house has mold in it. But for most people, the primary source of mycotoxins isn't household mold: it's diet.

You might think that avoiding moldy foods is a no-brainer. But mycotoxins are so prolifically dispersed throughout global agriculture that they are virtually unavoidable in the average modern diet. For example, commercially grown corn is typically heavily sprayed with pesticides that can cause a mutation in fungi that colonize corn. These mutated fungi grow in corn roots and pump toxins directly into the plant. Other common crops like barley, wheat, peanuts, and even coffee beans can also be notoriously high in mycotoxins. But it is important not to confuse "moldy" with "fermented." You are not necessarily exposed to mycotoxins if you eat fermented foods such as cheese, pickles, buttermilk, sour cream, and smoked fish. Sure, when consumed in high amounts, these foods can place you at higher risk for mycotoxin exposure, but many people remove moldy foods from their diet, keep eating fermented foods, and get well just fine.

You may have heard that mold or mycotoxin levels may be lower in organic foods, but the fact is that the mycotoxin content of a given crop depends on a variety of factors. For example, the amount of the mycotoxin deoxynivalenol in a product can depend on tillage practice, weather conditions, location of origin, and crop rotation. Indeed, while organic systems generally seem able to keep mycotoxin levels low, the available research doesn't indicate whether going organic reduces your risk of consuming mycotoxins. It's also important to know that candida—a fungus that's present in everyone but that can sometimes grow out of control—almost always plays a role in mold sensitivities, and for candida overgrowth, mold infection, and even Lyme disease, you should be eating a low-carb, low-sugar diet, because carbohydrates, particularly sugar and fruit, feed candida and many other fungal species.

Binders latch on to chemicals and toxins, such as bacteria, heavy metals, or mold, rendering them inactive and making it possible for the body to excrete them. Natural binders such as activated charcoal and clay have been used by both humans and animals for thousands of years to treat issues such as gas, bloating, stomach pain, and food poisoning, and also as a protocol during intestinal cleansing. They enhance the natural detoxification systems.

The following is a short list of some of the most popular binders:

Activated charcoal: In 1831, in a famous act performed in front of the French Academy of Medicine, a French physician consumed a lethal dose of the poison strychnine but suffered no deleterious effects because he also consumed charcoal at the same time. The clinical benefits of charcoal have been well researched since then. Activated charcoal has been shown to effectively absorb pesticides and herbicides, mold toxins, endotoxins, and more. It can also remove inflammatory molecules associated with a hyperactive immune response, such as interleukins and tumor necrosis factor, so it may be beneficial in calming an overactive immune system.

Bentonite clay: The use of bentonite clay dates back to early populations in the Andes, who carried balls of clay to consume as protection against poisons and toxins. It is particularly good at absorbing aflatoxin, a mycotoxin often found in peanuts, coffees, and grains, and it can also absorb pesticides, herbicides, and the cyanotoxins found in lakes polluted by algal blooms. It also has antibacterial properties and a healing effect on the lining of the gut.

Chitosan: Chitosan is created by enzymatic breakdown of chitin, a substance that forms the cell walls of fungi and exoskeletons of shellfish. In a book of medicine from the Ming Dynasty, it is written, "Break a crab shell, grind it, make a ball out of it, and eat it to treat anything that swells or grows." Chitosan promotes the growth of the good gut bacteria bifidobacteria and lactobacillus, and it can bind to bile salts that emulsify fat, so it can reduce fat absorption from a high-fat meal. It also binds and removes toxins present in bile salts, metals, polychlorinated biphenyls (PCBs), phthalates, and bisphenol A (BPA). It has also been shown to have protective effects against mercury-induced gene damage.

The good news is that research does indicate that antioxidants such as superoxide anion scavengers (enzymes that mop up free radicals in the body) can minimize the impact mycotoxins have on your body. Vitamin A, vitamin C, selenium, and glutathione are all good examples of antioxidants you can consume in food or supplements. Other strategies to eliminate mycotoxins include consuming binders such activated charcoal, sweating in a sauna, and eating garlic or supplementing with allicin, the active ingredient of garlic. Although many practitioners recommend high-dose methylation therapy via the use of methylated vitamins, usually delivered via IV, I do not. While it is true that the addition of methyl groups to molecules in the body can upregulate metabolic function and cellular efficiency, it may not be a good idea for those with a toxin or infection to use this type of therapy. This is because it is the mitochondria that recognize the presence of a toxin or infection due to a change in the electrical charge of the cell, and it is the mitochondria that then set off an orchestrated series of events to protect the cell. This includes halting methylation to protect the cell. If the cell is intentionally shutting down methylation when you get sick to protect itself, it certainly doesn't make sense to flood the body with a host of excess methyl groups.

In addition, if you have been significantly exposed to mold, there are certain healing steps that I recommend you take. The first is to address the limbic system, a group of structures in the brain that are particularly involved with emotion, including the amygdala, which is primarily responsible for how you process emotions. Signs that the limbic system region of the brain is

Silica: Silica bound to a thiol group (which is a special binding molecule containing sulfur and hydrogen) can be found in several supplements, including one made by Quicksilver Scientific. It delivers insoluble thiol groups that bind to and eliminate mercury and other heavy metals. The use of thiolated forms of silica dates back to the 1970s, when this compound was used to address mercury poisoning in Iraq. It performed even better than penicillamine, a common medical metal-chelating agent at the time. It is especially helpful in cases of mercury toxicity.

Aloe vera and acacia gum: Both aloe vera and acacia gum can ease the constipation that often occurs with the use of binders. Acacia gum contains dietary fiber that feeds the friendly bifidobacteria and lactobacillus bacteria in the gut, and it increases levels of butyrate, a short-chain fatty acid with anti-inflammatory effects that helps to heal a leaky gut. The bifidobacteria that the acacia feeds can lower endotoxin levels, normalize gut function, and reduce inflammation. Aloe vera has a soothing effect on the gut and has a long history of use for gastrointestinal disorders associated with inflammation, including peptic ulcers, gastritis, and inflammatory bowel disease.

There is no universal binder that works equally well on all toxins, so your best bet may be combining the binders listed here for a synergistic effect against any toxins. Dr. Joseph Brewer, one of the world's leading mold experts, has discovered that certain toxins are preferentially bound by certain binders. To be more specific, ochratoxins appear to be bound best by compounds such as cholestyramine and activated charcoal; aflatoxins are bound by activated charcoal and bentonite clay; trichothecenes are bound by activated charcoal, chlorella, and bentonite clay; and gliotoxins are bound by bentonite clay, *Saccharomyces boulardii* (a probiotic yeast), and N-acetylcysteine (NAC). A mold and mycotoxin test from a website like SurvivingMold.com can help pinpoint which toxins you have and therefore help you decide which binders to use.

For a list of good supplement options that include the binders listed above, see BoundlessBook.com/4.

being significantly affected by mold sensitivity or infection include severe anxiety, depression, despair, hopelessness, and depersonalization (feeling like you're not yourself), along with low energy, impaired cognition, and pain. One of the best methods for restabilizing the limbic system is a program designed by author and speaker Annie Hopper called Dynamic Neural Retraining, which uses mental exercises to rewire the limbic system (visit retrainingthebrain.com to learn more). Second, because the vagus nerve tends to become sympathetically overactive after mycotoxin exposure, I recommend a series of excellent exercises that have been developed by a body worker named Stanley Rosenberg, explained in his book *Accessing the Healing Power of the Vagus Nerve*. These exercises, which take about ten minutes a day to perform, can quiet the vagus nerve and the connecting cranial nerves. In conjunction with these exercises, I also highly recommend a form of therapy called osteopathic craniosacral work, which can be very effective for improving the vagal nerve tone (which increases vagus nerve activity). Osteopath James Jealous has a directory of practitioners trained in a particular form of this therapy on his website, jamesjealous.com.

If you're among the 25 percent of the population that possesses an immune response gene that prevents you from properly removing biotoxins from your body, mold becomes an even bigger issue because it circulates throughout your body and can result in a condition of biotoxin accumulation called chronic inflammatory response syndrome (CIRS), which you can test for through companies such as Life Extension or True Health Labs. If this is the case, you need to become hypervigilant not only about what you eat but also about the structures you go into, since up to 50 percent of buildings in the US are water-damaged.

To test for mold in your body, I recommend two options: (1) urine testing via the Real Time Laboratory or the Great Plains Laboratory, which will identify the specific toxins and mold strains that you have, or (2) the GENIE (Genomic Expression by Nanostring: Inflammation Explained) test from SurvivingMold.com, which is a newer and more comprehensive blood test that can identify unusual levels of gene activity associated with mold and mycotoxin exposure, failure of regulation of genes associated with CIRS, molds, mycotoxins, and more. In addition to the mycotoxin levels themselves, other biomarker clusters that can indicate some level of mycotoxin buildup include the following:

- high levels of antigliadin (AGA) antibodies
- low vasoactive intestinal polypeptide (VIP)
- high cortisol
- low vascular endothelial growth factor (VEGF)
- low melanocyte-stimulating hormone (MSH)
- high TGF beta-1
- high C4a
- high anticardiolipins (ACLA) antibodies
- low antidiuretic hormone (ADH)
- high matrix metallopeptidase 9 (MMP-9)
- high leptin

You might want to take 500 mg of oral glutathione twice daily for a week before a urine test for mycotoxins to make sure you get an accurate reading. This is because many people with mold or mycotoxin exposure have difficulty mobilizing these toxins, but using oral glutathione, 500 mg twice daily, for a week and then collecting the urine improves the diagnostic capabilities by mobilizing the toxins. So does sitting in an infrared sauna or a hot tub for ten to thirty minutes just prior to the urine collection—sweating mobilizes toxins too.

You can also take a free visual contrast sensitivity test at VCSTest.com, and this test—even in the absence of any blood or urine testing—can give you very good clues about your exposure to toxins, including certain species of mold and the mycotoxins they produce, along with parasites,

Smart Drugs

A smart drug is a medication used to treat a cognitive disorder like ADD. Sometimes these medications are designed to treat the disorder, but sometimes drugs intended for other conditions are used off-label to treat cognitive concerns. (An off-label use is anything that a drug hasn't been approved to treat by the FDA. For example, treating migraines with Botox injections, now a common practice, was considered an off-label use until the FDA approved Botox to treat migraines in 2010.) Please note that there are distinct differences between synthetic smart drugs and herbal or food-based nootropics, such as lion's mane mushrooms, *Ginkgo biloba* (ginkgo), or *Bacopa monnieri* (bacopa).

The synthetic chemical Adderall (amphetamine and dextroamphetamine) is one of the most popular smart drugs, with Provigil (modafinil) and Ritalin (methylphenidate) following close behind. These synthetic, stimulant-class smart drugs tend to produce significant spikes in neurotransmitters such as serotonin, dopamine, and norepinephrine, which can lead to neurotransmitter imbalances, drug tolerance, and habit formation. Drug tolerance is particularly dangerous because as your tolerance increases, you need more of the drug to notice its effects, and going without it can cause withdrawal symptoms. Higher dosages, in turn, can damage important physiological functions such as appetite, mood stability, and stress regulation.

heavy metals like mercury and lead, and the pathogens responsible for Lyme disease and its common coinfections, such as babesiosis, bartonellosis, ehrlichiosis, mycoplasma infection, or Rocky Mountain spotted fever.

In addition, because the symptoms of mold exposure and Lyme disease often overlap, it can be useful to test for Lyme as well, preferably using a test called the IGeneX Western blot. You can read even more about HLA and CIRS, along with testing for molds and mycotoxins, at SurvivingMold.com, and also in Dr. Neil Nathan's book *Toxic*. There is also a very helpful questionnaire that is surprisingly accurate at predicting the possibility of Lyme disease or Lyme co-infection (also known as multiple systemic infectious diseases syndrome, or MSIDS) at LymeActionNetwork.org.

HOW TO
EAT YOURSELF SMART

By avoiding foods that break your brain, you can combat and even reverse the damage caused by unhealthy eating patterns, mold, heavy metals, and endotoxins. But it's not just a matter of preventing damage—you can also eat yourself smart with the following four research-backed eating and nutritional strategies.

1. Pursue Ketosis

Ketosis is a metabolic state in which a certain amount of your body's energy supply comes from ketone bodies, by-products of burning fat. This stands in stark contrast to a state of glycolysis, in which blood glucose provides the primary source of energy. Generally, ketosis occurs when your body metabolizes fatty acids at a relatively high rate and converts those fatty acids into ketones.

True nootropics—natural, not synthetic, substances—on the other hand do not seem to carry the risks of tolerance development, habit formation, neurotransmitter imbalances, and impaired cognitive function. In fact, nootropics seem to protect and enhance the brain. The nootropic piracetam, discovered in the 1960s, and its relatives oxiracetam and nefiracetam can even reverse amnesia induced by electroconvulsive therapy and hypoxia, as well as reduce the effects of dementia.

If a drug is strongly felt on a consistent basis whenever you use it and it makes you high, wired, or sedated, it is acting more like a smart drug or performance enhancer and is likely not a natural nootropic. Nootropics are sustainable for long-term use, while smart drugs are not. If you have a prescription for Adderall or a similar stimulant, it is critical that you don't slip into overdosing, even a little, and people who take stimulant-class drugs without a prescription should be very cautious. Smart drugs do not support natural cognitive processes, can be toxic, and may depress or overstimulate the brain. I'll talk much more about nootropics and smart drugs in chapter 5.

The ketogenic diet was developed in the 1920s to reduce the frequency of seizures in epileptic children. Although they didn't fully understand the biological mechanisms, medical professionals at the time did know that elevated levels of ketones in the blood seemed to correlate with a significant decrease in epileptic episodes. Since then, ongoing research has revealed a variety of ways that ketosis improves brain function.

Although many people are aware that limiting dietary carbohydrates and eating slower-burning fuels such as healthy fats can help control hunger and reduce body weight via improved fat metabolism, it's less well known that the benefits of ketosis go much deeper, to a cellular level.

First, ketosis makes for healthier mitochondria, the driving forces of each cell in your body. When your mitochondria malfunction, they can't produce enough energy. As a result, tissues with high energy demands, such as muscles, the heart, and the brain, suffer, resulting in complications that can include blindness, deafness, movement disorders, dementia, cardiomyopathy (disease of the heart muscle), myopathy, renal dysfunction, and accelerated aging. Ketosis is effective at reversing mitochondrial dysfunction because it increases the number of mitochondria and the production of oxidative ATP, particularly in neurons. So by improving the number and energetic output of the mitochondria in your brain, you can significantly enhance cognition and protect yourself from neurodegeneration. (Incidentally, if this information about mitochondria intrigues you, I recommend you take an even deeper dive with the book *Mitochondria and the Future of Medicine* by Lee Know, which is one of the best scientific and practical books on mitochondria that I have ever read.)

Depending on your level of physical activity, after fasting for sixteen to seventy-two hours or after limiting your daily carb intake to 20 to 60 g per day, after two to three days, your remaining glucose reserves are insufficient for normal fat oxidation and for fueling your brain. At that point, the mitochondria in your liver begin to produce the three ketone bodies: acetone, acetoacetate, and beta-hydroxybutyric acid. These are derived from excess acetyl-CoA (a key molecule in the metabolism of proteins, carbohydrates, and lipids), which accumulates as you metabolize fats. This entire process of producing ketones is called ketogenesis. The ketone bodies are then converted into other compounds and metabolized into energy in your cells, including your neurons.

Ketone metabolism is known to create much lower levels of oxidative stress than glucose metabolism, resulting in reduced inflammation and improved mitochondrial health. This is especially important for your brain, since neurodegenerative disorders characterized by demyelination (degradation of the myelin sheath surrounding part of a nerve cell), such as multiple sclerosis, are thought to be heavily influenced by chronic inflammation. Research also suggests that fasting or a fasting-mimicking diet (such as a ketogenic diet or the use of exogenous ketone supplements) can improve neurodegenerative disorders by upregulating brain-derived neurotrophic factor (BDNF), which supports the continued growth and development of neuronal connections. A ketogenic diet has also been proven to facilitate the conversion of glutamate into the neurotransmitter GABA, which is important because chronically elevated glutamate levels can overstimulate brain cells and lead to neural inflammation.

Now don't get me wrong: I don't necessarily endorse a high-fat, low-carb ketogenic diet for everyone. But when it comes to your brain, ketones are the cleanest-burning fuel you can get, so a ketogenic diet, the use of exogenous ketones, and frequent periods of fasting (more on that in a moment) are all highly useful strategies to get into ketosis and achieve greater clarity, laser-like focus, and performance-grade cognition. One of the best and most comprehensive books I have ever read on ketosis is *The Keto Bible* by my friend Ryan Lowery and Dr. Jacob Wilson.

2. Fast

Earlier, I briefly alluded to fasting as a strategy for entering a state of ketosis. But fasting accomplishes far more than that and is, in fact, a potent way to both heal your brain and protect it from future damage. But before jumping into how fasting works, it is important to understand the distinction between fasting and caloric restriction.

Caloric restriction is an intentional reduction of your daily or weekly caloric intake. It works on a "calories in, calories out" basis, so that your energy output is greater than your energy input, which forces your body to burn stored fat for energy.

Fasting, on the other hand, especially intermittent fasting, does not necessarily require caloric restriction. It simply involves not eating for a given amount of time, and then eating within a limited period called a compressed eating window. You don't eat less; you eat less often. Indeed, even when I perform a twenty-four-hour fast, such as when I stop eating after dinner on Saturday and don't eat again until dinner on Sunday, I will often eat more than 2,500 calories for Sunday dinner, so there's no overall drop in calories. Similarly, my friend Todd White of Dry Farm Wines fasts every day until dinner and, although his metabolism is healthy and his weight is stable, often punishes an entire bottle of organic wine and an enormous slab of red meat, salmon, hollandaise sauce, mayonnaise, and other calorically dense and scrumptious foods for dinner.

Why is it important to make this distinction? Frankly, many lean, highly active people attempt to engage in frequent twelve-to-sixteen-hour intermittent fasts, regular twenty-four-hour fasts, or three-to-five-day fasts, and then they encounter thyroid downregulation, hormone depletion, low energy, and poor sleep because they are attempting to marry caloric restriction–based fasting with an extremely active, calorie-decimating lifestyle and a body that doesn't have a ton of energy stores to tap into.

Don't get me wrong: caloric restriction can certainly be good for you. An old Confucian principle that certain long-lived Asiatic people groups abide by is *"Hara hachi bu"*—"Eat until you are 80 percent full" (a loose translation). But fasting, especially short bursts of intermittent fasting, can be particularly effective for both losing fat and improving brain health and function without necessarily restricting calories (although fasting often naturally leads to a 20 percent to 30 percent daily caloric reduction). In other words, if you are overweight, obese, sedentary, or in need of giving your gut a serious break from calories, fasting can give you the benefits of restricting calories without actually restricting calories.

One of the ways that intermittent fasting improves brain function has to do with a process called neuronal autophagy, the intentional and healthy self-destruction of aging neurons to make room for new ones. Abnormal or restricted autophagic activity is associated with neurodegenerative diseases such as Alzheimer's, Parkinson's, Huntington's, and amyotrophic lateral sclerosis (also known as Lou Gehrig's disease). Frequent feeding, particularly on sugars and proteins, causes elevated insulin, which reduces neuronal autophagy, resulting in metabolic dysregulation and neurodegeneration. Intermittent fasts, especially fasts between sixteen hours and twenty-four hours long (such as a weekly twenty-four-hour fast) can significantly reduce insulin levels and allow the brain to engage in neuronal autophagy. Intermittent fasting also reduces inflammation, including neuroinflammation induced by the same lipopolysaccharides I discussed when introducing you to endotoxemia.

Entire books have been written on fasting techniques, including the excellent *The Complete Guide to Fasting* by Dr. Jason Fung and Jimmy Moore. But the most common, practical kinds of fasts are the 12-12 and 16-8 strategies. The 12-12 strategy involves twelve hours of fasting followed by a twelve-hour eating window. This is a relatively simple habit to get into on a daily basis, even for very active individuals, and it still allows you to get the neural benefits of fasting. A sixteen-hour intermittent fast can be even better because sixteen hours is the point at which cellular autophagy increases. But a word of caution: for very lean, active individuals (especially women), sixteen hours of fasting—even without caloric restriction—seems to be capable of causing hormonal imbalances and metabolic dysfunction.

3. Feed Your Gut Bacteria

The quality, quantity, and diversity of the bacteria in your gut have a profound influence on your brain. Dr. David Perlmutter explores this phenomenon in great detail in his book *Brain Maker: The Power of Gut Microbes to Heal and Protect Your Brain—for Life*, in which he explains, "These hundred trillion bacteria that live within your gut are so intimately involved in your brain at a number of levels. They manufacture neurochemicals, for example. Things like dopamine and serotonin. They manufacture important vitamins that are important to keep your brain healthy. They also maintain the integrity of the lining of your gut."

As I mentioned earlier, when your gut lining is compromised, the result is leaky gut syndrome. This increases systemic inflammation, which serves as a cornerstone for virtually all brain disorders, including Alzheimer's, multiple sclerosis, Parkinson's, and autism.

Dr. Perlmutter also writes about how gut bacteria are at the cutting edge of neurology research:

> *Being a brain specialist dealing with brain disorders, my whole career I've been stymied by not having really powerful tools to implement to bring about changes in individuals who have these issues. Now we're beginning to get those tools, and they are in the gut. Who knew? In neurology school, we didn't study the makeup of the gut bacteria and how that would ever influence the brain, and yet, this is leading-edge science. This is what our most well-respected researchers and peer-reviewed journals are talking about: not only are the gut bacteria fundamentally involved in brain health, but you can change the gut bacteria through interventions—taking probiotics and choosing to eat foods that are rich in prebiotics and to enhance the growth of good bacteria—and even more aggressive therapies [such as fecal transplants].*

While I don't think a fecal transplant is necessary to optimize your brain, there are gut bacteria–feeding strategies you can use to nourish and protect your microbiome and your brain.

Opt for whole, raw, organic, non-GMO foods that are friendly to the gut lining, such as bone broth, sprouted seeds, and cultured dairy products, along with fermented and cultured foods, like sauerkraut, kimchi, and kombucha, and fiber-rich prebiotic foods, like jicama, Jerusalem artichokes, garlic, and dandelion greens. It is important to note that pasteurized fermented foods often no longer contain living bacteria, so be sure that the products you purchase actually contain living microorganisms. Finally, one person's superfood can be another person's poison, and if you have a histamine intolerance, you should actually limit your intake of fermented foods and stick to a low-histamine probiotic such as Seeking Health's Probiota HistaminX.

4. Focus on Supportive Nutrients and Substances

In addition to the three dietary strategies above, you can also support your gut and brain by seeking the following compounds in both real foods and supplements.

CONJUGATED LINOLEIC ACID (CLA)

CLA is a fatty acid that can improve immune responses and may be helpful in protecting the brain. It is found in high concentrations in the meat and dairy of cows, sheep, and goats. Incorporate grass-fed, grass-finished beef or lamb or raw dairy products from those animals into your diet.

BUTYRIC ACID

Butyric acid, also called butyrate, is a fatty acid found in milk, cheese, and butter. It acts as an anti-inflammatory agent by inhibiting NF-kB activation in your colon. NF-kB regulates genes involved in immune inflammatory responses, so by shutting down diet- or microbiota-induced inflammation, butyrate helps minimize the effects of inflammation on your central nervous system. As with CLA, you can get more butyrate in your system by consuming grass-fed butter and other grass-fed dairy products.

GLUTATHIONE (GSH)

GSH plays a critical role in shielding cells and cellular molecules from damaging oxidants and facilitates the excretion of toxins from cells. It even helps to regenerate other antioxidants such as tocopherols and ascorbate to restore those antioxidants back to their active, nonoxidized state. To produce GSH, your body requires adequate protein intake. Your protein intake should range from 0.5 to 0.8 g per pound of body weight, which equates to about 85 to 136 g per day for a healthy 170-pound person. To enhance natural GSH production, consume foods that contain GSH precursors, including milk thistle, quality whey protein, arugula, broccoli, cauliflower, and kale, and foods that support methylation, such as avocado, lentils, liver, garbanzo beans, Brazil nuts, grass-fed beef, and spinach.

You can also supplement your diet with GSH via sublingual glutathione, liposomal glutathione, injectable glutathione, IV glutathione, or capsules, such as those from Jarrow or Almsbio. Sublingual and liposomal glutathione have been shown to be highly absorbable. Sublingual glutathione is placed under your tongue and taken up directly into the blood vessels there, allowing the glutathione to bypass digestion. Liposomes are small, membranous bubbles that are similar in structure to the membranes of your cells. By protecting the glutathione until it reaches its destination and merging easily with cell membranes, liposomes allow glutathione to be efficiently taken up. Effective doses of glutathione range from 250 to 300 mg daily, generally taken over the period of two to three months to achieve adequate levels.

CHARCOAL

I will readily admit that this doesn't have a great deal of research or science behind it, but several folks in the nutrition industry swear by carbon-rich supplements for decreasing neural oxidation and boosting brain performance. One of the simplest, most convenient sources of carbon is activated charcoal.

Activated charcoal is charcoal that has been treated with heat to enhance its potential as a toxin sponge—indeed, it can be used to soak up poisons that enter the digestive system. It also supports brain health by absorbing the toxins and heavy metals that can inhibit cognitive function and lead to things like brain fog, depression, and anxiety.

It is important to note that not all charcoal is created equal. For example, the charcoal briquettes often used for grilling contain toxins such as sodium nitrate (which can damage your cells and lead to the development of cancer cells) and trace amounts of lighter fluid. When they are burned, they emit carbon monoxide. It probably isn't a good idea to munch on this type of charcoal. Instead, look for activated charcoal that is specifically labeled as a dietary supplement, and be careful not to take it with other supplements or medications because it will significantly decrease the absorption of anything it's taken with.

DHA

DHA (docosahexaenoic acid) is an omega-3 fatty acid that's critical for brain growth in infants and proper brain function in adults. DHA deficiency is associated with fetal alcohol syndrome, ADHD, cystic fibrosis, phenylketonuria, depression, aggressive hostility, and adrenoleukodystrophy. That last condition is especially dangerous: it refers to the degradation of the myelin sheath protecting nerve cells. One study observed the effects of DHA supplementation on the memory and reaction times of young adults who had a low intake of omega-3 fatty acids and found that it improved both, particularly the episodic memory of the women and the working memory of the men. Another study revealed that DHA prevented aggression toward others from increasing in young students during times of mental stress. I've always wondered if this is why people who follow low-fat diets or who build up fatty-acid deficiencies tend to be, in my opinion, a bit more moody or aggressive.

DHA isn't difficult to incorporate into your diet. It is one of the primary oils in many species of shellfish and fish, such as shrimp, lobster, Dungeness crab, king crab, anchovies, salmon, herring, mackerel, tuna, and halibut. So to increase your DHA intake, you can increase your seafood intake or consume a high-quality brand of fresh, unoxidized fish oil—or both. I personally consume 10 to 15 g of fish oil on the days I don't eat fish. Of course, you should be very cautious eating fish if you suspect you have heavy metal toxicity, and you may even want to consider supplementing with krill oil (which is low in metals) instead or sticking to very small fish far down the food chain, such as anchovies, mackerel, herring, and sardines.

If you are allergic to fish or shellfish, DHA is also readily available in eggs and grass-fed beef. If you follow a vegan or vegetarian diet, you can still get DHA, but it does take a bit more effort and expense. Spirulina and chlorella contain moderately to highly bioavailable forms of DHA. You may have heard that seeds and nuts like flax seeds, hemp seeds, and chia seeds are also good sources of DHA, but the fact is, your body's ability to unlock those reserves and convert them into usable DHA is pretty low—some research has indicated that your body is actually incapable of deriving any DHA at all from seeds and nuts. However, some plants, such as brussels sprouts, are rich in short-chain omega-3 fatty acids, and while these are less potent than DHA, they also act as neuroprotectors and are beneficial for your cellular and brain health.

EPA

Like DHA, EPA (eicosapentaenoic acid) is an omega-3 fatty acid that's highly available in algae and oily fish, as well as in fish oil. EPA levels in the brain are typically 250 to 300 times lower than DHA levels, so it is not as critical for neuronal health, but it still plays a role in protecting your

Why Fish Don't Need Fish Oil

Sure, eating fish and consuming fish oil are excellent strategies for getting large amounts of absorbable EPA and DHA, but what about fish? Fish, especially nonpredatory fish that aren't eating smaller fish, don't really consume much fish oil, do they? So how do fish create EPA and DHA?

Fish produce an enzyme that converts the plants (particularly the algae) they consume into EPA and DHA. New research shows that humans who consume adequate amounts of these enzymes or precursors for these enzymes, along with important compounds such as omega-5, omega-7, omega-9, omega-11, gamma-linoleic acid, and conjugated linoleic acid, and supportive minerals such as zinc and magnesium, can upregulate their conversion of plant-based oils into EPA and DHA, thus lowering their need for large quantities of fish or fish oil. This is especially good news for plant-based eaters who want to get adequate essential fatty acids for the brain and nervous system.

In a nutshell, a properly structured diet should include saturated, monounsaturated, and polyunsaturated fatty acids along with phytochemicals, antioxidants, and minerals. This includes fish and roe, olive oil, grass-fed meats, seeds, nuts, organic vegetables, roots and tubers, and whole fruits. With this kind of balanced diet, the body has what it needs to produce much of its own EPA and DHA—just like fish!

The chart below provides a summary of the food sources of the fats and oils that should be included in the diet. As you can see, simply popping a few fish oil capsules each morning does not give the body the full spectrum of fats, enzymes, and minerals it needs for full brain and nervous system support (and indeed, excess omega-3 supplementation can actually down-regulate many of the pathways in the chart by competing with all the other forms of fatty acids!). Finally, new research shows that the curcuminoids in turmeric and curcumin may assist with the body's own natural formation of EPA and DHA.

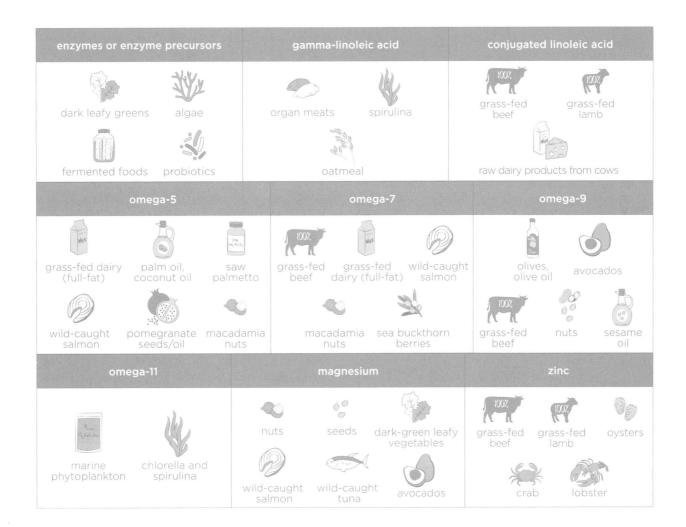

cells in general and your neurons in particular. EPA helps improve the strength of cell membranes and influences behavior and mood. It also acts as a precursor to eicosanoids, which are signaling and inhibiting molecules crucial in inflammatory and allergic reactions. Vegetarians and vegans sometimes try to get EPA by consuming terrestrial plants rich in ALA (another omega-3 fatty acid that I'll discuss more below), but it is important to note that the conversion rate of ALA to EPA is fairly low. Research suggests that only 2 percent to 10 percent of ALA is converted to EPA or DHA. While they are slightly pricier than fish oil and most plants, consuming spirulina or chlorella, or both, may be the most effective tactic.

ALA

ALA (alpha-linolenic acid) is a plant-based omega-3 fatty acid that cannot be synthesized in the human body: it must be obtained through food. Research suggests that ALA increases brain-derived neurotrophic factor, which plays a major role in maintaining neurons and improving learning and memory. ALA can be found in olives, extra-virgin olive oil, avocados, and walnuts. These Mediterranean diet–type fats can even provide benefits beyond those of anti-inflammatory omega-3 fatty acids. For example, olive oil primarily consists of a monounsaturated omega-9 fatty acid called oleic acid. Oleic acid possesses antioxidant properties that protect omega-3s from oxidation and is also a primary component of myelin sheaths.

Finally, the following whole foods are ideal to include in your brain-boosting diet.

AVOCADOS

The vitamin K in avocados helps prevent blood clots in the brain. In studies on diabetic rats, avocados exerted antioxidant effects on the brain and improved the function of brain mitochondria. Avocados have also been shown to improve spatial working memory and attention span.

BEET JUICE

Beet juice contains concentrated nitrates that decrease blood pressure and improve cognitive performance. In addition, the nitric oxide from beet juice helps increase neurovascular function and circulation to the brain. You'd have to eat at least three or four whole beets to get this same effect, and that amount of fiber, sugar, and calories can be difficult for some people's digestive systems to handle!

BLUEBERRIES, COCOA, VIRGIN OR EXTRA-VIRGIN COCONUT OIL

Blueberries, cocoa, and coconut oil all contain high levels of flavonoids and flavonols, which can help protect the brain from oxidative stress. Coconut oil can also prevent age-related memory loss and has medium-chain triglycerides, which give added protection against oxidative stress.

BONE BROTH

Bone broth contains high levels of glycine, a nonessential amino acid that can improve neurological function by enhancing memory.

BROCCOLI AND EGGS

Broccoli and egg yolks not only pair fantastically in an omelet but also contain choline, which helps improve both verbal and visual memory.

Simple Brain-Boosting Recipes

The following are a few tasty ways you can combine the foods you have discovered in this chapter.

- Slice an avocado, pour extra-virgin olive oil over the top, and add a pinch each of sea salt, black pepper, turmeric, and cayenne pepper, or a dash of fresh lime juice.

- Add avocado oil–based mayonnaise to a can of wild-caught salmon and wrap it all in a green lettuce leaf, a nori seaweed wrap, or a tortilla made of almond, coconut, or cassava flour.

- Mix flax seeds, chia seeds, and hemp seeds into grass-fed, organic plain yogurt and top with a sprinkling of organic blueberries, Ceylon cinnamon, and vanilla extract or liquid stevia drops.

- Smash an avocado, add salt and pepper, and smear it onto a green lettuce leaf or a tortilla made of almond, coconut, or cassava flour. Add organic, pastured scrambled eggs for a breakfast burrito.

- To avoid eating the inflammatory oils most restaurants use, bring a small container of extra-virgin olive oil when you travel or go out to restaurants to drizzle (or dump) on your salad or meal. I am notorious for showing up at restaurants with my own fancy oils and salts.

- Combine almond milk, sea salt, chia seeds, and liquid stevia drops in a mason jar and shake well. Chill the jar in the refrigerator overnight for a quick grab-and-go breakfast of chia pudding. Try adding nuts and seeds, such as walnuts and flax seeds, for even more healthy fatty acids.

- Chop up some kale, spread it in an even layer on a baking sheet, top with avocado oil, sea salt, and flax seeds or ground cashews, and bake at 275°F for about twenty minutes for nutty-flavored kale chips.

- Add a can of wild-caught sardines to a salad or a bed of zero-calorie, zero-carb shirataki noodles for a meal rich in protein and healthy fats.

KALE, SWISS CHARD, AND ROMAINE LETTUCE

The nutrients found in kale, Swiss chard, and romaine lettuce can be beneficial in preventing cognitive impairment and dementia.

OLIVE OIL AND WALNUTS

One of the minor constituents of olive oil that I haven't yet discussed is oleocanthal, which can reduce the neuron-damaging effects of ADDLs (amyloid beta–derived diffusible ligands, a protein found in many cosmetics, plastic products, and putties). These ADDLs can be a particularly nasty culprit when it comes to increasing Alzheimer's risk, and thus olive oil can have a preventative effect on Alzheimer's disease. Walnut extract can also help protect against ADDL-induced oxidative stress and cell death.

ROSEMARY

Rosemary extract, found in fresh rosemary or rosemary essential oil, possesses potent antioxidant properties. In particular, the antioxidant carnosic acid occurs in high levels in rosemary leaves and helps prevent chronic neurodegenerative diseases.

SALMON

Salmon is naturally high in omega-3 fatty acids and boosts the phospholipid bilayer that encases each neuron, thus strengthening the membranes of the cells in your brain. The fatty acids also strengthen the synaptic connections between neurons.

TURMERIC

Turmeric's active ingredient is curcumin. Research has shown curcumin to be an antioxidant and anti-inflammatory compound that improves cognitive function in people with Alzheimer's. It also enhances the uptake of amyloid-beta plaques by the cleanup crew of body's phagocytic white blood cells, resulting in improved neuroprotection and reduced inflammation in the central nervous system.

All these foods can be easily combined to make a variety of quick, easy, chock-full-of-fat meals. Also, pay close attention to chapter 14, in which diet customization and choosing the nutrition plan that is perfect for you will be covered in more detail.

THE LAST WORD

Congratulations: you are now equipped with a grocery list and food and supplement protocol for optimizing your brain and enhancing cognition.

Remember, to give your brain the fuel it needs, it's most important to seek out healthy fats from natural sources and avoid damaged, unstable fats (primarily in industrial oils, which sneak into a wide range of packaged and processed foods). You'll also prevent and repair damage to your neurons by limiting the following:

- Histamine- and oxalate-containing foods
- Glucose-fluctuating foods
- Artificially sweetened foods
- Condiments
- Trans fats
- Gluten
- Foods high in heavy metals
- Meals that are high-fat and high-carb
- Moldy foods
- Smart drugs

At the same time, you can support your brain by pursuing ketosis, fasting, feeding your gut bacteria, and seeking out supplements and foods that contain certain nutrients.

Keep in mind, the more clearly you can think, the faster you can react and remember information, and the more robust your nervous system, the more equipped you are to live a life of boundless energy each day.

ONE THING YOU CAN DO THIS WEEK

Each day this week, as you settle into healthy-fat consumption, your task is to incorporate the mighty avocado bowl into your diet. Take an avocado, slice it in half, and drizzle it (or drench it, if the spirit so leads you) with a high-quality, spicy, savory extra-virgin olive oil, then add sea salt and whatever other zests might titillate your taste buds, including turmeric, black pepper, or (one of my favorites) a slab of mouthwatering coconut manna. For a snack, eat half the avocado, or for a full, surprisingly satiating meal, eat the whole avocado on a bed of arugula or other dark leafy greens.

For citations for all the research studies mentioned in this chapter and a deeper dive into the topics of this chapter—including links to podcasts, blog posts, recommended tools and supplements, and much more—visit BoundlessBook.com/4.

Trenkle, Anthony E

8098
14094

Thursday, July 30, 2020   Bonnieee : update your

34835040313o

Trenkle, Anthony F
14608
Thursday, July 30, 2020
31183200405139   Boundless : upgrade your

LIMITLESS AND LUCY

NOOTROPICS, SMART DRUGS, AND PSYCHEDELICS

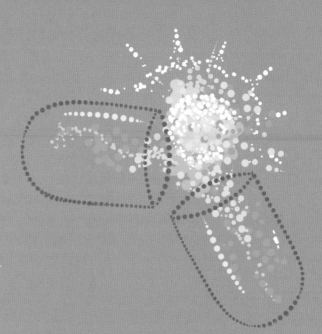

Breathing carefully, I clutched the Costco special edition family-size glass bottle of vodka and extracted 100 milliliters with a miniature glass pipette, which I then transferred into a small amber glass bottle. Then, with my nine-year-old son's tiny set of school scissors, I snipped exactly one-tenth of the blotter square of LSD I had ordered from a psychedelic drug website on the dark web the week prior—with a cloaked browser, of course, so the feds didn't come knocking at my door. I dropped the LSD into the bottle, gave it a thirty-second shake, and then placed it in the pantry next to my protein powder and creatine. I smiled. Within twenty-four hours, I would be ready to sample my first homemade, volumetric microdose of a drug reported to increase lateral thinking patterns, improve creativity, and massively boost productivity.

Why do I, a good Christian kid from the backwoods of Idaho, spend time in my kitchen mixing up LSD, psilocybin, ketamine, ibogaine, synthetic DMT tabs, and more—all while my children munch away at their scrambled eggs in the breakfast nook? And why do I, on cognitively demanding days, stir my cup of coffee with a nicotine-coated toothpick, sneak a heaping spoonful of powdered lion's mane mushrooms into my morning smoothie, or dump a packet of Chinese adaptogenic herbs into the pouches of my cheeks?

It all comes down to my investigation into how you can enhance your mind by combining ancestral wisdom and herbs such as bacopa and ginkgo with modern science and compounds like LSD and racetams.

Your coworker in the next cubicle could be achieving their hyperfocus via a microdose of LSD, a hit of huperzine, or a nicotine-infused arm patch. Words like *nootropic* and *smart drug* (yes, there is a difference) are quickly becoming household terms, especially due to all the recent media hype about their popularity with everyone from Silicon Valley CEOs to professional athletes to college students, along with the emergence of movies like *Limitless* and *Lucy*, popular TV shows such as *Wormwood* and *Hamilton's Pharmacopeia*, and unprecedented titles such as Michael Pollan's psychedelic exploration book *How to Change Your Mind*.

Why are these compounds so increasingly rampant? Think about how much sensory information we have to process each day. From big-city noise pollution to ringing phones, artificial lighting, and chemical-laden air fresheners inundating your senses, to electromagnetic fields piercing your brain, to the complicated new procedure you have to learn at work requiring fierce concentration, the human brain has to organize and cope with massive amounts of information, all while keeping you upright and sane.

The brain does indeed have incredible skills and unimaginable capabilities, but modern living creates unprecedented stress and sensory overload. Sensory overload has even been shown to cause irritability, anxiety, mood swings, depression, ADHD, fibromyalgia, PTSD, and chronic fatigue syndrome. So maintaining your ability to learn, process information, and form new neural connections is crucial for optimizing brain health, longevity, and, ultimately, boundless energy.

But you don't have to lock yourself in a dark, quiet room to protect your skull from the onslaught of stimuli. There are research-backed compounds that can amplify cognitive function, help your brain deal with sensory overload, get you through a period of sleep deprivation, and increase your creativity during an intense bout of work or study. When combined into "stacks" and taken in the correct doses, these compounds can very noticeably change how your brain performs—for the better, if used correctly. They impact receptor sites for neurotransmitters, alter levels of enzymes that break down neurotransmitters, change cell membrane structures, and control the movement of molecules in and out of the cell, improve blood flow to the brain, affect the development of neurons, and regulate hormones.

I have taken a deep dive in the wonderful world of smart drugs, nootropics, and psychedelics, and I have had the opportunity to interview some of the brightest minds in this unique field. In this chapter, I will spill the beans on it all, including how to navigate the oft-confusing world of smart drugs and nootropics, which are the best-of-the-best of the brain-boosting compounds I have used, and how to procure and microdose psychedelics.

I know you're probably chomping at the bit to discover how to microdose with psilocybin or ibogaine, or how to make that cup of coffee last a few hours longer without jitters, but before we dive into these intriguing topics, you have to understand the difference between a smart drug and a nootropic, as well as how to choose which one to take.

SMART DRUGS 101

Many people use the terms nootropic and smart drug as if they mean the same thing, but they're actually very distinct. All nootropics are technically smart drugs, but the opposite is not necessarily true. A smart drug is any substance that enhances memory, mood, concentration, or another aspect of cognitive function. Nootropics target the same functions, but by definition they must also be neuroprotective and nontoxic, and they are usually derived from natural, nonsynthetic sources. A Belgian pharmacologist named V. Skondia developed a medical definition for nootropics—they are compounds that meet all of the following criteria:

- have no effects on blood pressure or heart rate
- have no effects on EEG brain waves
- can pass through the blood-brain barrier
- have minimal side effects
- increase metabolism in the brain
- have been proven in clinical studies to enhance brain function

Dr. Corneliu E. Giurgea also proposed the following standards that focus more on the positive effects of nootropics. For a supplement to be considered a nootropic, it must do all of the following:

- enhance learning and memory
- enhance learned behaviors under conditions known to disrupt them
- protect the brain from physical or chemical injury
- enhance the tonic cortical and subcortical control mechanisms in the brain
- exhibit few side effects and extremely low toxicity
- lack the pharmacology of typical psychotropic drugs (such as motor stimulation and sedation)

For example, Adderall is a smart drug that doesn't qualify as a nootropic under either definition because it is a powerful stimulant that frequently causes negative side effects, such as high blood pressure and heart rate. There are many smart drugs on the market, the most well-known of which are the psychostimulants Adderall and Ritalin, both of which increase activity in the central nervous system. Other common, similar smart drugs are modafinil, ampakines, and L-deprenyl. Later in this chapter I'll examine specific nootropics and their uses, but first, let's look at how each of these smart drugs work and their benefits and potential risks.

Methylphenidate (Ritalin)

Methylphenidate was first used in medicine in 1960 to treat narcolepsy and attention-deficit/hyperactivity disorder (ADHD). It works by inhibiting the reuptake of dopamine and norepinephrine, which causes a flood of dopamine and norepinephrine in your synapses and amplifies the signals sent between neurons. These effects are similar to those of amphetamines (which I'll talk more about later in this section), which are synthetic, addictive, mood-altering stimulants used illegally in sports and legally as prescription drugs to treat children with ADD and adults with narcolepsy. It is incredibly easy to become addicted to methylphenidate. Misuse is shockingly prevalent, with students, biohackers, soccer moms, and busy executives popping it like candy.

Methylphenidate's side effects include insomnia, stomachache, headache, and anorexia. Overdoses (which may easily occur, because it can be difficult to estimate and regulate doses) can lead to agitation, hallucinations, psychosis, lethargy, seizures, tachycardia (rapid heart rate), dysrhythmia (irregular heart rhythms), hypertension (high blood pressure), and hyperthermia (high fever).

Methylphenidate is particularly dangerous for developing brains, such as those of children and adolescents, who are frequently prescribed the drug or, especially in the case of many teenagers and college students, use it without a prescription. The prefrontal cortex, which is responsible for cognition, personality expression, and rational decision-making, continues to develop well into the midtwenties. In the central nervous system, and particularly in the prefrontal cortex, dopamine levels must have a natural rise and fall for healthy rational thought processes (executive control) to develop. When methylphenidate is abused or used too frequently in rats, it can negatively impact this healthy cognitive development by keeping dopamine levels high. I have never used, nor do I plan to use, this smart drug.

Modafinil (Provigil)

The stimulant modafinil reduces fatigue and sleepiness. Its exact mechanism of action is not fully understood, but research suggests that, like methylphenidate, modafinil works by inhibiting dopamine reuptake, which keeps dopamine levels high. Research also suggests that this stimulates the hippocampus to release more of the neurotransmitter acetylcholine, leading to improved cognitive performance and memory.

Modafinil's risks are also similar to those of methylphenidate. Improper dosing or abuse of the drug may lead to the disrupted development of decision-making abilities and working memory in adolescents, warranting further research into modafinil's effects. Modafinil's effectiveness may also depend upon your IQ. Two university studies determined that in a test of attention span, modafinil improved cognitive performance only in the group with lower IQs.

While modafinil is safer than other stimulants because it has a milder effect on neurotransmitters, there are still risks associated with any kind of drug that affects dopamine. Keeping dopamine levels high can lead to addiction and, like the case of a pornography user who needs increasingly deviant porn to achieve the same results, can produce a resistance or reduced sensitivity to dopamine.

I keep a small emergency stash of modafinil in my pantry to call upon in the same way that a narcoleptic might use—to keep from falling asleep during a period of intense sleep deprivation, such as when I return home from an international flight at 3 a.m. and need to be at my children's school assembly at 8 a.m. But although I use it only one or two days out of every month, the energy it gives me does not feel natural, the potential for developing dopamine insensitivity concerns me, and I always have to make sure I get extra acetylcholine or choline from supplements and foods such as walnuts and eggs in order to avoid feeling very irritable when using this smart drug.

Amphetamines (Adderall)

Amphetamines are among the most powerful synthetic, stimulant-class smart drugs available and work by targeting dopamine, serotonin, and norepinephrine. These neurotransmitters are known as monoamines, and amphetamines block their uptake by clogging monoamine transporters. This leads to higher levels of monoamines in synapses, which causes the psychostimulant effects characteristic of drugs like Adderall.

Research has shown that amphetamines, even when used to treat neurological disorders like ADHD, can cause anorexia, weight loss, and insomnia. High doses can cause psychotic behavior, and even normal doses can produce symptoms of psychosis that range from short-term memory loss to visual and auditory hallucinations.

Ampakines (Alzheimer's drugs)

Ampakines are derived from the popular nootropic aniracetam, but they're chemically altered in a way that makes them act more like a smart drug. Their primary function is to bind to glutamate receptors. Glutamate is crucial for learning, memory, and synaptic plasticity (the adaptability of your neurons) and can bind with these glutamate receptors to enhance cognition. But when excess glutamate is produced and reacts with the receptors, the result can be excitotoxicity, cell death caused by toxic levels of excitatory amino acids. Research suggests that excitotoxicity plays a significant role in the development of neurodegenerative conditions like schizophrenia, delirium, and dementia.

Because ampakines bind to glutamate receptors, they block the uptake of glutamate and help prevent excitotoxicity, and research suggests that this minimizes the effects of conditions like Alzheimer's. But ampakines are now tightly regulated because if you exceed safe doses, you can cause neuronal damage from glutamate toxicity—the very neurodegeneration that ampakines are supposed to prevent!

Consumption of certain ampakines may also lead to a reduction in long-term synaptic depression (LTD), the process by which synapses are purposely weakened to avoid any plateaus in their efficiency. In other words, LTD gives your neurons and synapses a break so they can continue to develop and grow, and ampakines can keep this from occurring. Research suggests LTD is necessary for healthy synaptic plasticity, memory function, and motor skills. Granted, there is some debate about whether cognitive functions like motor skill acquisition actually depend on LTD, but if you were to take an excessively high dose of an ampakine, the overstimulation could suppress LTD and affect memory and motor skills.

L-deprenyl (Selegiline)

L-deprenyl, is used to treat patients newly diagnosed with Parkinson's, but it's also one of the darlings of the antiaging and smart drug communities. Monoamine oxidase inhibitors (MAOIs) like L-deprenyl are considered to be last-resort antidepressants and work by inhibiting the action of monoamine oxidase (MAO), an enzyme found in most tissues that promotes the oxidation and deactivation of monoamine neurotransmitters. Research suggests that MAO dysfunction is responsible for psychological and neurological disorders like Parkinson's, schizophrenia, ADHD, addiction, and depression. MAOIs help treat these conditions by lowering the elevated MAO levels.

Some research also suggests that L-deprenyl has some neurotrophic (neuron-stimulating) and neuroprotective effects in models of cerebral ischemia and stroke and, in rats, following traumatic brain injury. But it is critical to take the correct dose of L-deprenyl at the correct time. This is because when you take too much or take it too often, the drug loses its effectiveness. In fact, 40 mg per day provides no more benefit than 10 mg per day. Side effects are also a serious concern. L-deprenyl's potential side effects—especially at higher doses—include twitching and uncontrollable repetitive spasms in the tongue, lips, face, arms, and legs, blurred vision, chest pain, difficulty breathing, dizziness, irregular heartbeat, and irritability. In 17 percent of the cases in one study of the drug, the researchers had to stop treatment because of adverse side effects. I'm personally a bigger fan of several of the natural dopamine-modulating nootropics covered later in this chapter, including *Mucuna pruriens*, tryptophan, a good ole cup of coffee, and, yes, even nicotine.

Weighing the Risks and Benefits

Are you getting the impression that using synthetic stimulants to flood your brain with excess neurotransmitters may not be a good idea, especially when done frequently or in high doses?

Fact is, in small amounts, all these smart drugs can be relatively safe. But I am not convinced of their long-term safety or efficacy.

Sure, some are less risky than others, and these are increasing in popularity among biohackers and medical professionals. They are also popular among students, e-gamers, and athletes—among these groups, smart-drug doping is becoming more frequently banned. In academic settings and competitions, many of these compounds are now banned as performance-enhancing drugs. Yes, this means you could potentially get kicked off your university's chess club or debate team, or have your *Call of Duty* gaming title stripped if you're discovered to have modafinil in your system. But I would carefully consider the pros and cons of using any smart drugs as daily brain enhancers, especially in light of the safer alternatives you are about to discover: nootropics.

NOOTROPICS 101

So smart drugs are a modern, largely synthetic, and somewhat risky strategy for enhancing cognition. Proceed with caution. On the flip side, I would classify nootropics as the complete opposite: traditional herbs and extracts for cognitive enhancement, derived from ancestral practices and time-honored wisdom. Sure, it's possible to swallow too much St. John's wort or overdose on ginkgo and create the same neurotransmitter imbalances you could create with a synthetic smart drug, but it is far more difficult to harm your nervous system with a nootropic. And while you can get synthetic nootropics, even those are more natural and not as harmful as smart drugs because they don't alter neurotransmitters, cardiovascular function, or hormones quite as significantly.

Ayurvedic Nootropics

Traditional Indian and Chinese medical practitioners have tapped into the cognition-boosting effects of plants and herbs for at least five thousand years, since long before the first synthetic nootropic was created. Indian Ayurvedic medicine includes a group of nootropic plants called medhya rasayana, the four primary plants of which are mandukaparni, yashtimadhu, guduchi, and shankhpushpi. One of the most common supplements in Ayurvedic medicine is brahmi (otherwise known as bacopa, water hyssop, thyme-leaved gratiola, herb of grace, and Indian pennywort). Brahmi, which is most often called *bacopa*, is named after Lord Brahma, the creator god and originator of Ayurveda, and has been used for centuries to treat conditions ranging from pain and inflammation to epilepsy and memory dysfunction.

Bacopa's exact mechanism of action is not fully understood, but research suggests it promotes antioxidant activity and protects neurons in the prefrontal cortex, hippocampus, and corpus striatum against cytotoxicity (cell death) and DNA damage associated with Alzheimer's. These parts of the brain control several important functions: the prefrontal cortex is critical for rational, social, and personality behavior; the hippocampus is thought to be the seat of memory and the autonomic nervous system; and the striatum plays a role in the reward-associated release of pleasurable neurotransmitters such as dopamine. So the protective effects of bacopa help prevent the degeneration of many important cognitive faculties. An effective dose of bacopa ranges from 300 to 450 mg per day.

Ashwagandha, also called winter cherry, is another well-known Ayurvedic nootropic that can improve cognitive development, memory, and intelligence and reduce the effects of diseases like Parkinson's, Huntington's, and Alzheimer's. The optimal dose of winter cherry is 2 g three times a day, for a total of 6 g per day.

The lesser-known but highly effective aloeweed, one of four Ayurvedic herbs referred to as shankhpushpi, is also used to improve memory and intellect, as well as treat hypertension, epilepsy, and diabetes. Effective doses range from 20 to 40 g per day.

Celastrus paniculatus, also known as "intellect tree," is one of the more interesting Ayurvedic plants and one that I personally consume quite frequently as part of the supplement Qualia Mind. Traditionally, in India, *C. paniculatus* is taken in seed form, starting with ten seeds and working up to fifteen and finally twenty seeds. (On BoundlessBook.com/5, you'll find links to both whole seed and powdered seed forms.) But malkangni oil, derived from *C. paniculatus*, is also a good supplement. It can be used to enhance memory and intellectual capacity, improve dream recall, and induce lucid dreams. In one study performed on healthy rats, malkangni oil was shown to improve twenty-four-hour memory retention after a single dose, an effect accompanied by a reduction in monoamine neurotransmitters. This indicates a lower rate of loss of these neurotransmitters, which may help treat conditions like depression. In another study, malkangni oil administered for fourteen days reversed stress-induced spatial learning and memory impairment and restored working memory. In mice with memory deficits caused by the antinausea drug scopolamine, the oil has been shown to improve both spatial and fear memory (a type of conditioning through which an organism learns to avoid dangerous situations or events).

Traditional Chinese Nootropics

One of the most popular and well-known traditional Chinese nootropics is ginkgo, derived from the Chinese maidenhair tree. It is seen as a symbol of longevity and vitality, and research suggests that it can even stimulate the growth of new neurons. Research also suggests that ginkgo flavonoids, the main constituents of ginkgo extract, are potent antioxidants that have been shown to reduce the effects of Alzheimer's in mice as well as stabilize and improve the cognitive performance of Alzheimer's patients for six months to one year. Effective doses of ginkgo range from 120 to 240 mg taken one to four hours before a cognitively demanding task. To reduce age-related cognitive decline, consume 40 to 120 mg three times daily.

Another traditional Chinese brain-booster is danggui-shaoyao-san (DSS). Research suggests that DSS can induce angiogenesis (the growth of new blood vessels) and neurogenesis (the growth of new neurons), which makes it a potential treatment in ischemic stroke therapy. Research suggests that DSS also improves free radical–mediated neurological diseases such as Alzheimer's and Parkinson's, exhibits anti-inflammatory and antioxidant activities, and reduces cell death in the hippocampus. This promotes better moods, enhanced memory, and more balanced autonomic nervous system function. Currently, there is limited research on proper DSS dosing; for the most recent guidelines, visit BoundlessBook.com/5.

Vanillin

I absolutely love the musky, sweet smell and flavor of vanilla—but it's more than simply a flavor enhancer or perfume ingredient. Vanillin, the main component of vanilla (also found in ginger, allspice, capsaicin, and cloves), enhances cognition by boosting dopamine; brain-derived neurotrophic factor (BDNF), which supports the development of neurons; and a similar neuronal support factor, glial-derived neurotrophic factor (GLNF). Vanillin also has potent pain-killing and mood-supporting effects, and has been used traditionally as a treatment for inflammation, anxiety, and depression. The best way to prepare yourself a vanillin nootropic cocktail is to purchase organic vanilla bean powder and mix it into coffee or tea, or make your own vanilla extract: purchase organic vanilla beans (I prefer Madagascar vanilla beans, which have a rich and full flavor and aroma; avoid the tonka variety, as it can cause both liver damage and significant blood thinning), slice the beans in half, and soak them in vodka for four to six weeks to make your own vanilla tincture. This is far better than purchasing vanilla extract because most store-bought extracts contain artificial flavorings, corn syrup, and caramel color. Vanilla extract or powder is also a wonderful flavor addition to a cup of coffee.

Caffeine

Perhaps the most well-known and most widely used natural stimulant and neuroenhancer is—drumroll please—caffeine. Research suggests that caffeine can prevent memory deficits in experimental models of Alzheimer's and may even restore memory following impairment. In studies with college students, caffeine was shown to have particularly potent effects on memory improvement when consumed during students' nonoptimal time of day, early in the morning.

In nature, caffeine is never found in an isolated state, meaning that it is always found in a plant, such as tea leaves or coffee beans, that contains other compounds that enhance caffeine's effects, including cholesterols, polyphenols, and antioxidants. In fact, one study determined that caffeine alone does not account for the cognition-enhancing benefits of drinking coffee. Rather, the phytochemical content of coffee (which contains over a thousand different natural chemicals!) gives it potent antioxidant and anti-inflammatory properties that complement caffeine's neuroprotective effects on the central nervous system. Effective doses of caffeine range from 60 to 100 mg, which you can easily get from an 8-ounce cup o' joe.

A word of caution: Some people are slow caffeine oxidizers. These individuals carry copies of a gene called COMT that makes them more likely to produce high amounts of or have reduced turnover rates of a catecholamine class of neurotransmitters—which includes dopamine, epinephrine, and norepinephrine. For these individuals, a single cup o' joe can bestow some serious jitters, and multiple cups of caffeinated coffee are certainly not advised.

Nicotine

Although cigarettes have rightfully been vilified when it comes to health and longevity, nicotine itself—though best obtained some way other than sucking it through a cancer stick—has been shown to improve working memory. Research also suggests that oral consumption of nicotine improves memory consolidation during learning by increasing the density and efficiency of nicotinic acetylcholine receptors (nAChRs) in the cholinergic system, the part of the nervous system responsible for memory function. In addition, people suffering from cognitive deficits combined with a psychiatric condition (such as patients with schizophrenia) may enjoy even greater neuroprotection from nicotine consumption than healthy individuals.

Interestingly, nicotine's addictive potential and its cognition-enhancing benefits are inextricable: the processes are closely linked through the neurotransmitters they depend upon. Nicotine is addictive because it binds to nAChRs, which trigger the release of feel-good neurotransmitters like dopamine and glutamate, and your body responds by creating more nAChRs—and then you have to consume more and more nicotine to continue to feel its effects. When you attempt to quit, you experience withdrawal symptoms, and you have to smoke or consume some form of nicotine just to function normally.

But just as it plays a role in the action-reward cycle that creates nicotine addiction, dopamine also plays a role in enhancing a number of cognitive processes, such as working memory. It enhances cognition by acting on dopamine pathways and modulates addiction by acting on limbic pathways. These pathways are largely distinct—there may be some overlap, but not much—but nicotine stimulates strong dopaminergic activity in both.

Research has shown that while moderate doses of nicotine typically enhance cognition, high doses can inhibit cognitive performance. So when it comes to dosing nicotine, moderation and precision are key. Effective doses range from 2 to 4 mg administered over twenty to thirty minutes, a dose easily available in the form of nicotine gum or spray. Later in this chapter, I will fill you in on my own strategy for dosing and using nicotine.

One nifty trick I learned from my friend and health pioneer Paul Chek is that using a vaporizer in a nontraditional way can give you a dose of uplifting nicotine from organic tobacco and also provide a lung-based delivery for a host of compounds for either stimulation and relaxation, depending on the blend you pick.

For example, one pick-me-up blend I use in the Da Buddha vaporizer that sits on my desk combines organic tobacco, dried and ground green tea leaves, and a couple of drops of cinnamon oil or frankincense. For a more relaxing blend, I'll use an indica cannabis strain, dried and ground chamomile tea leaves, and a small sprinkling of lavender essential oil. It's fun to come up with your own recipes, but here are a few ideas to get your brain spinning:

- Peppermint leaves or oil, which improves blood circulation, raises alertness, and clears the lungs and respiratory passages

- Gotu kola leaves or extract, which sharpens memory and concentration

- Skullcap or hops, which act as mild sedatives and have a calming effect. (Skullcap is also good for headaches, which makes me wonder if that's why it's named that.)

- Wild oats, which reduce mental tension and anxiety

- Cloves, which reduce food cravings

- Primrose, which helps heal lung damage from smoking

- Chamomile, which acts as an antidepressant and promotes relaxation and sleep

- Ginger root, which is good for indigestion or stomach cramps, and makes a good digestif before meals

- Marijuana—indica strain for relaxation, sativa strain as a pick-me-up

Whatever you choose, be sure to select herbicide- and pesticide-free leaves and plants. I recommend the Da Buddha vaporizer because it offers a variety of temperature settings for the strains and blends that you choose.

Cannabidiol

Cannabidiol, or CBD, makes up about 40 percent of a cannabis plant. Unlike THC, the compound that produces psychoactive effects and is most often associated with the effects of marijuana, CBD contains potent medicinal properties that do not lead to a high or paranoia. Many forms of CBD are completely legal in most states and countries and are approved for use by most sports governing bodies. CBD has been shown to enhance focus, creativity, and mood and reduce general anxiety, social anxiety, chronic pain, stress, ADHD, insomnia, headaches, and inflammation.

Since CBD doesn't get you high and has far less addictive potential than THC, you can function quite well, reduce anxiety, maintain focus, and sleep better when consuming small daily amounts of CBD. But there is one caveat: CBD is not highly absorbable and needs to be blended with compounds such as curcuminoids or rendered more bioavailable for oral absorption. This means the most effective delivery mechanisms are vaping, a sublingual oil, or a capsule that has been blended with turmeric extracts. In addition, combining CBD and THC allows you to microdose marijuana for a mild cognitive edge without the lack of focus, increased appetite, or short-term memory loss associated with the high that THC tends to cause.

An effective dose of CBD begins at 10 mg. If you combine it with THC, blend it in a ratio of ten parts CBD to one part THC, or five parts CBD to one part THC (for example, 10 mg of CBD and 1 mg of THC). I recommend starting on the lower dosing end and slowly increasing the dose to find your optimal microdose. I have personally found 10 to 20 mg of CBD to help manage anxiety and stress and boost focus. Higher doses of between 30 and 40 mg can help you fall asleep more easily. In fact, I have taken doses as high as 100 mg before bed, slept like a baby, and woken up with no grogginess. CBD tolerances vary from individual to individual, and if you take it and notice nothing, I recommend you try more.

Traditional Nootropics from Around the World

Much to the chagrin of folks who argue that our ancestors would never have taken a supplement, especially one that affects cognition, the fact is many ancestral populations around the world have used nootropic plants for millennia.

For example, maca root has been used by indigenous Andean groups in South America for thousands of years. It is used to improve sexual function, memory, and learning as well as to reduce the effects of osteoporosis. Effective doses range from 1,500 to 3,000 mg.

Yerba mate is a tea made from a plant of the holly family (similar to mistletoe) and is consumed by many tribes across South America. It has been shown to improve cholesterol levels, protect the liver, and stimulate greater central nervous system activity. Effective doses range from 990 milliliters to 1.5 liters of tea per day.

Green tea is widely consumed in many cultures, especially in Asia, and is known to have potent health benefits due to its polyphenol content, especially the flavanols and flavonols. In cell cultures and animal studies, the polyphenols in green tea have prevented neurotoxin-induced cell injury. Green tea also has anti-inflammatory properties and, according to a study performed on mice, may delay age-related memory loss. It is safe to drink several cups of green tea per day, but it may be more efficient to take a green tea extract supplement to reach a daily dose of 400 to 500 mg of epigallocatechin gallate (EGCG), the primary active component of green tea.

Black ant extract is another fascinating nootropic. Powdered extract from the polyrhachis ant is an ancient Chinese tonic derived from ants that live up high in the mountains, often found among ginseng roots. This stuff has been named the "herb of kings," and for good reason: it contains a surprising amount of amino acids, vitamins, minerals, and antioxidants. In addition to containing high amounts of ATP, it also acts to modulate the immune system, build stress resistance, and even provide high amounts of ecdysterone, a growth hormone in insects that can have anabolic, muscle-building effects. Black ant extract is also extremely high in zinc, a mineral vital for muscle contractions, cellular growth and division, vision, the immune system, and libido. In my own personal experimentation with small amounts (½ to 1 teaspoon) of black ant extract, I've found it to be a perfect preworkout energy boost that also gives about four to five hours of focused energy and mental performance.

Then there's one of my favorites: lion's mane. Also known as the hedgehog mushroom, lion's mane is an edible fungus with a long history of use in traditional Chinese medicine. It is particularly rich in β-glucan polysaccharides, which are responsible for the neuroprotective and cognition-enhancing properties of this mushroom. Lion's mane increases nerve growth factor levels, which causes enhanced neuronal growth, neuron regeneration, and synaptic plasticity. It can also improve myelination, resulting in enhanced neuronal communication and nerve regeneration, improve memory, decrease neuronal excitability and excitotoxicity, protect neurons from inflammatory damage, and even reduce anxiety and stress. In clinical studies evaluating the effects of lion's mane on cognitive function, dosages from 750 mg up to as much as 5 g per day have been used.

Synthetic Nootropics

The realm of natural nootropics is accompanied by a family of synthetic nootropics not found in nature but synthesized in a laboratory, called racetams, which includes piracetam, aniracetam, oxiracetam, phenylpiracetam, and the anticonvulsant drugs levetiracetam and seletracetam. Most racetams act upon central nervous system receptors, neurotransmitters, the AMPA receptors responsible for fast synaptic transmission, and muscarinic receptors (interestingly, this is the same excitatory receptor that the fringe nootropic black ant extract acts upon).

Piracetam, one of the more popular racetams, directly enhances learning, memory, and attention, and it can, with no observed adverse side effects, restore cognitive performance in patients who have suffered cranial trauma, inflammation, strokes, and ischemic complications (loss of blood flow to a region) following coronary bypass surgery. It can also improve symptoms of delirium and reduce depression and anxiety. In adults, the standard dose of piracetam ranges from 1,200 to 4,800 mg divided into three smaller doses throughout the day.

Aniracetam has been shown to protect cells from the effects of glutamate excitotoxicity, resulting in an overall neuroprotective effect. While you may not be shoveling mouthfuls of glutamate down your hatch or eating cartons of MSG-laden Chinese food each night, aniracetam can help protect your brain from inflammation caused by other central nervous system irritants, such as herbicides, pesticides, and rancid oils. Effective doses of aniracetam range from a single 400 mg dose to two doses of 500 to 750 mg per day, taken with meals.

The following are some other popular synthetic nootropics.

NOOPEPT

The neuroprotector noopept can improve memory and attention and reduce depression and anxiety. Noopept acts similarly to racetams to improve overall brain function. Effective doses range from 10 to 30 mg per day.

PHENYLETHYLAMINE

Phenylethylamine can improve mood and increase attention and concentration. Known as the "love drug," it has also been shown to heighten feelings of arousal, excitement, and euphoria. There is little research that indicates an effective dose, but recommendations range from 300 to 1,000 mg per day.

URIDINE MONOPHOSPHATE

Uridine monophosphate enhances learning, memory, and overall cognitive function. Effective doses range from 500 to 1,000 mg per day.

PHOSPHATIDYLSERINE

Phosphatidylserine naturally occurs in high concentrations in the brain and has been shown to reduce stress, cortisol levels, and physical fatigue; improve ADHD and forgetfulness; and increase mental processing and memory. An effective dose is 100 mg taken three times daily, but anything over that may lead to adverse side effects such as insomnia.

HORDENINE HCL

Hordenine HCl occurs in high amounts in plants, such as barley grass, and is known to help burn fat and improve metabolism, and increase energy, alertness, and concentration. There is insufficient evidence to make any claim about dosage, but most supplements contain 30 mg to be taken two or three times daily.

VINPOCETINE

Vinpocetine protects the brain against toxins, increases blood flow to the brain, lowers inflammation, reduces fatigue, and increases attention, memory, and alertness. Effective doses range from 15 to 60 mg per day, best split up into separate dosages and taken three times per day, preferably with meals.

METHYLENE BLUE

More commonly known as "fish tank cleaner," methylene blue can be a potent mitochondria booster and cognitive enhancer—assuming you take a high-quality supplement free of common impurities like arsenic, aluminum, cadmium, mercury, and lead. But, quite inexpensively, you can purchase a relatively safe and proven cognition-enhancing form (albeit one that will turn your mouth Smurf blue for hours and sometimes irreversibly stain anything that it comes into contact with).

Methylene blue has been used to treat Alzheimer's, Huntington's, Parkinson's, and dementia, to prevent amyloid plaque buildup in the brain, and to restore mitochondrial function. In one clinical trial, methylene blue improved attention span, short-term memory, and memory retrieval from long-term memory. It has also been shown to increase memory consolidation (a process that maintains, stabilizes, and strengthens memories stored in the long-term memory) and even to have neuroprotective effects against brain inflammation and glutamate-induced excitotoxicity.

Effective doses range from 1 to 4 mg per kilogram of body weight, but more is not better, since excess use can lead to high levels of free radicals, oxidation, and inflammation. I personally use a low dose of methylene blue—80 micrograms—one to two times per week.

Understanding when and how to use these synthetic nootropics can be confusing. I recommend sticking to the research-backed stacks and supplements described later in this chapter, which intelligently and elegantly combine many of these nootropics in the proper amounts and ratios.

HOW TO ENHANCE THE EFFECTS OF NOOTROPICS AND SMART DRUGS

Certain compounds can enhance the effects of nootropics, smart drugs, and psychedelics (addressed later in this chapter) and even prevent the crash so often associated with such brain-boosters. These compounds, specifically the following six, work primarily by providing you with molecules and nutrients that can quickly become depleted as your brain works harder and faster. When you intelligently combine your nootropics, smart drugs, and psychedelics with choline donors, amino acids, adaptogens, neurovitamins, neurominerals, anti-inflammatories, antioxidants, and peptides, you can prevent many of the deficiencies, jittery side effects, and crashes that tend to arise with high, frequent doses of brain-boosters, as well as enhance and prolong the effects of your supplementation protocol.

1. Choline Donors

Choline is essential for brain development, detoxification, metabolism, muscle movement, digestion, and liver and gallbladder function. Choline donors work through different pathways in the nervous system to ensure your brain and body get adequate amounts of choline. When you are deficient in choline, you are more likely to crash after using a brain-booster, and the brain-booster itself may not work as efficiently. The following are the most potent choline donors.

CENTROPHENOXINE

Centrophenoxine protects the brain, enhances and improves working memory, and has antiaging and antioxidant effects. Effective doses range from one to three doses of 250 mg per day, but elderly individuals may respond better to three to six doses per day.

CITICOLINE

Citicoline combines choline and cytidine to reduce memory impairment, cognitive decline, and brain damage, and to improve learning and attention. Effective doses range from 1 to 2 g per day.

ALPHA GPC

Alpha GPC prevents cognitive decline, protects the brain, reduces inflammation, and increases attention span, memory, and growth hormone production (which may also slow down the effects of aging and help you lose weight). An effective dose is 400 mg three times per day.

2. Amino Acids

Amino acids are precursors to neurotransmitters and perform many physiological functions, such as repairing tissues, providing energy, improving mental and physical performance, and helping to grow or maintain muscle. The specific amino acids listed below are especially beneficial for the brain.

ACETYL-L-CARNITINE

Acetyl-L-carnitine can easily cross the blood-brain barrier and enhances cognitive processes such as memory, learning, and focus. It also improves brain-energy metabolism, reduces fatigue, and has potent antiaging and brain-protecting effects, and it can induce the production of more mitochondria, which increases energy production. Effective doses range from 500 to 1,500 mg per day.

N-ACETYL-TYROSINE

N-acetyl-tyrosine improves focus, motivation, memory, learning, and mood. Effective doses range from 500 to 2,000 mg per day.

Some research indicates that the effectiveness of tyrosine supplementation depends on proper neurotransmitter synthesis and function. This means your response to tyrosine may depend on the health of your neurotransmitters. (To get a sense of your own neurotransmitter status and how you can improve it, revisit chapter 1).

TAURINE

Taurine acts as an antioxidant and can improve memory, reduce anxiety, and promote sleep and relaxation. Effective doses range from 500 to 2,000 mg, although doses as high as 3,000 mg can be taken with little risk of adverse effects.

L-THEANINE

L-theanine is also an antioxidant with neuroprotective properties. It can improve mood, focus, and memory, reduce anxiety, and promote sleep and relaxation. Effective doses range from 100 to 200 mg daily. I have personally found that 400 mg in a cup of coffee can significantly reduce caffeine's side effects, such as excessive wakefulness or the jitters.

DL-PHENYLALANINE

DL-phenylalanine is a combination of two forms of the essential amino acid phenylalanine—the "D" form and the "L" form—and can easily cross the blood-brain barrier. DL-phenylalanine enhances mental alertness, mood, memory, and learning and reduces pain and depression. Effective doses range from 1 to 5 g per day.

As a word of caution, some people may not be able to handle phenylalanine due to a condition called phenylketonuria (PKU). PKU is a genetic disorder characterized by a deficiency of phenylalanine hydroxylase, the enzyme that breaks down phenylalanine. When excess phenylalanine accumulates, it can lead to growth failure, microcephaly (an abnormally small head, often due to poor brain development), seizures, developmental delay, severe intellectual impairment, and, in mild cases, a musty odor in the breath, skin rashes, hyperactivity, and anxiety.

There are less severe forms, such as variant PKU and non-PKU hyperphenylalaninemia, that are associated with a smaller risk of brain damage, and people with very mild cases of PKU may not even require treatment as long as they consume a low-phenylalanine diet. PKU can be easily detected with a simple blood test, and all states in the United States require a PKU test for every newborn—so if you live in the United States, you likely already know whether or not you have it.

ESSENTIAL AMINO ACIDS (EAAS)

The essential amino acids—histidine, isoleucine, leucine, lysine, methionine, phenylalanine, threonine, tryptophan, and valine—are essential because your body can't produce them on its own; you must consume them via diet or supplements. A balanced supply of EAAs is necessary for optimal brain function, and while there is limited information on the precise mechanisms by which different EAAs benefit cognition, research suggests that amino acids such as histidine and tryptophan are necessary for neurotransmitter function and neuronal signaling.

Rather than taking all of the amino acids listed above, you can try my shotgun approach, which is to take a blend of EAAs mixed in a precise ratio to make them as effective as possible. This is actually the exact ratio in the Kion Aminos blend that I personally formulate, which you can find at GetKion.com.

Bear in mind that you can overdose on EAAs: when dietary amino acid intake becomes too high, toxicities can arise. One of the by-products of both protein and amino acid metabolism is nitrogen, so if you consume too much protein, your body can enter a state of excessively positive nitrogen balance. When you have too much nitrogen in your body, ammonia accumulates, and ammonia accumulation can lead to neurotoxicity in the brain.

The recommended daily intake of protein for the average individual is 0.36 g per pound of body weight per day. This will maintain nitrogen balance for most healthy, not-super-active people. For hard-charging athletes, research suggests that there is not much benefit in exceeding 0.55 g per pound of body weight per day if you want to maintain nitrogen balance. For example, I weigh 175 pounds, so to maintain nitrogen balance, I would need to consume no more than 96.25 g of protein per day.

If you want to purposely exceed nitrogen balance, which can be an effective strategy to more rapidly gain muscle mass, research suggests that you don't need to eat more than 0.8 g of protein per pound of body weight per day. So if I wanted to put on muscle without causing excess nitrogen and ammonia accumulation to the point of toxicity, I could consume 140 g of protein per day. My personal EAA regimen is to consume 10 to 20 g per day via Kion Aminos, and twice that if I am injured or have a hard day of training. This reduces my muscle-building dietary protein intake to 100 to 130 g per day.

3. Neurovitamins

Many vitamins can enhance brain regulation and developmental processes and prevent damage to neurons. The following are the best vitamins to enhance any nootropic or smart drug you use.

VITAMIN B_1

Also known as thiamine, vitamin B_1 is best taken in the fat-soluble form benfotiamine, which increases energy, mood, and alertness and reduces pain and advanced glycation end products (compounds that accelerate brain degeneration). Research suggests that, since high doses of vitamin B_1 usually result in large amounts of unabsorbed B_1 being excreted, doses of 30 mg per day are sufficient. As a word of caution, alcohol can inhibit efficient absorption of vitamin B_1, so if you want the full benefits of vitamin B_1, limit or avoid alcohol on days you take vitamin B_1.

VITAMIN B_3

Vitamin B_3, when consumed in the form niacinamide, can reduce inflammation, anxiety, and age-related cognitive impairment. An effective dose is 15 mg per day, but people suffering from trauma, hypoxia, stress, or genetic mutations can benefit from higher doses. (For more details on a powerful antiaging form of vitamin B_3 called nicotinamide riboside, see page 532.)

VITAMIN B_5

Vitamin B_5's water-soluble form calcium pantothenate improves concentration, memory, and learning and reduces brain fog. Effective doses range from 500 to 1,000 mg per day.

VITAMIN B$_6$

When taken in the highly bioactive form pyridoxal-5-phosphate, vitamin B$_6$ increases mental and physical energy, prevents neuronal damage, and plays a role in memory formation, focus, motivation, and mood and sleep regulation. Effective doses are 1.5 mg per day for healthy women and 2 mg per day for healthy men, although women who are pregnant or lactating may need to take up to 2 mg.

VITAMIN B$_{12}$

When taken in the form methylcobalamin, vitamin B$_{12}$ can improve mood, memory, focus, and energy, and reduce anxiety, pain, and cognitive decline. Effective doses range from 1 to 2 mg per day.

VITAMIN C

Vitamin C in the form of ascorbic acid has antioxidant and neuroprotective effects, reduces fatigue, and improves mood and blood flow. Effective doses range from 90 to 150 mg per day.

VITAMIN D$_3$

When taken in the highly absorbable form called microencapsulated cholecalciferol, vitamin D$_3$ has powerful antioxidant and anti-inflammatory effects and delays brain degeneration and cognitive decline. Effective doses range from 1,500 to 2,000 IU per day.

Interestingly, many people have genetic factors, such as high pigmentation or interference with the conversion of cholesterol to vitamin D in response to sunlight, that prevent them from properly synthesizing vitamin D from sun exposure. A salivary genetic test such as the one offered by 23andMe is not enough to assess your genetic status for vitamin D production, so for deeper genetic insights, I recommend a more advanced salivary genetic panel, such as the Youtrients test at the DNA Company in Ontario, Canada (you'll find a link on BoundlessBook.com/5).

4. Adaptogens

Adaptogens are plant extracts that protect your body and brain from the effects of excess stress. A veritable Swiss army knife for your physiology, they have been shown to support neurogenesis, hormone production, and adrenal and HPA axis regulation, regulate cellular energy homeostasis, regenerate tissue, and improve learning and memory.

MUCUNA PRURIENS

Mucuna pruriens enhances mood, reduces anxiety and stress, protects the brain, stimulates sex drive, and increases focus and motivation. Effective doses range from 12.5 to 17.5 mg per kilogram of body weight per day.

COLEUS FORSKOHLII

Coleus forskohlii improves learning, memory, and mental stamina and reduces fatigue and inflammation. Effective doses are about 7.5 g per day for healthy women and about 9 g for healthy men.

RHODIOLA ROSEA (RHODIOLA)

Rhodiola improves mood, motivation, memory, and concentration and reduces fatigue and oxidative stress. Research suggests that daily rhodiola use as low as 50 mg can reduce fatigue, while safe neural enhancement occurs at 1,500 mg per day.

ACTIVAMP

ActivAMP, derived from *Gynostemma pentaphyllum*, is a form of ginseng root with antiaging and anti-inflammatory effects. It also improves memory and resistance to stress. Effective doses range from 100 to 500 mg per day.

5. Neurominerals

Neurominerals, like neurovitamins, are highly absorbable and can cross the blood-brain barrier to improve cognition. They are necessary for a host of physiological processes and, when combined, enhance each other's effects.

LITHIUM OROTATE

The neuroprotector lithium orotate preserves cognitive function, improves mood, and detoxifies the brain. Effective doses range from 5 to 150 mg per day.

MAGNESIUM THREONATE

Magnesium threonate is a more bioavailable form of magnesium. It improves learning, memory, sleep quality, and mood and reduces anxiety and the effects of neuropathic pain (pain caused by nerve damage). Research suggests that high doses around 600 mg per kilogram of body weight are effective.

ZINC PICOLINATE

Zinc picolinate, a more bioavailable form of zinc, is a powerful antioxidant, anti-inflammatory, and immune-system-boosting mineral that also helps improve memory, mood, and neuronal growth. Research suggests that the current recommended intake of zinc—8 to 14 mg per day—is effective at maintaining homeostasis. Mild zinc deficiency can be treated with two to three times this amount, and moderate to severe deficiency with four to five times this amount.

6. Anti-inflammatories and Antioxidants

These compounds specifically address oxidative stress and inflammation in the brain. They also support the transport and utilization of nutrients and regulate nervous system stimulation, hormonal secretion, and cholesterol levels. The best anti-inflammatories and antioxidants for the brain also tend to support mitochondrial health and cellular longevity (as will be discussed in more detail in chapter 19).

PQQ

PQQ reduces neurodegeneration and cognitive decline, promotes neuronal growth and survival, and improves sleep, energy, memory, and stress response. PQQ also has potent mitochondrial and antiaging properties (I'll talk more about that in chapter 19). An effective dose is 0.3 mg per day.

QUERCETIN

Quercetin, found in fruits and vegetables, can delay cognitive decline, protect neurons from toxins, regulate estrogen and androgen, and reduce inflammation. As a natural antihistamine, it's also been shown to stabilize mast cells (the immune cells that release histamines). Effective doses range from 50 to 150 mg per kilogram of body weight per day.

CURCUMIN

Curcumin is the active component of the spice turmeric. It possesses powerful anti-inflammatory and neuroprotective effects and can improve memory and mood, reduce oxidative stress and chronic pain, and delay aging. An effective dose is up to 8 g per day. Curcumin can be made far more absorbable by blending it with oils such as coconut oil or combining it with black pepper or the black pepper extract called piperine.

DHA

DHA is the omega-3 fatty acid most abundant in your brain. It has been shown to improve memory, learning, and mood and reduce oxidative stress, inflammation, and telomere shortening (a chromosomal indication of how fast you are aging). Effective doses range from 500 to 1,000 mg daily.

GREEN TEA EXTRACT

Green tea extract enhances learning abilities, memory, and blood flow, delays aging, and may reduce anxiety and chronic fatigue. When green tea extract is paired with quercetin and L-theanine, the cognitive effects become synergistic, meaning they enhance each other to produce a greater effect. Effective doses range from 50 to 500 mg per day, although higher doses have been associated with side effects like nausea.

BIOPERINE

Bioperine is derived from the black pepper extract piperine. It increases the absorption of other nutrients, has anti-inflammatory effects (especially when combined with curcumin), and increases motivation, focus, productivity, and reasoning skills, while stabilizing mood. An effective dose is 20 mg per day.

7. Peptides

No discussion of cognitive enhancement would be complete without addressing peptides, which are amino acid sequences designed to elicit certain effects—including slowed aging, fat loss, muscle gain, sexual enhancement, and better brain function—with laser-like specificity.

The peptide Semax is one of my favorite nootropic-like peptides. It was originally created in Russia during the 1980s with the express intention of improving cognitive function. In addition to stimulating the central nervous system, it works to modulate receptor sensitivity for a variety of neurotransmitters and brain chemicals, including acetylcholine, dopamine, serotonin, adenosine, and histamine.

In Russia, Semax is used as to prevent and treat circulatory disorders, including stroke. It is also used as a nootropic, specifically to enhance memory and control the negative effects of stress on cognitive function. It has been shown to protect the body and brain from various types of oxidative damage, and can enhance neurogenesis by increasing levels of BDNF.

Like most peptides, Semax is so potent that only small doses are needed to achieve the desired results. For most people, 0.5 to 1.0 mg per day is plenty. Because most peptides are very poorly absorbed when taken orally, Semax is usually taken as a nasal spray or subcutaneous injection. I have found that Semax combines quite well with the racetam family of nootropics (see page 95), and, in my own experience, a Semax-racetam or Semax-Qualia combo can give a good four to five hours of focused cognitive performance and focus without deleteriously affecting sleep or causing any type of anxiety or jitters.

For an even bigger boost in brain function, Semax works quite well when combined with the peptides Dihexa, Pinealon, and Cortagen (warning: you'll be awake and highly efficient for at least eight hours after using this peptide stack). It should be noted that many peptides, including Semax, are currently not approved by the FDA. This doesn't mean they're illegal to consume, but rather that they cannot be legally sold or advertised as "for human consumption." However, many physicians can and do prescribe this and other peptides, and I recommend visiting the International Peptide Society at PeptideSociety.org to find a physician who can work with you on an appropriate peptide protocol for your specific needs.

Peptides are best secured from a functional or integrative medicine physician who uses a good compounding pharmacy such as Tailor Made Compounding, although PeptideSciences.com offers relatively pure peptides and is the preferred source for many people who want to use peptides but can't get them from a doctor.

THE BEST BRAIN-BOOSTING STACKS

There are over a thousand websites and hundreds of reference guides chock-full of complicated methods for combining the compounds described in this chapter. There is a reason for this: as you have probably guessed by now, stacking nootropics can be far more effective than consuming a single, lonely nootropic in isolation. For example, adding choline or L-theanine to your morning coffee can make your brain feel fresh for hours. Mixing curcumin with black pepper can dramatically amp up the neural anti-inflammatory effects of both. And ultimately, a teaspoon of lion's mane mushroom extract just isn't as titillating as lion's mane blended with caffeine, L-theanine, nicotine, a touch of vinpocetine, and—for the brave soul—a tiny bit of psilocybin.

Take piracetam as another example. Piracetam has been shown to improve cell membrane function and act as a neuroprotector. When combined with other membrane stabilizers like choline and DHA, piracetam can improve and maintain efficient neuronal signaling, which improves cognition and reduces the risk of a crash after taking nootropics.

The supplement world is saturated with brain-boosting blends. It can be difficult to cut through the confusion and figure out what works and what could be a waste of time and money—or downright dangerous. So as you create your own stack, you must carefully think about your specific needs and goals.

If you want to reduce anxiety and depression but don't necessarily care to enhance your cognitive performance and don't need to get through a day of sleep deprivation, you could stick to a single nootropic that increases dopamine levels, such as *Mucuna pruriens* or tryptophan. If you want to reduce anxiety and depression while simultaneously improving your memory because you are studying for an exam, you could add bacopa to the *Mucuna* or tryptophan. Let's say you want to add long-term, lasting cognitive performance to the mix: in this case, you would add a racetam and, to avoid a crash, a touch of choline or DHA. It's a bit like creating a recipe, isn't it?

But if experimentation and using your noggin as an N=1 isn't your thing, I am going to spill the beans on the best stacks and done-for-you supplement blends I have personally used, the tried-and-true mixes that combine ultimate efficacy and safety with no nasty crashes or jitters.

1. Caffeine and Nicotine

Coffee and cigarettes have long been a popular combination. Think back to the 1950s image of a man in a tailored suit perfectly pairing his black brew with a cigarette hanging out the corner of his mouth as he enjoys the Sunday paper. Heck, there is even an Otis Redding song called "Cigarettes and Coffee" and a movie called *Coffee and Cigarettes,* which features Bill Murray, Tom Waits, Steve Buscemi, and Cate Blanchett partaking in their fair share of smoking and sipping.

Aside from the obvious pleasure some derive from this traditional combo, are there any benefits to simultaneously smoking and drinking coffee? One study in the *Journal of Epidemiology and Community Health* concluded that coffee may indeed provide protection against some of the damaging effects of cigarettes. In the study, researchers analyzed 497 men and women with confirmed cases of papilloma, carcinoma, and polyps of the bladder. All study participants, along with 1,113 control cases, were interviewed to determine their use of tobacco, exposure to secondhand smoke, and coffee consumption.

Turns out, when compared to smokers who regularly consumed coffee, smokers who didn't drink coffee had twice as much of the cell damage associated with tobacco use. In addition, the smokers who didn't consume coffee were up to seven times more likely to have these growths as nonsmokers. Regular smokers who drank coffee less than twice a week had double the chances of developing cancer than those who drank coffee more frequently. So ultimately, coffee-drinking cigarette-puffers have some health advantage over their smoking counterparts who don't drink coffee.

Of course, the antioxidant content of coffee may not be the only smoking savior. And no, it is not the tobacco and nasty chemicals in a cigarette that work the magic: as other studies have proved, it is nicotine. Nicotine is pretty powerful stuff, not only enhancing locomotive performance (ability to move with greater control and precision) and cognitive performance when combined with coffee but also ramping up exercise performance by 18 percent to 21 percent all on its own!

How do I pull off this stack? I suck on 1 mg nicotine toothpicks as I down a cup of coffee (the cinnamon flavor of the toothpicks blends quite nicely with a cup o' joe). I also keep a dispenser of 1.5 mg nicotine mints in my office. And, while I am not a fan of the artificial sweeteners they contain, I also keep a small stash of 2 mg nicotine gum in my fanny pack.

Of course, nicotine can be addictive. I recommend limiting yourself to no more than one or two toothpicks, or one or two mints or pieces of gum, per day, and only using them on more cognitively demanding days or, since nicotine is also a performance enhancer, prior to a workout. To enhance physical performance, consume 100 mg or more of caffeine and 2.5 mg or more of nicotine.

2. Caffeine and L-Theanine

Most people, especially slow caffeine oxidizers, find that they can eliminate the negative side effects of caffeine (such as jitteriness and headaches) by adding L-theanine to their caffeine source of choice. Research suggests that caffeine and L-theanine together can boost concentration, focus, and energy while reducing anxiety.

For this stack, use a ratio of four parts L-theanine to one part caffeine—for example, 400 mg of L-theanine with 100 mg of caffeine. You may want to start with a smaller dose, such as 200 mg of L-theanine and 50 mg of caffeine, then work your way up to find the best dose for you. (As a reference point, an 8-ounce cup of coffee has about 100 mg of caffeine.)

The beauty of this stack is that nature has already given us a perfectly packaged combination of caffeine and L-theanine in green tea, whether in the form of a cup of green tea, a bowl of matcha tea, or even a green tea extract supplement (green tea has less caffeine than coffee—about 25 mg per 8-ounce cup). Caffeine and L-theanine make a particularly convenient combination during those times when you don't want the excess stimulation of caffeine in isolation, such as a late-evening dinner or the latter stages of a workday, when a cup of coffee by itself might keep you awake too late into the night.

3. Caffeine, Tulsi, and Astragalus

Tulsi is one of the greatest calming adaptogens that exists, trusted and revered for centuries in Ayurvedic medicine and culture. Research suggests that tulsi can improve mood, support digestion, and promote stable energy levels. Because it is also an anxiolytic (meaning it reduces anxiety), tulsi, like L-theanine, helps reduce caffeine's overstimulating effects.

You can also blend tulsi with *Astragalus propinquus* (astragalus), which, in Chinese medicine, is a boundlessly invigorating herb that provides a stable source of energy. Astragalus contains an enormous variety of saponins, flavonoids, and polysaccharides and, when paired with antioxidant-rich coffee and tulsi, creates a match made in longevity heaven. For this blend, which I often make if drinking coffee in the afternoon, I am a fan of the Four Sigmatic Adaptogen Coffee, which contains coffee, astragalus, tulsi, and cinnamon.

4. Ginkgo, Bacopa, and Lion's Mane

This unique stack boosts mental focus, memory, learning, and cognitive performance while reducing anxiety and depression. I have found that it can significantly boost mental alertness for around six hours at a time without any jitteriness or irritability. It is important to allow a grace period of about twelve weeks of daily supplementation before you feel the stack's full potential, so don't expect immediate results.

A typical dose for this combination is 500 mg of lion's mane per day, 240 mg of ginkgo per day, and 100 mg of bacopa *twice* per day. Consider buying each ingredient in bulk to have enough to experiment with. If you do not experience positive results after twelve weeks, try adjusting the dose in small increments. For example, you can start by increasing your bacopa intake to 150 mg twice per day for a couple weeks. Just be patient: the result is worth the trial and error. Small amounts (between 100 and 200 mg) of the psychedelic psilocybin can enhance this stack.

5. Artichoke and Forskolin

Research suggests that artichoke extract supplements (made from the leaves of artichokes) possess potent antioxidant properties and reduce levels of blood-vessel-damaging cholesterol particles. Forskolin, derived from *Coleus forskohlii,* is one of the few compounds known to naturally boost cAMP (cyclic adenosine monophosphate), which reduces brain inflammation and strengthens the blood-brain barrier, and improve neural signaling in your brain.

I have experienced enhanced memory and word recall when consuming this stack. Tim Ferriss talked about it quite a bit in my podcast with him, specifically referencing its presence in the supplement CILTEP. Made primarily from artichoke extract and forskolin, CILTEP also contains vitamin B6, L-phenylalanine, and acetyl-L-carnitine. It is recommended that you take two to three capsules at the beginning of each day and to skip dosing one or two days per week to achieve optimal results.

6. Alpha GPC, AC-11, Bacopa, and Huperzine

This combination is found in the supplement Alpha BRAIN, created by my friend Aubrey Marcus at the company Onnit. According to a clinical trial conducted by the Boston Center for Memory, Alpha BRAIN has been shown to increase cognitive performance for healthy individuals and can potentially boost memory and learning capacity.

Alpha GPC has several benefits. It provides choline (which increases production of the neurotransmitter acetylcholine) and appears to support cellular membranes and reduce cognitive decline. AC-11 is derived from the rainforest herb *Uncaria tomentosa,* and research suggests that it may be able to help slow the development of cancer due to its DNA-repairing antioxidant properties. Bacopa is known to enhance memory and aid in treating dementia, Parkinson's, and epilepsy. Huperzine is derived from the Chinese club moss *Huperzia serrata.* Research suggests that it improves neurotransmitter levels and may also improve memory and protect neurons, making it a potential treatment for Alzheimer's and related conditions.

As a word of caution, a recent review of the scientific literature found that the quality of the evidence supporting the use of huperzine is low, so there is still debate over this particular nootropic. If you take a cholinesterase inhibitor like donepezil (Aricept), rivastigmine (Exelon), or galantamine (Razadyne)—which are all used to prevent or manage Alzheimer's—the Alzheimer's Association officially recommends not taking huperzine.

This stack seems to work best if you take it daily for about two weeks. After that, effects become more pronounced over time, so, as with the ginkgo, bacopa, and lion's mane stack, you need to let this blend build up in your system before you judge its overall effectiveness.

7. TianChi Chinese Adaptogenic Herb Complex

The list of herbs and ingredients in the supplement TianChi is far too long to include here, but it contains nearly every Chinese adaptogen and natural nootropic described in this chapter. So when it comes to a nonsynthetic approach to mental enhancement, this blend tops the list. All the herbs in TianChi are gathered from their native, wild environments or are organically grown, non-GMO, kosher certified, non-irradiated, and pesticide-free, then formulated in small batches by a Chinese herbal medicine practitioner in Oregon. The herbs are extracted in purified water and test free of heavy metals.

Most adaptogens in today's market are a standardized 5:1 extract, meaning that it takes five pounds of herbs to make one pound of extract. This is not always effective because some herbs may have to be extracted at a 10:1 ratio to actually be strong enough to be efficacious. The adaptogens in TianChi are extracted at a 45:1 ratio, making this one of the most potent blends available.

Strangely enough, I have found the brain-boosting effects of TianChi to be even more enhanced when consumed with beet juice or beet powder, probably due to beets' vasodilating effect. This is one of my favorite blends to mix up midmorning or midafternoon on an empty stomach for a clear-headed cognitive high. If you are trying to avoid anything even remotely synthetic, this is a good choice for you.

8. Qualia

Like TianChi, the nootropic blend Qualia is a shotgun approach, providing over forty-two different ingredients, including all the adaptogens, neurovitamins, amino acids, choline donors, anti-inflammatories, and antioxidants described in this chapter. Unlike TianChi, it also contains the synthetic nootropic noopept (which is about a thousand times more potent than piracetam) and a few other helpful ingredients, including curcumin, piperine, and caffeine. Qualia requires two daily dosing protocols: take the first dose on an empty stomach and the second with a meal.

For those who prefer to avoid any synthetic nootropics, get most of the natural compounds at a slightly lower price point (Qualia is admittedly quite expensive at $150), and get the benefits of the Indian plant *Celastrus paniculatus*, the manufacturer of Qualia, Neurohacker Collective, makes another supplement called Qualia Mind. For both ease of use and subjective efficacy, I prefer Qualia Mind.

Feeling overwhelmed? It is not as complex as you might think. At the end of this chapter, I will reveal what my weekly supplement schedule looks like. But first, I would be remiss not to mention the latest darlings of the mind-enhancing industry: psychedelics.

MICRODOSING PSYCHEDELICS

We are entering a new golden age of psychedelics. Microdosing with LSD, psilocybin, ketamine, and other compounds previously placed in the realm of party animals and rave enthusiasts is now commonplace for CEOs, Navy SEALs, and famous authors.

I am not going to focus on the ego-dissolving, trip-inducing effects of psychedelics, so if you are interested in learning more about that, I recommend reading *How to Change Your Mind*, by Michael Pollan. I will instead focus on microdosing, which involves ingesting tiny amounts of psychedelics to induce a noticeable and overall positive physical and mental effect.

My own experience with psychedelics has spanned several years of relatively high psilocybin and DMT doses for self-discovery once a quarter, weekly LSD microdoses for creativity and productivity (I take larger doses if I am both sleep-deprived and in need of hefty creative output), weekly or monthly psilocybin microdoses during holotropic breathwork sessions or hikes, ketamine microdoses during massages and sex, and ibogaine microdoses for a pre-workout or pre-sex boost.

When you take a microdose of a psychedelic, it is typically referred to as a subperceptual dose. Subperceptual doses do not have a significant impact on your ability to function normally, but the effects will be present in your mood and behavior. The lowest dose of a particular psychedelic that will produce a hallucinogenic effect is known as the threshold dose; since the goal is not to get a hallucinogenic effect, a microdose can be well below a psychedelic's threshold dose.

By integrating the correct doses of psychedelics into your weekly routine, you can achieve greater creativity, more energy, improved mood, increased focus, and better relational skills. There is a growing body of research that suggests that microdosing can improve depression, anxiety, PTSD, and emotional imbalance, help with alcohol and tobacco addiction, and mitigate ADD and ADHD behaviors.

Microdosing with Psilocybin

Psilocybin is naturally produced by more than two hundred species of fungi, otherwise known as "magic mushrooms." Research from archaeological evidence suggests that humans have used psilocybin mushrooms for over seven thousand years. I have personally found microdoses of psilocybin to be best for nature immersions, hiking, journaling, and self-discovery.

Psilocybin primarily interacts with the serotonin receptors in the brain and has been used in therapeutic settings to treat headaches, anxiety, depression, addiction, and obsessive-compulsive disorder. There is limited data to show any adverse drug interactions with the use of psilocybin,

Where to Buy Psychedelics

There are a variety of websites that sell psychedelics, but not all sources contain good-quality ingredients, nor is there any guarantee that the substance you purchase is not laced with undesirable compounds.

I have personally found the following three resources to be quite helpful when purchasing psychedelics or finding a quality source:

- The Third Wave (thethirdwave.co): This website offers a host of valuable information and downloadable pdfs on dosing, sourcing, safety, and techniques—and even an entire instructional course on microdosing.

- Reddit (reddit.com/r/psychedelics): Reddit contains many helpful personal anecdotes that are voted up or down by other users, and although it is rife with N=1 stories that may not apply to your specific situation, I've found it to be a helpful resource for discovering what DIY biohackers and psychedelic users are experimenting with in their own protocols.

- RealChems (RealChems.com): RealChems sources synthetic versions of 1P-LSD, ALD-52, ETH-LAD, AL-LAD, 4-AcO-DMT, and many other psychedelic and nootropic "research chemicals" that are "not sold for human consumption" (nudge, nudge, wink, wink).

For most of the psychedelic purchases you make online, you will need some form of cryptocurrency like Bitcoin and, in most cases, if you want to remain anonymous, a Tor browser or other cloaked browser.

and liver function, blood sugar, and hormonal regulation all appear to be unaffected during consumption. (However, to avoid any issues with significant neurotransmitter imbalances, it is best to avoid alcohol and serotonin-based antidepressants while taking any psychedelics.)

A psilocybin microdose ranges from 0.1 to 0.5 g. I highly recommend you start at the lower end of the dosing range with any of the psychedelics mentioned in this chapter. For psilocybin in particular, you can combine a smaller dose with lion's mane and niacin in a morning cup of tea for a very slight sensory boost without any distracting trip or gastric upset. Interestingly, blue lotus extract—which is commonly known as an aphrodisiac but can also result in a significant release of the psychedelic compound DMT (dimethyltryptamine) by the pineal gland—can be combined with psilocybin alone or the blend above for an even more pronounced effect that many describe as something similar to an ecstasy (MDMA) experience. Your pineal gland normally releases small amounts of DMT, but it is also found in some plants and can also be chemically synthesized, and when ingested in high amounts, it can result in a very noticeable, ego-dissolving psychedelic journeying effect, while smaller amounts have a pleasant nootropic effect. Blue lotus can upregulate your own production of DMT, or when taken with DMT, can magnify its effects. I purchase blue lotus for this purpose from Essential Oil Wizardry; you'll find a link at BoundlessBook.com/5.

Microdosing with LSD

Lysergic acid diethylamide, commonly known as LSD, is derived from a chemical in rye fungus. It was originally synthesized in 1938 to aid in childbirth and is widely known for its powerful hallucinogenic effects. It is less well known for what I use it for: inducing intense sparks of creativity when a merging of the left and right brain hemispheres is the desired goal, such as a day on which I need to do a great deal of creative writing or copywriting. It also works quite well for keeping you chugging along on a sleep-deprived or jet-lagged day.

Like psilocybin, LSD affects serotonin levels in the body. A dose of LSD dramatically increases levels of serotonin in the brain, which causes a feel-good dopamine release. Research suggests that LSD may also reduce blood flow to the control centers of the brain, which weakens their activity and allows for higher amounts of creativity and simultaneous use of both right and left hemispheres of the brain, allowing for a potent combination of analytical and creative thinking that would normally be difficult to tap into. This enhanced brain connectivity is likely why users experience increased creativity and unique thought patterns. Therapeutic effects of LSD include treating addiction, depression, anxiety, obsessive-compulsive disorder, cluster headaches, end-of-life anxiety, and resistance to behavior change. It also decreases reaction time, increases concentration and balance, decreases pain perception, and improves mood.

A typical LSD microdose ranges from 5 to 20 micrograms (not milligrams!). My own approach for dosing LSD—which I described at the beginning of this chapter—is called the volumetric dosing method. I buy blotter paper of LSD or P-LSD, then cut out a square of 100 micrograms with scissors and drop it into a 10-milliliter dropper bottle of vodka. I then know that a single drop of the liquid contains a neat 10 micrograms of LSD. This helps me avoid the inaccurate dosing so notoriously associated with simply cutting out a square of paper and placing it in your mouth. Interestingly, I have found that if you take slightly too much LSD, a small dose of CBD (between 10 and 20 mg) seems to take the edge off.

Microdosing with Ibogaine

Ibogaine is derived from iboga, an evergreen shrub native to the rainforests in central Africa whose root bark has high concentrations of psychedelic compounds. It has a rich history in the Bwiti religion in Africa and has recently found its way into Western medicine to treat drug addictions, improve physical energy and cognitive performance (in microdoses), and cause a surge in positive emotions.

To microdose with ibogaine, find a tincture or root bark form (the root bark form is usually encapsulated). If you use a tincture, find a source that has the root bark extracted into its purest form and combined with iboga alkaloids. A single drop of an iboga tincture equates to about a 0.5 mg microdose of ibogaine. In root bark form, an effective dose is 300 to 500 mg.

I have personally found ibogaine to be most useful before a workout or any effort that combines both mental and physical demands, such as tennis, basketball, or energetic sex. It will make you hyperactive and jittery if taken just before a day of desk work, which makes sense when you consider that African tribes traditionally whipped themselves into a frenzied pre-battle state on ibogaine.

Microdosing with Ketamine

Ketamine is a general anesthetic commonly used on animals but originally devised for and tested on humans (in fact, my paramedic brother commonly uses it on the patients he transports in the ambulance). Ketamine received notoriety as a party drug in the 1990s but is now is gaining momentum as a very effective treatment for depression. When administered as an IV infusion, it works very quickly on brain receptors and offers relief from depression symptoms in as little as twenty-four hours. In contrast, traditional antidepressants can take up to eight weeks to become effective and are accompanied by a host of negative side effects that ketamine doesn't seem to cause. These traditional antidepressants work by flooding neurotransmitters or blocking their reuptake in the central nervous system. But ketamine directly blocks glutamate and opiate receptors, both of which affect depression and pain responses, from being acted upon by neurotransmitters—resulting in a profound antidepressant effect without neurotransmitter desensitization.

Getting Started with Microdosing

For any of the psychedelic compounds discussed in this chapter, I recommend following the protocol laid out by James Fadiman in chapter 16 of his excellent *Psychedelic Explorer's Guide:*

- Consume a microdose of your chosen psychedelic twice per week for ten weeks.

- Allow two to three days between each microdosing day (for example, consume your microdoses on Wednesdays and Sundays).

- Write about your experience and be mindful of your expectations and desires.

- Especially in the early stages of experimentation, use the compound in a familiar or controlled setting.

- At the end of the ten weeks (or however many weeks you microdose), reflect on your experience and ask yourself, "Did I accomplish my purpose for microdosing?"

For one of the more comprehensive and insightful guides on microdosing, I also recommend Michael Pollan's book *How to Change Your Mind,* in which the author—an immersive journalist with little to no psychedelic experience—takes a deep dive into the world of psilocybin, LSD, DMT, and beyond.

Ketamine users have claimed, after as a little as a single session, to experience benefits such as increased compassion and sensitivity to others, an increase in overall joy of life, and a reduced fear of death. Ketamine is also quite popular in sensory-deprivation situations, such as float tanks—probably because it does such a good job deactivating the sympathetic fight-or-flight response and activating the parasympathetic nervous system, resulting in a better ability to let go of stressful, distracting thoughts and enter into a state of deep relaxation.

I personally had an extremely pleasant ketamine infusion experience at the offices of Dr. Matt Cook in San Jose, California, where I lay quietly on a table for two hours while experiencing a state of pure bliss. Upon completing the session, which also included music, meditation, and qigong, I felt light as a feather, as though I didn't have a worry in the world. What's more, my wife and boys both noticed that afterward I seemed more approachable, less worried, and more positive, particularly in stressful situations. For therapeutic purposes such as this, ketamine is most commonly administered in the dose of 0.5 mg per kilogram of body weight, but some people may respond to doses as low as 0.1 mg per kilogram of body weight, and others may require up to 0.75 mg per kilogram of body weight. I've also found ketamine to be very pleasant when used in an intranasal microdose of about 5 mg before sex (particularly because it increases sex drive and decreases inhibitions), and it also, probably because it can cause full-body relaxation, decreases pain perception and allows a massage therapist to dig a bit deeper into your muscles.

While I don't condone drugs as a replacement for spiritual disciplines, responsible use of ketamine is certainly a life-changing experience, particularly for people with depression or those wired to be hard-charging high achievers. (It should be noted that high-dose MDMA therapy can also be particularly effective for anxiety, depression, or ego dissolution, although I haven't yet tried it. However, my friend Tucker Max has, and his fascinating *Medium* article "What MDMA Therapy Did for Me" takes a deep dive into his experience.)

Should you decide to skip the IV infusion and DIY with oral ketamine, then please know that determining your ideal microdose can be tricky, so it is important to start below the recommended dose. If you are going to use it orally, taking ketamine sublingually is the most effective and direct route. A sublingual microdose of ketamine is about 0.75 mg per kilogram of body weight, although you can get a significant mood enhancement with as little as 0.2 mg per kilogram of body weight.

Never mix ketamine with any substance that depresses breathing, such as alcohol, opioids, or tramadol, as it is an extremely calming agent that can produce a heavy sedative effect if you are not careful or if you combine it with other sedative-like compounds. Finally, as with any psychedelic drug, a proper set (your mindset) and setting (your physical environment) is important, which is why I do not recommend any of the compounds discussed in this section, including ketamine, for a "party experience" if your goal is to instead engage in what I consider to be a more productive use of such compounds, particularly increasing introspection, creativity, productivity, or a deep, intimate connection with others.

Not the Usual Warning on Psychedelics

While writing this chapter, I was tempted to give you some warning or legal disclaimer about psychedelics. But here's the deal: these substances are becoming more commonly accepted and even legal. Recently, the FDA approved psilocybin for use in the treatment of depression. I predict that within the next decade, we will see many of these substances, which have had such a sullied reputation for so many years, become more and more legal, accessible, and, as consumers become more educated, safe.

I am often asked what supplements I take, why I take them, and if we really need supplements anyway. After all, if you follow a healthy lifestyle, I'll wager you probably eat plenty of plants, prioritize sleep, hydrate with filtered water (or, dare I say, at the risk of revealing my tinfoil hat, structured water), and expose yourself to the sun as much as possible.

In other words, you are, like me, what I would call a "healthy, woo-woo geek." You are an intelligent, well-informed person, you embrace your softer-side spirituality, and you pride yourself on your passion for health, nutrition, science, and fitness. Why would you need to take supplements for health, fitness, and longevity? Don't nutrient-dense food, good water, and clean living provide enough vitamins, minerals, and antioxidants?

I get it. There is a dizzying array of supplements to choose from, and the expense can add up fast. No one—including me—wants to spend their precious time counting and swallowing pills. Supplements can also be dangerous. I have dedicated entire podcasts to exposing the deceptive tactics that many supplement companies employ and have explored the host of unhealthy fillers that many supplements contain.

So why even consider supplementation? Let's begin with this: our modern, postindustrial, polluted, toxin-laden lifestyle demands more nutrients than food can provide.

That's right. The chronic stressors of modern life—ranging from exposure to heavy metals and synthetic chemicals to sensory overload—have been proven to increase your body's need for vitamins, minerals, and antioxidants, which are needed to shuttle toxins through detox pathways and prevent the formation of DNA-damaging free radicals. This means that even if you are eating clean, nutrient-dense food, you are likely not getting all the nutrients you need. There are five factors that contribute to the disconnect between the nutrients in our food and the nutrients we need.

1. **Nutrient-depleted soil:** Due to modern farming techniques and fertilizers, most soil today is relatively depleted of vitamins, minerals, and antioxidants. You may think that eating organic is the ultimate solution. While some research suggests that organically grown food contains more nutrients than nonorganic food, other research has concluded that there is no significant difference in nutritional content between the two. In addition, for most of human history (and

prehistory), our ancestors ate now-nearly-extinct, cellular (dense-cell-rich) carbohydrates in the form of foods like wild tubers, which provided essential prebiotics so that beneficial bacteria could flourish (in contrast to the refined acellular grains and white rice that compose most modern carbohydrates).

Cellular carbohydrates such as root tubers, fruits, leaves, and stems actually store carbohydrates in fiber-rich living cells that can remain intact during cooking. In contrast, processed and refined carbohydrates such as flour, sugar, and grains are "acellular" carbohydrates, because they lack intact cells. These modern carbohydrates not only create a scenario of nutrient deficiencies but also cause a void in cell-rich carbohydrates, which can lead to significant gut fermentation, blood sugar swings, and glycemic variability. A glance at a coffee shop display case or hotel breakfast bar that features bagels, muffins, and sugary cereals explains why many people need a snack a couple hours after breakfast to make it through the inevitable midmorning blood sugar crash. Blood sugar imbalances lead to chronic inflammation and may be responsible for up to 80 percent of modern diseases, including Alzheimer's disease. This is a roller coaster you definitely don't want to be on.

Similarly, the meat, eggs, and dairy products commonly found in grocery stores deliver fewer anti-inflammatory nutrients, such as omega-3 fatty acids, than those from wild or pastured animals. Most people eating a Western diet also consume an imbalanced ratio of omega-6 fatty acids to omega-3 fatty acids, further exacerbating chronic inflammation.

2. **Age-related declines in nutrient absorption:** Your ability to absorb nutrients from food decreases as you age. While growing children should absolutely be taking a multivitamin to support healthy tissue and bone formation, supplementation is equally important for older generations. Many medications used to treat age-related diseases, such as acid reflux and hypertension, also interfere with proper nutrient absorption, further increasing the need for supplements.

Then there is precious vitamin D. While there's no consensus on what constitutes sufficient vitamin D levels, it is safe to say that many Americans, especially aging Americans, who tend to spend more time indoors, do not get enough vitamin D. Even if we do our best to get sun exposure—whether it's taking a morning walk or eating lunch outside—it is rare to get as much sunlight and vitamin D as our outdoor-dwelling ancestors did.

3. **Poor food-handling practices:** Modern harvesting, shipping, processing, and storage techniques degrade the nutrient content of food. Plants grown with modern fertilizer may contain only 25 percent of the micronutrients of plants grown using more traditional farming methods, and nutrient content declines as they are shipped and sit on store shelves. It makes sense that a freshly picked apple is more nutritious than an apple bought in the winter at the supermarket, which was likely treated with 1-methylcyclopropene and could be up to ten months old (according to the FDA). And the preservatives used to maintain freshness could both impede the bioavailability of the food's nutrients and require your body to use more nutrients to process these synthetic additives.

4. **Pesticides, herbicides, and pollutants:** Our bodies are exposed to all kinds of toxins these days: pesticides, herbicides, and other chemicals in the modern food supply; polluted water; environmental contaminants from things like degraded plastic; and airborne pollutants like carbon monoxide, lead, and mercury. These synergistic factors vastly increase your need for extra vitamins, minerals, and nutrients, which combat the formation of free radicals and the toxins' attack on your metabolism and immune system.

5. **Exercise:** Because athletes and active individuals use more oxygen and energy than the average person, they need far more nutrients. Indeed, consuming only the recommended amounts of nutrients can actually limit your athletic performance. So if you engage in CrossFit WODs, Ironman triathlons, obstacle races, or heavy weight lifting, your nutritional requirements mean you need to take supplements.

You might be thinking that instead of taking supplements, you could simply ignore calories and eat more food to obtain nutrients. But there are scientifically demonstrated benefits to caloric restriction, including longevity. This is another reason supplements are crucial: they are a helpful boost for those of us who want to consume enough nutrients to function well but also want to live longer using strategies such as intermittent fasting, alternate-day fasting, and caloric restriction.

The assumption that previous generations didn't take supplements is not true. Ancient supplements include root, stem, and leaf teas, medicinal powders ground by mortar and pestle, and highly concentrated oil extracts. Just because these dietary supplements didn't look like capsules or oversized tubs of powders doesn't mean they weren't supplements. In addition, when harvesting wild plants, eating meat, and spending plenty more time in nature, our ancestors certainly consumed more dirt than we do now, and this soil contained a wide range of beneficial probiotics (some supplement manufacturers now produce products that are simply soil-derived probiotics!). Perhaps even more compelling is the fact that animals, ranging from insects to chimps, self-medicate and supplement by consuming specific compounds. For example, when some caterpillars get infected by parasitic flies, they eat poisonous plants to kill the invasive larvae. Ants fight off microbes and bacteria by adding spruce resin to their nests. Several animal species consume mud to counteract stomach upset, and animals of all kinds use plant medicine as their own rough approximation of supplements.

Ultimately, supplementing with vitamins, minerals, and even nootropics and psychedelics is a natural, time-honored way to enhance the body and brain. While many would argue that your brain should work fine on its own in our modern era, operating with flawless precision in the presence of clean food, pure water, sunshine, and fresh air, I beg to differ and have benefited highly from a bit of ancestral wisdom combined with better living through science.

If I could issue any warning, it would be this: Like synthetic smart drugs, psychedelics can cause a significant influx into the nervous system of neurotransmitters like serotonin and dopamine and, as a result, can cause addiction, tolerance, and neurotransmitter imbalances. So proceed with caution and, as the excellent book *Stealing Fire* by Steven Kotler and Jamie Wheal notes, use these compounds with more stoicism than hedonism.

Furthermore, I personally feel that anyone who strikes out upon a quest to "find themselves" via a hedonistic, ego-dissolving journey involving plant-based compounds such as ayahuasca, DMT, marijuana, psilocybin, or ibogaine should instead first engage in a comparatively stoic immersion in the spiritual disciplines of fasting, solitude, study, meditation, and prayer—even if that means delaying, say, a five-day trip to Peru for the alternative of a five-day solo journey into the wilderness near one's home. I suspect that many people will discover they can experience intense physical, mental, and spiritual breakthroughs via a bout of fasting, silence, and nature immersion, and that this experience can rival or even exceed any benefits derived from a plant-medicine journey.

Sure, it's far simpler to drink a tea or eat a mushroom cookie, hire a shaman to visit your New York City loft with some kind of special brew, and lie back, slip into a kaleidoscope of colors, and perhaps experience a new spiritual dimension. But I would challenge you to first tuck a journal under your arm and a tent into your backpack and venture into the forest for a few days of meditation and introspection with nothing but a bit of water, extra clothing, and your own mind. Journeying by yourself in a stoic setting like this should, in my opinion, be a prerequisite before any attempt to embark upon a psychedelic odyssey, which seems to have replaced the type of vision quests or rites of passage that humans used to experience as a core part of their passage into adulthood. This is likely one reason that so many of my acquaintances are on their forty-eighth ayahuasca trip and still haven't actually found a resolution for their struggles in life: they've never made an attempt to engage in a rigorous immersion in the spiritual disciplines first.

Don't get me wrong: I believe that everything on God's good earth was created for humans to intelligently use and derive benefits from. But in the same way that wine, honey, milk, and butter can be abused, so also can everything from St. John's wort to THC to mushrooms.

THE LAST WORD

When it comes to using chemistry, modern science, and ancestral wisdom to make your brain work better, there are obviously plenty of options. While I would urge you to use caution with smart drugs, I also encourage you to consider the use of both natural and synthetic nootropics to enhance both productivity and cognitive performance, and to also tap into the power of psychedelics for personal breakthroughs, creativity, and connectivity. While there's no substitute for quality sleep, brain-supporting food, and mitigation of environmental toxins and pollutants, experimenting with the stacks and supportive neurovitamins and neurominerals in this chapter can be a truly mind-altering and brain-bettering experience, particularly if you feel as though your brain could use a boost.

Are you feeling a bit of paralysis by analysis with all these mind-altering tactics? Does it seem like there are too many choices? Fear not: at right, I have laid out an example of how I personally weave all these compounds together into a week.

While you may not find yourself mixing an LSD homebrew in your kitchen anytime soon, a bit of better living through science may be exactly what you need to upgrade your productivity, creativity, and overall cognitive performance. You are now equipped with every shred of knowledge necessary to do so, whether you choose a risky smart drug approach, a natural nootropic approach, a synthetic nootropic approach, a psychedelic approach, or a blend of all four.

For citations for all the research studies mentioned in this chapter and a deeper dive into the topics of this chapter—including links to podcasts, blog posts, recommended tools and supplements, and much more—visit BoundlessBook.com/5.

Every day

I have a cup of black coffee every morning. If I consume coffee in the afternoon, I add tulsi and astragalus or L-theanine to it. If I am using coffee to help me plow through a demanding day or a period of sleep deprivation, I occasionally combine it with nicotine.

Monday, Tuesday, and Wednesday

I often take Qualia on these busier days when intense work demands arise, especially if I need faster word recall or brain processing speed (for example, if I am being interviewed for a podcast or speaking on stage). If I have been traveling or I am jet-lagged, I will include a dose of methylene blue to mitigate neuroinflammation.

Thursday

Thursdays tend to be less busy. I take TianChi if I need to gently boost blood flow and want to keep neural inflammation at bay. If I am doing more intense studying, reading, or memorizing, I will mix lion's mane into my coffee or drink the lion's mane straight with hot water or green tea.

Friday

This is a creative-writing, problem-solving, and brainstorming day. I often microdose with 10 to 20 micrograms of LSD in the morning to enhance the coordination between my left and right brain hemispheres.

Saturday

This is my off day. I consume no brain-boosters aside from a piping-hot cup of coffee.

Sunday

I devote Sundays to spiritual disciplines, personal exploration, and a hefty dose of neurogenesis. On these days, I use a more potent neuron-sprouting and ego-dissolving mix: a microdose of psilocybin blended with lion's mane extract and niacin. (If the niacin-induced skin flush and increased blood flow is too much for you, you can also use nicotinamide riboside, a form of vitamin B_3 that has similar effects without the flushing.)

ONE THING YOU CAN DO THIS WEEK

Never tried a nootropic before? This is your chance. C'mon. You know you're itching to. Go out this week and hunt down one of the nutrients, nootropics, or smart drugs from this chapter and use it, preferably on a cognitively demanding day.

I recommend adding a touch of lion's mane with a smattering of psilocybin and niacin to a morning cup of green tea to induce the sprouting of new neurons; 100 mg of L-theanine tossed into a cup of coffee to cause a slow, non-jittery bleed of caffeine into your system; or a nicotine toothpick during your next afternoon of hard work. I personally like to keep a few brain-enhancing options in my pantry and choose my own adventure based on the day's demands.

In chapter 19, I will revisit the notion of supplement stacks with a view to longevity, and these often overlap with many of the stacks in this chapter. You will find that when you arm your pantry with both brain-boosting and antiaging compounds, the effects of both seem to be magnified.

UPGRADE YOUR HEAD

BRAIN BIOHACKING GEAR, GAMES, AND TOOLS

Perched atop my indoor bicycle trainer and hammering away in preparation for the South Beach Triathlon in Miami, I reached toward my ears and switched on the high-tech Beats-by-Dre-esque headphones wrapped around my skull. Within seconds, invisible pins and needles dug into the top of my head, and for the next twenty minutes, the pinpricks increased in intensity. I tried to focus on pedaling harder while ignoring the perception that tiny aliens with acupuncture needles were attacking my cranium.

The headphones were no ordinary headphones but rather a special device designed for transcranial direct-current stimulation, or tDCS, of the nervous system. The result? Reduced perception of pain, increased skill acquisition and hand-eye coordination, and the ability to blast through a normally soul-crushing workout with relative ease.

Perhaps I am a masochist who has spent far too much time running through forests wielding my obstacle-racing spear, but, as a nerd at heart, I am enchanted with the concept of using electricity, sound waves, magnets, and a host of other biohacks to enhance my physical and mental performance. From shocking my gonads into better orgasms to putting magnets on my collarbone (and, admittedly, my nether regions) for better sleep and better sex to blasting my body with healing acoustics, if it is legal and safe, I have probably messed around with it—and, yeah, that includes running through electroshock cables in Tough Mudder races, covered in mud and with a dumb grin on my face.

So when I saw a *New Yorker* article entitled "For the Golden State Warriors, Brain Zapping Could Provide an Edge," I immediately perked up. Turns out the freakin' NBA professional basketball champions use tDCS to shock their heads before practice and games.

The headphones-like device the Warriors use is perhaps something you have heard of before. It is called the Halo Sport, and it was designed by a scientist named Dr. Daniel Chao, who had previously worked at a company that used brain stimulation to treat epilepsy. The original forms of tDCS involved attaching a couple of electrodes to a battery, sticking them to the user's head, and sending a tiny current—about five hundred to one thousand times lower than that used in electroshock therapy—through the brain. The current alters the excitability of your neurons, causing them to fire just a bit more quickly and readily, which makes skill-acquisition training more effective.

However, the Halo Sport is a bit of an upgrade from just a couple of electrodes and a battery. Instead, it is a fancy set of headphones that have electrodes strategically placed across the top, precisely positioned to send a current through an area of your brain called the motor cortex, the control center that sends commands to your muscles. The idea is that you put the headphones on for twenty minutes in the early stages of your workout or during your warm-up (or even before engaging in a left hand–right hand coordination activity, like playing a video game or a musical instrument) and activate the stimulation with the accompanying smartphone app. As you train, your brain delivers stronger, more synchronous signals to your muscles, allowing you to more quickly acquire a skill.

When I read the *New Yorker* article on the Golden State Warriors, I was already familiar with the concept of electric brain stimulation. I had heard the popular "9-Volt Nirvana" Radiolab podcast episode, in which Sally Adee, an editor at New Scientist, revealed that she discovered how to accelerate learning with tDCS at a Defense Advanced Research Projects Agency conference. In the episode, Sally found herself wielding an M4 assault rifle with a battery wired to her temple and discovering some pretty shocking (pun intended) improvements in her sniper skills. Incidentally, although the Reddit forum on building your own tDCS unit already existed, it exploded after the episode aired.

Back in 2013, I wrote an article about what was then a groundbreaking study in which Brazilian sports scientists used tDCS to apply a tiny electrical current to cyclists' motor cortex. The results were pretty darn impressive. After twenty minutes of real or placebo brain stimulation, the cyclists completed an all-out ride to exhaustion. Sure enough, the cyclists who underwent electrical stimulation experienced significantly lower heart rates, lower perceived exertion, and a 4 percent higher power output (that may sound small, but it is a huge improvement for a cyclist).

But even if you are not a professional athlete, you can now use tDCS and other brain-upgrading technology in the comfort of your own home. Let's say you have done a good job supporting your brain health. You avoid pro-inflammatory food, eat lots of omega-3 fatty acids and antioxidants, and perhaps even use a nootropic stack or microdose with a psychedelic. But you still want more. You want to live better through modern science, and you know there are tools that will help you achieve peak mental performance. You want to maximize your work productivity, be motivated to give every workout the focus it deserves, read faster, speak better, and operate in a way you never have before.

You're in luck. They may not be mainstream yet, but there are a host of safe tools that will enable you to increase blood flow to your brain, improve cognitive performance and skill acquisition, focus better during a workout, and even increase awareness and reduce stress.

6 TOOLS FOR BRAIN OPTIMIZATION

I personally use six proven tools that I have found to be the best of the best for catapulting your brain to the next level. Here they are, in no particular order.

1. Pulsed Electromagnetic Field Therapy

On my bedside is a tiny handheld unit called a FlexPulse, which I consider to be a portable "DJ for the brain." By adjusting the settings, I can use a 3 Hz frequency to lull my brain into a relaxed delta brain wave state, a 10 Hz frequency to generate focus-enhancing alpha brain waves, or a 23 Hz frequency to produce high-alert beta brain waves—or even a 100 Hz frequency for muscle repair (I'll talk about this more in chapter 12). The FlexPulse generates these frequencies in what is called a pulsed electromagnetic field, or PEMF. I have found that by placing the square pad of the unit directly on the hard occipital bone on the back of my head and securing it with a wrap-around sleep mask (often combined with the cranial electrotherapy stimulation described later in this chapter), I can knock myself out in no time at all for a perfect night's sleep or a quick nap.

PEMF therapy is not to be confused with the damaging EMFs (electromagnetic fields) you've no doubt heard about. Harmful EMFs and the therapeutic EMFs that PEMF devices generate are very different in their effects. All EMFs interact with tissue and biological systems, but while therapeutic EMFs support cellular communication and health, harmful EMFs negatively impact your body's functions.

The main distinctions between harmful and therapeutic EMFs involve characteristics of the waves themselves: wavelength, exposure time, and frequency. On the electromagnetic spectrum, PEMF devices produce long wavelengths and extremely low to very low frequencies. On the other hand, harmful EMFs have short wavelengths and high frequencies. For example, a 1 Hz PEMF frequency corresponds to a wavelength of about 100 million meters, which is more than 62,000 miles. (The earth's circumference is just 24,901 miles!) Alternatively, a harmful frequency of about 100 million Hz (which can be produced by your average microwave) has a wavelength of just one meter (about three feet).

FOUR CATEGORIES OF BRAIN WAVE PATTERNS

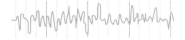

BETA (14–30 Hz)
- Concentration, arousal, alertness, cognition
- Higher levels associated with anxiety, disease, feelings of separation, fight or flight

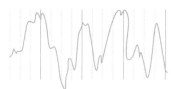

ALPHA (8–13.9 Hz)
- Relaxation, superlearning, relaxed focus, light trance, increased serotonin production
- Pre-sleep, pre-waking drowsiness, meditation, beginning of access to unconscious mind

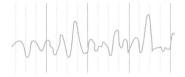

THETA (4–7.9 Hz)
- Dreaming sleep (REM sleep)
- Increased production of catecholamines (vital for learning and memory), increased creativity
- Integrative, emotional experiences, potential change in behavior, increased retention of learned material
- Hypnagogic imagery, trance, deep meditation, access to unconscious mind

DELTA (0.1–3.9 Hz)
- Dreamless sleep
- Human growth hormone released
- Deep trancelike, nonphysical state, loss of body awareness
- Access to unconscious and "collective unconscious" mind, greatest "push" to brain when induced with Holosync (see page 125)

PEMF therapy works by training your brain to produce particular electrical wavelengths. Your brain produces different electrical wavelengths throughout the day and night, including alpha, beta, delta, and theta brain waves. For example, when you are awake during the day and working, studying, exercising, or engaged in any other activity that requires focus, concentration, or alertness, you predominantly produce alpha and beta brain waves. During periods of sleep and some forms of meditation or relaxation, the brain shifts into higher delta and theta brain wave production.

When presented with a rhythmic stimulus, such as PEMF, your brain responds by synchronizing your brain's electrical activity to the rhythm, a process known as entrainment. Entrainment has the greatest probability of occurring if the PEMF is similar to frequencies found in nature. You are probably familiar with how compasses work: the earth produces an electromagnetic field that causes a compass needle to point toward magnetic north. But the earth also produces what are known as Schumann resonances, a set of low electromagnetic frequencies. The most well-known of these is the 7.83 Hz frequency, which is responsible for the benefits of grounding or earthing (a sleep- and recovery-boosting tactic I'll talk more about in chapters 7 and 12) and can also be used to mitigate many of the damaging effects of EMF.

You can control which wavelengths your brain produces by setting PEMF devices to those natural wavelength frequencies. For example, you can set the FlexPulse or EarthPulse to alpha mode prior to focused activities. You can use a device like the SomniResonance SR1 to enter a delta-wavelength state prior to sleep. You can use more powerful devices like the BodyBalance to expose your body to a mix of frequencies and even enhance the efficacy of nootropics and smart drugs. When used for cognitive performance, PEMF therapy has been shown to improve neuroplasticity and communication between brain regions. Research also suggests that high-intensity PEMF exposure can improve blood flow to the cerebral cortex, resulting in greater nutrient uptake by the brain.

While smaller devices like the FlexPulse and EarthPulse are a perfect introduction to the many therapeutic applications of PEMF, the ultimate PEMF device is a large unit—about the size of a massage table—from Pulse Centers called the Pulse XL Pro. Both Tony Robbins and I are huge fans of this massive, full-body setup, which you can use for everything from healing muscle sprains and reducing headaches to improving sleep onset (which is also known as a decrease in sleep latency, or an ability to fall asleep faster). Admittedly, this is an expensive option, but because of the power of the frequencies used, the device delivers potent benefits that work deep within your cells.

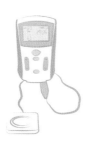

FLEX PULSE

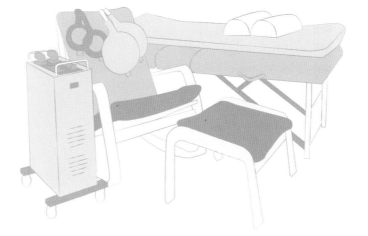

PULSE CENTER XL PRO

To understand how PEMF therapy works, you must first know why your cells—in both your brain and your body—require electricity. In his work with high-voltage discharges at the turn of the last century, Nikola Tesla, the inventor of alternating current, concluded that our bodies' tissues operate as energy-storing electrical condensers and that quite a lot of electrical energy can pass through them, surprisingly, without harm.

Many years later, beginning in the 1930s, Harvard physiology professor Harold Saxton Burr wrote ninety-three papers on his research showing that measurable electrical energy in organs is directly related to health. If the electrical energy was depleted or the charge across a cell membrane was too high or too low, tissue dysfunction followed, but if the electrical balance was restored, so was health.

Then, in his excellent book *Healing Is Voltage* (2010), Dr. Jerry Tennant wrote that cells are designed to operate at an electrical potential (charge separation) across the cell membrane of -20 to -25 millivolts. When your cells' voltage drops below that level, the result is chronic pain and disease. In other words, doctors need to start thinking like electricians, not just physicians. Tennant also describes how our acid-alkaline balance (pH) is also a measure of voltage. A normal human cell contains ample amounts of oxygen and operates at a pH of 7.35 to 7.45, which is the exact equivalent of -20 to -25 millivolts. (pH is linked to voltage because pH technically reflects the number of charged hydrogen ions—H+—per liter of solution.)

Today, the growing use of therapeutic PEMF devices is the result of the century-long evolution of research on using electrical current to affect self-healing and self-regulating cellular processes. While a direct-current stimulator, such a TENS unit or EMS device, uses electrodes that must make contact with the skin to interface with your nervous system and cells, a magnetic field generator can simply induce energy in a conductor (like your body's tissues) and do not require contact with the skin because no electricity actually touches you.

The greater the intensity of the pulse from a PEMF device, the more energy is delivered, and the greater the subsequent energy produced within your cells. It takes a fast-rising pulse with sufficient energy to create charge and voltage of sufficient depth in your body. A more expensive PEMF unit, such as Pulse Center's Pulse XL Pro, creates extremely high intensities, allowing for a depth of penetration far beyond other PEMF devices. These higher intensities of PEMF have been shown to induce significant increases in blood flow (sixty minutes of PEMF exposure results in about 20 percent greater blood flow). Mitochondrial respiration rate is also higher in cells exposed to PEMF, meaning these mitochondria produce energy faster. PEMF is most effective when the demand for ATP (cellular energy) is highest, when ADP levels are low and nutrients are not readily available—in other words, when you are hungry and exhausted. And the effects of PEMF pulsing on muscle mitochondrial respiration is still present as much as two weeks after exposure! PEMF also increases the number of mitochondria, similar to the increases caused by high-intensity interval training.

PEMF therapy also affects the immune system. Macrophages are some of the first responders of the immune system, protecting us from infections, bacteria, viruses, damaged-cell debris, and injury. One of the ways they respond is to engulf and devour offenders by means of a complex process called phagocytosis, which is similar to what happens during digestion in the acid environment of our stomachs. In one study, macrophages exposed to PEMF demonstrated a 56.2 percent increase in phagocytosis, devouring particles significantly faster and maintaining this advantage over unexposed macrophages for many hours after a single exposure.

Another study examined the effect of PEMF on the production of inflammatory markers associated with chronic disease and cancer, including tumor necrosis factor (TNF), transcription factor nuclear factor kappa B (NFkB), and the expression of the A20 (tumor necrosis factor-alpha-induced protein 3) in inflamed cells. Cells were exposed to PEMF at different frequencies to find out if any frequencies would affect the inflammatory response pathway. The study demonstrated that cells continuously exposed to PEMF at 5 Hz exhibited significant effects on the downregulation of TNF-alpha and NFkB and also showed a trend in the downregulation of A20. This means PEMF could be beneficial in modulating the immune response in the presence of infection.

When a cell's voltage is low, oxygen departs the cell, which lowers ATP production. PEMF increases circulation, thus providing more oxygen to the cell. PEMF also increases cell voltage, which raises pH and enables more oxygen to be dissolved within the cell for mitochondrial respiration. In this way, PEMF increases mitochondrial respiratory activity, resulting in more-efficient production of ATP by the cell's mitochondria. PEMF also increases the number of mitochondria, allowing for even more energy production in the cell. The increased energy output from a greater number of more efficient mitochondria enables each cell to accelerate recovery and perform its normal functions better. This leads to faster recovery, better resilience, and enhanced performance.

It's also important to note that when you have low cellular voltage, you have low pH, and low pH can create an acidic environment in which cancer can thrive. By using PEMF to create a more oxygenated environment, you can very likely lower your cancer risk. (You can read more about this phenomenon in Dr. Thomas Seyfried's book *Cancer as a Metabolic Disease: On the Origin, Management, and Prevention of Cancer.*)

I find it fascinating that early in the last century there was a huge debate about whether humans are electrical or chemical animals. With the discovery of antibiotics, a large part of the medical profession decided that we are chemical, which has led to our current state of medicine in which chemicals are the primary modalities used for treatment. But now, with the rise of chronic illnesses and an increasing understanding of the ways the human body is very much like a battery, smart functional-medicine practitioners are now beginning to incorporate electrical components such as PEMF into treatment plans.

Finally, a word of warning: very high intensity PEMF such as that produced by the Pulse Centers unit can kill bacteria, yeast, and fungus, and as a result, in some people it can cause a release of endotoxins. That can create an uncomfortable Jarisch-Herxheimer reaction, resulting in temporary nausea, headaches, and other flu-like symptoms. So it's best to ease yourself into any high-intensity use of PEMF if you have an infection or rampant inflammation.

2. Neurofeedback

I recently visited the Peak Brain Institute in Los Angeles for an advanced brain scan and brain-mapping system called quantitative electroencephalography, or QEEG, and I was shocked at what they discovered in my brain.

Dr. Andrew Hill, a UCLA-trained cognitive neuroscientist and lecturer, oversaw the entire protocol and discovered what he described as severe patterns of brain wave abnormalities and imbalances, including excess stressful beta waves, excess theta waves, and excess delta waves, with a significant lack of focus-enhancing alpha waves.

What does that mean? It suggests that I have a history of concussions and traumatic brain injury (caused by everything from football to mountain biking to kickboxing), as well as accumulated deficits of attention, increased distractibility, limited sleep potential, and suboptimal cognitive performance, all resulting from travel, exposure to toxins, excessive multitasking, and other lifestyle factors that plague hard-charging high achievers who perhaps too often put their noggin on the line.

Two months after the scan, I hopped on a plane back to LA and again ventured into the Peak Brain Institute for three days of intensive training. When I returned to Spokane, I had a briefcase packed with a laptop, electrodes, conducting gel, and all the other neurofeedback gear necessary to fix my brain. For the next three months, I trained for thirty minutes every other day using a style of neurofeedback I can best describe as meditation on steroids. My protocol involved flying a spaceship on the laptop with my mind. Each time my brain subconsciously shifted into unfavorable brain wave patterns, the spaceship would stop flying and the music generated by the neurofeedback software would fade away, very much like a cognitive slap on the wrist.

Neurofeedback training is a noninvasive form of central nervous system biofeedback. It involves placing electrodes on the scalp and works by encouraging certain brain regions, such as the frontal, parietal, temporal, and occipital lobes (the cortical brain regions), to raise or lower the amplitude and ratios of brain waves.

The electrodes produce a signal that is picked up by an EEG amplifier. These signals are fed into software, such as the spaceship-flying software, that gives the user some form of visual or auditory feedback or reward, like amplified music, more smoke exhaustion behind the spaceship, or progression to a new level, when the brain produces the desired changes in brain wave amplitude or frequency.

Which brain waves are affected depends upon the neurofeedback protocol you use. Some protocols affect alpha waves, while others affect beta, alpha/theta, theta, gamma, or delta waves. Under my protocol, every time I strayed into excess beta brain wave production, the spaceship slowed down or the music faded away, until my brain learned to avoid that particular pattern. So unlike peripheral biofeedback, such as practicing a handstand, neurofeedback is a largely involuntary process in which you shape the brain by giving it feedback only when it performs certain actions, like flying a spaceship.

Professional clinicians report that 90 percent of users notice significant positive results from neurofeedback training, which can be used for everything from reducing anxiety and stress to inducing faster sleep onset to resetting your marijuana or alcohol tolerance. (I know you are curious, so the answer is yes, my neurofeedback transformed me into a very cheap one-drink date.)

This type of protocol is slightly risky; it's not something for which you can download a free app on your smartphone. Every brain is different, so the single most crucial aspect of neurofeedback training is selecting the proper protocol. While the initial QEEG scan provides vital information about your brain, the training plan needs to be adaptive and iterative, based on how you personally respond to the training. This is why it is important to have the entire testing and training process overseen by a neurofeedback practitioner. Heck, when I did my three months of training with the Peak Brain Institute, Dr. Hill and I were text and email buddies nearly every day, and he now has a dedicated Slack channel, with overseas assistants who can handle off-hours questions.

Two of the longest, most immersive neurofeedback protocols are Biocybernaut (biocybernaut.com) and 40 Years of Zen (40yearsofzen.com). Practitioners claim that these protocols are the equivalent of several years of practicing Zen or meditation. During these programs, you spend a full week immersed in a combination of neurofeedback and brain wave entrainment. They are not for the faint of heart and are guaranteed to lighten your wallet. But they can permanently improve alpha brain wave production, thus enhancing creativity and focus for the rest of your life.

Many brain biohackers immerse themselves in these more intensive programs, and they are certainly good options if you have the time and money to dedicate to them. I personally prefer a handful of thirty-minute sessions each week in my own home, which is, I think, a far more sustainable approach, similar to engaging in short meditation sessions every day instead of doing one intensive ten-day Vipassana meditation course each year.

As a word of caution, neurofeedback can produce side effects, such as panic attacks, nausea, fatigue, sleep disturbances, and irritability. But if you follow the correct protocol with the correct electrode placements, most side effects are minor and short-lived, and they can even be quite informative to a neurofeedback practitioner. If you experience adverse effects, protocols can be adjusted to steer the brain in a different direction. But if you are training yourself with no supervision and no sense of what is actually happening in your brain, you can easily cause adverse effects, and if you continue engaging in unsupervised neurofeedback, these adverse effects can become permanent. So proceed with caution and the understanding that neurofeedback is indeed a powerful brain-enhancing strategy—when done properly.

Furthermore, it's important to understand that with neurofeedback, there are a wide variety of methods that each act in different ways to help your brain to function better, including the following:

- Z-score training
- LENS (low energy neurofeedback system)
- Low-frequency training
- Loretta training
- pROSHI
- NeurOptimal training
- CES (cranial electrotherapy stimulation)

These forms of neurofeedback all differ in subtle but important ways, and the average neurofeedback clinician spends many hours in training, often to learn just one specific method. This training includes how to properly position electrodes, which frequencies affect specific symptoms, and which protocols enhance certain areas, such as increasing memory, word recall, or athletic performance. Because of this, it's important not to "cowboy" neurofeedback on yourself with some random device you buy on the internet but to instead ensure that you work closely with a practitioner who is well versed in the protocol you've chosen for your specific needs. The website EEGInfo.com contains a good searchable directory to help you find a certified neurofeedback practitioner in your area.

3. Photobiomodulation

Scattered across the internet are several photos of me wearing a giant laser-light device on my head lighting up my skull like a Christmas tree, along with a nasal light probe shoved up my left nostril. The device, called a Vielight, operates on the principle of photobiomodulation, or PBM. I consider it to be the equivalent of a strong cup of coffee, most notably for the head.

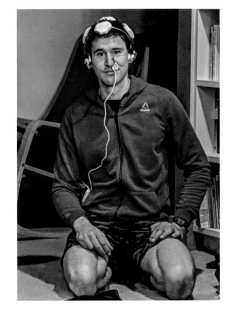

PBM can not only regulate or even reset your body's circadian rhythm, but it can also shut down inflammation in your brain and produce significant amounts of nitric oxide in neural tissue (NO acts like Viagra for your brain, dilating blood vessels to increase blood flow), boost oxygenation, and enhance memory function and cognition with a form of light called near-infrared light. In the past, you could only find PBM devices in a hospital or expensive clinical setting, but you can now purchase headset devices and have them delivered to your own home.

I consider the Vielight Neuro Gamma to be the crème de la crème of PBM devices, specifically for cognitive enhancement. It uses transcranial intranasal light exposure and includes a light-producing headset that you place over your skull and a small probe that you insert into your nostril. The Neuro Gamma pulses at 40 Hz and has been shown in controlled studies to provide an acute boost in cognitive performance that lasts several hours. If you are an experienced meditator, in seconds it can take you into an enhanced meditative state that would normally require hours to achieve. Elite athletes are also starting to use this type of device for enhanced reflexes and decision-making during competition. (I often pull a stocking cap over the headset so I can walk and move without jostling it too much.)

Via infrared light, the headset and probe stimulate blood capillaries in the nasal cavity, causing nitric oxide production and increased mitochondrial activity in neural tissue. Much of the nitric oxide produced not only is felt in your head but also crosses your blood-brain barrier into the rest of your body. This means you can use PBM to beat a hangover, assist with sleep regulation, boost blood flow before a workout, quell brain inflammation, and improve focus. The initial price point of a Vielight Neuro Gamma is a cool $1,750, but considering the potential of PBM to reverse or control conditions like dementia and Alzheimer's, I consider either the Vielight or some other way to expose your skull to near-infrared light waves—such as a Joovv device or near-infrared overhead lamp—to be worth the cost.

As with methylene blue, more is not better when it comes to PBM. You do not want to overstimulate the mitochondria in your brain, as this can result in harmful oxidation. I recommend using a Vielight once every forty-eight hours. The unit is preprogrammed for a twenty-five-minute treatment, after which it automatically turns off, so there is no risk that you will leave it on and forget to turn it off. Finally, most clinical literature indicates that light in the low-to-mid-800 nm to mid-600 nm range is the most beneficial (the Vielight Neuro Gamma operates at 810 nm).

4. Cranial Electrotherapy Stimulation

The original brain-biohacking wearable was an electric ray, also known as a torpedo fish. Yep, you read that right. In AD 46, the personal physician to the Roman emperor Claudius applied a live electric ray to the emperor's forehead to successfully relieve his migraines. Don't believe me? Check out the article I wrote entitled "Thousands of Years Before Modern Electricity, Ancient Romans Used Electrotherapy to Effectively Treat Neurological Conditions," which you'll find on BoundlessBook.com/6.

The electrotherapy was provided by the twitching underbelly of the enraged fish. It filled the patient's nose with its fishy scent and delivered an initially painful and then numbing electric shock (roughly the same pleasant voltage as a hair dryer dropped into a bathtub). "These are still the early days of wearable neurostimulation," an ancient tech blogger would have reported. "But on the bright side, the device, while possessing eyes and teeth, is at least conveniently wireless." Heh.

Today, we know that electrically stimulating the trigeminal nerve, which runs in part beneath the forehead, does suppress migraines. Indeed, the FDA approved the first wearable neurostimulation device to treat migraines in 2012, and the device's primary electrode is placed on the forehead. There are now several available devices that are far more comfortable than an electric ray. The type of brain stimulation they use is called "cranial electrotherapy stimulation" (CES), also known by the far less marketable term "electroconvulsive therapy" (ECT). They cause your body to release large amounts of dopamine and serotonin, resulting in a state of deep relaxation, no drugs required.

CES first came into use in 1938. The original CES user experience was significantly worse than having an electric ray placed on your head, as Jack Nicholson vividly demonstrated in the 1975 film *One Flew Over the Cuckoo's Nest*. That film effectively branded CES, and neurostimulation in general, for the next thirty years as something barbaric, despite the fact that anesthesia was widely used for CES procedures. In fact, since the 1970s, CES patients have quietly slept through their shock therapy and have woken up feeling better. But you wouldn't know that from the movie.

The 1970s also saw the rise of psychiatric medications, which provided a far superior user experience to CES—at least initially. This innovation inspired a small group of electrical engineers to partner with medical researchers to develop more discreet, noninvasive neurostimulation devices that delivered small, comfortable doses of electricity on a daily basis, as opposed to the infrequent, seizure-inducing doses of previous forms of CES. The idea was to achieve a sort of "user-experience parity" between a daily antidepressant pill and a low, daily dose of electricity. By the mid-1970s, several well-controlled published studies had validated small-dose, alternating-current electrotherapy for the treatment of depression, anxiety, and insomnia. A handful of devices emerged from these studies as something that doctors were willing to prescribe, and in 1976, the FDA ushered cranial electrotherapy stimulation devices into the modern era of federal regulation.

These early devices were often the size of small typewriters and were not well suited for home use, and none were successfully commercialized for the mass market. But by the 1980s, electrical engineers had developed a small, portable CES device that deployed two simple electrodes worn beneath a headband. Not only was the device easy and comfortable to use, but it generated multiple frequencies that allowed its alternating current to reach deep within the brain. The stimulation effectively dampened the brain's default mode network, a central region of the brain that is hyperactive during periods of stress.

CES has advanced far beyond early forms of therapy, and these devices are now available to anyone, even without a physician's prescription. The CES device I use is called a Circadia, and it works like gangbusters if I am agitated, frustrated, moody, or overwhelmed; if I'm having difficulty relaxing and quieting my mind; or if I have a headache, insomnia, jitteriness, or a tight jaw. A similar device is DAVID Delight Pro by Mind Alive, which features audiovisual entrainment (see below) in addition to CES. To settle down the brain or get a slight pick-me-up without the use of an electric ray, using a CES device is a handy strategy.

5. Brain Wave Entrainment

As you learned earlier in this chapter, brain wave entrainment involves using external stimuli to synchronize your brain's electrical activity. It is based on the fact that your brain tends to change its dominant electrical frequency to that of whatever dominant external stimulus it is exposed to. This allows you to enter different states of consciousness, such as deep relaxation or expanded awareness.

Audio and visual brain wave entrainment techniques are less targeted than neurofeedback but easier to use. During a brain wave entrainment session, you temporarily increase communication between your brain's right and left hemispheres, a process called hemispheric synchronization, which is similar to what you would achieve with a microdose of LSD or when learning a new skill.

Most brain wave entrainment devices use either an app or software that connects to the headphones, either through Bluetooth or through a wire connected to a smartphone or computer. There are also separate handheld devices that connect to headphones and eyewear. For example, brain wave entrainment apps use audio signals like binaural beats, and monaural tones are ideally used with headphones so that both ears receive the signal simultaneously. Others rely on isochronic tones, which are single tones that sound repeatedly, and do not require headphones. One of the most popular apps is Holosync, which entrains your brain into a delta brain wave state to reduce stress.

Other devices use artificial intelligence algorithms to create soundtracks that elicit focus, creativity, or relaxation by triggering specific brain wave responses; Brain.fm is one of the most popular. For sleep and relaxation, which is primarily what I use sounds for, I am partial to binaural beats combined with artificial intelligence, and for that, I use the white noise and binaural beats app SleepStream combined with Brain.fm. I often play the two simultaneously through noise-blocking headphones while I sleep. That may sound like a potent combination (and I'll describe it in more detail in chapter 7), but my head hasn't exploded yet.

Another effective approach is the use of audiovisual machines. These small, phone-sized devices use pulses of auditory and visual stimuli to alter brain waves. One of the better units is the DAVID Delight mentioned earlier, which also contains a built-in CES feature. I own one of these and have found it to be useful when I'm on an airplane or in another stressful environment and I want to block out all stimuli; when I don't have the time or ability to take a nap; and when I want to use a bit of better living through science to enhance focus or meditation. I consider it, from a sensory standpoint, to be the technological equivalent of a float tank.

Finally, there are entrainment-based headbands that can be used specifically for sleep, meditation, or relaxation. These headbands are made of soft, comfortable fabric that wraps around your head and contains sensors that detect and react to your sleep patterns. For example, when the sensors detect deep, delta slow-wave sleep, the speakers inside the headband play audio tones that increase the brain's production of delta brain waves. Currently, these headbands include the Dreem, Sleep Shepherd, and Philips SmartSleep. These devices also connect to apps that track your sleep data, send you tips for improving your sleep, and even gently wake you in the morning during your lightest sleep stage and in the time range you select. The bad part? Several of my colleagues and I have tested the electromagnetic fields coming from these devices, and they all— at least at this point, in terms of the limitations of the technology—produce very high amounts of dirty electricity (explained in detail in chapter 20) directly next to your head when they are communicating with a smartphone: the equivalent of holding a cell phone next to your head during the entire night. So be sure you are not wearing the device on your head when you sync it to a phone.

6. N-Back Training

If you see me, eyebrows furrowed and fumbling with my smartphone, waiting to board a flight, standing in line at the DMV, or waiting for a chiropractic adjustment, it is highly likely that I am using an n-back training app.

Available in free or inexpensive phone apps and computer software, n-back training involves increasingly difficult levels requiring recall of certain letters and numbers—and sometimes sounds. A University of Switzerland study and a German study demonstrated that just a few weeks of n-back training can increase executive function (the mental processes that enable you to plan, focus, recall instructions, and successfully multitask), along with the abilities to practice mental discipline, concentrate intently on one task while ignoring all else, mentally compartmentalize activities, direct attention with extreme specificity, and apply all creative energy toward one task until it's completed. In other words, n-back training induces the exact opposite of ADD symptoms. Considering their ease of use and affordability, I think everybody should have one of these apps on their computer, smartphone, or e-reader. In fact, if you want to introduce a child in your life to technology that can upgrade the brain, n-back training is a good choice.

Monday Through Friday

If you work at a desk, use a PEMF device in alpha brain wave mode in your office or home workstation. The device does not need to be touching your skin to work properly and can enhance your focus. To boost the focus-enhancing effects, pipe Brain.fm focus tracks through your speakers or headphones.

Duck away for a quick nap or recharge session using an audiovisual entrainment device like the DAVID Delight or a CES device like the Circadia, or simply grab the same PEMF device from your desk and switch it into a more relaxing delta brain wave mode.

Monday, Wednesday, and Friday

Do a round of head-boosting photo-biomodulation using a device like a Vielight.

Every Night

Use SleepStream, Brain.fm, or both to lull you into relaxing delta brain waves for a night of sleep. To boost the brain-relaxing effect, use a PEMF device in delta or theta mode.

Yearly

Do a stint of neurofeedback training, such as three months of Peak Brain Institute training at home or an immersive week in a program like Biocybernaut or 40 Years of Zen.

Saturday or Sunday

Play a round of n-back training. Keep an n-back app handy so you can toy around with it when waiting to board a flight, when you are stuck in line, or when you have a long ride in the back of a taxi or Uber.

THE LAST WORD

Perhaps you are thinking, "Couldn't I just do a crossword puzzle, play sudoku, or read a riddle book?" Sure. But while these brain exercises do help age-proof your brain and keep it functioning at peak capacity, none are as powerful as the methods described in this chapter. Should you want to go the simple route anyway, just know that to qualify as an effective brain exercise, an activity must present your brain with novelty, variety, and challenge.

In addition to crossword puzzles, brain aerobic books, new board games, and new mind-challenging sports such as ping-pong (did you know table tennis players are the smartest athletes on the planet, and, along the same lines, top chess players achieve longevity benefits similar to elite athletes'?), brain training can also include structured apps like Fit Brains or the Lumosity or Brainscape apps, which allow you to create your own flash cards and learning activities. To stay on the cutting edge of brain-hacking gear, I also recommend you check out Quantified Self (quantifiedself.com), an online community of people tracking their own N=1 experiments.

Should all this information be slightly overwhelming, I have included in this summary a practical sample week of brain training with the devices you have just discovered.

ONE THING YOU CAN
DO THIS WEEK

Pick one of the following tasks for this week:

- Download an n-back training app and commit to practicing for just five minutes per day for seven days in a row.

- If you don't mind spending money, buy one of the pieces of headgear described in this chapter. Your options include the Vielight Neuro Alpha or Gamma, Halo Sport, Circadia, or noise-blocking headphones combined with SleepStream or Brain.fm.

- Choose one activity that makes smoke come out of your ears, like learning a new song on an instrument (or learning a new instrument!), playing ping-pong or tennis, doing a crossword puzzle, or reading a book about a complex topic.

For citations for all the research studies mentioned in this chapter and a deeper dive into the topics of this chapter—including links to podcasts, blog posts, recommended tools and supplements, and much more—visit BoundlessBook.com/6.

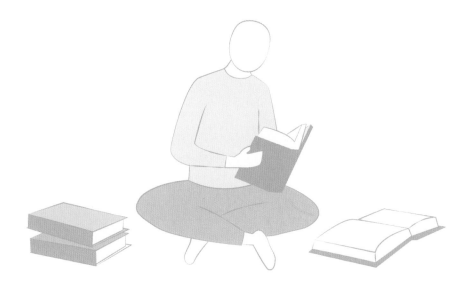

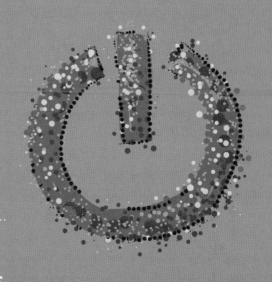

07

SLEEP

HOW TO FIX JET LAG, NAP LIKE A CHAMP, AND TRACK SLEEP CYCLES

Within five minutes of crashing into my dual-gel-layer mattress, I placed two tiny electrodes on either side of my head to lull my brain into a state of enhanced serotonin and dopamine production and cortisol elimination. Pumped into both ears via noise-blocking headphones were "sleep beats" that eased me into a delta brain wave state, along with AI-generated sleep sounds that "confused" my brain into being tired.

A small device on my collarbone sent a pulsed electromagnetic signal into my brain via the nerve plexus near my neck to generate even more delta waves. Because it had been a particularly stressful day, I placed a similar device near the occipital bone on the back of my head. On my bedside table, a nebulizing oil diffuser misted a lavender-rose-bergamot oil blend into the air, enveloping me in a sleep-inducing aroma. Surging under my body was 55-degree water generated by a small box next to my bed. I removed my blue-light-blocking glasses and, to enter a state of calm relaxation, replaced them with a luscious, silky wraparound sleep mask, which my wife had affectionately dubbed my "sleep princess mask."

Perhaps she is right. Maybe I am a sleep princess. But I will own it because I consider the emphasis I place on sleep quantity and quality to be crucial to much of my career, relationship, and athletic success. Sleep, as you'll learn in this chapter, is critical for cognitive function, focus, and self-control, and poor or insufficient sleep can cause everything from poor blood sugar control to inflammation to food cravings, poor recovery, and even depression.

While my pre-sleep routine may seem like a laborious flurry of unnecessary activities, it is actually a series of fully automated habits that takes me less than five minutes to complete. Sure, it has a lot of components, but I am a relentless self-experimenter and immersive journalist whose job involves testing what does and doesn't work for enhancing relaxation and deep sleep, and I don't expect everyone to go to such extremes. But small sleep-routine adjustments—such as optimizing your bedroom's nightly temperature or changing your brain wave frequencies with simple pieces of technology—can add up quite quickly and improve your health and productivity.

Fact is, since cracking the code on sleep with even the simplest methods in this chapter, my sleep quality has been shockingly good, whether I am curled up in a sleeping bag after a day of bowhunting in the mountains of Colorado or passed out on an airplane while flying to Dubai to speak to a roomful of antiaging docs. In this chapter, you are going to discover all these tactics—the tried-and-true, in-the-trenches techniques for enhancing sleep.

SLEEP 101

I sleep seven and a half to nine hours per twenty-four-hour period. Usually, I sleep seven to eight hours at night and take a twenty-to-sixty-minute nap during the day. When I hit this target, my workouts are better, my heart rate is healthy, my nerves are sharp, and my creativity and memory peak.

That may seem like a lot of sleep to you, but sleep is pretty darn important. If someone says he needs less sleep than the average person, 99 percent of the time he is lying to you or to himself, or both. Granted, not everyone responds to sleep loss the same way. Studies on twins have uncovered surprising genetic variations that may protect some people from sleep deprivation. For example, the p.Tyr362His variant of the BHLHE41 gene allows some people to maintain normal alertness and show limited signs of inflammation on less sleep. But this genetic variation is rare, and, as you will learn later in this chapter, most people need at least seven hours of sleep per night.

Even celebrities and athletes who don't sleep much—the "sleepless elite," like Barack Obama, Dean Karnazes, Martha Stewart, and Donald Trump, all of whom claim to sleep only four or five hours per night—are probably sacrificing something in other parts of their lives to get such small amounts of shut-eye. Somewhere in their work, creativity or memory is suffering. Somewhere in their body, inflammation is running rampant. Somewhere in a muscle or brain cell, regeneration is not occurring. This is the kind of biological damage you invite when you don't sleep enough, especially when you combine lack of sleep with intense physical or mental activity. In fact, if you don't sleep in a twenty-four-hour period, you will die sooner.

Okay, that may be a slight exaggeration. After all, nearly everyone has pulled an all-nighter at least once. While it can be an unpleasant experience, you can almost entirely recover from the damages of a lost night of sleep with a single night of eight or nine hours' sleep. (The strategies on the facing page will help.)

In Case You're Wondering

The introduction to this chapter may already have you curious about my pre-sleep tools. In order of appearance, they are:

- The Intellibed mattress
- The Circadia electrical stimulation device
- The SleepStream app
- The Brain.fm app
- The SomniResonance SR1 PEMF device
- The FlexPulse PEMF device
- The BodyBalance PEMF mat

- Lavender, rose, and bergamot essential oils from Young Living or Essential Oil Wizardry
- A nebulizing oil diffuser
- The chiliPAD
- Blue-light-blocking glasses
- The Sleepmaster sleep mask

Because I am an immersive journalist and biohacker, my methods and tools can change from month to month, but at the time of this writing, those are my biggest wins for sleep. You'll find links to all the sleep-enhancing tools mentioned in this chapter, along with constant updates to my relaxation, napping, and sleep routines, at BoundlessBook.com/7.

1. Stay Hydrated

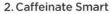

Your cells require both water and minerals to maintain the aqueous matrix in which they reside. In times of stress, such as after a night of poor or lost sleep, optimizing your cells' environment becomes even more important. When fighting through sleep loss, go out of your way to consume trace mineral drops, trace liquid minerals, quality sea salt (such as Colima sea salt), and plenty of water. This will also help control the raging appetite that sleep deprivation notoriously causes.

2. Caffeinate Smart

Don't overconsume coffee. Despite the exhaustion you may feel from sleep deprivation, consuming too much caffeine may reduce the quality of the next night's sleep. This will make you even more tired the next day, so that you have to drink even more coffee, and the cycle will continue.

One or two 8-ounce cups of coffee during the day will keep your eyes open without derailing your next night of sleep. Pass on the energy drinks and quad-shot caramel frappés, and prepare your caffeine wisely. Extra sugar means an extra-hard crash.

3. Move It

The best way to reset your internal clock is to get outside, catch some rays, and do some light aerobic exercise, whether it's yoga or a quick walk. The movement, light, and vitamin D will realign your circadian rhythm and eliminate some of your sleep-deprived anxiety. Incidentally, if you perform this routine in an overnight-fasted state, it will enhance your fat-burning capabilities for the rest of the day. (More on that in chapter 8.)

4. Eat Right

Your sleep cycle regulates your appetite. When you are sleep-deprived, your hunger hormone (leptin) levels will be high and your satiated hormone (ghrelin) levels will be low. Don't

opt for refined carbs and fats, which would make you more tired. Your goal is to achieve a slow, steady burn of energy. You can get this from foods that are high in protein, low in fat, and low on the glycemic index. Protein intake also increases the production of orexin, a hormone that keeps you awake and alert.

5. Buffer Immunity

When you are sleep-deprived, your immune system function declines and levels of pro-inflammatory compounds increase. Take 1,000 mg of activated charcoal to flush circulating toxins out of your system, and place four or five drops of oregano oil under your tongue to protect yourself against foodborne and airborne bacteria. To reduce inflammation and boost your immune system, you can also take 1,000 mg of curcumin (turmeric extract) after a night of poor sleep, especially one caused by a bout of alcohol-infused hedonism.

6. Nap Right

While there are certainly dangers that accompany regular polyphasic sleep—sleep in multiple shorter episodes, rather than in one large chunk—it can help you get through a brief period of sleep deprivation. The next time you're facing a long week of studying or you have an impending deadline to meet, try implementing a polyphasic sleep routine. It repairs your body about as much as possible without the proper seven and a half to nine hours of shut-eye that most people need. Get at least three hours of sleep per night, then take three twenty-minute naps throughout the day. This will remediate your lost night of sleep without destroying the next one.

If you really want to upgrade your nap with a highly effective (but admittedly expensive) biohack, I cannot recommend highly enough the NuCalm device, which combines specially programmed sounds that slip you in and out of conscious and subconscious states with a frequency bracelet and vagal nerve simulator. Initial studies of this device indicate that the Powernap function can simulate a full ninety-minute sleep cycle in just twenty minutes! Visit BoundlessBook.com/7 for a link to a fascinating interview I recorded with the inventor of the device.

But cumulative sleep loss is a different story. In one study, researchers constructed a cruel contraption that woke up rats as soon as they fell asleep. Using this contraption, it took an average of three weeks to kill a rat via sleep deprivation. Research also suggests that because sleep deprivation raises cortisol levels and inhibits neurogenesis, it eventually leads to brain damage.

For ethical reasons, researchers cannot reproduce these studies in humans. But by looking at human sleep disorders, you can get a clear idea of what happens when people don't sleep enough. For example, in people with fatal familial insomnia, progressively worsening insomnia caused by a genetic mutation, death occurs within a few months. The autoimmune disease Morvan's syndrome destroys the brain's potassium channels, leading to severe insomnia and, ultimately, death.

Sleep disorders also cause high blood pressure and heart disease and add $16 billion to national health-care costs per year. That doesn't even include the cost of accidents and lost productivity at work, which in America alone amounts to $150 billion per year. Remember the nuclear meltdown at Three Mile Island? The explosion and nuclear fallout at Chernobyl? The gas leak at Bhopal? The Zeebrugge ferry accident? The *Exxon Valdez* oil spill? These and many other industrial disasters have been directly linked to sleep deprivation.

Why is sleep deprivation so fatal? There are two main reasons. The first is that while you sleep, your brain reorganizes neural networks and cleans up cellular garbage, such as metabolic by-products. Throughout the day, even on the most boring day possible, you are consciously or

Does Self-Quantification Suck the Enjoyment out of Sleep and Exercise?

You may be wondering if an apparent obsession with self-quantification and biohacking is actually healthy. Should you quantify metrics such as exercise and sleep, or are there proven drawbacks? Are there hidden costs?

Turns out an article in the *Journal of Consumer Research* looked into this and reported on the results of six experiments on devices that measured activities such as walking or reading.

For example, in one experiment, researchers had 105 students color in shapes for a few minutes, then rate how much they enjoyed it. Those who got numerical feedback on their coloring (such as "You have colored one shape") colored more shapes, but they reported that they enjoyed it less.

In two other experiments, researchers gave one hundred people pedometers (step-counting devices) to wear through the day. Just like the coloring students, the people wearing the pedometers walked more than the people without pedometers but also reported enjoying the activity less, even when they didn't have access to the device's feedback and metrics. So it seems the mere act of wearing a device during an activity may take some of the enjoyment out of it.

In another experiment, three hundred students who read for a brief period of time while having their reading metrics recorded did, as you'd probably guess, read more than a control group, but the measured group

enjoyed the reading less, especially when they could see how many pages they had read (ahem: Kindle, anyone?).

The article in the *Journal of Consumer Research* hypothesized that this phenomenon occurs because measuring an activity can undermine intrinsic motivation to complete the activity. By drawing attention to the output rather than the process, constant measurement and quantification can make enjoyable activities feel more like work, thus reducing their enjoyment. The consequence of this can be decreased engagement in the activity and decreased subjective well-being.

So in summary: measuring something like exercise may make you exercise more but enjoy the exercise less. The same could potentially be said of sleep. Sure, you might quantify a good night of sleep, but did you wake up wondering about your sleep metrics rather than being grateful that you feel like a million bucks?

I'm not about to stop quantifying. But based on these findings, I've implemented some rules to keep quantification from ruining my enjoyment:

1. **I track, but I don't obsess.** I wear a self-quantification ring nearly every day, but I don't obsess over the results or run statistical evaluations on them daily. Instead, at the end of the day, I take a quick glance at just a few key metrics. Did I do a good job not sitting for unbroken periods longer than an hour? Did

subconsciously learning new things, memorizing facts or task processes, acquiring skills, and building memories through creative associations. By the end of each day, your brain is full of discrete pieces of information that have to be integrated with all the other information you have stored over your lifetime.

If this reorganization doesn't occur, your mind becomes a chaotic storehouse for cellular garbage and you run out of space for new memories. This affects nearly every function of your body that is governed by your central nervous system and causes the following:

- Poor heat regulation
- A decline in immune function
- Increased levels of cortisol, catecholamines, interleukin, C-reactive protein, and other stress and inflammatory hormones
- Imbalances in appetite- and blood-sugar-regulating hormones

This is why sleep deprivation makes it so freakin' hard to run, cycle, swim, race, or do a WOD, much less make it through a day of mentally demanding work. Your body is chock-full of inflammation, hormone imbalances, and blood sugar dysregulation and is operating well below peak capacity. Fact is, many people live much of their adult lives in this state, thinking it is completely normal to feel like a walking zombie.

I reach my daily goal of fifteen thousand steps? Was my heart rate or body temperature higher than it usually is, indicating excessive stress or overtraining? Then I move on, always reminding myself that it's more important to spend your time experiencing life, not analyzing it or staring at a screen that tells you how your life is going.

2. **I'm careful with electrical pollution.** As I discuss in my podcast episode "Is Bluetooth Radiation Dangerous?," I am careful not to put devices on my body that constantly emit a WiFi signal or a Bluetooth signal. I simply haven't seen enough research to feel confident that this type of constant exposure is safe or healthy in the long term.

3. **I listen to my body.** If a self-quantification device tells you that you exceeded your daily activity goals, you might be tempted to have a slice of cheesecake after dinner, even if you're not hungry. Or, if your device tells you that you got forty-five minutes less sleep than you normally do, you might be tempted to be tired or grumpy that day, even if you're really not that tired. So every morning, I'm always careful to take some quiet time to listen to my body and feel out what my energy levels really are, and when I have a day full of activity, I'm always careful not to stuff my face as some kind of reward or refueling effort and instead eat mindfully, asking myself whether I am actually hungry or whether I'm just having a knee-jerk reaction to technology.

4. **I recognize the value of intrinsic motivation.** Extrinsic motivation comes from knowing your ring or your bracelet is tracking what you're doing; somebody on social media is watching you; or there is some kind of event you've signed up for, like a triathlon, where people will see you try to achieve your goals. There's nothing wrong with that. But you need to recognize the value of intrinsic motivation, too. Intrinsic motivation arises from the experience of simply enjoying something—you get some kind of joy, some kind of satisfaction, some kind of feeling of competence from the activity. You're establishing a deeper connection with yourself, whether you're exercising or sleeping. So sometimes it is important to stop and, not necessarily remove your self-quantification device, but ask yourself whether you'd be enjoying and doing what it is that you're doing if it wasn't being quantified—focusing on not just the destination (like the achievement of fifteen thousand steps) but the journey (the sun on your face and wind on your skin as you take those fifteen thousand steps).

Okay, I'll step off my soapbox now. Don't worry about self-quantification ruining your life, but be careful with exposure to technology, obsessing too much, and forgetting to occasionally just unplug, listen to your body, and follow your intrinsic motivation. And if you find that exercise is no longer enjoyable or your sleep is becoming disrupted, try completely removing your device for a few days and see whether that changes things!

It is important to understand that the fix is not an easy day or a period of putting your feet up. Unlike rest or conservation of energy, neural repair requires your brain to be entirely shut off from input. This means you must be asleep for your neurons to recover.

The second reason you will die if you don't sleep is that sleep is the primary anabolic state of the human body. As you sleep, your body produces necessary growth hormone and testosterone, important muscle-repairing hormones that also enhance neural growth. The researchers from one study stated that these hormonal surges play a "crucial role in consolidating and enhancing waking experience." This is why you feel so damn good after a solid night of sleep. It is also why your body can take two to three times longer to repair and recover from physical exercise when you are sleep-deprived.

Sleep enhances not only neural and muscular repair but also adrenal gland function, liver detoxification, and immune system function. In fact, one of the leading causes of death in those sleep-deprived rats I mentioned earlier was bacterial infections resulting from a decline in immune function. New research shows that severe sleep loss jolts the immune system into a state of imbalanced hyperactivity, the same type of immediate response shown during exposure to stress. This is why I shake my head and feel sorry for people who brag about how little they sleep. They are shrinking their brains, shrinking their muscles, and making themselves sick.

YOUR CIRCADIAN RHYTHM DECODED

Before diving into the tactics that will prevent sleep-related health damage, it is important to understand the basics of circadian rhythm. Everything in the rest of this chapter will make more sense if you know what a twenty-four-hour cycle of sleeping and waking looks like, as well as how your body responds to factors like sunrise, meal timing, workout timing, sex, and sunset. As you read through this section, you will discover many of my own practical tips, so don't skip it because you don't like science. I promise to make it easy to understand!

Around 6:00 a.m., cortisol levels rise and, to wake you up, stimulate certain activities, such as increasing the heart rate and glucose uptake by the brain. At the same time, your body releases the hormone vasoactive intestinal polypeptide, fittingly called VIP. VIP stimulates actions associated with waking activity, such as vasodilation, increased contractility (strength of contraction) in your heart, and liver glycogenolysis (the breakdown of liver glycogen stores to elevate your blood sugar). All these activities result in more blood, nutrients, and oxygen being delivered to your brain, muscles, and other tissues.

VIP also relaxes the smooth muscles of your trachea, stomach, and gallbladder, allowing for a glorious bowel movement within two hours of waking. I have personally found that with a half teaspoon of the Ayurvedic herbal formula triphala at night and 400 mg of magnesium (in the form magnesium malate, found in the supplement MagSRT) with a piping-hot cup of black coffee in the morning, I can poop at around 8:30 every morning, two hours after I wake. VIP also promotes the secretion of ghrelin, the hormone responsible for making you hungry. If you have imbalances in ghrelin levels, which often manifest as cravings throughout the day, it is crucial to eat a meal within two hours of waking because a regularly timed breakfast helps reset your hormonal cycle. In this case, skipping breakfast to fast may do more harm than good (despite the benefits that accompany fasting and caloric restriction, which will be explored in depth in chapter 19).

Within your eyes and skin are cells known as photoreceptors, a type of light-sensitive neural cell. These photoreceptors turn light into electrical signals that trigger waking activity and regulate your circadian rhythm. By exposing yourself to sunlight in the morning, you can not only maximize cortisol's effects on your body but also stimulate your photoreceptors to enhance both your daily energy levels and your nightly sleep. The blue light that the sun produces in the morning interacts with your photoreceptors to improve alertness and mood, jump-start your circadian rhythm, and suppress levels of the hormone melatonin, which is responsible for making you feel tired. Morning sun exposure not only shifts your circadian rhythm back, allowing you to fall asleep more easily at your desired bedtime, but can even cause cortisol levels to decline earlier in the evening, so you don't have excessively high cortisol levels when you go to bed. To get these energy- and sleep-enhancing benefits, go for a simple twenty-to-thirty-minute morning walk, hike, or bicycle ride, or do a light yoga or breathwork session outdoors. In addition, as you will learn in chapter 8, doing these activities in a fasted state first thing in the morning will enhance your ability to burn fat for the rest of the day.

If you can't get morning sun exposure, you can still maximize cortisol's effects with light to moderate amounts of coffee, green tea, adaptogenic herbs such as the TianChi blend discussed on page 107, or blue-light-producing devices, such as the HumanCharger in-ear device and the Re-Timer glasses. If you opt for artificial light–producing devices, it is best to simulate natural sunlight as closely as possible by including red light exposure with a tool such as a Joovv red light photobiomodulation panel, a Clearlight infrared sauna, or a SaunaSpace red light bulb configuration (see chapter 13 for more information on all of these). But nothing is quite as effective as natural sunlight. This is why you may need little to no coffee in the summer but are a complete bear if you don't have your cup o' joe in the dark winter months. In an ideal scenario, while sipping my morning coffee, I use the HumanCharger and Re-Timer simultaneously for about twenty minutes, then use the bathroom and head outside for a twenty-to-thirty-minute aerobic exercise session in the sun (more on exercise timing later in this chapter).

From the time you wake up—which will vary significantly based on your chronobiology (that is, the genetic preset for your sleep-wake cycles)—until about 11:00 a.m., sex hormone levels peak (good to know if you want to sneak in a quickie before heading to work!). If you are male, and especially if you are under forty-five years old, you produce the most testosterone when you enter the first rapid eye movement (REM) sleep cycle each night and maintain a high production rate until you wake up. After you wake up, testosterone levels decline over the course of the day, with surges in secretion occurring about every ninety minutes. At the end of the day, testosterone levels reach their lowest point, and the cycle begins again when you enter your first REM cycle later that night. Like men, women have daily circadian rhythms, but they also have menstrual cycles that significantly impact their sleep and hormones. For example, hormonal fluctuations associated with the menstrual cycle increase slow-wave (deep) sleep and reduce REM sleep between ovulation and menstruation. Research suggests that women also experience a daily testosterone cycle similar to that of men, although women's testosterone levels cycle at a lower level. Since testosterone is responsible for stimulating sex drive in both men and women, if your libido is flagging, morning sex may help reset your circadian rhythm, especially if you have been having trouble sleeping later at night. Having regular sex in the morning signals your body to release more sex hormones at the ideal times of day, which is important because there is a direct correlation between sleep abnormalities and hormone imbalances.

Around 2:30 p.m., muscle coordination and reaction time peak, and around 5:30 p.m., cardiovascular efficiency, body temperature, protein synthesis, and recovery capacity peak, making these ideal times for intense workouts. When I have the luxury of choosing when to work out, I do my hard workouts in the late afternoon or early evening, finishing at least three hours before bedtime. This is why I encourage folks to do a light aerobic exercise session in the morning and save the hard interval or weight training for later in the day. Not only will it help align your circadian rhythms properly (especially if the morning session is in sunshine), but it will also enable you to perform at peak capacity during your heavy training sessions, enhance your fat-burning rate in the next morning's light aerobic exercise (as long as that exercise is performed in a fasted state), avoid excessively raising cortisol when cortisol is already high, and, if you fast for one to two hours following your afternoon or evening session, even equip you for a surge in growth hormone and testosterone. In addition, if you eat the majority of your carbohydrates in the evening (as I do), training hard late in the day ensures you are highly sensitive to insulin and carbohydrates and far less likely to experience excessive spikes in blood glucose or insulin while still allowing you to top off your energy stores for the next day's activities, and the surge in serotonin that occurs after carbohydrate consumption will help you sleep more soundly.

At sunset, your blood pressure and body temperature peak. While these are normal aspects of your circadian rhythm, I recommend taking a cold shower or cold soak to help your body naturally drop its temperature after you fall asleep (a concept addressed at the end of this section). From sunset to bedtime, which will also vary depending on your chronobiology, the hormones leptin and adiponectin are released to burn fat while you sleep. But high insulin levels, a sedentary afternoon, a high-calorie evening meal, and frequent grazing throughout the day all suppress the secretion of leptin and adiponectin, and even excessive nighttime light exposure can suppress leptin release. To maximize the fat-burning effects of these hormones, avoid high calorie intake in the afternoon and evening or perform a hard workout in the afternoon, and limit your exposure to your smartphone, e-reader, TV, and laptop after sunset. To enhance adiponectin release, you can also take 300 to 500 mg of magnesium before bed. Incidentally, moderate amounts of coconut oil, MCT oil, nut butters, seeds, nuts, and even fructose from raw honey do not significantly spike insulin and may be consumed late in the evening.

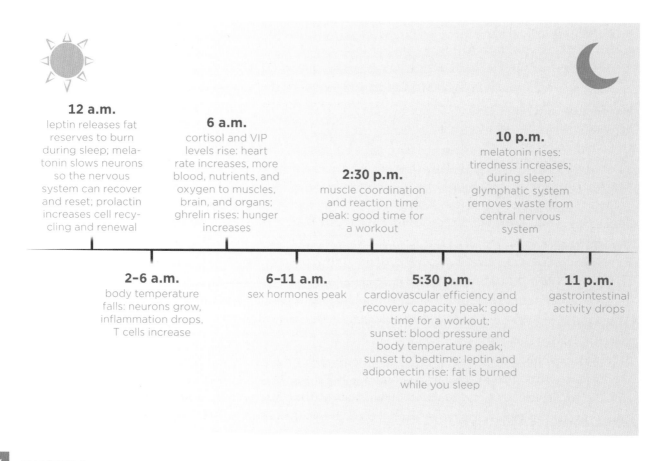

12 a.m.
leptin releases fat reserves to burn during sleep; melatonin slows neurons so the nervous system can recover and reset; prolactin increases cell recycling and renewal

2–6 a.m.
body temperature falls: neurons grow, inflammation drops. T cells increase

6 a.m.
cortisol and VIP levels rise: heart rate increases, more blood, nutrients, and oxygen to muscles, brain, and organs; ghrelin rises: hunger increases

6–11 a.m.
sex hormones peak

2:30 p.m.
muscle coordination and reaction time peak: good time for a workout

5:30 p.m.
cardiovascular efficiency and recovery capacity peak: good time for a workout; sunset: blood pressure and body temperature peak; sunset to bedtime: leptin and adiponectin rise: fat is burned while you sleep

10 p.m.
melatonin rises: tiredness increases; during sleep: glymphatic system removes waste from central nervous system

11 p.m.
gastrointestinal activity drops

Around 10:00 p.m., your body starts secreting the hormone melatonin. Melatonin makes you feel tired by turning off waking brain activity to allow for neural repair and by pulling oxygen and hormones away from the rest of your body. But blue light from your TV, laptop, smartphone, e-reader, and bright household light bulbs can inhibit the production of melatonin, so it is crucial to minimize your exposure to these light sources. You can also use blue-light-blocking glasses, screen dimmers, sleep masks, blue-light-free light bulbs, and blackout curtains to reduce the amount of blue light you are exposed to.

The protein agouti also peaks around 10:00 p.m. Like ghrelin, agouti can stimulate your appetite if leptin levels are suppressed. You can probably see how easy it is to settle into a vicious cycle of poor sleep, weight gain, and cravings: Late-night snacking causes blood glucose fluctuations and elevates insulin levels. This, in turn, suppresses leptin and reduces leptin sensitivity. Leptin levels are then too low to counteract agouti, so you get hungry when you are supposed to be sleepy. Then you eat, insulin levels spike again and suppress leptin, and agouti levels rise even more, and the cycle continues to deteriorate. Sound familiar?

As noted earlier, the exact time you fall asleep will significantly vary depending on your individual chronobiology, but no matter your chronobiology, while you sleep, your glymphatic system becomes active. Like the lymphatic system, the glymphatic system is a drainage network, but it's localized in your brain and spinal cord. Just as your muscles and other tissues accumulate metabolic and inflammatory by-products from normal daily function, your central nervous system can also accumulate by-products and even toxins that, if not removed by the glymphatic system, can result in a state of neurotoxicity. Glymphatic system activity in the brain peaks during slow-wave NREM sleep. A PEMF machine set to delta mode can help improve glymphatic function by allowing you to enter deeper NREM states even faster. Research also suggests that consuming omega-3 fatty acids can improve glymphatic drainage, and, surprisingly, so can your sleeping position (lying on your right side appears to be best). (I'll go into more detail about glymphatic drainage in chapter 17.)

Around 11:00 p.m., gastrointestinal activity declines, so you don't have to poop until the morning. Around 12:00 a.m., leptin enters the hypothalamus in the brain. This is critical from a metabolic standpoint because when leptin enters the hypothalamus, your fat reserves are released. As you sleep, your core temperature falls, and your body has to maintain a set point of warmth. Leptin in your hypothalamus stimulates your mitochondria to produce heat. Just as cold thermogenesis activates brown adipose tissue to burn fat, a good sleep cycle allows leptin to properly enter your hypothalamus, which, in turn, allows your mitochondria to burn fat.

Also around 12:00 a.m., melatonin enters an area of the brain called the suprachiasmatic nucleus and reduces your neuron-firing rate. This slows down your brain, allowing your nervous system to recover and store the day's information. As melatonin peaks, prolactin is also released. A deficiency in prolactin, often found in postmenopausal women, can cause weight gain, reduced brain activity, and high levels of inflammatory cytokines associated with lack of recovery and chronic pain. On the other hand, balanced prolactin levels increase the recycling of cells, the renewal of cells, and the creation of new cells, and promote the release of growth hormone. Research suggests that melatonin is actually responsible for stimulating the release of prolactin, so the same blue-light-elimination strategies for enhancing melatonin secretion will also allow prolactin levels to rise.

Between 2:00 and 6:00 a.m., your core body temperature falls, allowing for neural repair, neural growth, reduced inflammation, and an increase in T cells (the killer cells of your immune system). For your core body temperature to drop, you need to have been asleep for about six hours. So unless you are genetically programmed to be a night owl (more on that later), if you go to sleep at, say, midnight, your body won't be able to repair itself as well. To support my body's temperature fluctuations, I sleep on a device called a chiliPAD (also known as an Ooler), which circulates cool water at my chosen temperature of 55 degrees beneath my body during the night, and I keep my home at about 63 to 65 degrees.

This temperature drop signals your body to produce cortisol at around 6:00 a.m. Then you rinse, wash, and repeat the process of healing your body and building new neurons. Pretty cool, huh? Are you convinced that sleep is important?

WHAT'S YOUR CHRONOBIOLOGY?

My friend Dr. Michael Breus—the author of the book *The Power of When* and a man who's been dubbed, appropriately enough, "America's Sleep Doctor"—is famous for making quite popular the previously little-known fact that not everyone operates at peak physical and cognitive capacity with the recommended 10 p.m.–to–6 a.m. sleep routine.

Sure, I personally feel like a rock star when I am in bed at or slightly before 10:30 p.m. and wake up between 6:00 and 6:30 a.m., but that is because I am, in the words of Dr. Breus, a "Bear" chronotype, along with about 50 percent of the world's population. What does this mean exactly?

Every person has an internal clock that impacts several aspects of his or her physiology, such as sleeping, waking, cognition, and digestion. This clock is called the primary circadian pacemaker, and it's located in the suprachiasmatic nucleus of your brain. Sure, you can control when you sleep, wake, and eat, but your internal clock has a built-in preset for these things based on your genetics. This means that there is a perfect time for everything from exercise to sex to creative work, and when you synchronize your activities with your biological clock, your entire life flows better.

Not every clock keeps the same time, which you probably know if you have heard of "early birds" and "night owls." Traditionally, psychologists and sleep doctors determined chronotypes using a "morningness-eveningness" questionnaire, but after more than a decade of working as a sleep doctor and recognizing the high variability in ideal sleep-wake patterns among his patients, Dr. Breus developed a far more comprehensive and accurate questionnaire (available at ThePowerOfWhenQuiz.com) that sorts people into one of four chronotypes, named for animals: Dolphin, Lion, Bear, and Wolf.

From an evolutionary standpoint, this variation in chronotypes seems to make sense: since our ancestors lived in groups, having a variety of natural sleep and wake times meant that someone was awake to ensure security for the group at all hours. It is also quite interesting to note the chronotype distribution in the average population:

Dolphins: 10 percent
Lions: 15 to 20 percent
Bears: 50 percent
Wolves: 15 to 20 percent

The fact that more people are Bears explains current office and school hours, along with somewhat regular breakfast, lunch, and dinner times and the oft-recommended—in everything from *Reader's Digest* to *Prevention* magazine to *Men's Health* and *Women's Health* magazines—"bed by ten, up by six." This can be pretty damn frustrating if you are not a Bear, especially since you can't change your chronotype. Your chronotype is determined by your PER3 gene; a longer PER3 gene means you tend to be an early riser, and a shorter one means you tend to be a late riser.

The Ideal Routine for Every Type of Person

According to psychologist and sleep specialist Dr. Michael Breus, there are four different chronotypes, or a person's internal clock and rhythm.

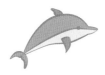

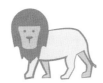

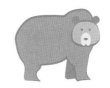

DOLPHIN	**LION**	**BEAR**	**WOLF**
Dolphins are light sleepers and are often diagnosed with insomnia.	Lions tend to wake up early with lots of energy. By early evening, they're exhausted.	Bears' internal clocks track the rise and fall of the sun. They need a full 8 hours of sleep a night.	Wolves have a hard time waking up early and are most energetic in the evenings.

DOLPHIN

6:30 a.m.
Wake up and exercise.

7:30 a.m.
Eat breakfast.

9:30 a.m.
Have coffee.

10 a.m.–12 p.m.
Brainstorm and work on creative projects.

12 p.m.
Eat lunch.

1–4 p.m.
Walk around the block if you're feeling tired.

4–6 p.m.
Work on intellectually demanding tasks. Send professional emails.

6 p.m.
Meditate or do yoga.

6:30–8 p.m.
Eat dinner.

10:30–11:30 p.m.
Turn off all screens. Take a hot shower/bath. Read a novel.

11:30 p.m.
Go to sleep.

LION

5:30 a.m.
Wake up and eat breakfast.

6–7 a.m.
Do planning and big-picture thinking. Meditate.

9–10 a.m.
Have coffee.

10 a.m.–12 p.m.
Hold meetings.

12 p.m.
Eat lunch.

1–5 p.m.
Brainstorm and journal.

5–6 p.m.
Exercise.

6–7 p.m.
Eat dinner.

10 p.m.
Turn off all screens.

10:30 p.m.
Go to sleep.

BEAR

7 a.m.
Wake up and do a few minutes of exercise.

7:30 a.m.
Eat breakfast.

9–10 a.m.
Plan your day.

10 a.m.
Have coffee.

10 a.m.–12 p.m.
Work on difficult tasks. Send professional emails.

12 p.m.
Take a walk, eat lunch, and take another walk.

2:30–2:50 p.m.
Nap or meditate.

3–6 p.m.
Make phone calls and send emails.

6–7 p.m.
Exercise.

7:30 p.m.
Eat dinner.

8–10 p.m.
Brainstorm.

10 p.m.
Turn off all screens.

11 p.m.
Go to sleep.

WOLF

7–7:30 a.m.
Wake up with two alarms. Jot down your thoughts.

7:30 a.m.
Eat breakfast.

8:30 a.m.
Do a few minutes of outdoor exercise.

9 a.m.
Plan your day.

11 a.m.–1 p.m.
Have coffee. Take care of busywork.

1 p.m.
Take a walk and eat lunch.

4–6 p.m.
Hold meetings and present your ideas to coworkers.

6–7 p.m.
Exercise.

8 p.m.
Eat dinner.

11 p.m.
Turn off all screens. Meditate. Take a hot shower.

12 a.m.
Go to sleep.

Ultimately, the classic advice that everyone should wake up early to be successful is just not true, and neither is the recommendation that everyone should go to bed before midnight (I have personally been at fault for recommending just that to folks who are obvious Dolphins or Wolves). Rather than forcing yourself to adhere to the recommended sleep, wake, productivity, and creativity times dished out by books written for a broad, general market, perhaps it is better to determine your unique chronotype and design your schedule to take advantage of your natural rhythms.

Should this seem like you will have a miserable life going to bed at 8:00 p.m. while your friends are just heading out to dinner, or sleeping in until 10:00 a.m. and getting fired from your job, please know that although your chronotype is genetic, you can indeed make some shifts in your activities to move it around just a bit. If you were born a Lion, for example, you will never naturally be able to stay up as late as a born Wolf. But by adjusting the timing of meals, exercise, caffeine intake, and exposure to artificial and natural light, you can make microadjustments to thrive in any society. In addition, your chronotype changes through childhood, adolescence, adulthood (twenty-one to sixty-five), and old age. (My grandmother, who used to go to bed at 11:00 p.m. and rise at 7:00 a.m. to serve me bagels with cream cheese, progressed to going to bed at 1:00 a.m. and sleeping in until 10:00 a.m.)

Finally, if you want to determine your ideal circadian rhythm activities and chronobiology with an even more precise alternative to Dr. Breus's quiz, you may be interested in an app designed by Dr. Satchin Panda, myCircadianClock. The free app is part of Dr. Panda's project to use smartphones to advance research on biological rhythms in the real world, and it will help you track daily behaviors, such as eating, sleeping, moving, and taking supplements and medications. Data that you share through the app is used as part of a research study to help researchers understand how the daily timing of behaviors influences health, and the app provides personalized insights into your daily rhythms. Just don't use it in bed without donning your blue-light-blocking glasses.

THE STAGES OF SLEEP

In 1929, scientists invented the electroencephalogram (EEG), which records brain activity. EEG recordings showed for the first time that sleep is a dynamic behavior, one in which your brain is highly active at times and not simply "turned off," as was previously thought.

Over time, sleep studies using EEGs (and other instruments that measure eye movements and muscle activity) revealed two main types of sleep. These two types of sleep are defined by characteristic brain wave patterns in a sleeping person's brain and the presence or absence of eye movement. These two main types of sleep are rapid eye movement (REM) sleep and non–rapid eye movement (NREM) sleep.

REM sleep (also known as stage 4 sleep) is a unique phase of mammalian sleep characterized by random movement of the eyes, low muscle tone throughout the body, and vivid or lucid dreaming. This phase is also known as "paradoxical sleep" and sometimes "desynchronized sleep" because of its physiological similarities to a waking state, including rapid, low-voltage, desynchronized brain waves—basically a combination of alpha brain waves and beta brain waves.

The Stages of Sleep in One Night

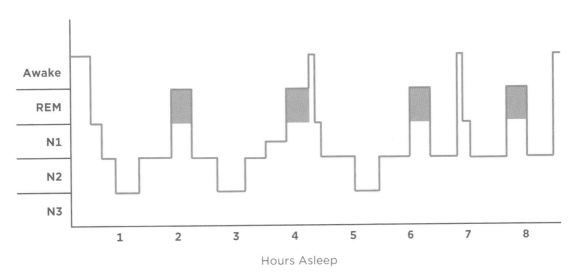

Hours Asleep

Source: Kimberly A. Babson and Matthew T. Feldner, eds., Sleep and Affect: Assessment, Theory, and Clinical Implications (New York: Academic Press, 2015).

During a typical night of sleep, you usually experience about four or five periods of REM sleep, which are quite short at the beginning of the night and longer toward the end. The first REM episode typically occurs about seventy minutes after falling asleep, and the rest of the episodes are about ninety minutes apart. REM sleep typically occupies 20 to 25 percent of total sleep in adult humans, or about one and a half to two hours of a full night's sleep. If you're using a sleep-tracking device, that's the percentage you should be shooting for.

NREM sleep is best defined as any sleep not recognizable as REM sleep. NREM consists of three separate stages: stage 1, stage 2, and stage 3, also known as N1, N2, and N3. N1 and N2 are typically classified as light sleep, and N3 is classified as deep sleep.

N1 (stage 1), often referred to as "drowsy" sleep, is the lightest sleep, on the border between sleep and wakefulness. Your muscles are alert and active, and your eyes slowly move back and forth and may open and close. This is when your brain wave activity transitions from more unsynchronized beta and gamma waves with frequencies of 12 to 30 Hz and 25 to 100 Hz, which are typical of the waking state, to slower, more synchronized alpha waves at a frequency of 8 to 13 Hz and, finally, to 4 to 7 Hz theta waves.

Typically, you don't dream in N1 sleep, but because your muscles are still active, you may suddenly twitch or jerk during short microawakenings as wakefulness gives way to slumber. During this time, which lasts about ten minutes, you may hear sounds and conversations, but you are unwilling to react or respond. This stage should ideally consume about 5 percent of your time asleep.

During N2 (stage 2), muscle activity declines and your awareness of your surroundings fades. Stage 2 brain waves are primarily theta waves, but N2 sleep is distinguished by two traits: (1) sleep spindles, which are short bursts of 12 to 14 Hz brain waves (known as sigma waves) lasting about half a second each, and (2) K complexes, which are short, high-voltage negative peaks followed by slower complexes called "positive complexes," and, finally, another negative K complex peak; each complex lasts one or two minutes. These sleep spindles and K complexes suppress your response to external stimuli, helping to protect your descent into slumber and promote sleep-based memory consolidation and information processing.

You spend more time in N2 than in any other sleep stage: ideally, you should spend 45 to 50 percent of your time asleep in N2. The total of N1 (ideally 5 percent) plus N2 (ideally 45 to 50 percent) is what a sleep-tracking device like the Oura ring quantifies as total light sleep and should be around 50 to 55 percent on a sleep quantification reading.

Finally, N3 (stage 3) is variously known as "deep sleep," "delta sleep," or "slow-wave sleep." It's characterized by delta brain waves with a frequency of around 0.5 to 4 Hz. During N3, your awareness of your surroundings declines even more, so that you're unaware of sights, sounds, or any other external stimuli. Your breathing rate, heart rate, brain temperature, blood pressure, and neural activity all reach their lowest levels. You're more likely to dream during this stage than in any other NREM stage, and you may also experience parasomnias like sleepwalking, night terrors, and talking in your sleep. During N3, memory consolidation and information processing also occur.

If someone tried to wake you up, they'd have more difficulty during N3. If you did wake up, you'd likely feel very groggy, and it would take you about thirty minutes to break away from sleep inertia and reach normal levels of mental performance. Many new alarm clocks and self-quantification devices sync to your phone or cause a vibration or alarm to occur during the point in the morning when you are *not* in this stage of sleep (I think that's a quite handy feature).

N3 sleep should ideally make up around 15 to 20 percent of your total sleep time.

Okay, so let's review what kind of percentages you should be looking for when analyzing your sleep data:

Awake time should be 1 to 5 percent
REM sleep should be 20 to 25 percent
Light sleep (N1 + N2) should be 50 to 55 percent
Deep sleep should be 15 to 20 percent

To go through all the stages of sleep takes about ninety minutes, and you should ideally go through four to five of these sleep cycles during any twenty-four-hour period. A twenty-to-sixty-minute nap can actually quite closely simulate a cycle similar to the ninety-minute cycles you go through during a night of sleep.

I'm not even going to pretend that I track my sleep cycles every night. I'm not that anal. (I don't count my calories every day, either.) I did log my sleep cycles for one month to determine the quality of my sleep, just as I counted my calories for one year to get an idea of how many calories are in the foods I eat. But if you are anything like me, once you have an idea of how your lifestyle choices affect your body, you can't waste precious time testing and tracking. Think of tracking as a temporary educational tool.

The tool that I have found to be most useful is an easy-to-use ring called the Oura, which tracks sleep time, sleep stages, sleep onset latency, nighttime sleep temperature, and a host of other sleep parameters. It can even be placed into airplane mode before sleeping if you want to reduce your Bluetooth exposure (which I recommend). You can find a few podcasts and articles I've done on this device on BoundlessBook.com/7.

HOW MUCH SLEEP
DO YOU REALLY NEED?

Age, genetics, environment, and differences in daily physical and mental strain can all cause significant variations in the ideal amount of sleep.

The National Sleep Foundation (NSF) has general guidelines based on their relatively up-to-date research (see the table at right), but these guidelines do not account for the significant chronobiological variations that occur from person to person.

But you can at least get a basic idea of sleep needs from the NSF guidelines. For most adults, not only is sleeping fewer than seven hours per night associated with reduced alertness and increased risk of chronic disease, but sleeping more than nine hours per night is also associated with an increased risk of chronic disease and even a shorter life span! That's right: more sleep is not necessarily better.

However, physical activity significantly affects sleep requirements: the more active you are, the more sleep you need. In my experiences with triathletes, UFC fighters, and NBA players, athletes who must perform at elite levels need ten to twelve hours of sleep per twenty-four-hour period, and the typical CrossFitter, marathoner, cyclist, or exercise fanatic needs seven and a half to nine hours of sleep per twenty-four-hour period. Here are some of the more interesting statistics on sleep in athletes and exercise enthusiasts:

- Maximum bench press drops by twenty pounds after four days of sleep restriction.
- With proper sleep, tennis players see a 42 percent increase in hitting accuracy.
- Sleep loss causes an 11 percent reduction in time to exhaustion, meaning you get tired faster when exercising.
- Perceived exertion increases 17 percent to 19 percent after thirty hours of sleep deprivation.

There are also other effects of sleep restriction on performance indicators. The T cells of your immune system become hyperactive, and levels of leukocytes, neutrophils, monocytes, natural killer cells, and pro-inflammatory compounds increase. You become less sensitive to insulin,

Three Simple Changes for Better Sleep

After reading the Ayurvedic medicine and lifestyle book *Change Your Schedule, Change Your Life,* I began to incorporate three primary practices from that book that drastically improved my sleep quality:

1. Go to bed at the same time each night, preferably before 10:30 p.m. (although the best bedtime for you will depend on your chronobiology).

2. Do some light exercise before breakfast.

3. Avoid eating a mega-meal for dinner and instead make lunch the largest meal of the day.

I suspect that these three ancestral Eastern medicine rules primarily apply to the 50 percent of the population who fall into Dr. Breus's "Bear" category and may not apply to other chronotypes, but they have worked quite well for me, and many Ayurvedic physicians frequently recommend them.

Sleep Needs by Age

Newborns (0–3 months)	14–17 hours
Infants (4–11 months)	12–15 hours
Toddlers (1–2 years)	11–14 hours
Preschoolers (3–5)	10–13 hours
School-age children (6–13)	9–11 hours
Teenagers (14–17)	8–10 hours
Younger adults (18–25)	7–9 hours
Adults (26–64)	7–9 hours
Older adults (65+)	7–8 hours

Source: "How Much Sleep Do We Really Need?," National Sleep Foundation, www.sleepfoundation.org/articles/how-much-sleep-do-we-really-need.

which results in poor blood sugar regulation and weight gain. Levels of cortisol, epinephrine, norepinephrine, and dopamine increase, resulting in an overstimulated sympathetic nervous system, elevated heart rate, poor recovery processes such as muscle protein synthesis and digestion, and reduced amounts of IGF-1, growth hormone, and testosterone. You also experience increased psychological stress and have an increased risk of suffering from anxiety or depression.

If you are moderately or highly active or regularly compete at a high level, it may take you around forty-five minutes to fall asleep, compared to the fifteen to twenty minutes it takes the average well-rested person. You may also have trouble getting enough sleep, even with naps, especially when going through periods of heavy training and leading up to a competition. A study of 632 high-performance athletes showed that over 65 percent of them exhibited sleep alterations the day before a competition, and other research suggests that the figure is as high as 80 percent.

Sleep restriction is a significant injury risk factor and is accompanied by notable reductions in neuromuscular control and proprioception (your coordination and awareness of your movements). The increase in proinflammatory cytokines noted above is likely why sleep-deprived athletes have high rates of upper respiratory tract infections. Long-term sleep restriction causes a progressive reduction in maximum and submaximum strength in a host of different exercises, and restricting sleep can also reduce the respiratory rate and time to exhaustion in maximum incremental exercise tests. In other words, the more active you are, the more sleep deprivation is going to hurt you, because you will be unable to perform at peak capacity and recover fully.

When I interviewed renowned sleep coach Nick Littlehales, who has helped professional athletes, including the soccer stars of Manchester United and Real Madrid, sleep better for more than thirty years, he explained how he developed an unorthodox approach to help shift workers, elite athletes, and hard-charging high achievers get enough sleep. Rather than tracking the total number of hours slept per twenty-four-hour period, Littlehales and his athletes focus on achieving a certain number of ninety-minute sleep cycles.

In Littlehales's system, which he details in *Sleep: The Myth of 8 Hours, the Power of Naps, and the New Plan to Recharge Your Body and Mind*, each ninety-minute block of sleep is equal to one sleep cycle. Two sleep cycles require three hours of sleep, three cycles require four and a half hours, and so on.

Even if you can't get a strict seven to nine hours of sleep per night, you should try to achieve thirty-five cycles per week (five cycles per night, on average), and try not to get any fewer than thirty cycles. I have found that this approach comes in handy when I am traveling, working hard, or going through a period in which I can get only, say, four to five hours of sleep per night Monday through Friday. By tossing in a few extra naps (conveniently, as little as twenty minutes of daytime napping equates to a full ninety-minute sleep cycle) and slightly longer nights of sleep on Saturday and Sunday, I can still achieve at least thirty sleep cycles for a seven-day period. You can quantify your sleep cycles using a device like the Oura ring, which is what I personally use.

Most people perform best on seven to nine hours of sleep per twenty-four-hour period. If your schedule doesn't allow that, shoot for thirty to thirty-five sleep cycles per seven-day period. Incidentally, there is no rule that you must sleep between 10:00 p.m. and 6:00 a.m. I recommend taking Dr. Michael Breus's quizzes and checking out Dr. Satchin Panda's circadian research to identify the sleep-wake cycle that works best for you.No matter what sleep-wake cycle you decide on, food, supplements, and exercise can have a profound effect on your sleep. Even small adjustments to these factors can help you fall asleep faster, get more restful sleep, and weather the effects of poor sleep better.

FOOD, SUPPLEMENTS, AND EXERCISE

Over the past decade, I have had the privilege of interviewing some of the world's top sleep researchers, sleep doctors, and sleep experts on my podcast. I have learned a host of practical, scientifically proven tips to enhance sleep, especially when it comes to the nature and timing of your exercise, food, and supplements. In this section, I will reveal my primary tactics for hacking each of these aspects of your circadian rhythm.

Food

The following six guidelines can help you customize your diet for better sleep.

1. SEEK OUT SLEEP-ENHANCING FOOD.

Research suggests that certain foods have a profound beneficial effect on sleep. For example, fatty cold-water fish like salmon and mackerel contain high amounts of vitamin D and omega-3 fatty acids, essential nutrients for regulating serotonin and sleep. Consuming fruit can also improve the quality of your sleep, likely because of the slow release of energy from fructose and the satiating effect of water and fiber. I am personally a fan of small, dark berries, "ugly" and slightly bitter or sour grapefruit or apples, and wild fruits. These all tend to be higher in phytonutrients and fiber than their domesticated counterparts (like the perfect, juicy apples and pears at your local supermarket, which may be up to ten months old!). One study demonstrated that consuming two kiwis an hour before bed for four weeks significantly increases sleep quality and quantity. Other research suggests that tart cherries improve sleep because they raise melatonin levels.

So if you want to sleep better, a simple but potent dinner would be a wild-caught salmon fillet topped with a tart cherry sauce or sliced kiwi, along with roasted vegetables for satiating fiber and a bit of white rice to boost serotonin secretion. For dessert, try a giant spoonful of coconut oil topped with a dab of almond butter, a pinch of sea salt, and a drizzle of raw honey. This combination will provide a slow release of energy as well as minerals to regulate blood pressure and cortisol levels.

Do You Need More Sleep as You Age?

There is some debate surrounding how sleep requirements change with age. Some research suggests that adults over the age of fifty do not require as much sleep as younger individuals. But other research suggests the opposite, claiming that older adults need just as much sleep as they did when they were younger and that they just have a reduced ability to get that sleep. Indeed, the Sleep Foundation states that once you reach the age of eighteen, your sleep needs stay pretty consistent for the rest of your life: about seven and a half to nine hours per night (just remember that the timing of these hours will depend upon your chronotype—see page 138).

Nine changes in sleep habits can occur as you age:

- Advanced sleep timing, in which you both go to bed and wake up earlier

- Longer sleep onset latency, which means it takes longer to fall asleep

- Overall shorter sleep duration

- Increases in deep-sleep interruptions, such as frequent forays into light-sleep stages

- More-fragile sleep, so that you are awakened more easily by noises and lights

- Less slow-wave (deep) sleep

- Increases in lighter NREM sleep stages, which is less restorative than deep NREM sleep

- Shorter and fewer sleep cycles

- More time spent awake throughout the night

Over the age of fifty-five, a propensity toward daytime napping increases, and many older adults report daytime sleepiness so severe that it interrupts their plans.

So how do you know if you are getting enough sleep in your later decades? If you're getting five to six hours of sleep and can function normally, with few or no adverse effects on cognition and physical energy, then you are probably getting enough sleep. It may simply be that your genes and personal chronobiology allow you to get by on the sleep changes associated with aging or that your level of physical activity is low enough that you don't have high sleep requirements. In addition, research suggests that when deep slow-wave sleep is suppressed in a sleep lab, older adults do not exhibit a significantly increased need for deep sleep, suggesting that the "pressure to sleep" decreases with age. But if you feel tired and sleepy throughout the day, then you likely need to take steps to improve your sleep quality and quantity. The following are distilled, ready-to-implement tactics to help you do just that.

Take melatonin: Melatonin is a hormone that's responsible for making you feel tired. When the sun starts to set, the falling light stimulates your optic nerves to send a signal to your master body clock, the suprachiasmatic nucleus (SCN). The SCN then sets off a chemical cascade that results in the secretion of melatonin.

The problem is that melatonin production declines as you age, so supplementing with melatonin is an effective way to combat age-related sleep deprivation. Many melatonin supplements contain up to 5 mg, but you only need 0.3 to 0.5 mg to enjoy the hormone's sleep-inducing benefits.

2. PAY ATTENTION TO THE GLYCEMIC CONTENT OF YOUR FOOD.

If it takes you a long time to fall asleep, consume any high-glycemic-index carbohydrates, such as rice, bananas, or baked potatoes, or anything else that spikes blood sugar, at least four hours before bed (although I don't recommend consumption of high-glycemic-index carbohydrates at all, unless during or after a workout). Avoid sweet desserts after dinner and instead consume your nightly bar of dark chocolate or bowl of coconut ice cream when you are in a more insulin-sensitive state, such as after a workout. If you do have desserts, try to squeeze in a ten-to-thirty-minute postprandial (after the meal) brisk walk. You can also swap your regular desserts for coconut oil topped with almond butter, sea salt, and honey. Avoid frequent snacking in the late afternoon and evening, and limit dinnertime carbohydrates to lower-glycemic-index sources like dark, leafy greens and sweet potatoes.

Reduce your exposure to artificial light: Before artificial light allowed people to stay up working past sunset, the body clock followed the rising and setting of the sun. The blue light emitted by the sun stimulates waking activity, and as those wavelengths fall and red light wavelengths increase closer to sunset, you respond by becoming more tired. But most artificial light sources (like that $1,100 iPhone in your pocket) produce high amounts of blue light and can disrupt this natural cycle. Blue-light exposure acts, in part, by suppressing melatonin secretion, which is quite useful in the morning but does you no favors in the evening. Fortunately, with tools such as blue-light-blocking software for computer monitors, blue-light-blocking glasses, red incandescent light bulbs installed in your bedroom, and much more, you can minimize the effects of artificial light. In chapter 20, you will discover an extremely detailed explanation of how to do this.

Use PEMF to enhance slow-wave sleep: Research suggests that one of the underlying mechanisms of age-related sleep deprivation is a reduction of the slow brain waves produced during the first three of the four sleep stages. So an effective strategy to help you fall asleep and stay asleep is to use a pulsed electromagnetic field (PEMF) device. These devices can be set to delta brain wave mode. As you lie in bed with the device underneath your mattress, your sheets, or anywhere touching your body, your brain waves will synchronize with the pulses given off by the device. This will help ease you into a deep, slow-wave sleep state.

Avoid stimulants in the afternoon: While certain populations, like southern Italians and Sicilians, can drink coffee late in the day and still get a good night's sleep, you might not respond to afternoon stimulants so well, especially if you don't carry the same fast-caffeine-oxidizing genes as these folks. The effects of stimulants like caffeine can linger in your system for up to six hours, preventing you from falling asleep or waking you up in the middle of the night when the stimulant finally wears off and the subsequent hypoglycemia kicks in.

So should you find yourself turning to caffeine for an afternoon pick-me-up, make sure you incorporate supplements to reduce caffeine's propensity to disrupt sleep at night when consumed in the afternoon—chapter 5 includes many examples and suggestions. For example, if you consume caffeine later in the day, pair it with L-theanine, using a 1:4 caffeine-to-L-theanine ratio: if you consume 100 mg of caffeine (roughly the amount in an 8-ounce cup of coffee), consume it with 400 mg of L-theanine. Smaller doses of L-theanine, around 100 to 200 mg, can take a bit of the edge off caffeine, but you may need more as you age, especially if you just have to have that post-dinner espresso.

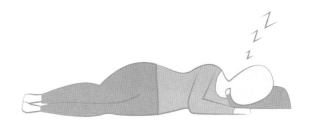

Golden Milk Bedtime Elixir

This delicious drink aids your digestion, relaxes an amped-up nervous system, and helps you get in the mood for a night of restful sleep.

- ½ cup full-fat coconut milk
- 1 teaspoon ginger powder, or 2 tablespoons ground fresh ginger
- 1 teaspoon turmeric powder, or 2 tablespoons ground fresh turmeric
- ¼ teaspoon ground nutmeg
- 4 whole peppercorns, crushed
- 2 or 3 drops organic liquid stevia
- 1 teaspoon coconut oil
- Pinch of ground cinnamon (optional)

1. *Place all the ingredients except the coconut oil and cinnamon in a saucepan over medium heat and bring to a simmer, then turn the heat down to low. Simmer for 5 minutes, then remove the pan from the heat and allow to cool for 5 minutes.*

2. *Strain the cooled liquid through a fine-mesh strainer or cheesecloth into a glass or mug. Add the coconut oil. Sprinkle with ground cinnamon if desired for additional flavor.*

3. HAVE A LIGHT DINNER.

Even though American culture is structured around huge evening dinners, don't make it a habit to consume large meals right before bed. High-calorie meals consumed before bed may excessively spike blood glucose and insulin levels, particularly if the meal is high in protein and carbohydrates (more on both of those in a moment) and will inhibit the release of the fat-burning hormones leptin and adiponectin. Push yourself away from the table when you are 80 percent full and take a twenty-to-thirty-minute postdinner stroll to assist digestion and control blood sugar. If you do eat a large meal, take a cold or lukewarm shower to cool your core body temperature, eliminate pesky meat sweats, and enhance deep sleep.

4. CONSUME ADEQUATE PROTEIN.

Research suggests that consuming adequate protein can significantly improve sleep quality. Your body breaks down protein into amino acids, which serve as the primary building blocks of neurotransmitters. One of these amino acids, tryptophan, is found in high concentrations in protein-rich sources like turkey, chicken, red meat, eggs, fish, spirulina, almonds, and pumpkin seeds. Tryptophan is necessary for your body to produce the neurotransmitter serotonin and the hormone melatonin, so make sure you eat enough of these protein sources to enhance your sleep quality and quantity.

You can slightly increase the level of tryptophan in your brain by consuming carbohydrates along with these protein sources. Indeed, research suggests that, rather than turkey consumption alone, high amounts of carbohydrates are partly responsible for the drowsiness that follows Thanksgiving dinner. This is because carbohydrates promote the release of insulin, which shovels all amino acids *except* tryptophan into muscle or fat tissue. As a result, you have more tryptophan than other amino acids in your blood, so the amino acid transporters in the blood-brain barrier are shuttling more tryptophan into your brain. Once it's in your brain, tryptophan is synthesized into serotonin and melatonin, and you become tired.

You should aim to consume at least 0.55 g of protein per pound of body weight per day, and if you have sleep problems, increase that to up to 0.7 to 0.8 g per pound. A healthy 160-pound man would need about 112 g of protein per day, and a healthy 110-pound woman would need about 70 g. If you are doing any cyclic caloric restriction, increase your protein intake throughout the day on lower-calorie days. For a low-calorie option, I am a huge fan of supplementing with essential amino acids (EAAs) and have found that many people on calorie-restricted diets respond quite well to 10 to 20 g of EAAs per day.

5. CONSUME ADEQUATE CARBOHYDRATES.

If you wake up frequently during the night, you may be one of those folks who are so active that they need more carbohydrates to ensure they don't have middle-of-the-night episodes of hypoglycemia (low blood sugar).

On extremely active days, I personally consume 100 to 200 g of slow-release carbohydrates, such as legumes, amaranth, quinoa, millet, and even sweet potatoes. Many fat-lovers—folks who are just a bit too orthorexic about their diets—are concerned that this will take them out of ketosis (the metabolic state of primarily burning fat). Fact is, it will. But based on my own blood and breath ketone testing and that of my clients, a fat-adapted person will reenter ketosis by the morning. In addition, unless you are managing a disease like epilepsy or multiple sclerosis, when it comes to optimizing recovery, fat-burning, and cognitive function, regular nights of deep, restorative sleep trump being in ketosis 24-7. (I'll talk much more about ketosis in chapter 14.)

6. LIMIT YOUR SATURATED FAT INTAKE.

Your evening meal should contain only low to moderate amounts of saturated fat. If you often feel like you have a brick in your stomach after dinner, don't overdo it on the marbled meat, butter, coconut oil, and MCT oil. This is particularly important if you consume the coconut oil dessert described earlier after dinner. The fat in the coconut oil is the maximum amount of saturated fat you want to consume in the evening, especially if you consume meat or fish at dinner.

Supplements

There are hundreds of sleep supplements on the market, but research has shown that certain compounds are more effective than others in improving sleep onset latency, wake times, and deep-sleep percentages. For example, there are a diverse array of nutrients that influence the synthesis of serotonin and melatonin. In this section, I'll identify these and other nutrients that can help you maximize your sleep.

TRYPTOPHAN

When tryptophan accumulates in your blood, it crosses the blood-brain barrier and is converted into 5-hydroxytryptamine (5-HT), a precursor of serotonin. 5-HT is also a precursor of melatonin in your pineal gland and causes lethargy and drowsiness. Consuming protein sources rich in tryptophan, such as whey protein, increases tryptophan levels by up to 130 percent, significantly increasing brain levels of serotonin.

If you consume close to the protein recommendations above and eat your carbohydrates at dinner, you probably don't need to take supplemental tryptophan. Should you need to supplement tryptophan, research suggests that 1 g improves both the quantity and quality of sleep.

B-COMPLEX VITAMINS

In addition to serotonin and melatonin, your body produces vitamin B_3, or niacin, from tryptophan. It may be beneficial to take supplemental niacin so that less of the tryptophan you consume is used to synthesize it and more is used to synthesize serotonin. Vitamin B_9, or folate, and vitamin B_6, or pyridoxine, also help convert tryptophan into serotonin. Vitamin B_{12}, or cobalamin, helps synthesize melatonin; supplementing with B_{12} is particularly important for vegetarians because it is primarily found in animal foods. Most good multivitamins contain B-complex vitamins. I personally prefer the Thorne multivitamin, which includes a p.m. dose that contains both B-complex vitamins and other relaxing, cortisol-reducing compounds.

MAGNESIUM

Magnesium helps convert 5-HT into N-acetyl-5-hydroxytryptamine, a precursor to melatonin. The most absorbable forms of magnesium are magnesium citrate, glycinate, taurate, and aspartate, although magnesium that is bound to malate, succinate, or fumarate is also effective. Magnesium carbonate, sulfate, gluconate, and oxide are the cheapest, most poorly absorbed forms, so I recommend avoiding them.

Effective doses of magnesium range from 200 to 500 mg. As a word of caution, consuming more than 1,500 mg per day of magnesium can result in loose stools and disaster pants—or, in this case, disaster blankets.

ZINC

Research suggests that a zinc deficiency reduces melatonin levels. Perhaps this is why many athletes, who are often zinc deficient, swear by the 1-2-3 compound found in supplements called ZM— zinc monomethionine aspartate, magnesium aspartate, and vitamin B_6. As for me, since I tend to get my magnesium and vitamin B_6 from other sources, I turn to a source of zinc that is ten times higher in zinc than even the mighty shellfish: black ant extract.

MELATONIN

Melatonin is a hormone secreted by the pineal gland (provided you aren't exposed to too much artificial light at night) that produces a sedative or hypnotic effect, especially with high-dose supplementation. Doses as high as 60 mg are often used to treat sleep disorders or, in my case, as a potent "cure" for jet lag. (Warning: a 60 mg melatonin dose can induce significant morning grogginess and ideally should only be used the first night after crossing multiple time zones.) But keep in mind that side effects of chronic heavy melatonin use include headaches, nausea, daytime drowsiness, and even nightmares.

Most research suggests doses of 0.3 to 12 mg to improve sleep. A more natural way to increase melatonin levels and avoid drowsiness is to take a 0.3 mg microdose at night or increase tryptophan levels via the methods mentioned earlier.

L-THEANINE

The amino acid L-theanine is most commonly found in green tea leaves but can also be taken as a supplement. It can significantly reduce stress and increase relaxation without causing drowsiness, most notably when combined with a source of caffeine (such as an afternoon cup of coffee) that would normally disrupt sleep.

Research suggests that L-theanine crosses the blood-brain barrier in about thirty minutes and improves mental relaxation without loss of alertness by acting directly on the central nervous system. Once it crosses the blood-brain barrier, it reduces sympathetic nervous system activity, improves post-stress relaxation, lowers blood pressure, and reduces cortisol levels and anxiety. I recommend starting with a dose of 100 to 200 mg. If you consume it with a caffeine source like coffee, consume it at a 1:4 caffeine-to-L-theanine ratio. So if you consume 100 mg of caffeine, consume 400 mg of L-theanine.

VITAMIN D

Vitamin D deficiency is strongly associated with nonspecific musculoskeletal pain, chronic pain, and hormone deficiencies. Chronically low vitamin D levels are also associated with poor sleep and may contribute to the development of obstructive sleep apnea and associated cardiovascular disease. Risk factors for chronically low vitamin D levels include dark skin tone, obesity, limited sunlight exposure, pregnancy, chronic anticonvulsant use, chronic steroid use, intestinal malabsorption syndromes, and, as in my case, a genetic inability to properly synthesize vitamin D from sunlight.

Typical vitamin D doses range from 2,000 to 4,000 IU per day. Doses should always be taken with 100 to 150 mcg of vitamin K_2 to limit the risk of high blood calcium levels. I prefer the Thorne Vitamin D/K liquid blend for a quick and easy source in the correct ratios.

SUPPLEMENTING FOR SPECIFIC CONCERNS

Finally, author Stephen Buhner, in books such as *Secret Teachings of Plants* and *Plant Intelligence*, has written extensively about herbal approaches for better sleep in people who have mold, mycotoxin, and Lyme issues (all discussed at length in chapter 4). For this purpose, he especially notes the benefits of Chinese skullcap root, pulsatilla, greater celandine, and motherwort. In conditions of nervous system damage or being stuck in "fight-or-flight" mode, valerian, kava kava, and passionflower, along with the homeopathic remedies PSY-stabil, viscum, aconite, and Somcupin, can be beneficial, as can 5-HTP (5-hydroxytryptophan), L-tyrosine, Fibroboost, and GABA.

Exercise

You probably won't be surprised to learn that sleep quantity and sleep onset latency both improve with physical activity. In this section, you will discover how to optimize your workouts to enhance your sleep.

PERFORM LIGHT AEROBIC EXERCISE EARLY IN THE MORNING.

Research suggests that thirty minutes of moderate-intensity aerobic exercise at 65 percent of maximum heart rate attained at VO_2 max prior to breakfast is highly beneficial for enhancing sleep. Indeed, exercise can cause circadian-phase-shifting effects that are perhaps as potent as bright light. So before breakfast, perform some light aerobic activity for twenty to forty-five minutes. This activity won't amplify high cortisol levels in the morning, won't spike your appetite so much that you face-feed the rest of the morning, and will leave enough glycogen in the tank for a harder workout later in the day.

The simplest way to achieve this is with a brisk, thirty-minute sunshine walk. Walk to work and eat breakfast there, walk the dog, or walk the kids to school—you get the idea. I am also a huge fan of going for a relaxing swim in cool or cold water or performing a thirty-minute yoga session in my sauna.

COMPENSATE FOR ANY EARLY-MORNING HARD TRAINING.

Training hard in the early morning can damage your sleep patterns, so if you must perform your intense workout in the morning, take strategic naps during the day (such as a twenty-minute post-lunch siesta) and implement more sleep hygiene practices at night, such as low artificial-light exposure, a cool room, noise elimination, and low amounts of work and stress.

WHEN POSSIBLE, SAVE HARD WORKOUTS FOR THE AFTERNOON.

Research suggests that longer workouts (up to two and a half hours long) between 2:00 and 6:00 p.m. at 50 percent to 80 percent of VO_2 max can drastically improve sleep. In an ideal scenario, you should save any hard, high-volume workouts for the afternoon or early evening. You gain the most benefits when you do your hard workouts three to eight hours before bedtime, so try to wrap up your session by, say, 7:30 p.m. at the latest if you want to go to bed at 10:30. In fact, thirty minutes of high-intensity exercise at 85 to 90 percent of maximum heart rate done to exhaustion three to four hours before bedtime can increase sleep efficiency and reduce sleep onset latency.

COMBAT SLEEP DEPRIVATION WITH AEROBIC EXERCISE.

Research suggests that either long sessions of aerobic exercise or intense ten-minute bouts done every two hours during a sleep-deprived day can partially alleviate sleepiness during periods of sleep restriction. In other words, do one long-and-slow session, such as a nature hike, or several short-and-fast sessions, such as a quick series of kettlebell complexes or a few rounds on an Assault AirBike every two hours.

CALM YOUR NERVOUS SYSTEM FOLLOWING EXERCISE.

Exercise increases your body temperature (which has an inverse relationship with sleep quality) and sympathetic nervous system activity for several hours afterward. Perhaps this is why deep, relaxing breathwork or a lukewarm or cold shower after your workout can enhance sleep. For the ultimate treat, I am a fan of warm magnesium salt baths. If I have time, I will even go so far as to drag a near-infrared light panel called a Joovv into my bathroom to enhance the mitochondria-boosting effects of the magnesium.

MY OWN ROUTINE FOR BETTER SLEEP

Ultimately, I get the best sleep when I perform twenty to thirty minutes of easy morning exercise in as much natural light as possible in a fasted state prior to breakfast. Then, I perform a hard thirty-to-sixty-minute workout in the late afternoon or early evening, which I always follow with a quick cold shower or, if time permits, a magnesium bath with near-infrared light exposure. In my experience, this is a potent one-two exercise combo for enhancing sleep, combined with a little biohacked invention from yours truly.

SOUNDING AND GROUNDING

Common sleep hygiene recommendations include practices like sleeping in a dark room, avoiding electronic light-producing devices while in bed, and keeping your room at a cool temperature. But two often-underemphasized aspects of sleep hygiene have been big wins for me in the sleep department: sound and the ground.

If you live in a noisy neighborhood or near an airport, or if a train passes by your house at midnight, 2:00 a.m., and 5:00 a.m. every night, then you may need some help blocking out the noise. In this case, you can use a wraparound sleep mask combined with earplugs to block out light and sound. Or you can use soft, side-sleeper-friendly headphones, such as SleepPhones, and listen to a white-noise app like SleepStream, Brain.fm, or Pzizz to "silence" sirens, airplanes, and barking dogs. (Or, if you are like my mother, you can also use the sounds of whale song, the appeal of which I have never quite understood.) Many of these apps have been specifically formulated to lull you to sleep and include options such as meditation tracks, gentle piano, ocean waves, rain, and, of course, whales.

But managing sound for better sleep can go way beyond white noise and earplugs: you can use sound and music to alter your brain waves for deep relaxation. Remember from chapter 6 that brain wave entrainment is the practice of bringing your brain wave frequencies in sync with an externally produced frequency. When you're asleep, meditating, or deeply relaxed, delta and theta brain waves dominate, and with a brain entrainment device that emits sounds at the right frequency, you can bring your brain waves from focused and alert alpha and beta brain waves to relaxed delta and theta brain waves.

The sound frequencies typically used in brain wave entrainment are called binaural beats. Binaural beats are two tones close in frequency that are played together, one in each ear. As both sounds encounter the brain, they combine for a frequency that's the difference of the original frequencies. For example, a 495 Hz audio tone in one ear and a 505 Hz audio tone in the other ear together create a 10 Hz tone. That's perfect if you're seeking alpha brain waves, but for delta brain waves, you'd want the difference between the two frequencies to be closer to 3 Hz.

How can you use binaural beats to improve sleep? I recommend the Pzizz app or the SleepStream app, both of which produce relaxing sounds combined with binaural beats. Alternatively, you can use the AI-generated sounds on the Brain.fm app, which does not produce binaural beats per se but instead "confuses" the brain into producing delta brain waves. This app, as well as the SleepStream app, can also be used to enhance focus or creativity, depending on the selected setting.

HOW BINAURAL BEATS WORK

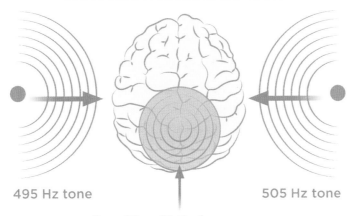

495 Hz tone   505 Hz tone

Resulting 10 Hz frequency

You can also use Dr. Jeffrey Thompson's Delta Sleep System tracks or Michael Tyrrell's 2Sleep tracks, both of which you can play as background music in your bedroom to lull you to sleep. I recommend placing a speaker on either side of your bed so that your brain is exposed to a balanced sound from your left and right, or using "sound furniture," such as the HUMU sound-conducting pillow.

Then there is grounding, which is so important for releasing accumulated positive ions from your body. Also known as "earthing," grounding is the practice of exposing your body to the natural magnetic frequencies produced by the earth. When you have your feet firmly planted on the ground, you come into contact with negative ions, which are produced by turbulent, crashing water, such as waves at the beach and waterfalls, and in forests, mountains, and other places affected by rainstorms or thunderstorms. When you are exposed to negative ions, your body releases positive ions that accumulate via cellular metabolism. Accumulated positive ions reduce the natural electrochemical gradient across your cell membranes. This gradient is responsible for allowing compounds in and out of your cells, so when excess positive ions disrupt the gradient, they also disrupt cellular metabolism and increase inflammation.

I spend about 90 percent of my time grounded, whether by going barefoot, wearing grounding shoes or sandals, sleeping with a grounding device under my mattress, or wearing a grounding wristband. This may seem strange, but grounding is one of the best sleep hacks I know.

In addition to wiggling your toes in the dirt each day, you can use a mattress or mat wired to the earth through an outlet to tap into the earth's negative ions and natural magnetic frequency. These devices are called grounding mats and have been used by professional athletes, including Tour de France riders between grueling race stages, to enhance sleep and recovery.

An even more potent grounding technique is to use small devices or large beds that emit the same magnetic frequency as the earth. Two portable, user-friendly devices that can be placed on or near your body or under your mattress are the FlexPulse and the EarthPulse. You can also use the SomniResonance SR1 device, which is placed directly on your collarbone to send a delta-brain-wave-inducing signal via the brachial plexus from your shoulder up to your brain. Then there is the Biomat pad, which will set you back several thousand dollars but beats the pants off most grounding or earthing mats because it also produces infrared heating light. Finally, there are the larger BEMER mats, BioBalance mats, and Pulse Center beds, all of which can be used for recovery, hormone production, injuries, headache elimination, and a host of other health-enhancing effects.

What about grounding shoes or sandals? I personally wear a brand called Earth Runners. Black plugs made from a carbon-rubber compound are placed in the sole under a weight-bearing part of your foot. The plugs, designed to conduct a free flow of negative ions from the earth to your body, allow you to become grounded when you walk on grass, sand, soil, or even concrete.

For more information on grounding, watch the documentary entitled, fittingly enough, *The Grounded*. It tells the story of Haines, Alaska, where lives were changed and health dramatically improved after people adopted a practice of grounding as part of an experiment. I highly recommend that you add this film to your must-see list. Dr. James Oschman, the scientist behind much of the research in the film, has stated that grounding is "probably the most important discovery since penicillin."

And for a deep dive into the science and best practices for grounding and earthing, I highly recommend the book *Earthing*, by Clint Ober, Stephen T. Sinatra, and Martin Zucker.

TRAVEL AND SLEEP

My Five-Step Airplane Sleep System

Let's face it: with the dry air, cabin pressure, poor food, inadequate water, and enormous doses of dirty electricity, frequently flying on airplanes is one of the worst things you can do for your sleep. I get plenty of complaints from folks about how hard it is to sleep on airplanes, but the fact is I can sleep quite well on just about every flight. How? Every time I fly, I implement the same potent sleep routine:

1. **Request a window seat.** It is far easier to sleep when you can lean your head against the airplane wall.

2. **Consume a serving of reishi mushroom extract,** such as two packets of the Four Sigmatic blend. This will allow you to sleep without waking up drowsy, especially when combined with 20 to 40 mg of CBD.

3. **Use a J-shaped travel pillow.** These inflatable pillows are the highest-rated travel pillows on Amazon (the brand I use is Travelrest). They work especially well for side sleepers when combined with the window seat trick, but they also work when you are stuck in an aisle or middle seat.

4. **Eliminate noise.** Use foam earplugs combined with Sony or Bose noise-blocking headphones.

5. **Eliminate light.** Wear a full wraparound sleep mask to eliminate exposure to overhead lights or TV screens.

That's it! Go forth and sleep like a baby on your next flight (for anyone who has sat next to a baby on an airplane, I apologize for the poor analogy).

How to Manage Jet Lag like a Champion

It doesn't matter how fancy your compression socks are or how many bodyweight squats and calf raises you do in the back of the airplane. When you are on that plane, you are inside a tiny metal tube that's being bombarded by solar radiation and that's completely disconnected from the earth's natural magnetic field. You are also exposed to WiFi signals (often available during the entire flight), people talking on their phones and checking email (which happens for the entire gate-to-takeoff and landing-to-gate phases), dehydration from altitude, dry filtered air, toxin-laden airplane food, bad water, airborne pathogens, and—if you are traveling across multiple time zones—jet lag.

Jet lag sucks, as all frequent flyers know. The symptoms include longer sleep onset latency (especially if you are flying east), early wake times (especially if you are flying west), interrupted sleep, poor cognitive performance, fatigue, headaches, irritability, and problems with digestion, such as indigestion, constipation, and even reduced interest in and enjoyment of food.

Jet lag is a chronobiological issue that occurs when you travel across multiple time zones. The day-and-night cycle of your destination isn't what you're accustomed to, so your body clock isn't in sync with the destination's time. The problem is exacerbated because eating, sleeping, hormone regulation, and body-temperature-variation patterns also do not correspond to what you are used to. Not much beats flying for radiation exposure, full-body inflammation, free radical production, reduced recovery, and inhibition of important biological processes like protein synthesis.

I don't know about you, but when I am traveling and have to perform at peak capacity, often just hours after my flight touches down, I simply can't afford the full-body damage and loss of fitness that can occur every time I hop on a flight to a race or conference. What can you do about it? You are about to discover nine-plus ways to beat jet lag.

1. PRACTICE GROUNDING.

Grounding, as explained earlier in this chapter, is the practice of exposing your body to the natural magnetic frequencies produced by the earth. Grounding becomes most effective after flying, since hurtling forty thousand feet above the planet in a metal tube is about as disconnected from the earth as you can get.

How do you ground yourself when traveling? As soon as I land at my destination, I make it a point to put on a pair of special shoes called Pluggz or sandals called Earth Runners, both of which have built-in carbon plugs that allow for grounding without being barefoot. In fact, I often go outside in just my bare feet (yes, I am the guy in spandex or a Speedo doing barefoot yoga in the grassy lot behind the hotel). I also use the PEMF devices discussed earlier, set at about 7 to 10 Hz, to achieve a grounding effect when simply lying in bed, and I travel with a lightweight grounding mat that I can easily place under the sheets on any hotel bed. For the most concentrated exposure to negative ions, you can swim in the ocean or take a walk after a lightning storm (lighting infuses the surface of the earth with a high number of negative ions).

2. GET LIGHT EXERCISE.

Research suggests that exercise can regulate circadian rhythms. As lousy and miserable as you may feel training after a day or two of international travel, the sooner you can vigorously move after arriving at your destination, the sooner you will bounce back from jet lag and normalize your circadian rhythm.

You don't have to do a killer WOD or an epic run when you get to your destination. If I am feeling a bit blah after traveling, my top three exercise choices are walking (barefoot or in grounding shoes or sandals if possible) in the sunshine or on a beach, swimming (preferably in cool or cold water), and outdoor barefoot yoga. Finally, for each sedentary hour on an airplane, I do fifty air squats near the back of the plane or in any other open space I can find.

3. AVOID STIMULANTS UNTIL YOU ARRIVE.

To reduce jet lag, it is a relatively common recommendation to limit the consumption of caffeine, alcohol, and nicotine. Because these chemicals overstimulate the central nervous system and have the potential to disrupt an already disrupted circadian rhythm, I absolutely agree and do not go near caffeine or any other CNS stimulant while en route to my destination. But once you arrive at your final destination, these same compounds can work wonderfully to keep you awake until it is officially bedtime in your new time zone.

4. TAKE MELATONIN.

When I've traveled across more than three time zones, before going to bed my first night at my final destination, I consume 60 to 80 mg of melatonin (yep, that's a lot!) to reboot my circadian rhythm. This seemingly insane amount of melatonin was prescribed by a cancer physician friend of mine to help his patients deal with pain at night, and upon learning this from him, I gave it a few tries as a jet lag hack. It works, but you will need to say a prayer that your hotel, hostel, or home doesn't catch fire, because you will be extremely groggy. Melatonin is also a natural anti-inflammatory, so it will help reduce the inflammation that occurs during air travel.

5. DRINK LOTS OF WATER.

You become dehydrated when sitting in the dry cabin air of an airplane, so a crucial part of overcoming jet lag is drinking enough water. I have experimented with a very high water intake and have found that it helps quite a bit compared to the disappointingly tiny water cup handed to me by the flight attendant every couple of hours.

I drink close to 16 to 20 ounces of water, nearly a full bottle, each hour and feel a distinct difference in sleep, mood, and energy upon landing. Just make sure that, if you are in a middle or window seat, your aisle-based seatmate is spry and willing to move every time you need to pee, or you can politely ask to switch seats. Find water boring? Travel with a small bottle of organic stevia and add it to club soda or sparkling water to create a cream soda–esque experience. As a word of caution, consuming 16 to 20 ounces of water per hour may cause hyponatremia (water intoxication), so I recommend that you consume trace liquid minerals or electrolytes with each bottle.

6. TAKE A COLD SHOWER.

Cold showers reduce inflammatory cytokine levels, activate brown adipose tissue to burn fat, and induce a hormone response, particularly by causing a high release of adrenaline. I have gone so far as to go into an airline lounge in the airport for a ten-to-fifteen-minute cold shower during a long layover. I also take a two-to-five-minute cold shower in the hotel when I arrive at my final destination. Finding a nearby spa allows you to take things to the next level, as you can do hot-cold contrast therapy with several rounds of dry sauna exposure followed by a cold plunge or cold shower. (For you frequent travelers, I highly recommend Banya 5 in Seattle or AIRE Ancient Baths in New York City.)

Splashing lots of cold water in your face can also help, but it is not nearly as effective as immersion or showering. Cold showers also dilate your blood vessels because they release more nitric oxide, and the subsequent increase in glucose and oxygen uptake by your organs and muscles can dramatically reduce jet lag.

7. CONSUME CURCUMIN.

Curcumin, which is found in turmeric and curries as well as in concentrated supplement forms, is a potent antioxidant when taken on an empty stomach both before and after flying. It easily crosses the blood-brain barrier and shuts down inflammatory cytokines in neural tissue and may even boost testosterone and growth hormone production.

Upon landing at my final destination, I take about 1,000 mg of curcumin from a highly absorbable source, such as Meriva, which is found in many supplements, like the Thorne multivitamin. A meal with curries and sulfurous vegetables (think broccoli and cauliflower), such as tandoori chicken at a good Indian restaurant, can work wonders for jet lag.

8. SEEK OUT SULFUR

Sulfur-rich foods are excellent antioxidant precursors and help reduce the inflammation that can occur when flying. Sulfur is found in broccoli, cauliflower, garlic, onions, and brussels sprouts. Of course, if you opt for sautéed garlic and onions preflight, you may need to brush your teeth afterward (unless you plan on creating enemies during the flight). Supplements containing sulfurous compounds, such as glutathione, N-acetylcysteine, MSM, or DMSO, can be even more effective than sulfurous foods. But if you squeeze a few meals with these foods into the days leading up to your flight and just after, you will feel much better when you travel and be less likely to suffer immune system deficits.

For an even more potent dose of antioxidants, you can take a cocktail of (or get an IV with) glutathione, astaxanthin, selenium, vitamin E, CoQ10, N-acetylcysteine, vitamin C, and alpha-lipoic acid. Animal studies have shown that a large dose of antioxidants like this can reduce the oxidative stress caused by the radiation experienced during airline travel, as can taking a large dose of DHA, chlorella, or spirulina before flying and even loading with 50 mg of the supplement pycnogenol three times daily during your entire trip.

9. GET A HIT OF OXYTOCIN.

Oxytocin is a potent hormone that lifts your mood and acts as an antioxidant, antidepressant, and anti-inflammatory. It's naturally released after sex and during childbirth and breastfeeding, but you can supplement with an oxytocin nasal spray dose of about 10 to 21 IU per day, so you can get an oxytocin fix any time and any place, including while you are traveling.

In addition to using a nasal spray, you can hug someone or, while it is slightly less effective, warmly shake someone's hand. Bodily contact will cause your brain to release low levels of oxytocin. So when you get to your destination, find the first person who is okay with it and give him or her a big, loving bear hug. Or do some partner carries up the stairs at the hotel (which, incidentally, makes a great travel workout). Just brush your teeth first if you used the garlic-and-onions trick.

10. USE THESE ADDITIONAL TRICKS AND TIPS.

In addition to the nine tactics above, there are plenty of other tricks you can use to feel amazing when you hop off your flight:

- Stand up and stretch for a couple of minutes for every hour you sit. My favorite stretch is called the Core Coil, which was invented by my friend David Weck. You'll find a video of it on BoundlessBook.com/7.
- Wear full-body graduated compression gear. I recommend the shirts by AlignMed.
- Bring your own food. I personally carry EnergyBits or RecoveryBits spirulina and chlorella tablets combined with macadamia nuts and high-quality coarse sea salt, like Colima sea salt. Ketone salts and ketone esters are also fantastic anti-inflammatories to use during travel (you will discover why in chapter 19).
- Travel with Omica Organics vanilla- or butterscotch toffee–flavored liquid stevia to add to club soda or seltzer water for more flavor (trust me, it will taste like a delicious vanilla cream soda) and to help keep hunger at bay.
- Travel with Hammer, Nuun, or GU electrolyte tablets to add to water or dissolve in your mouth like a salty-sweet lozenge (I adopted the latter habit during Ironman triathlons).
- Smear the inside of your nostrils with sesame oil or olive oil to keep your nasal passages moisturized in the dry cabin air.
- Use the light-producing Re-Timer glasses and the HumanCharger in-ear light device on your first morning at your final destination, especially if you know you will be indoors for much of the day or you won't be able to get any sunshine.

10 TIPS FOR
CONQUERING THE NAP

Napping is one of the most potent ways to combat accumulated sleep loss. I personally nap for twenty to sixty minutes per day, usually by curling up on my infrared Biomat and putting on my NormaTec compression boots for a post-lunch siesta. By dividing my day in two with the equivalent of one sleep cycle's worth of deep sleep, this nap effectively gives me two days of productivity squeezed into one.

Research suggests that following sleep restriction, a thirty-minute nap significantly improves athletes' performance in speed trials. Research also suggests that naps can improve cognitive processes that are dramatically affected by sleep restriction, which may enhance highly complex motor skills and prevent exercise-induced injuries.

Siestas are particularly rich in slow-wave (deep) NREM sleep, which is why a nap significantly increases alertness, creativity, recall, and memory in the second half of the day. Naps also help reduce waking blood pressure and improve cardiovascular health. If you miss a good night of sleep, a well-timed nap can help you dig your way out of a sleep-deprivation hole. On the other hand, poorly timed naps (in the late afternoon or evening) can actually worsen insomnia and reduce alertness later in the day, so curling up for a nap before dinner is usually not a good idea. Here are my top ten dos and don'ts for conquering the nap.

1. DON'T USE AN ALARM CLOCK UNLESS YOU HAVE TO.

Why shouldn't you use an alarm clock? I am a fan of the disk and RAM (random-access memory) metaphor. Think of the brain and its sleep cycles as a PC. During the day, while learning information, you store new data in temporary RAM. During NREM sleep, you write the data down to the hard disk. During REM sleep, you organize the data, sort it, and build new neural connections.

This cycle repeats until all RAM data is neatly transferred to the disk for long-term use and your RAM is clear for the next day. Upon waking up, you reboot the computer. But if you reboot too soon with an alarm clock, you may leave your disk fragmented. Your data access will be slow, and your thinking will be confused. Some of the data may not even get written to the disk, as if you had never stored it in RAM at all. There are also the biological implications of using an alarm clock. Like a slap in the face or a bucket of cold water, an alarm clock quickly wakes you up and causes an immediate, unnatural release of adrenaline and cortisol.

Fact is, after a while, you don't really need an alarm clock. Once you begin a healthy napping habit, your body will naturally wake up in twenty to sixty minutes. If you must use an alarm clock, use one that gradually wakes you up, such as the SunRise Alarm Clock, the Sleep Time by Azumio iPhone app, or the Sleep as Android app for Android phones. Alternatively, the chiliPAD can be programmed to circulate warm water under your body at the time you'd like to begin waking up, which can also be an effective strategy for gradually waking without a blaring alarm clock.

2. DO TIME YOUR NAP.

It's best to take your nap when you are the least alert, which is seven to eight hours after you wake up in the morning. For example, I wake up at 6:00 a.m. and have my best naps around 1:00 p.m. Research suggests that anytime between 11:00 a.m. and 3:00 p.m., which is seven to eight hours after waking for most people, are good times to nap.

3. DON'T DRINK COFFEE OR CAFFEINATED DRINKS BEFORE YOUR NAP.

It is a myth that if you drink caffeine before a nap, the caffeine will hit your bloodstream as you wake up. Even tiny amounts of caffeine can significantly disrupt sleep quality, especially if you metabolize caffeine quickly.

4. DO SLEEP MORE AT NIGHT IF YOU FIND YOURSELF TAKING LONG NAPS.

If you nap for more than an hour and a half, you probably are not sleeping enough at night, or you have some adrenal imbalances that you need to address.

5. DO AVOID STRESS FOR AN HOUR OR TWO BEFORE NAPPING.

I try to schedule my lowest-stress activities for right before my naps. For me, this typically means office and household duties, like rearranging my desk, cleaning the garage, reading, writing, or eating lunch—definitely not doing phone consults or responding to emails.

6. DON'T EXERCISE IMMEDIATELY BEFORE YOUR NAP.

Naps can assist with exercise recovery, but try to finish working out at least forty-five minutes before your nap.

7. DO EAT BEFORE YOUR NAP.

Don't go down for a nap hungry, as hypoglycemia can disrupt sleep. This is why a post-lunch siesta can be so effective.

8. DON'T FORCE IT.

If you try napping for a month and simply can't nap no matter what, don't worry about it. Go back to your regular sleep routine and look at the free-running sleep information on BoundlessBook.com/7.

9. DO HAVE A NAPPING RITUAL.

Whenever possible, nap at the same time of day and perform the same pre-nap sequence of activities each day (for example, work, exercise, shower, eat, and nap in that order each day).

10. DON'T USE ALCOHOL OR SEDATIVES TO INITIATE A NAP.

A couple of glasses of wine at lunchtime will cause you to wake up sluggish and fatigued. Instead, I have found that a couple packets of Four Sigmatic reishi mushroom elixir, two or three capsules of an adaptogenic herb supplement called Inner Peace, or 5 to 10 mg of CBD will help me settle down for a nap without causing grogginess later.

THE LAST WORD

The science and logistics of sleep are incredibly important, and the host of tools, hacks, and strategies for optimizing sleep can be dizzying and confusing. But I have made a concerted effort to distill into this chapter the most effective sleep-optimizing strategies.

Should you want to take an even deeper dive into sleep, I recommend a gold mine of a website: SuperMemo. I spent nearly a month poring over it and finding many well-researched ideas for this chapter. It includes everything from advanced sleep hacks to the best timing for naps to instructions for perfecting free-running sleep. It is a lot of information, but it will satisfy your inner sleep geek and fill in any gaps in your understanding.

In addition, there are several fantastic sleep books that I think everyone who sleeps (that's you, right?) should own and read:

- *The Power of When*, by Dr. Michael Breus
- *Change Your Schedule, Change Your Life*, by Dr. Suhas Kshirsagar
- *Sleep: The Myth of 8 Hours, the Power of Naps, and the New Plan to Recharge Your Body and Mind*, by Nick Littlehales
- *Why We Sleep: Unlocking the Power of Sleep and Dreams*, by Dr. Matthew Walker
- *The Circadian Code: Lose Weight, Supercharge Your Energy, and Transform Your Health from Morning to Midnight*, by Dr. Satchin Panda
- *Lights Out: Sleep, Sex, and Survival*, by Dr. T. S. Wiley

In the meantime, congratulations! You have conquered boundless energy of mind and are fully prepared to achieve whole and balanced boundless energy of body. In the next several chapters, you will discover potent strategies for building muscle, improving your cardiovascular system, and boosting longevity, fat loss, and recovery, so you can create a sound body to carry your optimized mind.

ONE THING YOU CAN DO THIS WEEK

Each morning this week, preferably within a couple of hours of waking, expose your eyes, ears, skin, or entire body to as much natural sunlight or blue light as possible (just ten to twenty minutes counts!). Each night, eliminate as much artificial light exposure as you can by wearing blue-light-blocking glasses (or, in a pinch, sunglasses), limiting screen time, or installing blue-light-blocking software on your electronic devices. Alternatively, try reading a paper book instead of staring at a screen.

> For citations for all the research studies mentioned in this chapter and a deeper dive into the topics of this chapter—including links to podcasts, blog posts, recommended tools and supplements, and much more—visit BoundlessBook.com/7.

LEAN AND MEAN

HOW TO BURN FAT FAST WITHOUT DESTROYING YOUR BODY

"Dude, you photoshopped your head on that body." I shook my head and smiled proudly as my friend Gerad stared up at the framed photo in my office—a photo of me standing wide-legged onstage with a giant creatine-fueled grin on my face as I held a double biceps flex pose.

"You were really at three percent body fat?"

I nodded. "Two hundred fifteen pounds and three percent body fat."

It's true. As a competitive bodybuilder, I spent three years cracking the code on burning massive amounts of fat tissue without wasting away into malnourished, muscle-depleted oblivion. Copious amounts of time spent in advanced nutrition, anatomy, physiology, biochemistry, and pharmacology science classes at the University of Idaho combined with a hefty dose of time spent lurking on bodybuilding forums taught me how to chisel my body and brain into fat-loss ninjas. Following my short-lived bodybuilding career, I proceeded to spend the next decade immersed in an equally unhealthy body-abusing sport: Ironman triathlon, in which I continued to decipher body-composition optimization in pursuit of the perfect power-to-weight ratio (including the most successful fat-burning strategy I have ever discovered, revealed later in this chapter).

But my approach to fat loss is not just influenced by my time in the bodybuilding and Ironman trenches. It also takes a deep research dive into the science of what works for safe, effective, and lasting fat decimation—strategies that go far beyond the sage, age-old advice to move more and eat less. Sure, fat loss and the attainment of a sexy, lean body begin with getting off your butt, moving more, working out, and slowly lowering the supersized dark chocolate bar away from your gaping maw. But when it comes to losing fat fast, staying shredded, ripped, and toned year-round, and getting to the weight you want—without two-a-day workouts and being cold and starving all the time—there are potent strategies that fly under the radar.

For example, take the flawed concept that, while you can add more fat cells to your body, you can never get rid of them. This dogma, commonly accepted in the fitness and diet industry, dictates that if you have ever had excess weight or bits of undesirable adipose tissue on your waist, hips, and butt, then the fat cells never disappear, even with weight loss—they just shrink. These fat cells, smaller in size but not in number, then lurk in the wings for the next time you mess up and eat a few too many bites of steak or an extra scoop of ice cream, at which point those calories are doomed to get shoveled directly into the eager, waiting fat cells.

But this isn't true. I realized this when I interviewed physician and nutritionist Dr. Cate Shanahan on my podcast. Dr. Shanahan explained that if you eliminate just one notorious biological variable present in most people eating a standard Western diet, then you can not only lose fat but also kill existing fat cells and transform them into more metabolically active tissues, such as brown fat and even stem cells, making yourself more resistant to future weight gain. What is this variable?

It's not excess calories. It's not chocolate. It's not, to the chagrin of diet-book authors worldwide, gluten. It's not refined carbohydrates or saturated fat.

It's inflammation.

That's right: inflammation—particularly from exposure to a toxin-laden environment, consumption of heated and rancid vegetable oils, a stressful lifestyle, and sleep deprivation—can make fat cells resistant to dying. Inflammation promotes insulin resistance, which, in turn, causes higher levels of insulin to accumulate in your blood. In response to this excess insulin, your body reduces the metabolism of stored body fat. So to achieve lasting fat loss, you have to shut down inflammation. This chapter will explain the best way to do that. But before you learn how to beat inflammation-induced weight gain, you have to understand the basic mechanics of fat loss.

FAT LOSS 101

Where does all the fat go when you lose weight? Most fat-loss books and so-called weight-loss experts, physicians, dietitians, and personal trainers will tell you that fat is converted to energy or heat, but actually, this would violate the law of conservation of mass—mass, in an isolated system, is neither created nor destroyed. Fat also isn't pooped out or turned into muscle.

Instead, you breathe away fat.

That's right: your lungs are the primary excretory organs for weight loss. Here's how it works: Any excess carbohydrates or protein that you eat, even that half stick of butter you drop into your piping-hot cup of coffee, are converted into triglycerides, a type of fatty acid, and stored in the lipid droplets of fat cells (adipocytes). Excess dietary fat, meanwhile, undergoes lipolysis (the breakdown of fat) followed by re-esterification to allow it to be stored in adipocytes. People who want to lose weight while maintaining muscle and other important tissues are, biochemically speaking, attempting to burn through the triglycerides stored in adipocytes. These triglycerides are composed of carbon, hydrogen, and oxygen atoms. Triglycerides can only be broken down when these atoms are unlocked through a process known as oxidation, which requires oxygen.

Researchers found that for 22 pounds of fat to be oxidized, 64 pounds of oxygen must be inhaled. The oxidation results in about 61 pounds of carbon dioxide being excreted via the breath and about 24 pounds of water being excreted via urine, feces, breath, and sweat.

Thus, your lungs are the primary excretory organs for fat loss. Now stick with me here on the math: Each breath contains a little over 0.001 ounce of CO_2, of which about 0.0003 ounce is carbon. So a total of 17,280 breaths during the day (an average of 12 breaths per minute, a normal resting rate) will rid the body of at least 0.32 pound of carbon, with roughly a third of this fat loss occurring while you are completely inactive—assuming you get about eight hours of sleep per night.

How do you replace all that carbon you breathe out? Unless you have a horrible habit of munching on charcoal rocks or decide to overdose on charcoal capsules, the only significant carbon sources I know of are dietary carbohydrates, proteins, and fats.

So from as simple a standpoint as possible, losing fat means consuming less carbon than you have exhaled. If you were to spend a day doing nothing but sleeping for eight hours, resting for eight hours, and performing light activities that double your resting metabolic rate for eight hours, you would exhale about 7 ounces of carbon. Substituting one hour of rest per day with one hour of moderate exercise, such as hiking or cycling, increases your metabolic rate about seven-fold. This removes an extra 1.5 ounces of carbon from the body, increasing the amount of carbon exhaled by around 20 percent, from 7 ounces to 8.5 ounces.

 (sleep x 8 hrs) + (rest x 8 hrs) + (light activity x 8 hrs) = **7 oz carbon**

 (sleep x 8 hrs) + (rest x 7 hrs) + (light activity x 8 hrs) + (moderate exercise x 1 hr) = **8.5 oz carbon**

Problem is, weight loss can easily be offset by eating. A single 100 g muffin, for example, provides about 20 percent of the average person's daily energy requirement. This means physical activity as a weight-loss strategy is foiled even by relatively small quantities of food. So what is the most effective, albeit traditional and boring, solution to this conundrum? Simple: move more and eat less.

Congratulations, you now know as much about the true mechanisms behind weight loss as the average biochemistry student. But let's say you are already eating less and moving more. You are—theoretically at least—engaging in enough physical activity to breathe off more than enough carbon, and the scale still isn't budging. What gives?

You are about to discover sixteen reasons why you are not burning fat, why you may be resistant to weight loss, or why you are piling on pounds, and exactly what you can do to turn yourself into a fat-burning machine.

16 REASONS YOU CAN'T BURN FAT

When you're having trouble moving the needle on your weight, the answer isn't necessarily dieting or exercising more. If you're already active and eat healthy, then it's time to consider whether one or a combination of the sixteen factors below may be impeding your weight loss.

1. Inflammation

Remember the common belief that fat cells never go away? That simply isn't the case. There is something you can do to annihilate those fat cells, and that is to rid yourself of inflammation.

Before I jump into the nitty-gritty, let me emphasize that not all inflammation is bad. Acute inflammation is a natural biological reaction to stressors. For example, when you cut yourself, the area surrounding the cut becomes inflamed as your immune system and regenerative processes respond to prevent infection and quickly heal the cut. Acute inflammation also occurs when your muscle fibers are broken down and then rebuilt after a hard workout.

But when you overload your body with physical and mental stress to the point that it produces a constant stream of inflammatory chemicals, you can cause chronic inflammation. A combination of increased transforming growth factor beta signaling and a reduction in certain BMP-like signaling pathways promotes inflammation and can lead to adipose tissue dysfunction in obesity. Matrix metalloproteinases, enzymes that remodel the extracellular matrix (the network of molecules outside cells that give them support and structure) and regulate white blood cell movement, can also cause inflammation when their blood plasma activity gets too high. High levels of vascular endothelial growth factor, which aids in the growth of new blood vessels, are correlated with inflammation and obesity.

Genes can also play a role in chronic inflammation. For example, the enzyme nitric oxide synthase is involved in nitric oxide (NO) production, and while some NO is good, nitric oxide synthase hyperactivity can lead to excess NO, which can increase meta-inflammation, a state of low but chronic inflammation in immune and fat cells. Many genetic and epigenetic factors can contribute to this process, which is often called "NOS uncoupling." Rather than making nitric oxide, NOS uncoupling produces superoxide free radicals, particularly reactive ions that can contribute to the destructive path of inflammation. (You can get a genetic analysis from the company StrateGene to determine if you have a predisposition to NOS uncoupling.)

Another gene related to inflammation is the NFE2L2 gene, which manages the expression of Nrf2, a protein that helps protect against oxidation. If Nrf2 is not working properly, your body won't handle iron properly, and it may make excess free radicals. Often, people with variants in their NFE2L2 genes suffer from inflammatory conditions that nothing seems able to resolve. Functional genetic testing can help determine whether you have issues with this gene. Fortunately, there are some natural substances, such as sulforaphane (found in broccoli), resveratrol (found in the skins of grapes and in certain berries), bacopa, milk thistle, and turmeric, that support healthy Nrf2 activity and thereby reduce inflammation. (To determine if you have an issue with Nrf2-related inflammation, I recommend you connect with Dr. Bob Miller at TOLHealth.com for his genetic analysis, because this pathway is one of his specialties.)

There are more chemicals, enzymes, and factors involved in inflammation, but you get the idea: chronic inflammation is systemic and affects the entire body.

The biggest and most underemphasized cause of chronic inflammation is rancid oil. Oil that has been exposed to high temperatures or high pressures causes a one-two whammy of inflammation and insulin resistance. Polyunsaturated fats, which are especially prone to becoming rancid, are found in canola, safflower, peanut, and sunflower oils, which are commonly used in restaurants and in popular comfort foods from french fries, pizza, and chicken wings to mac 'n' cheese, packaged sushi, and trail mix. When polyunsaturated fats become oxidized and rancid, they promote the production of toxic substances in your arteries, which, in turn, promote chronic inflammation throughout your entire body. So the number one tactic for turning your body into a fat-decimating factory is to cut out those oils and replace them with healthy fat sources, such as coconut oil, extra-virgin olive oil, avocado oil, and macadamia nut oil.

Many nutritionists claim that the greatest inflammation-inducing aspect of any diet is sugar. But compared to rancid oils, glucose, fructose, sucrose, and other sugars are not all that inflammatory, as long as they are quickly metabolized. Sure, in massive quantities, such as half a dozen bananas a day, a stack of pancakes for breakfast, or multiple stops each day at the coffee shop baked goodies section, these sugars can cause serious issues (in a moment, I'll explain how fluctuating blood glucose levels can prevent you from losing weight). But overheated, overpressurized oils are inflammatory even if they are metabolized.

A second major cause of inflammation that is not addressed often enough is chronic stress. Continual, constant stress—from working way too much, PTSD, a tragic event, relationship issues, poor breathing patterns, frequent travel, and many other sources—can cause your brain to become overexposed to excitatory neurotransmitters such as glutamate and your limbic system to become stuck in fight-or-flight mode. The limbic system is a complex system of nerves and networks in the brain that controls basic emotions such as fear, pleasure, and anger and basic drives such as hunger and sex. As the limbic system becomes overstimulated, your immune system can become hyperactive and begin to see many foods and supplements as foreign invaders, resulting in a cytokine cascade and systemic inflammation, especially in type A, hard-charging, high achievers, who may also be acetylcholine-dominant (see page 14). This type of inflammation responds very well to breathwork, yoga, meditation, sleep, relaxing exercise, and other stress-mitigating strategies.

No discussion of inflammation would be complete without discussing cell danger response (CDR). CDR is the metabolic response to danger that protects cells and their hosts—including you, the human host—from harm. When you encounter chemical, physical, or biological threats that surpass your cells' ability to handle the accompanying emotional, exercise, or chemical stress, CDR kicks into gear. At that point, your cells become drained of resources necessary for functional capacity, which produces a number of changes in cell function, including electron flow, membrane fluidity, protein folding, metal detoxification, vitamin availability, oxygen consumption, and carbon and sulfur resource allocation.

When CDR first kicks in, it causes the release of metabolic intermediates like ATP, ADP, ROS, and oxygen, all of which can trigger an inflammatory response. Once the stressor has been eliminated, your body activates anti-inflammatory, regenerative mechanisms to counteract CDR and undo the damage. But if you experience chronic CDR from chronic stress, it disrupts your gut microbiome and metabolism, impairs organ system function, leads to behavioral changes, causes a decline in fat loss and muscle synthesis, promotes chronic disease, and triggers your body to release a harmful steady stream of inflammatory cytokines.

So what can you do about CDR? The most important treatment strategy for dealing with this "stuck" inflammation is to identify the emotion, traumatic event, infection, or toxin responsible for the response and treat it thoroughly. Treatment usually requires a combination of supplements, dietary and activity changes, and nutritional adaptogen therapies, and the best course of action is to meet with a functional medicine practitioner well versed in the syndrome. I highly recommend that you read the book *Toxic* by Dr. Neil Nathan, and look up the work of Dr. Robert Naviaux at Naviaux Lab (naviauxlab.ucsd.edu) to find solutions for CDR that has arisen due to emotional trauma, exercise overtraining, chemical stress, mold or mycotoxin exposure, or any other major life stressor that may have left you in a constantly activated "fight-or-flight" mode.

2. Glycemic Variability

Meet the elephant in the room that affects a host of longevity and chronic disease parameters, as well as fat loss: glycemic variability (GV). This term refers to the level and intensity with which your blood sugar fluctuates. GV accounts for hypoglycemic periods, postprandial rises in glucose levels, protein converted into sugar from a mess of steak or bacon and eggs (a process known as gluconeogenesis), and even blood sugar increases from stress or cortisol. (Shockingly, when I run 24-7 tests of my blood glucose levels via the continuous blood glucose monitor that is implanted into my tricep, the highest my blood glucose ever gets is after my big morning cup of coffee, due to the cortisol release and the subsequent dumping of liver glycogen into my system.)

GV is such a crucial component of your physiology that the brilliant surgeon and respected longevity physician Dr. Peter Attia said, in an interview on the eight keys to longevity, that "the name of the game is glucose disposal. Can you maintain a low average level of glucose and a low variance of glucose and a low area under the curve of insulin?" (The "area under the curve of insulin" refers to the amount of insulin displacement that occurs over the course of a day.)

If GV gets out of control and your blood sugar gets too high, your body has two choices: either shovel the sugar into your muscles and liver or store it in body fat. So if your energy expenditure throughout the day isn't high enough to convert blood sugar into potential energy in your muscles, you are going to gain fat tissue. Below, you will find six ways to prevent that from happening and even get rid of the carbohydrate-related body fat you already have. But first, you should understand one important fact: *sugar in your food isn't always bad.*

Yeah, you read that right.

Although sugar is demonized by waistline-conscious health nuts and elite athletes, sugar is not the menace it is made out to be. Every form of sugar—whether from bread, rice, bananas, yams, plantains, Mexican Coke, or coconut milk ice cream—is converted to glucose or triglycerides, both of which can be burned as energy if you are in a caloric deficit. You run into problems when you consume too much sugar, consume it too frequently, consume too much protein, or consume too much food overall.

You'll notice that the list of examples above includes foods that many people don't think of as high in sugar and may even consider healthy—bananas, yams, and plantains, for instance. But these are sources of sugar, just as donuts are. So now that you understand that you might be on a high-sugar diet even if you don't consume a lot of what would be recognized by most people as sugar, here are my six most effective strategies for controlling your blood sugar.

STRATEGY #1: STRENGTH TRAINING

Research suggests that when you strength train, you increase your ability to drive glucose into muscle tissue. Strength training decreases blood glucose levels and increases insulin sensitivity, even if you're lifting weights that are only 30 percent of your single-repetition maximum weight (1RM). This means you can control blood sugar, upregulate sugar transporters, and reduce the storage of sugar as fat with relatively light bodyweight exercises, such as push-ups, air squats, and lunges.

STRATEGY #2: PRE-BREAKFAST FASTED CARDIO

Research has shown that exercising before breakfast, particularly in a fasted state, is a potent strategy for controlling blood sugar. Incidentally, this is also an Ayurvedic strategy described in books like Suhas Kshirsagar's *Change Your Schedule, Change Your Life.* (I'll talk more about Ayurvedic medicine in chapter 15.)

One study assigned a group of participants to train in the morning before eating, drink only water during training, and then eat a large breakfast after training. Despite eating a large breakfast, the group's participants gained almost no weight, and their metabolic rates increased, so that they more efficiently burned the energy they consumed later in the day. So get a little training in before having your gluten-free muffin or creatine smoothie or handful of fish oil pills.

STRATEGY #3: POSTPRANDIAL WALKS

A Japanese study divided participants into three groups and had each group either sit, stand, or walk after a meal. They found that low-volume, easy walking for thirty minutes after a meal kept the concentration of fat in the blood 18 percent lower than sitting or standing after a meal. So not only should you exercise before breakfast in a fasted state, but you should also go on an easy twenty-to-thirty-minute walk immediately after dinner. And yes, I personally count dancing, having sex, playing backyard badminton, chasing the kids, or doing yard work as "walking."

STRATEGY #4: STANDING

While walking is more effective than standing after a meal, standing is much more effective than sitting. One office study found that standing for 180 minutes after lunch instead of sitting for the same amount of time reduced post-lunch blood sugar spikes 43 percent. Another study found that alternating between standing and sitting every thirty minutes throughout the workday reduced blood sugar spikes by 11.1 percent on average. So even during a day at the office, you don't have to work out to control blood sugar. The trick is not to sit down for the entirety of your workday and to hack your office environment so you stay physically active all day long (more on that in chapter 11).

STRATEGY #5: PLANTS, HERBS, AND SPICES

For those times when you can't exercise, you are forced to sit down for most of the workday, you have an eleven-hour flight, or you just want some extra help with blood sugar management, you can consume plants, herbs, and spices that help keep blood sugar stable. Some notable examples include Ceylon cinnamon, *Gymnema sylvestre*, berberine, rock lotus (a.k.a. shilianhua or stone lotus), and bitter melon extract. These are all potent, natural ingredients and compounds that can decrease the length and intensity of blood glucose spikes and prevent diabetes.

STRATEGY #6: FIBER

Anaerobic bacterial fermentation breaks down dietary insoluble fiber into short-chain fatty acids (SCFAs). About 95 percent of the SCFAs in your body are composed of either acetate, propionate, or butyrate. Research has shown that acetate inhibits the conversion of glucose to fatty acids in the liver. This reduces the accumulation of fat in adipose tissue and the liver and improves blood sugar management. Propionate improves glucose tolerance and insulin sensitivity (interestingly, propionic acid, of which propionate is the conjugate base, can inhibit gluconeogenesis in the liver and is also derived from the fermentation of fiber). In mice, butyrate has been shown to prevent and treat diet-induced insulin resistance by increasing insulin sensitivity, allowing the mice to metabolize glucose better.

You can find dietary insoluble fiber in foods such as nuts, sweet potatoes, yams, dark leafy greens, and legumes. If these foods cause gas, bloating, or other GI issues for you, you can also approximate the same effects by getting into a state of ketosis or by using ketone supplements such as beta-hydroxybutyrate (BHB) salts.

Walking, standing, fasted cardio, a little weight training, a few common herbs and spices you can obtain at your local health food store, and some extra fiber are all it takes to prevent the glycemic variability that holds many people back from fat loss and achieving the body they want.

Is Insulin Always Bad?

I personally don't engage in extreme carbohydrate restriction or a strict low-carb, high-fat ketogenic diet, because I want to maintain healthy insulin levels. Like cortisol, insulin is often vilified, but it's actually a superhormone that performs a host of functions beyond shoving excess sugar into fat cells. In fact, insulin performs several important jobs that have nothing to do with glucose—jobs that are performed far less efficiently if carbohydrates are excessively restricted.

SKELETAL MUSCLE METABOLISM: Insulin is critical for protein metabolism in muscle tissue and performs anabolic and anticatabolic actions—meaning it's crucial for muscle growth and repair. It increases the rate of transport of amino acids into muscle tissue, making them available for muscle protein synthesis. It also reduces muscle protein breakdown.

THYROID FUNCTION: The hormone thyroxine (T4) is produced in the thyroid gland and is then converted into the more active hormone triiodothyronine (T3). This process is upregulated by insulin and is significantly decreased during periods of excessive caloric or carbohydrate restriction.

BONE HEALTH: Cells called osteoblasts create new bone tissue and remineralize existing bone matrix by secreting hydroxyapatite crystals. Insulin increases osteoblast activity, proliferation, differentiation, and survival while also increasing collagen synthesis to improve connective tissue integrity.

HEALTHY IMMUNE RESPONSES: When insulin is elevated, immune cells become more stable. Insulin activates immune cells called neutrophils (the first line of defense during infection or injury) and other immune system sentinel cells. It even enhances the effectiveness of natural killer cells, which destroy infected or cancerous cells. It also activates helper T cells, which assist with immune attacks, and regulatory T cells, which modulate immune responses and prevent autoimmune diseases.

Conversely, blocking insulin can reduce the proliferation and migration of regulatory T cells. This is why high insulin levels can be inflammatory and at the same time insulin resistance or constantly suppressed insulin levels are associated with autoimmune issues and the suppression of the immune system.

CENTRAL NERVOUS SYSTEM HEALTH: Insulin can cross the blood-brain barrier and bind with receptors in different areas of the brain. For example, it can bind to receptors in the hypothalamus and hippocampus, where it regulates hunger and energy balance and even increases cognitive functions such as neuroplasticity, learning, and memory. Poor insulin signaling in the brain is associated with cognitive impairment, dementia, and Alzheimer's disease.

Insulin also protects against neuroinflammation by binding to receptors on microglial cells, the brain's resident immune cells. When insulin is low in the brain, the level of inflammatory cytokines in neural tissue increases. In people with particularly low insulin levels, this is often treated with intranasal insulin supplementation.

HORMONE REGULATION: Insulin acts with insulin-like growth factor 1 and follicle-stimulating hormone to increase estrogen and testosterone production. It also decreases levels of sex hormone binding globulin, which binds to testosterone and estrogen in the blood and renders them inactive. This means that, to a certain point, higher insulin levels give you more sex hormones and improve their bioavailability. Insulin also interacts with cortisol, growth hormone, and glucagon, as well as neurotransmitters like dopamine, serotonin, and melatonin.

For all these reasons, I make sure that I consume natural, healthy amounts of carbohydrates, particularly in the evenings on my more physically active days.

3. Cortisol and Stress

When you are stressed, your body releases hormones such as cortisol that turn on functions that are essential for your immediate survival, such as higher blood pressure and rapid decision-making, while inhibiting nonessential functions, such as immune function, digestion, and protein synthesis. This is helpful if you need to handle an acute stressor (like a looming deadline or an obstacle race), but it is also the reason why chronic stress restricts your ability to shed that extra weight around your midsection. Cortisol acts by suppressing insulin secretion, inhibiting glucose uptake into your cells, and disrupting insulin signaling to muscle tissue. That means that chronic stress directly causes insulin resistance, which then leads to weight-loss resistance, increased inflammation, dyslipidemia (elevated blood fat and cholesterol levels), and hypertension.

I have coached many clients, especially lean, hard-charging, type A men, who were already addressing many of the other factors mentioned in this chapter but still couldn't eliminate that last bit of belly fat. Once they learned how to manage stress and reduce cortisol, the extra belly fat often vanished, much to their surprise and satisfaction. (The other adjustment that achieves a similar effect is the complete elimination of processed sugar.) Even exercise, when performed in excess, can leave you chronically stressed and with elevated cortisol levels. And overtraining does not just happen to athletes—you may be in this category if you are not recovering properly (see chapter 12), you undernourish your body, or you fail to get quality sleep.

Other stressors that spike cortisol include the following:

- The death of a loved one
- Relationship or personality conflicts and sexual frustrations
- Losing a job
- Academic stress or continuing educational pressure
- Emotions such as boredom, hunger, anger, depression, fear, and anxiety
- Toxins and pollutants from your food or environment
- Excessive heat, cold, or humidity (including some harebrained decision to take a thirty-minute ice bath every day or blast yourself with a ninety-minute hot yoga class five days a week)
- High altitude or poor oxygen availability (including shallow chest breathing)
- Poorly designed, restrictive, or uncomfortable clothing and shoes
- Psyching yourself up too frequently (like engaging in Wim Hof fire-breathing at the beginning of every activity, from waking to working out to making an important call)
- Pressure to perform and constant attention from social media
- Lack of encouragement or love from others

One of the best ways to know if you are chronically stressed is to measure your heart rate variability (HRV). HRV is the variability in the amount of time between each heartbeat and can be used to track your nervous system health and recovery status. When the parasympathetic "rest-and-digest" nervous system is activated, it releases acetylcholine to induce a low heart rate and a state of relaxation. Your HRV will be highest at this point, so a high HRV indicates a low state of stress.

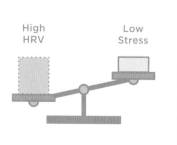

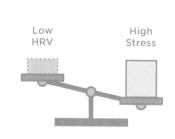

If you are not well-rested, the normal, healthy beat-to-beat variation in your heart rhythm falls. Abnormal variation can indicate a serious stress issue, especially if you see consistently low HRV values (my personal red flag is any HRV value below 80, unless I'm training very hard for a competition and am in an overreached state) or values that jump around from day to day (70 one day, 90 another day, 60 the next day). Tracking your HRV allows you to see if you are overstressing your body, producing excess cortisol, or becoming resistant to weight loss. In chapter 12, I'll explain how to track HRV quickly and effectively and how to interpret your numbers.

In my experience, low HRV primarily arises from a poor diet, poor breathing, relationship and work stress, overtraining, poor air quality, excessive artificial light exposure, electrical pollution from WiFi and Bluetooth signals, or impure water. When I addressed each of these variables in my own life over years of cleaning up damage, I achieved a consistent HRV of 90 every day, except on days when I was purposely training hard for a race or competition.

4. Sleep Deprivation

Only about 35 percent of all Americans get the recommended amount of sleep every night—between seven and nine hours—and many get less than six hours. Sleep deprivation has severe effects on the human body and weakens the immune and nervous systems so much that you become vulnerable to diseases and neurodegeneration. When it comes to fat loss, research has shown that getting between four to five hours of sleep per night causes insulin resistance and high glycemic variability, leading to diabetes, appetite cravings, and weight gain in people who would otherwise be healthy. Scarier yet is that all it takes to cause this type of damage is a single night of partial sleep.

Sleep deprivation is known to raise cortisol levels, reduce glucose tolerance, and increase sympathetic nervous system activity. One study found that, in addition to reducing insulin sensitivity and glucose tolerance, sleep deprivation reduces levels of the satiety-inducing hormone leptin and increases levels of the hunger-stimulating hormone ghrelin. So not only does sleep deprivation reduce your ability to metabolize glucose, but it also makes you want to consume more sugar and hedonistic, vegetable-oil-laden snack foods. This is why it is so easy to grab a second helping at the buffet or fail to stroll by a vending machine unscathed when you are sleep-deprived. (To understand even more about the link between sleep and weight gain, I highly recommend you read Dr. Satchin Panda's *The Circadian Code* and Dr. Matthew Walker's *Why We Sleep*.)

5. Snacking and Postworkout Calories

When I was bodybuilding, it was well known in the "mass gain" community that one of the best strategies for piling on the pounds was to arrive at work with a container of yogurt, a couple of Tupperware containers of lean chicken with rice and broccoli (bricken!), a couple of ziplock plastic bags of almonds, a handful of energy bars, and a premade protein shake, and consume all of this gradually over the course of the day. Sure, by lifting heavy weights morning and night for a couple of hours at a time, I would convert most of this food to muscle, but this type of grazing is also a fantastic strategy to pile on body fat, especially if you don't spend your life pumping iron in a gym.

The theory that you need to eat six small meals throughout the day to keep your metabolism elevated is a myth that I am guilty of having preached to many of my fat-loss clients. But it has long since been debunked by science. While digestion does produce a thermic effect that increases your metabolism, the bump is slight.

Frequent snacking increases glycemic variability and prevents you from getting the gut- and longevity-boosting benefits of fasting. It also keeps your blood sugar levels elevated and shifts your metabolism into sugar-burning mode, which does not allow your body to tap into its stored fats for fuel. In fact, there is no evidence that eating more than three meals per day boosts your metabolism, helps you lose weight, or aids in appetite control. On the other hand, if you eat only two or three meals per day in what is called a compressed eating window, your body burns fat and releases more antiaging and growth hormones. So eating six small meals per day may be worse for your waistline than eating two or three larger meals spread throughout the day.

The belief that you will enter "starvation mode" if you don't eat frequently is also false. It takes about three days of complete fasting or up to four weeks of extreme caloric restriction for your body to downregulate metabolism and thyroid activity. Research has shown that short-term fasts, such as daily, overnight twelve-to-sixteen-hour fasts, will actually increase your metabolic rate due to an increase in norepinephrine, one of the hormones that signal fat cells to break down. You don't necessarily have to reduce your caloric intake, especially if you are an active individual. The trick is to eat less often, not to eat less. (For all the details on calculating how many calories you should eat, visit BoundlessBook.com/8.)

Another common myth is that you need to shove some protein and carbs in your mouth or grab a Jamba Juice immediately after a workout. The idea behind eating right after finishing a workout is to maximize muscular adaptations, repair damaged tissues, and rapidly shuttle glycogen into muscle for ample anabolic growth during a limited window of maximum carbohydrate absorption (twenty minutes to two hours after training). But in every study looking at the benefits of immediate postworkout eating, participants ate after exercising in a fasted state, usually to exhaustion—and frankly, most of us are not jumping out of bed to exercise for 90 to 120 minutes with no fuel. So unless you want to gain significant mass (like if you are a high school or college football player trying to get to the next level by putting on 20 pounds), as long as you have eaten at some point prior to working out, there is no need to drop everything to slug down that postworkout protein drink. Your blood levels of amino acids and stored carbohydrates will still be elevated from any eating done prior to your workout—meaning that for a 5 p.m. visit to the gym, your body can metabolize your breakfast or lunch for fuel. In fact, occasionally waiting a couple of hours after you exercise to eat may boost growth hormone and testosterone levels. Unless you are performing two-a-day workouts within an eight-hour window each day, there is no need to drop the barbell and hustle to your gym bag for a shiny, wrapped recovery snack.

6. Not Moving Enough

Whether I am standing, lunging, kneeling, sitting, leaning, or in any other position I frequently adopt during a day of work, I stop every twenty-five to fifty minutes for a two-to-five-minute break of an activity such as kettlebell swings, a quick stroll up the stairs, jumping jacks, or a handful of burpees. Heck, I even pull over my car during road trips to do a hundred jumping jacks for each hour of driving, duck into the bathroom at restaurants for forty air squats in a stall, and do elaborate stretch routines at the back of airplanes.

I don't do this because I am a hyperactive freak who is addicted to exercise. Rather, as you have already learned, weight loss requires an expenditure of energy greater than the intake of energy through your diet. The brutal truth is that for most people, sitting for eight hours a day does not expend enough energy to counterbalance breakfast, lunch, dinner, and snacks, no matter how much exercise is performed at the beginning or end of the day. Even in people who exercise, habitual sedentary behavior is associated with metabolic syndrome, increased risk of obesity, type 2 diabetes, cardiovascular disease, and premature mortality. When you are regularly sedentary for extended periods, your blood sugar levels go haywire because a low level of physical activity causes unfavorable changes in insulin signaling, glucose transport, and the activity of lipoprotein lipase, the primary enzyme responsible for breaking down fats.

The solution? Move more, especially when you are at work, which is when people tend to move the least. Even in a traditional cubicle-based office, it is not difficult to duck away to the bathroom for air squats, the parking lot for jumping jacks, or the stairwell for stair climbs.

Research suggests that the effects of being sedentary, including insulin resistance, are partly independent of the amount of time spent in moderate- and vigorous-intensity physical activity. In other words, if you spend the majority of your day sitting down or just standing there with your knees locked, that hour you spend at the gym isn't doing you many metabolic favors. Sitting and even static standing may even place you at risk for heart issues during exercise, because a hard workout at the end of the day then becomes an attempt to force blood through "kinked" vessels.

Remember this: while a formal workout at the beginning or end of the day is not necessary for weight loss, *low-level physical activity throughout the day is*. (For details on how to turn your office into a calorie-decimating workstation, visit BoundlessBook.com/8.)

7. Too Much Exercise

Not only do you not lose weight when you don't move enough, but you also don't lose weight when you move *too much*. That may not be what you want to hear in an era of self-fulfillment and self-identity through exercise, with hard-core CrossFitters trying to stay on the whiteboard, Navy SEALs inspiring housewives to get up at 4 a.m. to crush the day and go to the pain cave, and a physical culture all about zero days off, no pain no gain, balls to the wall, and going HAAM (google that one if you're curious).

Don't get me wrong. I am not opposed to going to the pain cave, consistently going to the gym, and exercising more than the average person (especially if you are trying to climb your own Everest, such as training for a triathlon or a Spartan Race or, well, Mount Everest). But excessive exercise can lead to elevated levels of cortisol and inflammation, and we now live in an era of overtrained, inflamed folks with hormonal dysregulation and cortisol coming out their ears.

To gain strength, you have to tear muscle fibers by lifting moderately heavy weights, which tells your body that it needs to build more muscle in that area. To tear your muscle fibers, especially if you are already a trained individual, you have to push your muscles past their comfort levels. So to get stronger, you must lift weights beyond what you can comfortably handle. Increasing endurance involves a similar approach: you must encounter exhaustion and push the borders of your stamina to build everything from red blood cells to new mitochondria. But you don't need to do this every day. Indeed, consistently difficult daily training is accompanied by serious physiological complications. One study concluded that severe overtraining leads to immune system damage, fatigue, mood disturbances, physical discomfort, sleep difficulties, and reduced appetite. Even during the recovery stages of this study, fatigue and immune system deficits persisted if individuals pushed themselves to the brink of overtraining.

The fix? Take days off. Take more days off if you are older. Most hard-charging high achievers under forty benefit from at least one day of rest and recovery per week, and most folks over forty benefit from two to three such days. This doesn't mean couch and dark-chocolate-face-stuffing time. It just means you scratch your "I must make my body better" itch via activities such as sauna sessions, easy yoga, a cold soak, a massage, some trampolining, a nice hike (not the one with a brutality rating of five stars on your smartphone trails app), or anything else that allows you to enhance your body without beating it to shreds.

8. Chronic Cardio

No gym these days seems complete without a whole room or hallway dedicated to the rat-on-a-wheel glory of treadmills, stationary bikes, elliptical trainers, and—my favorite—steppers. But cardio tends to be vastly misunderstood as a fat-burning tool, and there is even an ongoing debate between meatheads and endurance junkies over what good or harm cardio does. The general belief among park joggers is that running melts fat off the belly like butter, while those who eschew cardio say it can harm your heart and even make you *more* fat.

The truth is a bit more nuanced than "cardio is good" or "cardio is bad." Cardio does not directly make you fat, especially since the daylong low-level physical activity I endorse in this chapter could technically be classified as cardio.

But cardio is not risk-free—especially the type that involves long marathon-training death marches, multihour cycling sessions, and the excessive, draining slog on the lineup of cardio machines at the gym. For example, legendary ultramarathoner Micah True died in 2012 at fifty-eight years old during a typical "easy" twelve-mile run. Considering that he could run as many as a hundred miles in a single day, twelve miles should have been nothing. But upon autopsy, his heart was found to be enlarged and scarred, and his death is now believed to be due to Phidippides cardiomyopathy, which is caused by chronic, excessive endurance exercise. Named for a Greek messenger who died after running more than 175 miles in two days, Phidippides cardiomyopathy is characterized by a heart that is enlarged and scarred, and is accompanied by elevated cardiac risk biomarkers such as troponin and natriuretic peptides, along with small patches of cardiac muscle damage that can be responsible for heart arrhythmias and even sudden death.

Unless you consistently run extreme distances, it is unlikely you need to worry about suffering (or pronouncing) Phidippides cardiomyopathy. But True's death (as well as many other such instances detailed in my last book, *Beyond Training*) illustrates that long bouts of cardio, while they may significantly improve your endurance, are not necessarily the best for your health—or your waistline. In fact, one of the problems that many endurance athletes become frustrated with is an inability to shed fat.

The reason for this is simple: endurance training and chronic cardio create a state of extreme metabolic efficiency. When you engage in aerobic exercise, your body wants to work as efficiently as possible while producing the greatest amount of physical output. So if you're performing long cardio sessions with increasing volume and frequency, your body will attempt to shed unnecessary, excess weight and store usable energy it can draw on during these sessions. Do you know what weight is more or less unnecessary when you run, because of its need to be carried and cooled? *Muscle.* And do you know what's a great source of stored, usable energy for cardio? *Body fat.* So when you perform increasingly grueling death marches, your body gets rid of muscle and stores fat to prepare for each bout of cardio, while also downregulating anabolic hormones such as testosterone and growth hormone, as these are paradoxical to extreme endurance efficiency. To see what I mean, perform a Google image search for "sprinter vs. marathoner" or "sprinter vs. long distance runner" and compare the body types—many marathoners, especially recreational marathoners, even have a visible paunch of fat at the waistline and lower belly.

To make matters worse, since muscle tissue mobilizes stored fat, especially when you are resting, the less muscle mass you have, the less fat you tend to burn. In addition, your body will eventually adapt to endurance cardio and burn energy more efficiently, which means that when you launch into a cardio session, you will use less and less of your stored body fat. Unless you reach the training volume of hard-core endurance athletes like Scott Jurek, Dean Karnazes, Timothy Olson, and other cardio junkies who often perform cardio in excess of four hours a day (which isn't necessarily good for your heart, time management, or productivity), chronic cardio won't do much to help you reach your weight-loss goals. Indeed, research suggests that aerobic exercise and cardio are only effective when you are both overweight and new to exercise.

So if you are already active, you should engage in short, high-intensity interval cardio sessions and also switch cardio modes frequently, meaning that if you do three intense cardio sessions per week, you could alternate between swimming, cycling, and running. One study found that after twenty weeks of training, the participants who performed HIIT (high-intensity interval training) lost more body fat than those who engaged in steady-state endurance training (like long, slow treadmill runs). HIIT is also effective in the prevention and management of insulin resistance and type 2 diabetes. Most HIIT sessions last about thirty minutes at the most, so you are getting a lot more bang for your buck than if you were to spend an hour tooling along on a treadmill.

9. The SAID Principle

The SAID principle is one of the first principles I learned in my undergraduate exercise physiology courses. It stands for "specific adaptation to imposed demands," and it basically states that your body will eventually adapt to the demands you place upon it. If running is your only form of cardio or push-ups are your only form of upper-body training, eventually, your body will become so adapted to those demands that it burns fewer calories and experiences fewer gains in response to the stimuli. As a result, you see fewer and fewer results from the tried-and-true exercise regimen that seemed to work so well for twelve weeks.

Perhaps there actually is something to adopting the latest workout fad found in the last health magazine you read ("Get the Six Day Beach Body You Deserve with These 12 Body Weight Moves!"), then dropping it for an entirely new routine once the next magazine arrives in your mailbox a month later ("Norwegian Volume Training for a Better Butt!"). Sometimes the best workout plan is the one you are not currently doing. Not only that, but the best time of day to work out is often whatever time of day you are not currently working out, the best length of time for an HIIT cardio workout is anything shorter or longer than what you are currently doing, and the best sport for shedding pounds is whatever sport you are not currently playing. Sure, you do want some consistency and a reliable routine that keeps you motivated, but if the scale isn't budging, sometimes randomness and variety are the answers.

The following are five specific modifications you can make to minimize the effects of endless repetition.

MODIFICATION #1: COMBINE EXERCISES

If your regimen includes a lot of weight lifting, you can combine many lifts into highly dynamic movements. If your current routine has you performing a set of squats and a set of shoulder presses, for instance, you can shock your muscles by combining the lifts into one single squat-to-shoulder-press movement. You can also do lunges and curls, vertical jumps and push-ups (a burpee), or medicine ball lift-and-throws.

MODIFICATION #2: IMPLEMENT ACTIVE REST PERIODS

Rather than resting between weight-training sets, do a thirty-, sixty-, or ninety-second cardio boost. For example, between sets of pull-downs or presses, run to the stationary bike and sprint for a minute. The metabolic demand of your workout will completely change. (This is my usual workout mode at hotel gyms because of the potent combination of strength and cardio training.)

MODIFICATION #3: TAKE IT OUTSIDE

Instead of your usual forty-five-minute jaunt on an elliptical, grab a set of dumbbells or a weighted backpack and hit the hiking trails. The unpredictability and undulation of a hiking trail can significantly increase physical demands and throw your body new curveballs.

MODIFICATION #4: CHANGE THE CENTER OF GRAVITY

If you usually use a barbell for your lunges, switch it up and try using dumbbells, kettlebells, or a medicine ball instead. Don a weighted vest or weighted backpack during a walk. For a cable exercise, move the cable up or down a few notches and come at the movement from a new angle. The altered weight positions and angles will force your body into an entirely new metabolic situation.

MODIFICATION #5: WORK OUT AT A DIFFERENT TIME OF DAY

Been working out in the morning for the past few years? Throw your body for a loop and hit the gym an hour before dinner. The whole workout will feel entirely different. If you normally exercise after lunch, turn lunch into a nap session and hit the gym for an early-morning workout instead. The only folks for whom this trick isn't such a great idea are those suffering from poor sleep: exercising at random intervals throughout the day isn't so great for your chronobiology.

These are just a few ways you can switch up your workouts and minimize repetition. When in doubt, follow this rule: *Don't go for more than four weeks without significantly changing a specific staple of your exercise program.*

10. Not Enough Exposure to Cold

It might surprise you to learn that not all fat is created equal. When most people think of fat, they think of the bad fat that accumulates around the belly, waist, hips, butt, and thighs. But that's just the tip of the fatberg. Bad fat is known as white adipose tissue (WAT, or white fat). This is stored energy that sits there waiting for you to mobilize it, providing, in the meantime, a bit of insulation and organ cushioning.

In contrast, brown adipose tissue (BAT, or brown fat) is primarily located around the sternum, clavicle, and rib cage and generates heat by directly mobilizing the energy stored in white fat. This process is known as nonshivering thermogenesis (commonly referred to as "cold thermogenesis") and occurs in the mitochondria of BAT cells when calories are turned into heat instead of ATP.

The hypothalamic and stem regions of the brain cause an upregulation of the sympathetic nervous system when they are activated by a sensation of cold. Please note that it is quite cool (ha!) that BAT uses calories to create heat rather than ATP because this means that cold drains your gas tank the same way fasting does.

There is also another type of fat called beige fat. Beige adipose tissue is BAT that, after cold exposure, appears within white adipose tissue. This process is known as the browning of white adipose tissue. But functionally, there is no difference between the metabolic activity of brown fat and beige fat, so the distinction pretty much comes down to location.

The key takeaway is that cold exposure stimulates brown fat to burn white fat, so one of your primary fat-burning techniques should be daily cold thermogenesis. In addition to daily cold showers at no more than 55 degrees Fahrenheit, a weekly cold soak for about twenty minutes in an ice tub, and frequent forays from the sauna to the cold and back, I use actual cold gear, especially in the summer, to enhance the formation of BAT. For example, the Cool Fat Burner vest wraps around your upper torso and activates the BAT in those regions, while the Cool Gut Buster enhances the formation of metabolically active beige fat around the waistline.

Strike, Stroll, Shiver

For two decades, from my days of ripped bodybuilding glory to lean triathlon speed, I have relied upon one daily, simple yet elegant fat-loss technique that has never failed me or the clients I train for everything from the elimination of morbid obesity to competition stage readiness. It is my most potent 1-2-3 fat-loss technique, and I call it "Strike [as in "hunger strike"—aren't I clever?], Stroll, Shiver."

1. Strike: This first step is optional, but it will give you an added fat-burning bonus: prior to "Stroll," step 2, consume a cup of coffee or green tea to help mobilize fatty acids and slightly boost your metabolic rate. It has to be plain-Jane coffee or tea—no sugar, no cream, no MCT oil, no butter—but you can add a couple of capsules of a blood sugar stabilizer such as berberine or bitter melon extract, a shot of apple cider vinegar, or a teaspoon or two of Ceylon cinnamon or cayenne extract to enhance its fat-burning effects even more. Just remember: no calories. If you are concerned about losing muscle or you are attempting to gain significant lean muscle mass, you can also consume 10 to 20 g of essential amino acids as well, which will provide a small anabolic effect without significantly spiking blood glucose or insulin.

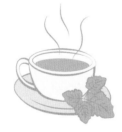

2. Stroll: As soon as you wake up, before you eat anything—before you sit down to breakfast or make yourself a smoothie or pour butter into your coffee or jump into your emails or take a shower—do a ten-to-forty-minute light aerobic session. Do this while you are still in a fasted state, which will allow your body to tap into its own fat for fuel. (Having coffee or tea per step 1 won't break your fast.) Choose a simple exercise you can perform 24-7, 365 days a year, such as a walk in the sunshine (bonus: morning vitamin D and circadian rhythm alignment!), an easy yoga session, walking the dog, riding your bike, a leisurely swim, or even a

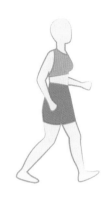

sweat in a dry or infrared sauna. Choose anything that's light, easy, aerobic, conversational, and low-stress. It won't cause a significant release of cortisol, it won't completely exhaust you for the day, it will still allow you to perform a hard workout later in the day, and it won't make you feel famished and want to devour every breakfast item in sight afterward. But it will jump-start fat-burning.

3. Shiver: Complete your "stroll" and dive straight into two to five minutes of exposure to anything cold. Any of the cold thermogenesis tactics in chapter 2 count, including a hot-cold contrast shower, a dip into a cold river or lake, a cold bath, or even donning cold thermogenesis gear such the Cool Fat Burner or Cool Gut Buster vest (the latter can be worn for forty to sixty minutes as you work, commute, clean the garage, or eat breakfast). This step will not only help strip inflammatory white adipose tissue off your belly but also increase your metabolically active brown adipose tissue, which will further enhance your capacity to burn fat.

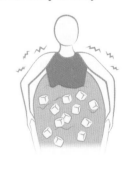

That's it! I stick to this strategy year-round, including on Christmas Day and Thanksgiving, and it is one of the biggest fat-loss game changers I have ever utilized. It also fits nicely into the simple category of "move more and eat less," with a few extra hacks thrown in.

11. Hormonal Imbalances

Endocrine disruption and hormonal imbalances can occur when you're as young as your early twenties and can be caused by exposure to chemicals such as pesticides and plasticizers; external stress such as relationship or financial problems; internal stress such as viruses, heavy metal accumulation, and blood sugar swings; dietary contaminants; deficiencies in critical micronutrients; lack of sleep; and poor digestive health. When hormones are disrupted, metabolism slows down, appetite rages, and inflammation manifests.

Although both men and women struggle with hormonal imbalances, women seem to have more trouble with imbalances that specifically cause resistance to fat loss. For example, the hormone estrogen is higher in women and promotes cell division, cell growth, and, in excessive amounts, the formation of fat tissue. Women also naturally produce more progesterone, which protects against such excessive fat growth. Problem is, progesterone production declines much faster with age than estrogen production, so between ages thirty and fifty, a woman can develop estrogen dominance. At that point, fat rapidly accumulates and becomes much harder to lose. Of course, men can also experience similar age-related issues as testosterone falls and estrogen rises.

There are steps you can take to minimize the effects of hormonal imbalances. But first, it's best to determine whether a hormonal imbalance is causing weight-loss resistance. Some blood tests give you a snapshot view of your hormone levels at a single moment, but you can test for hormonal imbalances that occur throughout a twenty-four-hour cycle with the DUTCH urine test, which I'll talk more about in chapter 16.

If you do find hormonal imbalances after receiving the results of your DUTCH panel, or if you suspect a hormonal imbalance is keeping you from losing weight, you can make some lifestyle and dietary changes to mitigate the damage.

HORMONE STRATEGY #1: EAT MORE CRUCIFEROUS VEGGIES

Cruciferous vegetables include broccoli, cauliflower, brussels sprouts, and cabbage. They contain indole-3-carbinol, an antioxidant that metabolizes excess estrogen.

HORMONE STRATEGY #2: FILTER YOUR WATER

Heavy metals and chemicals like fluoride (which is actually a registered insecticide and rodenticide) found in drinking water can damage the endocrine system. You can eliminate these metals and chemicals by installing a drinking water filtration system, such as a reverse osmosis filter, in your home. Unless you want to add trace liquid minerals to your water afterward, be sure to get a unit with a built-in remineralizer to refortify the water with good minerals like calcium, magnesium, and potassium.

HORMONE STRATEGY #3: USE GLASS OR STAINLESS-STEEL PRODUCTS INSTEAD OF PLASTIC

Chemicals that interfere with hormones, like BPA, can seep from plastic bottles and cups into your drinking water or food. My friend Anthony Jay has written a book called *Estrogeneration* that specifically addresses how plastic exposure affects estrogen, and I recommend reading it if you want to learn more about how environmental factors are affecting hormones and harming health. (Chapter 20 also includes plenty of potent environmental-hacking strategies that will significantly reduce your exposure to endocrine disruptors such as BPA.)

12. Exposure to Toxins and Chemicals

Three-letter-acronym toxins like PCBs, DDT, DDE, and BPA have been found in extremely high concentrations in human fat tissue and cause significant metabolic damage, hormonal imbalances, and even more fat storage.

Toxins are shoveled into adipose tissue by your body to protect other functional tissues and the internal organs. If you store too many toxins and nondegradable chemicals in fat tissue, you will have a much harder time losing weight, no matter how much you exercise or how much clean food you eat or how much cold exposure you get. But this is also why a rapid fat-loss regimen often results in skin rashes, zits, and diarrhea: as you mobilize fat, you also mobilize the toxins it contains. The toxins then cause other symptoms unless they are dealt with via a detox protocol.

Filtering your water and using glass or stainless steel instead of plastic are great ways to minimize toxin and chemical damage. You can also take steps to minimize uncomfortable side effects, such as irritability and inflammation, that can occur as chemicals and toxins get mobilized from fat and released back into your blood system. A full spectrum of whole-food antioxidant sources can be incredibly beneficial in eliminating the free radicals and oxidants that cause cellular damage and accelerate aging. Plus, if you get some of your antioxidants from plant sources such as dark berries and leafy greens, then you will also get fiber in your diet. Fiber acts like a sponge and can soak up toxins from your system as they are released. For this reason, while on any fat-loss regimen, you should aim for roughly 35 to 60 g of fiber per day from organic produce, berries, and a limited amount of larger fruits, seeds, and nuts. (There are more details and guidelines for dealing with toxins in other chapters: chapter 4 includes a list of foods and ingredients high in antioxidants, as well some supplemental antioxidants; chapter 13 explains how to detox your body; and chapter 20 explores detoxing your home from invisible chemicals in air and water.)

13. Food Allergies and Intolerances

If you have a food allergy, then you probably already know it. Food allergies are accompanied by severe symptoms such as throat swelling or respiratory distress—as you may know from a friend who needs to be within a stone's throw of an ambulance if he so much as sniffs a peanut.

An allergy occurs when your immune system misidentifies a protein as harmful and mounts an emergency response. Some proteins or protein fragments, such as those found in peanuts or shellfish, are resistant to digestion, and in people with an allergy, the proteins that don't get broken down during digestion are tagged by an antibody called immunoglobulin E. This fools the immune system into thinking that the protein is an invader, so your immune system attacks it and triggers an allergic reaction. The subsequent effects can include hives, shock, severe drops in blood pressure, respiratory distress, and anaphylactic reactions. As you can imagine, weight gain is not your primary concern if this happens—simply staying alive is the higher priority.

In contrast, a food intolerance is much more subtle and can happen because of a number of physiological deficiencies, such as insufficient levels of the liver enzymes that dissolve fructose, or low levels of the enzyme lactase, which can lead to an intolerance of unfermented dairy products (the fermentation process involved in making, say, yogurt tends to significantly reduce levels of lactose). Gluten intolerances are also common, although many people who believe they have gluten issues may have an entirely different problem. Most gluten-containing foods also contain gliadin. If you have a subclinical sensitivity to gliadin, consuming these foods can cause an inflammatory response in the small intestine (I'll talk plenty more about this in chapter 13). This is more common in people of Northern European and Eastern European descent.

The symptoms of all these food intolerances can be similar to those of food allergies, but they're not as pronounced. But both allergies and intolerances involve an inflammatory response, which can lead to weight gain if you consistently consume foods you can't tolerate.

Cyrex Laboratories offers what I consider to be the best food intolerance panel. Rather than giving you a frustrating and inaccurate laundry list of foods you are never supposed to touch again, it identifies an accurate, targeted list of foods to remove from your diet, without an annoying false positive list of foods you're not allowed to eat (more on why this is the case in chapter 13). Cyrex's approach to testing for reactivity to cooked, processed, and raw foods sets the laboratory apart from its competitors because once a food is heated to 118 degrees or more, its protein structure and potential for triggering an antigen reaction may change. For example, a person's inflammatory response to cooked chicken may be far different than the response to raw chicken. As a result, the Cyrex Array 10-90 test minimizes the risk of missing reactivity or generating false positives in response to common foods, and Cyrex's Comprehensive Food Immune Reactivity Panel—although expensive at close to $1,000 and only available by a physician's order—is even more informative because it combines tests for wheat and gluten cross-reactivity with tests for over 180 different food antigens. (In addition to simply avoiding foods you don't tolerate well, there are many things you can do to fix your gut once damage has been done, as I'll explain in chapter 13.)

14. Micronutrient Deficiencies

If you have spent any time trying to balance your diet, you have undoubtedly heard the term *macros*, which refers to the three macronutrients: protein, carbohydrates, and fats. While these are crucial nutrients, they don't even begin to cover all the vitamins, minerals, and other micronutrients that your body needs to function at a basic level. Research has shown that specific micronutrient deficiencies are associated with weight gain and obesity. Among these micronutrients, the most significant are vitamin D, chromium, biotin, thiamine, and antioxidants. Deficiencies in these can prevent fat loss via mechanisms that include altered insulin gene transcription, amplification of intracellular insulin signaling, and changes to glucose and amino acid metabolism. Metabolism and weight loss are also negatively affected by deficiencies in magnesium, boron, vitamin A, vitamin K_2, and choline.

Micronutrient deficiencies can be caused by digestion issues or, because many of these micronutrients are fat soluble, fat deficiencies and malabsorption. How much of which micronutrients a person needs varies from person to person (a diversity that I first discovered in Roger Williams's *Biochemical Individuality* and that I'll talk more about in chapter 13). For example, some people have higher rates of excretion of micronutrients than retention, and people with tuberculosis have far greater needs for vitamin C and vitamin A. While it is unlikely that you have tuberculosis, you get the idea: different people have different nutritional requirements.

Due to this nutritional diversity, it is worth investing in a laboratory test to determine whether or not you are deficient in any micronutrients. A comprehensive micronutrient test measures a host of vitamins, antioxidants, minerals, and amino acids in your blood to determine sufficiencies and deficiencies. My recommendation is the Genova ION (Individual Optimal Nutrition) Profile with 40 Amino Acids nutritional analysis, which can also help identify nutritional deficiencies that may be causing chronic diseases, sleep disruption, or cognitive decline.

15. Hypothyroidism

The thyroid gland produces hormones that regulate metabolism. It secretes thyroxine (T4) and triiodothyronine (T3), which influence the metabolic rate of lipids, cholesterol, glucose, and proteins within the cells throughout your body. When the thyroid becomes underactive, it results in a condition called hypothyroidism, which can often result in weight gain.

What causes hypothyroidism? In adults, it can be caused by deficiencies in iodine and selenium, but it can also occur as a birth defect known as congenital hypothyroidism. Excess stress can cause disorders of the hypothalamus that reduce levels of T3 and T4. Long-term caloric or carbohydrate deprivation can also reduce thyroid activity. As you can imagine, when you combine hard exercise, a busy work life, and lack of sleep, the thyroid takes a big hit. For example, the lowest thyroid activity I have ever experienced was when I was a skinny, carbohydrate-restricting Ironman triathlete, and the only factor saving me from the stereotypical endurance athlete "muffin top" was my extreme level of physical activity.

If you suspect you have hypothyroidism, you can get a comprehensive blood test for thyroid activity or a resting metabolic rate (RMR) test to evaluate whether your metabolic rate is too low. If you do identify thyroid-related issues, you can first, as ironic as it may seem, consider slowing down. Overtraining is one of the key contributors to weight-loss resistance. Back-to-back days of weight lifting or empty miles of the same ho-hum pace, limited recovery days, and the absence of recovery weeks are all tough on your thyroid function. In addition, you can seek out nutrient-dense, thyroid-supporting foods: seaweed and dulse for iodine, Brazil nuts, shellfish, and oysters for selenium, and coconut oil for proper thyroid conversion and metabolism in the gut.

16. Lack of a Regular Eating Schedule

Research suggests that for some people, maintaining a regular eating schedule can improve the metabolic response to meals. So if you are having trouble losing weight, rather than skipping breakfast some days and eating it on others or having dinner late some nights and early the other nights or shifting from restaurant to restaurant for your lunch choices, you should establish far more consistent meal patterns. Heck, I have had clients who shed pounds simply by eating the same meals (a smoothie for breakfast, a salad for lunch, meat or fish and vegetables for dinner) at the same times day in and day out for a few months.

Women seem to benefit most from this type of regularity. In one study of healthy lean women, an irregular meal pattern resulted in lower postprandial metabolism than a regular meal pattern. In another study, lean women who ate meals on a regular schedule had better insulin sensitivity and improved blood fat levels. In yet another study, this time of healthy obese women, regular mealtimes increased postprandial thermogenesis, insulin sensitivity, and blood lipids, putting the women in a state more conducive to weight loss.

Some folks can thrive on an erratic eating schedule. But for many people, irregular meal times seem to significantly lower the metabolic rate compared to eating at regular meal times. The result can be dysregulated appetite and altered metabolism. If you don't have a structured eating schedule and you are having trouble losing weight, try eating at the same times every day for a while, and try to keep the volume and nature of the meals relatively consistent.

THE LAST WORD

This chapter talked a lot about different factors that can prevent you from losing weight and how to reverse those negative effects to get the body that you desire. But before you go waltzing off into the sunset with your physique toolbox, expecting to attain a perfect, shredded body, there is something you should understand: *everybody is different, and so is every body.*

Even if you aren't satisfied with your physique according to the subjective beauty standards thrown at you in magazines and pop culture, it may be the case that your body has reached its ideal weight. You may not like to read this, and it may not seem fair, but you can reach a state of healthy homeostasis even if you have a higher-than-desired body fat percentage. If you are doing everything right, if you have nailed every element in this chapter, and you still can't seem to lose more weight, you might have to accept the fact that you have reached your healthy homeostasis and you just weren't designed to have veins in your abs or striated lats or skinny calves. And that's okay—own those thick legs!

Excessive exercising and dieting with an orthorexic approach to life while beating your body to smithereens with fat-loss biohacks is certainly not going to shift you into maximum fat-burning mode or shrink your waistline. In fact, it is more likely to downregulate vital components of having boundless energy, such as relationships, satisfaction, and happiness.

So accept the fact that you have a unique body. Inject light levels of physical activity or mild discomfort into the day, stand while you work, take cold showers, avoid sitting for long periods of time, engage in deep diaphragmatic breathing, implement intermittent fasting, and use the other unconventional fat-loss techniques that will enhance not just fat loss but health. Then simply be satisfied and happy with the body you have been blessed with.

ONE THING YOU CAN DO THIS WEEK

Since I said earlier that this is my favorite fat-burning technique, you probably saw this coming: tomorrow morning, perform "Strike, Stroll, Shiver," the potent 1-2-3 fat-loss technique you discovered earlier in this chapter. First, consume some caffeine in the form of coffee or tea (if desired, take a few other choice supplements, such as bitter melon extract). Second, perform ten to forty minutes of light, fat-burning aerobic activity. Finally, take a two-to-five-minute cold shower. That's it! If you make this practice a staple in your life, it will help keep you lean year-round. (See page 177 for more details on these steps.)

For citations for all the research studies mentioned in this chapter and a deeper dive into the topics of this chapter—including links to podcasts, blog posts, recommended tools and supplements, and much more—visit BoundlessBook.com/8.

SEXY FOREVER

HOW TO BUILD FUNCTIONAL MUSCLE FOR LIFE

30, 29, 28, 27, 26 . . . Sandwiched between music producer Rick Rubin and author Neil Strauss, I struggled against a giant Nautilus machine in the basement of eighty-five-year-old Don Wildman's Malibu home, churning out reps in what *Esquire* magazine had dubbed "The Hardest Workout in the World": a puke-inducing two-hour suffer-fest that Don performs three times per week, humbling younger fitness enthusiasts like myself.

Afterward, as I lay flat on my back recovering on the carpet of Don's basement, I pondered which was more difficult: the workout I had just completed, the three hours of ultimate frisbee I'd played with sixty-five-year-old primal godfather Mark Sisson, the extreme isometric ARX Fit workout with eighty-year-old longevity icon Art De Vany, my underwater pool workout with seemingly ageless big-wave surfer Laird Hamilton, my rock-tower-building workout in the desert with fifty-seven-year-old Paul Chek, or my four-hour sauna foray with the crazy, sixty-seven-year-old Finnish inventor and fitness icon Vessi Jalkanen.

In adventures like these and many more, I have picked up quite a few tips. For example, want to know how to reverse nearly forty years of aging? It's simple: *lift heavy stuff.*

In this chapter, you will learn why lifting heavy stuff could be one of the most potent tactics for defying age. In fact, details from the latest in muscle-building and muscle-maintenance research make this chapter your ultimate guide to preserving youth and building lean, functional muscle in the cleanest, most efficient way possible.

I will delve into fascinating twin studies on antiaging and weight lifting, the best type of muscle fiber to possess, a single gene that turns on muscle-building and antiaging pathways, how to stop the average loss of 6 pounds of muscle per decade, the type of exercise that beats the pants off cardio and aerobics, how to turn your cells into tiny muscle-building machines, and much, much more.

We will also venture out of the whitewashed lab with its petri dishes and into the real world. After all, the important question is whether strength training, load bearing, and powerlifting can truly make you live longer, and this chapter will give you the best antiaging secrets from some of the fittest old people on the face of the planet.

A fit body is a sound physical dwelling for boundless energy. You will leave this chapter equipped to get the body you want quickly, safely, and without spending oodles of hours in the gym.

LONGEVITY AND LIFTING 101

Muscles become smaller and weaker with age via a process called sarcopenia. Research suggests that a key part of this decline occurs in your muscle cells' mitochondria, the primary engines of energy production. A 2007 study demonstrated that six months of progressive resistance training, otherwise known as "lifting heavy stuff," made the gene expression of aging mitochondria appear to be significantly younger. During this study researchers discovered that men at an average age of seventy were able to improve strength by approximately 50 percent. The strength-training seniors closed the strength gap between themselves and men who were nearly forty years younger, taking it from 59 percent to 38 percent. That is an improvement of almost 36 percent in a mere six months. Muscle biopsies from the study showed a remarkable reversal of the expression profile of 179 genes associated with age and exercise. Genes that are downregulated with age were upregulated with exercise, while genes that are upregulated with age were downregulated with exercise.

The researchers reported: "Healthy older adults show a gene expression profile in skeletal muscle consistent with mitochondrial dysfunction and associated processes such as cell death, as compared with young individuals. Moreover, following a period of resistance exercise training in older adults, we found that age-associated transcriptome expression changes were reversed, implying a restoration of a youthful expression profile."

Yes, you read that right: when it comes to mitochondria, strength training reversed nearly forty years of aging! But exercise doesn't only affect mitochondria. It also promotes the growth of fat-burning fast-twitch muscle fibers and even protects DNA from the wear and tear of aging by acting on telomeres, the end caps of DNA molecules.

Why Telomeres Matter

Telomeres cap the chromosomes in your cells and protect them from damage. As you age, telomeres wear out and shorten from repeated cell division, oxidative stress, and inflammation, eventually leaving your cells' chromosomes unprotected. When your telomeres disappear, the wear and tear begins to cut into your genes, your cells become damaged, and soon they are discarded.

Here's how it works: when a cell prepares to divide, the double helix of a DNA strand inside the chromosome is unzipped, leaving the genes open so they can be copied. But the telomere at the ends of the chromosome can't be completely copied, so once the DNA has

been copied, a little bit of the telomere gets snipped off. The telomere theory of aging dictates that as cells divide and proliferate, the telomeres become shorter and shorter until they disappear. At this point, the rest of the chromosome can't be copied; the cell is now incapable of replicating itself, so it simply ages.

Oddly enough, this phenomenon doesn't seem to happen to everyone. A group of researchers in Sweden recently discovered that some people's telomeres don't get shorter through cell replication; in fact, they can even get longer over time. It could be that those people have robust, built-in cellular antiaging mechanisms, or they could have an early sign of cancer (for example,

In another study, scientists measured telomeres in twins to determine the effects of exercise on aging. The researchers hypothesized that, from a biological standpoint, telomere lengths might be able to tell them how old someone is. They had 2,401 twins (2,152 women and 249 men, aged eighteen to eighty-one) fill out questionnaires on physical activity level, smoking status, disease status, and socioeconomic status, and extracted DNA from participants' blood samples.

What did the researchers find? Telomere lengths decrease with age. No surprises there. But both women and men who were physically active had longer telomeres than their sedentary counterparts, even after adjusting for age, weight, diseases, socioeconomic status, and smoking. In addition, the subjects who performed more than three hours of vigorous physical activity per week had longer telomeres than subjects ten years younger.

These results indicate that people who don't put heavy physical loads on their bodies may be biologically ten years older than active people of the same chronological age. Since the subjects were identical twins, this effect isn't due to genes but rather to a lifestyle factor: exercise. When one twin exercised significantly more than the other, they had longer, more durable telomeres.

In yet another study, researchers found that replacing slow-twitch (type I) muscle fibers with stronger fast-twitch (type II) muscle fibers produced a significant reduction in both fat mass and insulin resistance. The researchers examined genetically engineered mice that contained a muscle-growth-regulating gene called Akt1 that could be turned on and off by the researchers.

Activating the Akt1 gene caused the mice to grow type II fibers without exercise (this is important to note, since mice don't lift weights that well, even when commanded to by scientists in white lab coats). When the Akt1 gene was turned on, the mice adopted the characteristics of a lean and powerful sprinter or weight lifter. When the gene was turned off, the mice reverted to type I muscle fibers and became more obese and insulin resistant with no change in diet.

The researchers reported that, "remarkably, type II muscle growth was associated with an overall reduction in body mass, due to a large decrease in fat mass. In addition, blood tests showed that these mice became metabolically normal [with no insulin resistance]. This work shows that type II muscle doesn't just allow you to pick up heavy objects; it is also important in controlling whole body metabolism. It appears that the increase in type II muscle fiber orchestrates changes in the body through its ability to communicate with other tissues."

The key takeaway from this study is that when you have more slow-twitch muscle fibers, which develop when you engage in chronic endurance exercise, you gain fat more easily. When you have

the potential for uncontrolled DNA replication), or it could be something we simply don't know about yet.

Even though the science is young, a simple blood test allows you to determine your telomere lengths and track the effectiveness of any antiaging tactics you implement. An example of an at-home test is Teloyears. A functional medicine physician can also oversee a slightly more accurate Spectracell analysis. In chapter 19, you will discover much more about telomeres and how to keep them from shortening, along with an intriguing enzyme called telomerase.

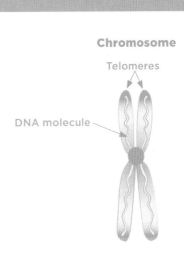

Chromosome

Telomeres

DNA molecule

Hefty bouts of chronic cardio and endurance exercise don't do you many fat-loss favors. But do long bouts of aerobic exercise provide any benefits? Is it all bad for your heart, as many scientists and weight-training junkies claim?

A series of studies have revealed that endurance exercise is actually quite effective at preserving telomere lengths, which may help slow aging (see page 183). For example, one study found that ultrarunners' telomeres were 11 percent longer than those of non-runners, which corresponds to a sixteen-year reduction in biological age. Another, more recent study found that people who exercised the most had biological aging markers that appeared nine years younger than those who were sedentary. But how much cardio do you have to do to see telomere benefits? Do you really have to go out and run ultramarathons?

Researcher Larry Tucker of Brigham Young University has investigated this question and published three relatively recent studies on telomeres. Tucker analyzed data from nearly six thousand adults and examined their telomere lengths and physical activity patterns. Those who exercised did indeed have longer telomeres, but only those who exercised the most. Even after adjusting for differences in demographics and lifestyle, the high-physical-activity group's cells were almost nine years younger than the sedentary group's cells. There were no significant differences in telomere lengths between the sedentary, low-activity, and moderate-activity groups. This means that to get the benefits of running, you have to engage in the highest amount of activity. Based on his research, Tucker recommended a threshold of about thirty minutes of cardio five days per week for women and forty minutes of cardio five days per week for men.

While these studies didn't account for time spent strength training and didn't have a control group of people who performed HIIT training or heavy lifting, they do suggest that not all chronic cardio is harmful. This makes sense when you consider the high levels of low-intensity physical activity done throughout the day in many centenarian and hunter-gatherer populations.

Now, a recent study revealed that there really is not a law of diminishing returns when it comes to cardiovascular fitness and mortality. But this shouldn't be interpreted to mean that there's no ceiling to the amount of exercise you can benefit from, which is how popular media interpreted this latest research, making claims such as "New Study Shows You Can't Exercise Too Much" and "There's No Such Thing as Too Much Exercise." At first glance, this study does indeed appear to bust the myth that chronic cardio is bad for you and contradict the U-shaped curve of endurance training showing that a certain amount is good, but more is not better. It appears that the results do suggest that the more you train, the longer you'll live. But this study didn't actually measure time spent training. Instead, the study subjects were given treadmill stress tests to determine their cardiovascular fitness, and then they were divided into different tiers of fitness based on the results. As you can imagine, everything from genetics to training efficiency to cardiovascular health could drastically affect these results, and they in no way imply that the more you train, the better. All we can really infer from this study is that higher levels of cardiovascular fitness predict greater longevity.

more fast-twitch muscle fibers, you burn fat faster and can more quickly achieve the body you want. Do you know what builds fast-twitch muscle fibers? That's right: strength training.

Beyond the age of thirty, we lose approximately 6 pounds of muscle mass per decade. These studies indicate that strength training may be critical in the fight against aging, obesity, and related ailments, such as diabetes, heart disease, stroke, hypertension, and cancer.

Finally, a study on strength training looked into reports of abnormally short telomeres in the skeletal muscle of athletes with exercise-associated fatigue. The goal of the study was to determine whether chronic hard exercise might negatively impact muscle telomere lengths.

The researchers compared telomere lengths of powerlifters who had trained for an average of eight years against those of healthy, active subjects with no history of strength training. There was no abnormal shortening of telomeres in the powerlifters. In fact, the powerlifters' telomeres were significantly longer than those of the control group and were positively correlated to the powerlifters' individual records in the squat and dead lift. In other words, the stronger the power-lifter was, the longer his telomeres were.

These results indicate that long-term strength training is not associated with abnormally short telomere lengths and that the heavier the load on your muscles, the longer your telomeres. And remember that, from a longevity standpoint, big, bulky, bodybuilding-esque muscle can be inferi-or to compact, wiry, explosive, powerlifting-esque muscles. Makes even more sense now, eh?

LIFTING HEAVY STUFF CAN MAKE YOU LIVE LONGER

Do Some Sports Make You Live Longer?

Let's get this out of the petri dish and into the real world. Can strength training and powerlifting actually make you live longer?

A recent study showed that older adults who met twice-weekly strength-training guidelines had lower odds of dying. This study was the first to demonstrate such an association in a large, nationally representative sample over an extended period, particularly in an older population.

Sure, previous studies had found that older adults who were physically active had a better quality of life and a reduced risk of mortality. There's a lot of research suggesting that regular exercise is associated with health benefits that include a reduced risk of early death, cardiovascular disease, diabetes, and cancer.

However, this study on the effects of strength training on mortality in older adults was a bit of a bigger deal. Researchers analyzed data from the 1997–2001 National Health Interview Survey (NHIS) as well as death certificate data through 2011. The NHIS collects data on health, disease, and disability in the United States from a nationally representative sampling of all fifty states and the District of Columbia. The 1997–2001 survey included more than thirty thousand adults aged sixty-five and older.

The researchers found that during the survey period, more than 9 percent of older adults reported at least twice-weekly strength-training sessions. They then followed the participants for fifteen years through death certificate data from the National Center for Health Statistics' National Death Index to get a long-term view of the association between strength training and mortality.

What did they find? *Older adults who engaged in strength training at least twice a week had 46 percent lower odds of death for any reason than those who did not.* They also had 41 percent lower odds of dying from cardiac problems and 19 percent lower odds of dying from cancer.

When it comes to sports and mortality, the research is quite interesting. One study led by Oxford University and published in the *British Journal of Sports Medicine* looked at eighty thousand people over the age of thirty to find out what effects different types of sports have on longevity. It turns out that people who play racquet sports (such as tennis or racquetball) on a regular basis can reduce their risk of dying prematurely by 47 percent. The next most beneficial exercise was swimming, which reduced the risk of dying prematurely by 28 percent, followed by cycling at 15 percent. Running, football, and rugby did not seem to impact longevity. But while the benefits of basic physical activity and aerobic exercise are well established, there is less research on strength training—although researchers have demonstrated the benefits of strength training for diabetes, osteoporosis, lower back pain, and obesity, and smaller studies have observed that greater muscular strength is associated with lower risks of death.

Older adults who met strength-training guidelines were, on average, slightly younger (closer to sixty-five, the minimum age for the survey) and were more likely to be married white males with higher levels of education. They were also more likely to have healthy body weights, engage in aerobic exercise, and abstain from alcohol and tobacco. But when the researchers adjusted for these demographic variables, health behaviors, and health conditions, the results remained the same. Even after the researchers controlled for physical activity level, people who practiced strength training seemed to enjoy a greater mortality benefit than those who reported physical activity alone.

This groundbreaking study provided substantial, statistically significant evidence that strength training in older adults is beneficial for slowing the effects of aging.

WHAT KIND OF WEIGHT TRAINING IS BEST?

Lest you rush to the gym salivating to engage in the ultimate antiaging, muscle-toning routine and launch into an Arnold Schwarzenegger–esque workout, I do have one reminder for you: bigger muscles aren't always better.

Compact and explosive muscle beats out pure muscle mass for slowing aging. The healthiest muscles are those found on a wiry physique of modest size, capable of exerting a lot of force over a short period. Sure, you can certainly get strong and muscular doing CrossFit-esque workouts that require maximum dead lifts in two minutes, or ungodly amounts of snatch reps, or bodybuilding workouts that have you doing bicep curls until you are bleeding out the eyeballs—but when it comes to maximizing longevity, those approaches are unlikely to be sustainable. Remember, you want to be able to maintain strength and muscle in an uninjured state when you are forty, sixty, and eighty years old. For this, especially if you are just getting started or want the minimum effective dose of strength training, I recommend performing two specific workouts each week.

The first workout is a super-slow lifting protocol similar to that described by Dr. Doug McGuff in his book *Body by Science*. For twelve to twenty minutes, perform a few multijoint exercises with relatively heavy weights, doing each rep over thirty to sixty seconds. The workout should include the following:

- An upper-body push (e.g., overhead presses, push-ups, chest presses)
- An upper-body pull (e.g., bent or upright rows, lat pull-downs, pull-ups)
- A lower-body push (e.g., leg presses, squats)
- A lower-body pull (e.g., dead lifts, Romanian dead lifts, lower back extensions, reverse hyperextensions)

Why is this type of workout so darn effective? The first benefit is that performing reps very slowly has low injury-producing potential. In addition, a recent study coauthored by Dr. McGuff highlights how super-slow resistance training to muscular failure results in the same type of cardiovascular adaptations caused by a long run. These adaptations include a better ability to buffer lactic acid, increased mitochondrial density, and even better blood pressure.

The second workout is a high-intensity bodyweight circuit designed by researchers to maintain strength and muscle in as little time as possible (a workout later featured in the *New York Times* as "The Scientific 7-Minute Workout"). Each exercise below is to be performed for thirty seconds, with ten seconds of rest between exercises. Aside from the wall sits, you should perform these exercises as explosively as possible. The exercises are these:

- Jumping jacks or burpees
- Wall sits
- Push-ups or clapping push-ups
- Crunches or knee-ups
- Step-ups or lunge jumps
- Squats or squat jumps
- Dips
- Planks
- Jump rope, stair sprints, or running in place with high knees
- Lunges or lunge jumps
- Push-ups with rotation (at the top of the push-up, alternately raise your arms and point them straight up)
- Side planks

If you want the minimum effective dose of strength training that will help you find the sweet spot between longevity and muscle, you can get away with as few as two strength workouts per week—one with slow, controlled heavy lifting and one with high-intensity bodyweight movements.

In chapter 10, you will discover a done-for-you two-week training schedule that works to improve the cardiovascular system, build mitochondria, increase metabolic efficiency, and more.

Can You Really Build Muscle with Bodyweight Training?

The conventional ways to build muscle are to perform big, compound lifts, such as squats and dead lifts, or to combine the super-slow approach and fast, explosive approach. But those aren't the only methods for gaining size and strength. Contrary to popular belief, you can gain muscle by performing more reps with light weights or even your own bodyweight.

One study on the effects of high reps and low reps on muscle growth compared sets performed with weights at 80 percent of one-rep maximum (1RM) to complete muscular fatigue with sets performed with weights at 30 percent of 1RM to complete muscular fatigue. Turns out that the weight of the load is not important. Instead, what matters is whether a muscle is worked to complete fatigue. This study demonstrated that high reps and light weights can stimulate just as much muscle growth as low reps and heavy weights. So you can, for example, build chest muscles by doing a few sets of high-rep push-ups to complete failure. This is a potent tactic if you are stuck in a hotel or living room, or if you have no access to bars and plates and still want to build muscle.

In another study, super-slow lifting at 55 percent to 60 percent of the participant's 1RM increased both muscle thickness and maximal strength just as much as standard-speed lifts performed at 80 to 90 percent of the participant's 1RM. In yet another study, both heavy lifts of eight to ten reps and light lifts of eighteen to twenty reps activated the genes involved in muscle growth. Research has also demonstrated that twenty-five to thirty-five reps with lighter weights leads to the same gains in muscle size as eight to twelve reps with heavier weights. Even in seasoned weight lifters, twenty to twenty-five reps with a light weight leads to the same muscle growth as eight to twelve reps with a heavy weight.

Ultimately, if you want to add muscle mass as fast as possible, you should either lift heavy weights or use super-slow training. But you can still build muscle with light weights and high reps—and, incidentally, research suggests this approach is particularly effective when training legs.

WHY BIGGER MUSCLES AREN'T BETTER

Do you ever try to move fast? No, I mean *F-A-S-T*. When was the last time you were at the gym and tried to hoist a barbell over your head as explosively as possible? When was the last time you were running on a treadmill or riding a bicycle and moved your legs so fast that your brain hurt trying to keep up?

Fact is, when it comes to optimizing the performance of your nervous system and cementing the connection between your brain and the rest of your body, it doesn't really matter how heavy you lift or how much muscle you build.

Sure, strength training and muscle building are fantastic tools for aesthetics, symmetry, musculoskeletal development, and even slowed aging—fundamental goals that will be addressed in later chapters. But when it comes to optimizing your brain and nervous system, recruiting more muscle fibers faster, enhancing nerve-firing speed, and optimizing brain-body coordination, it is far more important to focus on fast, explosive movements.

I was first exposed to the extreme benefits of moving fast when I interviewed a well-known sports performance coach named Nick Curson. Nick, the creator of a training system called Speed of Sport, trains some of the best UFC and NFL competitors on the planet. Rather than giving enormous weights to the men and women he coaches, he instead has them move light loads and their own body weight as freakin' fast as they possibly can. As a result, his athletes are incredibly explosive and functional and don't walk around with relatively useless slabs of extra muscle mass.

There is also a direct link between your power-to-muscle-mass ratio and your longevity. What does that mean? It means bigger muscles aren't always better. Instead, when it comes to slowed aging and longevity, your ability to quickly recruit muscle fibers seems to matter most. I became aware of the fascinating truth about why bigger muscles aren't necessarily better when I spoke with author Paul Jaminet on my podcast about his theory that a smaller muscle capable of exerting more force is healthy muscle, while a gargantuan but relatively weak muscle is an unhealthy muscle.

To understand how large muscles—muscles that are big and bulky but don't necessarily produce much explosive force—may be unhealthy, look at cardiomegaly, enlargement of the heart. When heart tissue is incapable of exerting as much force as it should, the heart often grows larger to compensate. Those who have cardiomegaly, including exercise enthusiasts, often die an early death because the heart has to work so hard to support its own bulk. In the same way, old-school bodybuilding techniques or other exercise styles that are designed to produce pure mass, rather than force, can potentially damage your health. Indeed, Paul cited a study on guinea pigs that showed that lower muscle mass and higher muscle-force capacity, which is found in powerlifters and anyone training more for power and speed than for strength and size, could actually be associated with longevity.

In other words, the healthiest muscle *strength* gains might come with only small muscle *size* gains, because larger muscles take far more energy to carry and cool and require far more antioxidants for repair, recovery, and mitochondrial activity. It is well established in exercise science that muscle contractions lead to elevated levels of reactive oxygen species (ROS) in skeletal muscle, and although these highly reactive molecules are beneficial for normal cell signaling, when in excess, they have many deleterious effects, particularly because they contribute to a net inflammatory state. So if your goal is the ultimate combination of performance, aesthetics, and longevity, what you should pursue are functional, efficient, powerful muscles rather than unnecessary pounds of excess muscle mass. You should also take into consideration the fact that the more muscles you have, the more calories you must consume to maintain (or build) that muscle—which flies in the face of the proven science that moderate caloric restriction can enhance a variety of health factors, including, most notably, longevity. After all, when was the last time you saw a professional bodybuilder eating once a day? If you watch any Netflix video about a professional bodybuilder, half the show will typically involve their shoveling massive plates of food down their gaping maws. I personally experienced this when I had to eat 5,000 to 7,000 calories per day as a 215-pound bodybuilder.

The fact that excess muscle mass negatively impacts longevity is backed up by data on growth hormone (GH) and insulin-like growth factor 1 (IGF-1), which both play an intricate role in the aging process. GH, which is secreted by your pituitary gland, stimulates the production of IGF-1. In fact, the growth-promoting effects of GH result from IGF-1, which stimulates the proliferation and survival of cells.

Now don't get me wrong: these compounds are certainly beneficial. IGF-1 released in response to GH is anabolic and promotes the growth and repair of skeletal muscle. IGF-1 also acts as a neurotrophic factor in the brain, promoting neurogenesis (the growth of new neurons) and the survival of existing neurons, along with better cognitive function. Activities like exercise or a thirty-to-sixty-minute sauna session can induce GH release and, therefore, IGF-1 release.

On the other hand, research suggests that lower levels of GH and IGF-1 result in increased longevity. For example, mice, worms, and flies that are genetically engineered to be deficient in GH or IGF-1 live nearly 50 percent longer. Research also suggests that the overexpression of GH in mice, worms, and flies causes up to a 50 percent shorter life span, mainly due to kidney and liver dysfunction. Ultimately, the key is to find the sweet spot for GH, which doesn't necessarily include the use of GH injections.

Research has also associated variations in the gene that encodes for IGF-1 receptors (which reduce IGF-1 levels) with a significantly longer life span in humans. This is likely because reduced IGF-1 levels increase the expression of genes involved in stress resistance, especially resistance to oxidative stress. So in the same way that having too much muscle mass increases antioxidant needs, so do excessive levels of GH and IGF-1.

Fact is, research suggests that pure muscle mass does not increase longevity. Instead, longevity is more heavily correlated with muscle quality and the ability of the muscle to support daily functional activities such as walking, sprinting, and lifting heavy stuff, all of which positively impact insulin resistance, fat-burning rates, mitochondrial density, mobility, muscle fiber type, and strength.

So when it comes to muscles, bigger is not the same as better. In simple terms, the greater the proportion of a muscle's contractile tissue to its noncontractile tissue, the greater the amount of force it can produce for its size and the greater its muscle quality. In addition, higher-quality muscles developed for performance rather than size also have increased mitochondrial density and more energy-producing capacity per pound of muscle. Perhaps this is why many professional bodybuilders die young or suffer from chronic, inflammation-related diseases. The healthiest muscles are those found on a small, wiry, powerful physique with modest size but a high force-producing potential and the ability to summon significant amounts of power and speed. To build these muscles, you have to recruit more muscle fibers, enhance nerve-firing speed, and optimize speed and power. You are about to learn how to do just that so you can move like a cat, sprint like a cheetah, spring like a tiger, and achieve a sweet spot that gives you enough muscle for a better brain and body but not so much muscle that you reduce your life span.

Should You Get Growth Hormone Injections?

Injecting GH is becoming an increasingly popular therapeutic tactic for stimulating muscle growth, improving wound and bone fracture healing, improving sleep quality, and enhancing longevity, although the general consensus in antiaging medicine is that excess GH may shorten life span because it makes the body too anabolic. But the story behind how GH is processed may give you a new understanding of whether GH is really capable of shortening, not lengthening, life span.

Here's how it works: Whether GH is injected intravenously or produced naturally by the pituitary gland, upon introduction to the bloodstream, it travels to the liver and switches on the production of nine proteins. Two of these proteins are IGF-1 and IGF-2, but the rest are known as binding proteins and have a wide range of health effects. For example, binding protein 1 (BP1) reduces the risk of cardiovascular disease. When you are deficient in BP1, you experience impaired cardiovascular function and an increased risk of heart attack. Meanwhile, a BP2 deficiency leads to reduced insulin sensitivity and increased risk of diabetes. BP4 has strong anti–colon cancer factors and increases apoptosis—programmed cell death, which clears the way for healthy new cells. BP5 stores IGF-1 and transports it to the bone to support bone health, and BP6 improves neural function, neuroprotection, and neurogenesis.

Then there's BP3, the most commonly tested-for binding protein, which is a significant carrier of IGF-1 and mitigates the risk of cancer. The Melbourne Collaborative Cohort Study found that small increases in the levels of BP3 induces a 48 percent reduction in colon cancer. This is because BP3 absorbs IGF-1, which stimulates cell reproduction and therefore could, if not properly bound, increase the risk for cancer.

So what this means is that if you have cancer or a higher risk of cancer, using a GH therapy—which will increase IGF-1—may encourage the cells carrying a cancer-causing genetic mutation to replicate, increasing your risk of cancer growth.

Within your cells, a protein called p53 acts as a regulatory mechanism for cancer: it determines whether a mutation-carrying cell is reproducing, and when it finds one of these cells, p53 tries to fix the mutation. If it fixes it, then all is good. But if it can't, p53 turns on the production of BP3, which absorbs IGF-1 so that it can't stimulate cell reproduction. This, in turn, reduces the chance of the mutation spreading.

All these binding proteins are stimulated by GH, which means that GH does have a significant impact on longevity and long-term health. This also means that the presence of IGF-1 isn't necessarily an issue—the

problem is how it's handled and removed when levels get too high, particularly by your binding proteins.

In other words, if your binding protein levels are inadequate during a GH protocol, which would likely be due to low antioxidant intake, a diet void in wild plants, or lack of proper supplementation with nutrients such as quercetin (which is particularly potent at increasing binding protein levels), it is indeed highly possible that a GH treatment may be increasing your risk of cancer.

In addition, there are other reasons I am not convinced that the current antiaging infatuation with GH injections is a healthy practice. While I am a fan of incorporating lifestyle strategies to increase GH, such as intermittent fasting (particularly the fascinating research by Dr. Jason Fung showing that GH levels climb 200 to 300 percent with one day of fasting and remain elevated for up to forty-eight hours!), heavy lifting, and adequate protein consumption, I just haven't seen enough data to prove that GH is particularly effective or safe (although I'd love to see studies done on folks who are both using GH and implementing these strategies).

For example, to evaluate the safety and efficacy of GH in healthy older people, one team of researchers reviewed thirty-one GH studies. The dose of GH varied considerably among these studies, and the duration of therapy ranged from two weeks to a year, but each dose did succeed at boosting levels of IGF-1 (which, as you now know, reflects the level of GH) by 88 percent.

Compared to the subjects who did not get GH, the treated individuals gained an average of 4.6 pounds of muscle and shed a similar amount of body fat. But unfortunately, the GH-injected individuals also experienced a high rate of unpleasant side effects, such as fluid retention, joint pain, breast enlargement, and carpal tunnel syndrome. Other research suggests that GH injections induce an increased risk of cancer in general and prostate cancer in particular.

The data on GH for performance is unimpressive as well. Because GH is banned in most sanctioned sports, scientists have been unable to evaluate GH in many real-world conditions. But they have conducted randomized clinical trials that administer GH or a placebo to athletes and then measure body composition, strength, and exercise capacity in the lab. It turns out that after receiving daily injections for an average of twenty days, subjects who received GH increased their lean body mass, but this did not translate into improved performance. GH did not produce any significant increases in strength or exercise capacity. In addition, the subjects who received GH were more likely to experience fluid retention and fatigue.

2 NONTRADITIONAL WAYS TO BUILD AND MAINTAIN MUSCLE

The prevailing thought among exercise enthusiasts is that if you stop training for a certain period, you will lose muscle strength and mass. So far, this chapter has addressed the most traditional ways to build and maintain muscle: lifting weights and doing bodyweight exercises. But there are other ways you can maintain muscle, even if you are injured or can't make it to the weight room or a home gym.

1. Electrical Muscle Stimulation (EMS)

You have no doubt seen the as-seen-on-TV ads for the special electrodes you attach to your abs to magically get a six-pack. Known variously as electrical muscle stimulation (EMS), neuromuscular electrical stimulation, or electromyostimulation devices, these contraptions use electrical impulses to directly stimulate motor neurons and cause a muscular contraction. (A TENS unit, which also uses electrical impulses, is good for managing pain, especially in the lower back, but stimulates only surface neurons.)

Your brain sends electrical impulses through your central nervous system to fire your muscles. EMS circumvents the brain, allowing for deep, intense muscular contractions without taxing your nervous system, joints, or tendons. Fact is, your muscles don't know the difference between a voluntary contraction and an electrically induced one—they just recognize the stimulus. The contractions can be quick, with longer pauses between contractions, or they can last as long as seconds and sometimes minutes at a time.

To use an EMS device, you place the electrodes on your skin at each end of the target muscle. The device usually has four channels with lead wires, and each wire is connected to two pads. Small amounts of current run from one pad to the next to complete a circuit, using your muscle tissue as a conduit. The current runs at specific frequencies and pulse durations (usually microseconds) that stimulate the motor neurons within the circuit. The muscle fibers innervated by the motor neurons then contract, and you start twitching. There are three ranges of EMS frequencies, each of which activates one of the three types of muscle fibers: slow twitch, intermediate fast twitch, and fast twitch.

For several years, I used EMS only for recovery, but now I use it for full-body strength-training and explosive strength-training sessions. It is particularly effective for nervous system training if you practice deep, diaphragmatic breathing at the same time. I even use EMS in cars and on airplanes—in fact, I am writing this very sentence on an airplane with a Marc Pro attached to my sore calves.

I own a Compex Sport Elite for portable EMS-based muscle training and use my Marc Pro for EMS-based recovery sessions. I also own what I consider to be the Cadillac of EMS units: the NeuFit, which can simulate a 600-pound squat! As a word of caution, when done properly, a full-body NeuFit session gives you hypertrophy and results in rapid muscle growth but will leave you pretty sore for the next five to seven days.

Tricks of the Trade: The Best Portable Muscle-Building Tools

The fittest folks I know can make training portable and have no excuses for not staying fit as road warriors, jet-setters, and family-reunion attendees. Indeed, one of the secrets to maintaining an effective, functional strength program is the ability to work out any time at any place. Not every hotel is going to have a good gym (can you say "squeaky elliptical trainer and dusty dumbbells"?), and not every friend or relative you visit is going to have equipment. Having a few key items on hand that I can pack into my travel bag and pull out in a park, airport, basement, or backyard allows me to stay in professional-athlete shape despite spending up to three weeks of every month on the road.

One of my most versatile, portable tools is a suspension trainer. There are many suspension trainers available, including the ever-popular TRX, and several of the new models, such as the GoFit, Ignite, and KBDuo, are made with pulleys, wheels, and bungee cords that make a suspension trainer workout even more versatile. But I prefer a simple, no-frills model you can attach to a door frame in a hotel or house, the bars at a playground, or the stairwell of an airport. You can then perform suspended pull-ups, planking exercises, lunging balance moves, and a host of other movements. This is crucial, because most portable workouts include plenty of push-up variations, but aside from lying on your back under your hotel room coffee table and attempting to do pull-ups on the edge of the table, or trying to dead lift your entire bed, there's a notable lack of pulling options in most travel scenarios. Sure, you can do push-ups on any floor and box jumps onto a bed, but you can't exactly do pull-ups on most objects without breaking something. I'll sheepishly admit that I have broken a few hotel desks and door frames attempting to use them as pull-up and horizontal rowing devices.

In an era of sitting and hunching over computers and phones, it is crucial for your shoulder and back health that you pull as much as or more than you push during a workout. The added benefit of pulling is enhanced grip strength, which is correlated with longevity, shoulder health, and overall physical brute strength, and a suspension trainer will allow you to work your grip even in the absence of a barbell or pull-up bar. In a pinch (pun intended), another trick is to keep a Captains of Crush hand grip strengthener in your purse, laptop bag, or other travel gear and train your grip while driving, waiting in line, talking on the phone, or sitting on an airplane.

Another item you will always find in my travel kit is an elastic band, which I began using over a decade ago while cycling through Italy with my wife and simultaneously training for a bodybuilding competition. She would lie in bed each morning laughing at me as I'd bang away at curls, overhead presses, tricep extensions, and sideways band walks, but the band helped me maintain and even build slabs of muscle, fueled by gelato and pasta. I still use an elastic band to this day, although I have since upgraded to a fancy band system called the X3 Bar (see chapter 11 for more details). Conveniently, these bands can also be used for the type of joint traction you'll read more about in chapter 17.

Finally, no portable exercise kit would be complete without Kaatsu bands, also known as blood flow restriction (BFR) bands or occlusion training bands, long used as potent training tools by elite athletes, law enforcement agencies, militaries, and Japanese martial artists.

Much like a tourniquet, a Kaatsu band (the name is a mash-up of the Japanese words for "additional"—ka—and "pressure"—atsu) places pressure around your upper arms and legs. This reduces blood flow from your extremities back to the heart, so that your limbs become engorged with blood, filling ordinarily unused capillaries and mobilizing extra muscle fibers while also raising the concentration of lactic acid in the blood. These effects trick the brain into thinking the body is undergoing a massive workout and even trigger the pituitary gland to produce additional growth hormone. (Visit BoundlessBook.com/9 for a few Kaatsu training tools.)

When you combine Kaatsu training with bodyweight exercises, a suspension strap, or an elastic band, you can create a massively effective yet wonderfully simple workout.

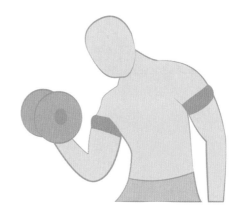

A sample on-the-road workout for me includes:

- BFR bands wrapped around my arms and legs
- A 2-minute burpee warm-up
- 10 suspension strap pull-ups
- 10 suspension strap push-ups
- 1 minute of jumping jacks
- 10 elastic band sideways shuffles
- 10 elastic band squat-to-overhead presses.
- 1 minute of sitting down on the floor and standing up as many times as possible (a surprisingly difficult and highly functional exercise)
- 10 elastic band upright rows
- 10 suspension strap lunges for each leg

Repeat three to five times through with minimal rest. Include the burpee warm-up in each round for an additional challenge.

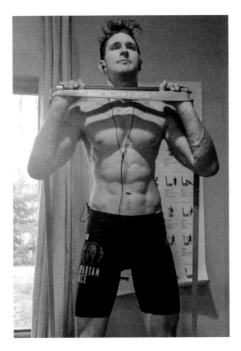

Another favorite workout of mine, if I have access to a gym, is to perform back-to-back supersets for each muscle group, following each superset with two minutes of cardio performed as hard as possible. A sample workout would include:

- 2 minutes on a cardio machine such as an elliptical trainer, bike, rowing machine, or stairmill
- Chest press to failure—8 to 15 reps
- Row to failure—8 to 15 reps
- 2 minutes on a cardio machine
- Squat or leg press to failure—8 to 15 reps
- Dead lift or leg curl to failure—8 to 15 reps
- 2 minutes of cardio
- Shoulder press to failure—8 to 15 reps
- Lat pull-down to failure—8 to 15 reps
- 2 minutes of cardio
- First core exercise of choice to failure, such as side plank rotations
- Second core exercise of choice to failure, such as lower back extensions

Repeat three to five times through with minimal rest.

If you follow BenGreenfieldFitness on Instagram, you will find plenty more workouts to try, as I'm often posting creative travel workouts I do when I'm on the road.

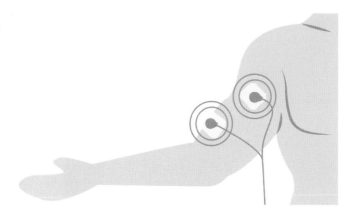

While an EMS device certainly isn't going to help you burn enough calories or fat to give you an Adonis-like six-pack, it can provide a significant boost in cardiovascular and musculoskeletal fitness. (For more tips on how to incorporate EMS into a training session, read my blog post "How to Use Electrical Muscle Stimulation to Enhance Performance, Build Power and VO$_2$ Max," linked to on BoundlessBook.com/9.)

2. Heat Stress

You can prevent the loss of muscle strength and mass by using a dry sauna, wet sauna, or infrared sauna. Heat stress prevents muscle loss by triggering the release of heat shock proteins (HSPs), which eliminate free radicals, support antioxidant production, and repair misfolded, damaged proteins in muscle tissue. Research suggests that the HSPs rats produce when they experience heat stress are associated with 30 percent more muscle regrowth compared to a control group. In fact, one HSP—HSP70—is associated with longevity, suggesting that heat stress may also have significant antiaging effects.

Proper levels of growth hormone are also crucial for muscle repair and recovery. Research suggests that two twenty-minute sauna sessions separated by a thirty-minute cooling-off period can double growth hormone levels. Two fifteen-minute sauna sessions at an even warmer temperature separated by a thirty-minute recovery period resulted in a fivefold increase in growth hormone levels. If you combine heat stress and exercise, it induces a synergistic increase in growth hormone. This is why I often do isometrics, yoga, push-ups, and squats in my infrared sauna (on BoundlessBook.com/9 you'll find a link to a sample sauna workout that I perform).

Sauna exposure also increases blood flow to skeletal muscles and helps fuel them with glucose, amino acids, fatty acids, and oxygen while removing metabolic by-products like lactic acid and calcium ions. Sauna exposure can even build new red blood cells at a rate similar to illegal performance-enhancing drugs like EPO. (My blog post "Ten Scientifically Proven Reasons I Am Addicted to a Daily Sauna" has more on how to build and maintain muscle via heat stress: BenGreenfieldFitness.com/saunascience.)

I will readily admit that for fast muscle growth and muscle maintenance, there is no substitute for lifting heavy stuff or exposing your muscles to time under tension. But if you don't have access to exercise equipment or have movement or injury limitations, you can also build and maintain muscle with strategies such as bodyweight or low-weight training and EMS and sauna therapy.

Unlike a long cold soak, which can blunt the hormetic effects of exercise, you can use a sauna postworkout to get even more benefits out of your training while also increasing blood flow and decreasing recovery time.

ENTER 6 OF THE FITTEST OLD PEOPLE ON THE PLANET

Hopefully, by now you are convinced that if you aren't lifting heavy stuff, you should be. But when it comes to staying as fit and sexy as possible as you age, lab-based science is one thing and personal, in-the-trenches, real-world experience is quite another. I find it fascinating to study and even exercise with some of the fittest old people on the face of the planet to see exactly what they are doing.

I recently read an article from Vice entitled "The Healthiest Old Person on the Planet Explains How to Stay in Shape," in which we meet a man named Charles Eugster, who began lifting weights at eighty-five and lived to be ninety-seven years old.

Charles became a decorated British sprinter in his late eighties and into his late nineties. He held world records in the 200-meter indoor and 400-meter outdoor sprints, as well as British records in the 60-meter indoor, 100-meter outdoor, and 200-meter outdoor sprints. This is all pretty impressive, considering that most guys his age could barely walk across the street without stumbling over the curb (if they were even still alive!).

Charles was also a bodybuilder, public speaker, writer, rower, wakeboarder, entrepreneur, and fashion designer who planned his own line of elderly couture. He even claimed that some of his white and gray hairs turned brown! While I am skeptical of that last claim, I do know this: he certainly seemed to have cracked the code on how to stay fit as you age.

Let's delve into the secrets of Charles Eugster and five other extremely fit old people, shall we?

Can Seniors Get Stronger?

Many fitness enthusiasts and athletes believe that at around fifty to sixty years old, you lose your ability to get stronger. But the fact is, while you do lose muscle mass as you age, you can stave off the age-related loss of strength. According to a study in the *Journal of Strength and Conditioning Research*, beyond the age of sixty-five, you can—contrary to popular belief—make significant strength gains.

The study put a group of men in their midthirties and a group of men in their midsixties on the same strength-training programs. For ten weeks, twice per week, the men performed five sets of eight to fourteen repetitions of leg press and leg extension exercises, with one to two minutes rest between sets. The researchers measured the leg strength and lean muscle mass of both groups before and after the training period. While the older men, unlike the younger men, didn't gain any muscle mass in their legs, their strength training did indeed lead to significant strength gains in their one-rep-maximum leg presses.

So if you are over sixty, don't worry about losing your ability to get stronger. Perform a full-body strength-training workout a couple of times a week. Don't mess around with light weights and high reps, which don't seem to be effective for seniors. Choose a weight that allows you to perform a maximum of fifteen reps per exercise (but preferably less). For the simplest solution, just implement the super-slow training routine on page 188 one to two times per week and stick with it for a few months. You will be surprised by the results.

Antiaging Tip #1: Eat Real Food (Charles Eugster)

Sure, Charles lifted weights, which is crucial for maintaining muscle mass and hormone levels as you age and can reduce the rate at which telomeres shorten. But regarding his diet, he said in his interview with Vice:

> Variety is key. I start every day with a protein shake because, as you get older, your protein synthesis no longer functions as well. I avoid sugar and eat lots of meat, especially fat. I've been on a fat trip lately. Fat! Piles of fat. Yet, I was in a supermarket the other day and was perplexed to find yogurt with zero fat. What on earth is that? The idea of the nutrition pyramid where, at the top, is a little fat and meat, and at the bottom a lot of carbohydrates, is, excuse me, bullshit. Humans are so unbelievably stupid that we have begun to tinker with food. Our theories of nutrition have resulted in a pandemic of obesity. Can you imagine a hunter-gatherer enjoying a low-fat yogurt? Let me tell you this, too: I read a report recently which said that a fatty diet also increases your drive.

If, like Charles, you have Northern European ancestry, it is highly unlikely that that you can eat modern fat-free and low-fat foods, live a long time, and look good doing it. There are certain populations who, due to genetics, salivary amylase production, and hormonal responses to carbohydrates, may be able to get by on less fat (more on this in chapter 14). But they are still not eating modern "frankenfoods."

Antiaging Tip #2: Learn New Stuff (Laird Hamilton)

The last time I hung out in Kauai with fifty-four-year-old big-wave surfer Laird Hamilton, who is still just as spry and quick-moving as the twentysomething surfers he puts to shame on huge waves around the world, Laird highlighted one of his best antiaging secrets: keep learning new stuff.

Laird's garage is a testament to this philosophy. It is chock-full of unique toys that Laird has invented to attack ocean waves in new ways. It is also packed with skis, snowboards, Jet Skis, foil boards (one of the most fun "flying" experiences you will ever have if you can hunt one down), balance-training devices, and all manner of different tools to force his brain and muscles to maintain neurons and build new ones. People often ask me why I delve into everything from archery to snowboarding to spearfishing to obstacle course racing to kickboxing to ukulele playing, and this is one of the biggest reasons why!

Indeed, renowned neuropsychiatrist Dr. Daniel Amen has shown that this concept is key to maintaining youthfulness. He has identified specific areas of the brain that are challenged by different tasks:

- The prefrontal cortex is improved by meditation, language games like crossword puzzles and Scrabble, and strategy games like chess.
- The temporal lobes are improved by memory games and learning musical instruments.
- The parietal lobes are improved by juggling, map reading, and logic games like sudoku.
- The cerebellum is improved by dancing, yoga, tai chi, and coordination games like table tennis.

In his book *Change Your Brain, Change Your Life,* Dr. Amen also includes breathing techniques to calm inner turmoil, antidepression tips, antianger diet tips, focus-enhancing strategies, and problem-solving techniques. I have incorporated one of his recommended meditation techniques into my custom yoga routine:

- Touch your thumbs to your index fingers while chanting "saa."
- Touch your thumbs to your middle fingers while chanting "taa."
- Touch your thumbs to your ring fingers while chanting "naa."
- Touch your thumbs to your pinkies while chanting "maa."

The first time through, repeat the sounds out loud for two minutes, then whisper them for two minutes, repeat them silently for four minutes, whisper them again for two minutes, and finish by repeating them out loud for another two minutes. Then sit quietly for one to two minutes.

Antiaging Tip #3: Lift, Move, Sprint (Mark Sisson)

My friend Mark Sisson, aged sixty-five, probably possesses the finest set of six-pack abs you have ever seen on anyone, much less on a guy his age. What's his secret? Rather than engaging in long, slow chronic cardio, he instead does short, fast, all-out sprint workouts at least once a week, all year long. He doesn't overdo these and recommends performing such workouts (ultimate frisbee, high-intensity treadmill intervals, or hard uphill cycling) once every seven to ten days.

He also performs intense sessions of heavy, full-body weight lifting one to three times per week for seven to thirty minutes. Finally, he avoids any long, unbroken periods of sedentary time by using tactics like treadmill workstations and relaxing paddleboard sessions.

Lift, move, sprint. Pretty simple concept, eh? You can learn more about Mark's philosophies and daily habits in a podcast interview I conducted with him (visit BoundlessBook.com/9 for the link).

Antiaging Tip #4: Do Epic Things (Don Wildman)

Ten years ago, I read an *Esquire* magazine article entitled "The Hardest Workout in the World." In it, the author outlined then-septuagenarian Don Wildman's grueling, intense, multistage weight-training workout, dubbed the Circuit. The first time I ventured into Don's home gym in Malibu to do the Hardest Workout in the World, I thought it would be a piece of cake. After all, if a seventy-five-year-old could do it three times a week, I would surely be able to manage it, too! When I crawled out of the gym almost three hours later with lactic acid oozing out of my pores, I was thinking a bit differently. My body was feeling the aftershocks of Don's challenge for several days.

Don, who recently passed away at the age of eighty-five, not only performed this epic workout up until his death but also went mountain biking on difficult trails for miles every single day and enjoyed stand-up paddleboarding, big-wave surfing, and even helicopter snowboarding. These may seem like scary, daunting tasks, but Don still did them, and he certainly lived life at a much more exciting level than 99 percent of his peers and stayed incredibly fit doing it. So what epic or scary event or workout can you add to your calendar this week, this month, or this year?

Antiaging Tip #5: Train Eccentrically (Art De Vany)

The ripped, eighty-year-old Art De Vany, one of the founders of the ancestral fitness movement, gets away with extremely short weight-training episodes of just fifteen minutes per day by using an exercise strategy called "eccentric training." This potent workout method results in not only a significant antiaging effect but also an increase in growth hormone and testosterone levels. In a podcast episode with Tim Ferriss, Art explained his approach.

Eccentric training is also known as "negative training" because it refers to the lengthening or lowering portion of a lift, during which the muscle tends to become more stressed and stimulated compared to the concentric, positive, lifting phase of an exercise. To perform a negative dead lift, for example, you set the bar at a certain height—maybe on weight-lifting blocks, as if you were already halfway through the movement—then grab the bar, step back, and lower it to the ground. Since the human body can handle up to 1.75 times more weight eccentrically than concentrically, this type of training allows you to load your muscles with an amount of weight you couldn't normally lift. This, in turn, stimulates a more powerful adaptive response to the slight muscle tearing that occurs with weight lifting. The proven benefits of eccentric training include improved injury rehabilitation, reduced risk of injury, increased gains in strength, stronger connective tissue, and improved muscle function. Research even shows that eccentric training can double stem cell counts in your muscles without exhausting them. As stem cells divide and proliferate, some remain in the stem cell niche, which is where stem cells reside within specific tissues—in this case, the skeletal muscle. But others exit the niche to assist with tissue healing and the anabolic response to training. The stem cells that exit, known as "satellite cells" or "mesenchymal-like stem cells," are crucial for muscle regrowth after any exercise. By doubling these counts, eccentric training promotes faster muscle regrowth.

Art uses this style of training for about ten to fifteen minutes every day. Even if he doesn't have a spotter, he uses different machines and will load up a weight he can handle with both arms or legs, push through the first part of the movement, then finish the movement using only one arm or leg as he slowly lowers back to the starting position. He claims that every muscle group can reap incredible benefits from this style of training, especially muscles related to posture, since they need to have the endurance to keep you upright all day.

One of Art's other posture exercises involves standing with your back to a wall, slightly arching your lower back, keeping your head and shoulders back against the wall, and then walking away from the wall without collapsing your spine or neck—rather than lowering your head to look forward, look over your cheekbones while maintaining your posture.

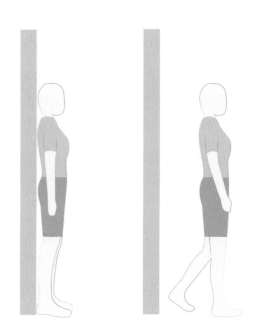

Finally, Art doesn't work every muscle group every day. He alternates muscle groups throughout the week, making certain to hit each group a couple times every seven days. With this training method, he ensures that he remains injury-free and that his muscles are lean, long, quick, and not too big.

Antiaging Tip #6: Stay Supple (Olga Kotelko)

In the fascinating book *What Makes Olga Run? The Mystery of the 90-Something Track Star and What She Can Teach Us About Living Longer, Happier Lives,* we meet Olga Kotelko, a senior track star who has since passed away but who, at the time the book was published, held over twenty-three world records in track and field, seventeen of which were in the aged-ninety-to-ninety-five category.

When I read the book, one of the biggest takeaways for me was that Olga didn't beat up her body without going out of her way to recover and stay supple. She instead woke up in the middle of every night, grabbed an old, empty wine bottle beside her bed, and gave herself a full-body, foam-roller-style massage on all her fasciae, muscles, and joints.

Whether you book a weekly or monthly massage or do short, daily foam-rolling routines like the metabolic mobility routine on my YouTube channel at BenGreenfieldFitness.com/metabolicmobility (which I do once or twice per week), you will find that deep tissue work can keep muscle soreness, cranky joints, poor movement, and other issues we accept as normal in seniors at bay. And yes, you can do this type of massage even when you travel, with no more equipment than a hard plastic (e.g., Nalgene) or glass water bottle wrapped in a t-shirt or a pillowcase and a common lacrosse ball (read Kelly Starrett's *Becoming a Supple Leopard* to see what I mean).

What They All Have in Common: Regularity

Finally, I would be remiss not to note that, when studying the habits of these fit old people and many others, I have discovered that routine often trumps novelty.

Mark Sisson paddleboards and plays ultimate frisbee every week. Paul Chek lifts heavy rocks in his homemade rock garden each morning (listen to my podcast with him to see what I mean—see BoundlessBook.com/9). Laird Hamilton performs thrice-weekly underwater pool workouts. My über-fit sixty-six-year-old Finnish friend Vessi swims naked each morning and hits the sauna each night. Sure, the SAID ("specific adaptation to imposed demands") principle does dictate that you must constantly switch up your workouts to keep getting stronger and faster. But in order to remain injury-free, establish a sustainable program, and reduce decision-making fatigue, many of these folks do the same routines day in and day out. They throw in the occasional gritty adventure, new workout, or unpredictable sport, but there is always some semblance of routine.

The True Causes of Heart Attacks

If you are worried that heavy lifting or hard exercise will give you a heart attack, allow me to introduce you to Thomas Cowan, MD, who is, in my opinion, one of the most brilliant minds in modern holistic medicine. He expertly blends ancestral wisdom and modern science to make meaningful changes in human health.

Dr. Cowan has been a three-peat guest on my podcast and was featured on an episode entitled "Why Your Heart Is Not a Pump (And What Most Doctors Don't Know About the True Cause of Heart Disease)." During the episode, we discussed the fact that the current understanding of heart disease as a problem originating in blood vessels is completely wrong. Rather, heart disease is rooted in sympathetic nervous system overload, mineral deficiencies, and an unwillingness to treat the vessels in your body more like the roots and vessels in a plant. Dr. Cowan informed me that one clue to understanding why bypass grafting and stent placement have not eliminated cardiovascular problems comes from the work of the Italian pathologist Giorgio Baroldi.

In his groundbreaking book *The Etiopathogenesis of Coronary Heart Disease: A Heretical Theory Based on Morphology*, Baroldi, who had performed autopsies on heart attack patients for forty years, observed that only 41 percent of these patients had significant stenosis (plaque buildup) in the artery leading to the affected area of the heart. In fact, 50 percent of these stenoses developed after the heart attack occurred.

These results suggest that approximately 80 percent of heart attacks have some other cause than a blocked artery. It is no wonder that, in most cases, unblocking arteries—no matter how thoroughly or carefully done—does not resolve the heart disease.

In his book *Human Heart, Cosmic Heart: A Doctor's Quest to Understand, Treat, and Prevent Cardiovascular Disease*, Dr. Cowan suggested three other causes of heart attacks—also known as myocardial infarctions, or MIs. He asserted that we must address these causes not only to prevent and treat angina, unstable angina, and heart attacks but also to avoid heart attacks during heavy physical exertion.

1. Autonomic nervous system imbalance: Heart rate variability testing, which assesses autonomic nervous system activity, suggests that many patients who have an MI have reduced parasympathetic nervous system activity in the days, weeks, and months leading up to the MI—that is, the parasympathetic nervous system, which is responsible for bodily functions at rest (what's often called "rest-and-digest" mode), has been downregulated. Most MIs result from a combination of chronically low parasympathetic activity and a temporary stressful event like a hard workout. Decreased parasympathetic activity (or decreased parasympathetic tone) is a consequence of chronic stress, diabetes, hypertension, smoking, and a lack of physical activity. In other words, if these factors are present in your life, think twice about doing hard physical activity until you have addressed them and the other issues below.

2. The problem isn't coronary arteries: Typical anatomical drawings of the heart suggest that all of the blood flow to the myocardium (the middle layer of the heart muscle) goes through the three major coronary arteries. While these arteries are certainly important, the heart possesses a rich supply of blood vessels that make up its microcirculation. So the heart is perfectly well suited to do its own bypass in the event of chronic disruption of blood flow through one or more of the coronary arteries. This is why thousands, maybe millions, of Americans are walking around with coronary arteries greater than 90 percent occluded and yet have no symptoms whatsoever. The body, using its robust capillary network, has done its own bypass, and the heart therefore still has a good blood supply.

It is only in cases of chronic diseases like diabetes that MIs occur. One of Dr. Cowan's primary points during our interviews was that an adequate intake of good, clean water, preferably in the form of structured water, and a high intake of a full spectrum of minerals (such as calcium, phosphorus, zinc, magnesium, potassium, and trace minerals) support the heart in its regular circulatory activity. So regardless of who you are, and especially if you have a history of cardiovascular disease or risk of heart attack, be careful with heavy lifting and hard exercise if you are dehydrated, drink subpar municipal water, or don't have an adequate mineral intake.

3. Metabolic acidosis: Perhaps the most important and most overlooked reason people suffer heart problems is the production and buildup of lactic acid in heart tissue. When the heart finds itself in a stressful situation and its mitochondria can't produce enough energy, it undergoes what is called a glycolytic shift and begins to ferment sugar for fuel. Once this shift occurs, lactic acid accumulates in the surrounding tissues. Lactic acid also accumulates in your skeletal muscles when you exercise, but, unlike skeletal muscles, your heart muscles can't relax, so lactic acid continues to accumulate, and the buildup eventually leads to angina or chest pain.

The lactic acid also leads to a lower pH in the heart, which prevents calcium from entering myocardial cells and inhibits the contraction of heart muscle fibers.

Eventually, cell death occurs in the surrounding tissue, and this is called an MI.

To address this issue, Dr. Cowan highly recommends a little-known medication called strophanthus (also known as ouabain), commonly called "the insulin of the heart." Research suggests that strophanthus improves parasympathetic nervous system function and cardiac microcirculation and converts lactic acid into pyruvate, the heart's preferred fuel. (If you are interested in learning more about strophanthus, check out "The Insulin of the Heart" on my website—there's a link at BoundlessBook.com/9—which includes an article Dr. Cowan wrote about this fascinating plant.)

Finally, no discussion of the true causes of heart attacks would be complete without mentioning takotsubo cardiomyopathy. The idea behind this phenomenon is that you are far more likely to die of a heart attack caused by chronic anxiety or a poor relationship than of a heart attack caused by squatting, deadlifting, or running a marathon.

Takotsubo cardiomyopathy, also known as stress cardiomyopathy, occurs due to a sudden and temporary weakening of the heart muscle, often triggered by emotional stress, including the death of a loved one or a breakup. Takotsubo cardiomyopathy is often referred to as "broken heart syndrome" and is a well-known cause of lethal ventricular arrhythmias, ventricular rupture, and heart failure.

So what's the final verdict when it comes to heart attacks and exercise?

Eliminate chronic stress, keep yourself well-hydrated, consume adequate minerals, ensure your heart is not constantly burning glucose as fuel, and fix any weak or broken relationships in your life. Your heart will then be far more likely to respond well to a difficult workout.

THE LAST WORD

I absolutely dig the idea of playing football with my grandkids when I'm ninety, freediving when I'm ninety-five, and hunting an elk when I'm one hundred. By implementing the muscle-building tactics in this chapter, along with the antiaging secrets of some of the fittest old people on the face of the planet, you can equip yourself with a body that will allow you to do the same. After all, if you want to live a long time, I suspect you want to look as good as possible, even if modern society thinks you should be sitting in a rocking chair at a nursing home watching *Seinfeld* reruns.

ONE THING YOU CAN DO THIS WEEK

Take an upper-body bodyweight exercise, such as a push-up or pull-up, and a lower-body bodyweight exercise, such as a lunge or squat, and perform the movements as slowly as you possibly can—it should take at least thirty to sixty seconds to get to the top of one rep and thirty to sixty seconds to return. Repeat to total exhaustion. This technique, known as eccentric, negative, or super-slow training, is a fast-track method to build strength and mass. For an additional bonus, do this workout with BFR bands or a Kaatsu training device.

For citations for all the research studies mentioned in this chapter and a deeper dive into the topics of this chapter—including links to podcasts, blog posts, recommended tools and supplements, and much more—visit BoundlessBook.com/9.

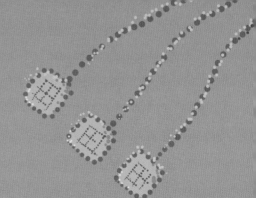

FITNESS DECODED

THE ULTIMATE BLUEPRINT FOR A PERFECT BODY

"You ready?"

I nodded and gulped. The guy in the polo shirt and glasses standing next to me flipped the green switch in his hands, and suddenly my abs—covered in a Christmas-light-esque array of blinking electrodes—exploded into an intense contraction that shook my body from head to toe.

For a painfully long two minutes, he continued the stimulation with the fringe Russian muscle-recruitment device, then finally switched it off and, smiling, stepped away. I wiped the beads of sweat from my forehead and stared down at my quivering ab muscles, now forming a neat, tight six-pack.

"Dang."

"Yeah, and tomorrow you're going to feel like you did a thousand crunches."

When it comes to extreme exercise efficiency, this machine—which can simulate a 600-pound squat with just a few flimsy electrode pads—ranks right up there with the hyperoxic training device in my office, the mountain-incline treadmill in my garage, the industrial-size vibration plate in my basement, and the enormous pulley-piston-driven ARX machine my wife forced me to build an entirely new shed in the forest to accommodate.

But frankly, while chapter 11 will teach the voracious go-getter with deep pockets and a passion for biohacking how to find the funnest, fanciest exercise tools that exist, the truth is that you don't need to empty your wallet or spend oodles of time cracking the code on getting the body you want.

Suppose you want to live as long as possible. Suppose you also want to look as good as possible doing it. Suppose you want to maximize your hormone balance, drive, fertility, strength, power, and cardiovascular capacity. Suppose you want to step back, investigate every shred of exercise research, and inject only the most effective strategies into your life—not to prepare for masochistic suffer-fests like triathlons, marathons, obstacle races, or other feats of physical endurance, but rather to maximize longevity and look good naked.

Whether we're looking at total caloric intake, exercise, sunlight exposure, protein consumption, or work habits, we often think we have to do way more than we need to in order to get the results we want. Why crank out those extra reps or put in those extra hours if you don't have to? After all, failing to heed the minimum effective dose can often cost you money, time, and mental real estate.

Sure, if you want to do an Ironman triathlon or a multihour obstacle race or compete at the CrossFit games, you need to put some extra work into sport-specific, occasionally soul-crushing training. But all that volume isn't necessarily good for you, and it certainly isn't necessary for extending your life span.

The first section of this chapter will reveal the minimum effective dose of exercise. You will discover the truth about how much exercise you really need to live a long time, with the approach that traditional Chinese medicine considers to be the ultimate way to be boundless: a balance of easygoing yin and hard-charging yang. You will also find a done-for-you exercise program you can do for the rest of your life at any time and in any place while maintaining the sweet spot between health, performance, and longevity.

THE MINIMUM EFFECTIVE DOSE OF EXERCISE

In 2015, the *New York Times* published an article entitled "The Right Dose of Exercise for a Longer Life." The article discussed the results of two studies that investigated how much exercise you need to get longevity benefits. But before jumping into those results, it is important to note that rather than being controlled or randomized, these studies relied upon the participants' memory recall of their exercise habits. Like diet studies that rely on memory recall of meals, these kinds of studies can be prone to human error. But they can still give us important information.

The first study found that people who did not exercise at all faced the highest risk of early death. Those who exercised a little—not meeting the current American Heart Association guidelines of 150 minutes per week, but at least doing something—reduced their risk of premature death by 20 percent. Those who performed 150 minutes of moderate exercise per week enjoyed a 31 percent lower risk of dying than those who never exercised.

But the greatest benefits came to those who exercised moderately, mostly by walking, for 450 minutes per week—a little more than an hour per day. These people were up to 39 percent less likely to die prematurely than those who never exercised.

Even more interesting is the fact that after 450 minutes per week, the longevity benefits of exercise plateaued but never significantly declined. Those who performed ten times or more the recommended exercise dose never really got any extra benefits than those who exercised at a dose closer to the recommended guidelines. While their risk of dying young did not increase, they also did not get significantly healthier from a longevity standpoint, suggesting that an excess of easy, aerobic exercise isn't going to hurt you, but it also isn't going to provide any further decrease in mortality risk.

The second study reached a similar conclusion but focused more on exercise intensity. The results stand in stark contrast to studies that suggest that frequent strenuous exercise might contribute to early mortality. Not surprisingly, this study found that meeting exercise guidelines significantly reduced the risk of early death, even if that exercise was as moderate as walking.

But those who engaged in occasional vigorous, high-intensity exercise saw an additional reduction in mortality risk. People who spent up to 30 percent of their weekly exercise time in vigorous activities were 9 percent less likely to die prematurely than people who exercised at a moderate intensity for the same amount of time. People who spent more than 30 percent of their exercise time doing strenuous workouts gained an extra 13 percent reduction in early mortality risk compared to those who never broke through that intensity barrier. Even the few people in the study who engaged in the greatest amounts of intense exercise had no increase in mortality risk.

At this point, you may be wondering what qualifies as moderate and what qualifies as vigorous. Moderate-intensity aerobic exercise raises your heart rate and makes you sweat. You'll know if you're working at a moderate intensity if you can't sing a song during a workout but you can still talk. Vigorous-intensity aerobic exercise makes you breathe hard and fast, makes your muscles burn, and significantly increases your heart rate. If you are working at this level, you won't be able to say more than a few words without pausing for a breath.

What's the ultimate takeaway from these two studies? Researcher Klaus Gebel, who led the second study, said, "Try to reach at least 150 minutes of physical activity per week and have around 20 to 30 minutes of that be vigorous activity." He also noted that a larger dose of exercise, for those who are so inclined, did not seem to be unsafe.

All this research suggests that you need at least twenty minutes of structured exercise per day if you want to live a long time—assuming, of course, that you do not spend the rest of the day sitting down. But it is one thing to live a long time and another thing entirely to look as good as possible doing it. Frankly, no matter what "looking good naked" means to you, you are going to need a bit more than a blanket recommendation to perform at least 150 minutes of physical activity per week and have about 20 to 30 minutes of that be vigorous activity.

If you want low-enough body-fat levels to be cut but high enough levels to optimize hormones and fertility, enough muscle mass to be strong and aesthetic but not so much that you become a cancer-prone bodybuilder, and enough cardiovascular fitness to be venous and vibrant but not so much that you are overtrained, you need the minimum effective dose of exercise to achieve cardiovascular fitness, muscular endurance, strength, mitochondrial density, metabolic efficiency, and stamina.

GET FIT, LIVE A LONG TIME, AND LOOK GOOD NAKED

There are six aspects of training that you need to incorporate into your longevity protocol to balance aesthetics, fitness, and longevity.

1. Cardiovascular Fitness

DEFINITION

Cardiovascular fitness is defined as the maximum amount of oxygen you can utilize, an amount called VO_2 max (also known as maximal oxygen consumption, maximal oxygen uptake, peak oxygen uptake, or maximal aerobic capacity). This is simply your maximum rate of oxygen consumption during intense exercise, and it's highly correlated overall fitness, health, and longevity.

HOW TO DO IT

A 2014 study found that the minimum effective dose for maintenance of cardiovascular fitness is five four-minute high-intensity rounds at 87 to 97 percent of your maximum heart rate, with approximately four minutes of rest or low activity after each round to allow you to recover sufficiently.

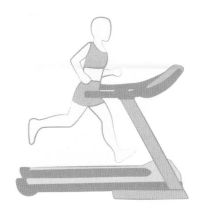

TAKEAWAY

For the minimum effective dose of cardiovascular fitness, perform five intense four-minute interval training sessions with full rest periods, such as five four-minute efforts on a bicycle, with each effort followed by four minutes of very easy pedaling. Do these once every two weeks.

2. Maximum Muscular Endurance and Aerobic Capacity

DEFINITION

Your maximum muscular endurance is, as the name suggests, the maximum amount of work your muscles can endure, and your maximum aerobic capacity is the maximum amount of time you can "do battle" while keeping your force output high.

HOW TO DO IT

For muscular endurance and aerobic capacity, nothing beats Tabata sets: four minutes of going all-out for twenty seconds, resting for ten seconds, and repeating. In one study, participants performed one four-minute Tabata session with a single exercise four times a week for four weeks. Exercise choices included burpees, mountain climbers, jumping jacks, and squat thrusts, but you could also engage in treadmill or outdoor running, rowing, kettlebell swings, or indoor or outdoor cycling.

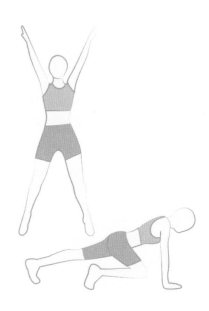

Compared to four thirty-minute steady-state treadmill exercise protocols per week in the control group, the Tabata group (which, if you do the math, was performing just sixteen minutes of exercise per week) saw massive gains in both aerobic capacity and muscle endurance. (You'll find more research on Tabata training on BoundlessBook.com/10.)

TAKEAWAY

Most studies use two to four Tabata sessions per week. I recommend performing two Tabata sessions per week, especially if you are doing everything else recommended in this chapter.

3. Ideal Strength-to-Muscle-Mass Ratio

DEFINITION

You want to be able to muster massive amounts of strength in small, tightly packed groups of muscle fibers—in other words, you want hard, wiry, explosive muscle. Bigger muscles aren't necessarily better. You should instead focus on maintaining some muscle mass while ensuring that the muscle is as functional and strong as possible.

HOW TO DO IT

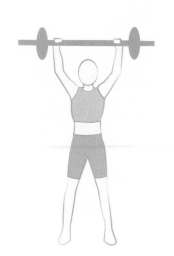

The best way to achieve the ideal strength-to-muscle-mass ratio was detailed back in chapter 9 and involves just two workouts per week.

The first workout is a super-slow lifting protocol as described by Doug McGuff in his book *Body by Science*. Perform twelve to twenty minutes of a few multijoint exercises with extremely slow, controlled lifting (thirty to sixty seconds per rep) and relatively high weights. The protocol should include:

- An upper-body push (e.g., overhead press, push-ups, chest press)
- An upper-body pull (e.g., bent or upright rows, lat pull-downs, pull-ups)
- A lower-body push (e.g., leg press, squats)
- A lower-body pull (e.g., dead lifts, Romanian dead lifts, lower back extensions, reverse hyperextensions)

The second workout is a high-intensity bodyweight circuit program called the seven-minute workout, designed by a pair of researchers to maintain strength and muscle in as little time as possible. Perform each of the following exercises for thirty seconds, with ten seconds of rest between exercises. Do each exercise as explosively as possible, trying to perform as many reps as possible in the thirty seconds (aside from an exercise like the plank, which is an isometric hold).

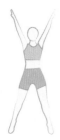

Jumping jacks or burpees

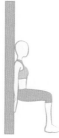

Wall sits

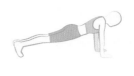

Push-ups or clapping push-ups

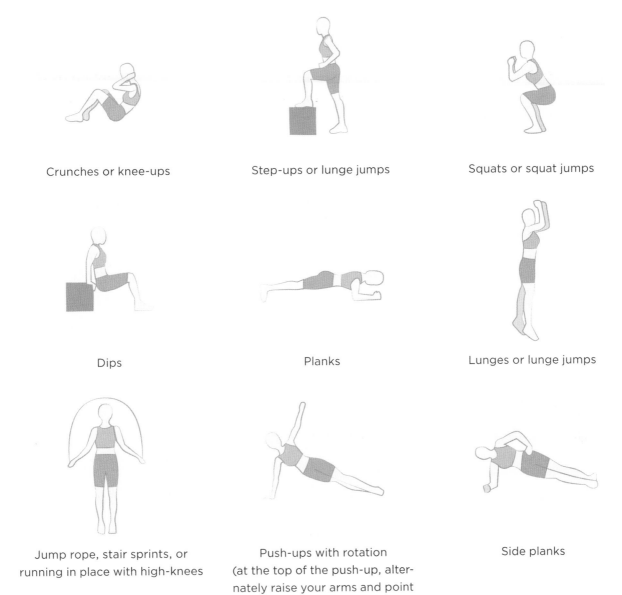

Crunches or knee-ups

Step-ups or lunge jumps

Squats or squat jumps

Dips

Planks

Lunges or lunge jumps

Jump rope, stair sprints, or running in place with high-knees

Push-ups with rotation (at the top of the push-up, alternately raise your arms and point them straight up)

Side planks

SUMMARY

Do two strength workouts per week—one with slow, controlled heavy lifting and one with high-intensity bodyweight movements.

4. Maximum Mitochondrial Density

DEFINITION

Mitochondria are the power plants of your cells. They are responsible for producing ATP, your body's primary form of cellular energy. Mitochondrial biogenesis is the creation of new mitochondria, and increasing mitochondrial density means packing the maximum number of mitochondria into your muscles so you can metabolize more fat and glucose.

VO$_2$ Max and Aging

In 1965, a group of researchers in Dallas enlisted five healthy twenty-year-old men to spend three straight weeks in bed for what would become one of the most well-known studies ever performed: the Dallas Bed Rest and Training Study. As you may imagine, the five participants had lost their physical fitness by the end of the study, with their VO$_2$ maxes plummeting by 27 percent.

Thirty years later, the men had gained an average of 50 pounds and their body fat percentages had doubled. But when researchers tested their VO$_2$ maxes, they had only dropped by 11 percent from their healthy twenty-year-old levels! In other words, a few weeks of bed rest was far worse than aging when it came to a crucial marker of fitness.

These findings are backed by research from Norway that has shown, with robust statistical evidence, that someone in his fifties can have the same level of fitness of someone in his twenties. The key, of course, is exercise—specifically how much and how intense.

The study analyzed data on 4,631 men and women pulled from Norway's biggest health database. These individuals had undergone laboratory tests to check their VO$_2$ maxes (the results represent the world's largest database of objective VO$_2$ max measurements). The database allowed researchers to compare fitness markers with cardiovascular risk factors and other assessments of overall health. This gave them the statistical data to back up what prior studies have suggested: age isn't everything when it comes to fitness.

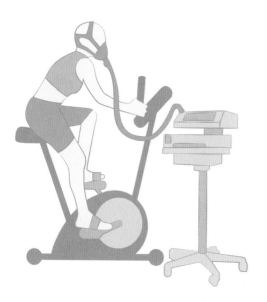

The researchers found that exercise intensity was far more important than exercise duration when measuring VO$_2$ max. The researchers also examined the benefits of high-intensity exercise, specifically interval training. During interval training, you perform four or more short periods (usually about four minutes long) of high-intensity exercise and engage in active rest between each burst of activity. This kind of interval training is especially effective and efficient for staying fit as you age.

The researchers also found that women whose VO$_2$ max measurement was below the median were five times more likely to have a cluster of cardiovascular risk factors than those with the highest VO$_2$ max scores. For men below the median, the risk was even higher: they were eight times more likely to have a cluster of cardiovascular risk factors than those with the highest VO$_2$ max scores.

In addition, the researchers discovered that women whose VO$_2$ max was below the median had a fivefold increase in cardiovascular risk factors than the women who had the highest VO$_2$ max scores.

The study concluded, "Even if you were highly active at a young age, you have to keep being active to get the health benefits from it." Turns out one of the best ways to do that is to perform at least one VO$_2$-max-boosting workout every one to two weeks.

I personally do a single VO$_2$ max session each week, usually with a stationary bike set up next to my LiveO2 adaptive contrast training machine (a method of delivering supplemental 100 percent oxygen, a strategy detailed in chapter 11). First, I perform two four-minute sets at my maximum sustainable pace and at full hypoxia, with four minutes of recovery at full hyperoxia between each set (the LiveO2 has a feature that allows you to alternate between hyperoxia and hypoxia with one simple sliding switch). I then repeat the process, with the next two four-minute sets done at full hyperoxia and the rest periods done at hypoxia. In a second session during the week, I do a mitochondrial workout with the same setup, but with four all-out thirty-second efforts and four-minute rest periods between them. The first two thirty-second efforts are at hypoxia with four-minute hyperoxic rest periods, and the next two are at hyperoxia with four-minute hypoxic rest periods.

HOW TO DO IT

Research suggests that a workout consisting of four thirty-second all-out cycling sprints significantly activates mitochondrial biogenesis in the skeletal muscle of humans. Three sets of five four-second treadmill sprints with twenty seconds of rest between sprints performed three times per week has the same effect. Similarly, workouts of four to six thirty-second bouts of all-out sprint cycling with four minutes of rest in between, done three times a week, also improves important components of mitochondrial health.

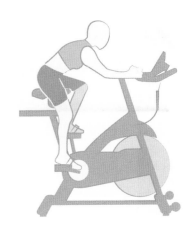

SUMMARY

When it comes to maximizing mitochondrial density, all you need are short, intense sprints. Tabata sets will cover most of your mitochondrial bases. But if you have time to spare after your strength or endurance workouts, perform a few brief, intense sets of sprints, such as five four-to-thirty-second sprints. Yes, you read that right: these sprints can be as short as four seconds.

Alternatively, once every one to two weeks, perform four to six thirty-second rounds of all-out sprint cycling with four minutes of rest after each round.

5. Optimized Fat Burning, Metabolic Efficiency, and Blood Sugar Control

DEFINITION

Optimizing these aspects of your health means maximizing your body's ability to generate ketones and burn fatty acids for fuel while avoiding frequent fluctuations in blood sugar.

HOW TO DO IT

Turning yourself into a fat-burning machine comes down to implementing the following tactics:

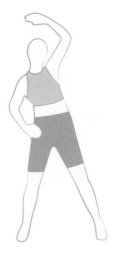

- Perform a short aerobic workout as many mornings during the week as possible, preferably in an overnight fasted state.

- Avoid frequent snacking.

- Save all your carbohydrates for the end of the day, and until then eat high amounts of healthy fats with moderate amounts of protein.

- Stay physically active all day long—use a standing workstation and take jumping jack or walking breaks.

- Become more resilient by engaging in cold thermogenesis and sauna therapy.

SUMMARY

Start each day with ten to thirty minutes of light, fasted-state activity (such as yoga, walking the dog, or doing yard work), take at least one cold shower per day, visit the sauna at least once per week, consume only nutrient-dense carbohydrates like sweet potatoes and dark, leafy greens, and be as active as possible all day long. You can even control blood glucose fluctuations with a simple fifteen-minute walk after the day's main meal. And, of course, go back and review chapter 8 if necessary.

6. Maximum Stamina

DEFINITION

Stamina is the ability to move at low to moderate intensity for ninety minutes or longer. Around the ninety-minute mark, your muscle and liver glycogen stores run out, and your body has to burn fat for fuel.

HOW TO DO IT

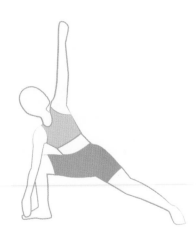

Stamina isn't necessary for looking good naked or living a long time, but I like to know that if I had to, I could hunt down an animal, ride my bicycle to a nearby city, hike over a mountain range, or survive a zombie apocalypse—similar to how our ancestors were able to engage in persistence hunting for many hours or days, often with limited food and water. But contrary to popular belief among marathoners and triathletes, building stamina does not require a two-to-three-hour death march every weekend. The human body is quite capable of moving for long periods and requires only brief stamina-training forays.

Once or twice per month, do something like a backpacking trip, long bike ride, Bikram yoga session, or anything else that combines endurance, mental focus, and low-to-moderate-intensity physical activity. Try to do this in a fasted state or with minimal fuel on board, such as ketones, amino acids, and electrolytes.

SUMMARY

Unless you sign up for something like an obstacle race, century ride, triathlon, or marathon, stamina training is not necessary. But if you want to add the stamina feather to your cap, get out and do something that takes ninety minutes or more at least once per month. If you want to challenge yourself, you could even make that session a triathlon, 5K, Spartan Race, or any other crazy fitness adventure, like rafting or rock climbing. The rest of your physical endurance will be built simply by avoiding long periods of sedentary time.

The Bottom Line

That's it! Once you put all these tactics together, combining fitness, longevity, and aesthetics is not too daunting. Your program to optimize your physique and life span should include the following:

- Five intense four-minute intervals, one session every two weeks
- Two to three Tabata sets per week
- One twelve-to-twenty-minute super-slow strength session per week
- One seven-to-fourteen-minute high-intensity bodyweight workout per week
- A short series of sprint bursts one to three times per week, such as five four-second all-out sprints broken up by twenty-second rest periods
- A fasting protocol (check out chapter 19 for more information) and limited snacking
- Low-level physical activity all day long
- One ninety-minute or longer stamina session once or twice per month

When you do the math, this program requires no more than thirty to sixty minutes per day to get fit, look good naked, and live a long time. Just remember that what I have described above is not designed to turn you into a super-athlete. It is designed to give you a fantastic body and a long life.

THE LAST WORD

I have woven all these tactics together in done-for-you programs that provide videos, exercise instructions, daily workout routines, and anything you may need. These courses will help you eliminate the guesswork involved in optimizing your life span and fitness, and help you to unlock boundless energy without excessively beating up your body.

The first course is called, fittingly enough, the Look-Good-Naked Longevity Plan and is available on the online portal TrainingPeaks. You can also find it in a downloadable PDF format. In both versions, all the information from this chapter is laid out on a weekly calendar that you can print and sync to your computer and phone. During the eight-week program, I give you daily, step-by-step instructions for the exact muscle-training, fat-burning, cardiovascular, and mobility protocols that maximize every second you spend exercising. Whether you want to look good naked, get massive gains in fitness, or both, you can wash, rinse, and repeat this eight-week cycle throughout the year. A link to the TrainingPeaks version and the PDF is available at BoundlessBook.com/10.

In addition, I recently hosted a film crew at my home for an entire week. The crew, representing a company called MindValley, filmed an entire quest for beauty and longevity enhancement and wove each of the principles you have just discovered into that quest. You will find this quest on BoundlessBook.com/10.

Finally, on that same URL, you can find a morning routine that I specifically designed to accompany this book and to give you boundless energy for the entire day. It can be modified to last anywhere from fifteen to thirty minutes, depending on your amount of available time. In the meantime, if you are drooling to dive into one of my routines right away, check out the sidebar for a sample perfect two weeks of training. This sample includes all the elements from this chapter structured in a protocol that should take no more than forty-five minutes per day.

ONE THING YOU CAN DO THIS WEEK

As you have learned, the body responds quite favorably to short, all-out bursts of activity followed by long rest periods. The next time you get on a treadmill, bicycle, elliptical trainer, or any other exercise machine, do a brief warm-up, then go as hard as humanly possible for thirty seconds. Rest for four minutes by moving slowly. Do this four times through. That's it. That's the whole workout. Our workout programming often becomes too complex, and research proves that this is the type of exercise that gets safe and fast results.

> For citations for all the research studies mentioned in this chapter and a deeper dive into the topics of this chapter—including links to podcasts, blog posts, recommended tools and supplements, and much more—visit BoundlessBook.com/10.

WEEK 1

COLD THERMOGENESIS

Choose 5 to 7 days this week and complete the following 5-minute showering protocol in a fasted state: 10 seconds of warm water followed by 20 seconds of cold water, 10 times through.

In addition, choose one day and do either a 10-minute ice-cold shower or 15 to 20 minutes of full-body cold-water immersion

DAY 2

Workout 1:
Morning Fasted Fat Burning

Before breakfast, perform 20 to 30 minutes of light cardio: yoga, fast walking, cycling, the elliptical, swimming, or hiking. The goal is to burn fat and lean up. You can drink a cup of plain black coffee or tea before this, but don't consume any calories until you are done. If you can't perform this cardio in the morning, do it after dinner and don't eat anything afterward.

Workout 2: Swim Hypoxic Sets (optional)

Perform a 500-meter warm-up. Then swim 12 rounds of 25 meters each. During each round, do not breathe, or keep breathing to a minimum. Recover for 10 seconds, then repeat. Swim as smoothly as you can—you don't need to sprint. See what changes in technique and fluidity you can make to conserve energy and oxygen.

Workout 3: The 7-Minute Workout

Perform each exercise for 30 seconds with 10 seconds of rest between exercises. One round takes about 7 minutes, but, if time allows, I recommend doing 2 or 3 rounds. Be sure to use good form on each exercise.

- Jumping jacks
- Wall sits
- Push-ups
- Crunches
- Step-ups
- Squats
- Dips
- Planks
- Running in place with high knees
- Lunges
- Push-ups with rotation
- Side planks

DAY 1

Foundation Training

You will need the book *True to Form: How to Use Foundation Training for Sustained Pain Relief and Everyday Fitness* by Dr. Eric Goodman to do this properly. Go through each of the ten foundation exercises in the book just once (it will take you about 10 to 15 minutes), with a focus on perfect form.

Tabata Sets

Perform a 10-to-15-minute warm-up, then complete 8 rounds of 20 seconds of a single exercise (burpees, jumping jacks, mountain climbers, kettlebell swings, squats, treadmill running, cycling, rowing machine—you choose) with 10 seconds of rest between rounds. Go at an all-out, maximum-intensity pace each round. Cool down with nasal breathing and easy aerobic movement for 5 to 10 minutes.

DAY 3

Workout 1: Metabolic Mobility
(The Ultimate Foam Roller Routine)

At each station, make 20 to 30 passes with the foam roller. Making one pass means you go up the muscle group and back down.

- **Station 1:** Perform 10 burpees. Foam-roll the Achilles tendon and calf on your right leg.
- **Station 2:** Perform 10 burpees. Foam-roll the Achilles tendon and calf on your left leg.
- **Station 3:** Foam-roll your right hamstring. Perform 20 forward and backward high leg swings with your right leg.
- **Station 4:** Foam-roll your left hamstring. Perform 20 forward and backward high leg swings with your left leg.
- **Station 5:** Perform 10 burpees. Foam-roll the outside of your right hip.
- **Station 6:** Perform 10 burpees. Foam-roll the outside of your left hip.
- **Station 7:** Foam-roll the IT band on your right leg (located on the outside of your thigh). Perform 20 side-to-side leg swings with your right leg.
- **Station 8:** Foam-roll the IT band on your left leg. Perform 20 side-to-side leg swings with your left leg.
- **Station 9:** Perform 10 burpees. Foam-roll the adductors (on the inside of your thigh) on your right leg.
- **Station 10:** Perform 10 burpees. Foam-roll the adductors on your left leg.
- **Station 11:** Perform 50 jumping jacks. Foam-roll your back from bottom to top.
- **Station 12:** Perform 50 jumping jacks. Foam-roll your entire right shoulder complex.

- **Station 13:** Perform 50 jumping jacks. Foam-roll your entire left shoulder complex.
- **Station 14:** Perform 10 burpees. Foam-roll your neck (back, left side, right side).
- **Station 15:** Perform 10 burpees. Foam-roll the front of both quads.

DAY 4

Workout 1: Morning Fasted Fat Burning

Before breakfast, perform 20 to 30 minutes of light cardio: yoga, fast walking, cycling, the elliptical, swimming, or hiking. The goal is to burn fat and lean up. You can drink a cup of plain black coffee or tea before this, but don't consume any calories until you are done. If you can't perform this cardio in the morning, do it after dinner and don't eat anything afterward.

Workout 2: Super-Slow Routine

For this workout, view the video on BoundlessBook.com/10, which lays out the exact routine to perform.

DAY 6

Workout 1: Morning Fasted Fat Burning

Before breakfast, perform 20 to 30 minutes of light cardio: yoga, fast walking, cycling, the elliptical, swimming, or hiking. The goal is to burn fat and lean up. You can drink a cup of plain black coffee or tea before this, but don't consume any calories until you are done. If you can't perform this cardio in the morning, do it after dinner and don't eat anything afterward.

Workout 2: Mitochondrial and Metabolic Sprints

Do an all-out, maximum-intensity sprint on a rowing machine, bike, or elliptical (kettlebell swings, lunge jumps, or squat jumps can be used as a substitute if necessary) for 4 rounds of 30 seconds with 4 minutes of active rest between rounds. Active rest can be walking, easy jogging, or easy cycling. Finish with five 4-second all-out sprints, with 20 seconds of rest between sprints. (For more on the science behind these two forms of sprinting, visit BoundlessBook.com/10.)

Workout 2: Tabata Sets

Perform a 10-to-15-minute warm-up, then complete 8 rounds of 20 seconds of a single exercise (burpees, jumping jacks, mountain climbers, kettlebell swings, squats, treadmill running, cycling, rowing machine—you choose) with 10 seconds of rest between rounds. Go at an all-out, maximum-intensity pace each round. Cool down for 5 to 10 minutes.

DAY 5

Workout 1: Tabata Sets

Perform a 10-to-15-minute warm-up, then complete 8 rounds of 20 seconds of a single exercise (burpees, jumping jacks, mountain climbers, kettlebell swings, squats, treadmill running, cycling, rowing machine—you choose) with 10 seconds of rest between rounds. Go at an all-out, maximum-intensity pace each round. Cool down with nasal breathing and easy aerobic movement for 5 to 10 minutes.

Workout 2: Sauna

Spend 20 to 40 minutes (as long as you can tolerate) in a dry sauna. Focus on deep breathing, box breathing (four count in, four count hold, four count out, four count hold), occasional yoga moves, and stretches.

Drink water in moderation (as little as you can get away with). Finish up with a cold shower. It is fine for your heart rate to get high during this session and for it to feel a bit uncomfortable.

DAY 7

Workout 1: Deep Breathing & Yoga

Engage in deep, nasal belly breathing during a morning yoga routine, which, for this particular day, should ideally last 45 to 60 minutes. Try to do this routine in the sunshine to amplify vitamin D levels. If that isn't an option, use a brightly lit room. Focus on your breath.

The yoga routine you follow is up to you. Whatever routine you perform, you should preferably perform it alone. My top recommendation is Gaia TV and any of their 45-to-60-minute relaxation routines. No power or calorie-blasting yoga! Many of the Rodney Yee DVDs are also good.

Workout 2: Morning Fasted Fat Burning

Before breakfast, perform 20 to 30 minutes of light cardio: brisk walking, cycling, the elliptical, swimming, hiking, or anything else you can perform while maintaining an easy, conversational, aerobic pace. The goal is to burn fat and lean up. You can drink a cup of plain black coffee or tea before this, but don't consume any calories until you are done. If you can't perform this cardio in the morning, do it after dinner and don't eat anything afterward.

Hot-Cold Contrast

Alternate between a 5-minute cold shower, cold soak, or easy cold-water swim (the water must be 55 degrees or less) and a 10-minute dry sauna or wet sauna session. Cycle between these for as long as possible, preferably for 30 to 45 minutes, which would allow you to perform two or three cycles.

WEEK 2

COLD THERMOGENESIS

Choose 5 to 7 days this week and complete the following 5-minute showering protocol in a fasted state: 10 seconds of warm water followed by 20 seconds of cold water, 10 times through.

In addition, choose one day and do either a 10-minute ice-cold shower or 15 to 20 minutes of full-body cold-water immersion

DAY 2

Workout 1: The 7-Minute Workout

Perform each exercise for 30 seconds with 10 seconds of rest between exercises. If time permits, attempt to do 2 or 3 rounds. Use good form on every exercise.

- Jumping jacks
- Wall sits
- Push-ups
- Crunches
- Step-ups
- Squats
- Dips
- Planks
- Running in place with high knees
- Lunges
- Push-ups with rotation
- Side planks

Workout 2: Morning Fasted Fat Burning

Before breakfast, perform 20 to 30 minutes of light cardio: brisk walking, cycling, the elliptical, swimming, hiking, or anything else you can perform while maintaining an easy, conversational, aerobic pace. The goal is to burn fat and lean up. You can drink a cup of plain black coffee or tea before this, but don't consume any calories until you are done. If you can't perform this cardio in the morning, do it after dinner and don't eat anything afterward.

Workout 3: Swim Hypoxic Sets (optional)

Perform a 500-meter warm-up. Then swim 12 rounds of 25 meters each. During each round, do not breathe, or keep breathing to a minimum. Recover for 10 seconds, then repeat. Swim as smoothly as you can—you don't need to sprint. See what changes in technique and fluidity you can make to conserve energy and oxygen.

DAY 1

Workout 1: Tabata Sets

Perform a 10-to-15-minute warm-up, then complete 8 rounds of 20 seconds of a single exercise (burpees, jumping jacks, mountain climbers, kettlebell swings, squats, treadmill running, cycling, rowing machine—you choose) with 10 seconds of rest between rounds. Go at an all-out, maximum-intensity pace each round. Cool down with nasal breathing and easy aerobic movement for 5 to 10 minutes.

Workout 2: Foundation Training

Go through each of the ten Foundation exercises in the book *True to Form* by Dr. Eric Goodman just one time with a focus on perfect form.

DAY 3

Workout 1: Tabata Sets

Perform a 10-to-15-minute warm-up, then complete 8 rounds of 20 seconds of a single exercise (burpees, jumping jacks, mountain climbers, kettlebell swings, squats, treadmill running, cycling, rowing machine—you choose) with 10 seconds of rest between rounds. Go at an all-out, maximum-intensity pace each round. Cool down with nasal breathing and easy aerobic movement for 5 to 10 minutes.

Workout 2:
Metabolic Mobility (The Ultimate Foam Roller Routine)

At each station, make 20 to 30 passes with the foam roller. Making one pass means you go up the muscle group and back down.

- **Station 1:** Perform 10 burpees. Foam-roll the Achilles tendon and calf on your right leg.
- **Station 2:** Perform 10 burpees. Foam-roll the Achilles tendon and calf on your left leg.
- **Station 3:** Foam-roll your right hamstring. Perform 20 forward and backward high leg swings with your right leg.
- **Station 4:** Foam-roll your left hamstring. Perform 20 forward and backward high leg swings with your left leg.
- **Station 5:** Perform 10 burpees. Foam-roll the outside of your right hip.
- **Station 6:** Perform 10 burpees. Foam-roll the outside of your left hip.
- **Station 7:** Foam-roll the IT band on your right leg (located on the outside of your thigh). Perform 20 side-to-side leg swings with your right leg.
- **Station 8:** Foam-roll the IT band on your left leg. Perform 20 side-to-side leg swings with your left leg.
- **Station 9:** Perform 10 burpees. Foam-roll the adductors (on the inside of your thigh) on your right leg.
- **Station 10:** Perform 10 burpees. Foam-roll the adductors on your left leg.

- **Station 11:** Perform 50 jumping jacks. Foam-roll your back from bottom to top.
- **Station 12:** Perform 50 jumping jacks. Foam-roll your entire right shoulder complex.
- **Station 13:** Perform 50 jumping jacks. Foam-roll your entire left shoulder complex.
- **Station 14:** Perform 10 burpees. Foam-roll your neck (back, left side, right side).
- **Station 15:** Perform 10 burpees. Foam-roll the front of both quads.

DAY 5

Workout 1: Tabata Sets

Perform a 10-to-15-minute warm-up, then complete 8 rounds of 20 seconds of a single exercise (burpees, jumping jacks, mountain climbers, kettlebell swings, squats, treadmill running, cycling, rowing machine—you choose) with 10 seconds of rest between rounds. Go at an all-out, maximum-intensity pace each round. Cool down with nasal breathing and easy aerobic movement for 5 to 10 minutes.

Workout 2: Sauna

Spend 20 to 40 minutes (as long as you can tolerate) in a dry sauna. Focus on deep breathing, box breathing (four count in, four count hold, four count out, four count hold), occasional yoga moves, and stretches.

Drink water in moderation (as little as you can get away with). Finish up with a cold shower. It is fine for your heart rate to get high during this session and for it to feel a bit uncomfortable.

Workout 3: Foundation Training

Go through each of the ten Foundation exercises in the book *True to Form* by Dr. Eric Goodman just once with a focus on perfect form.

DAY 6

Workout 1: 4-Minute HIIT with 4-Minute Rest Periods for VO$_2$ Max

Complete five rounds of intense 4-minute intervals. Go at the maximum pace you can maintain without compromising on form. Take a 4-minute easy, aerobic, active rest period between each round. You can run, bike, swim, use the elliptical, or row. You'll find more information on the effectiveness of this routine on BoundlessBook.com/10.

Workout 2: Morning Fasted Fat Burning

Before breakfast, perform 20 to 30 minutes of light cardio: brisk walking, cycling, the elliptical, swimming, hiking, or anything else you can perform while maintaining an easy, conversational, aerobic pace. The goal is to burn fat and lean up. You can drink a cup of plain black coffee or tea before this, but don't consume any calories until you are done. If you can't perform this cardio in the morning, do it after dinner and don't eat anything afterward.

DAY 4

Workout 1: Super-Slow Routine

For this workout, view the a video on BoundlessBook.com/10, which lays out the exact routine to perform.

Workout 2: Morning Fasted Fat Burning

Before breakfast, perform 20 to 30 minutes of light cardio: brisk walking, cycling, the elliptical, swimming, hiking, or anything else you can perform while maintaining an easy, conversational, aerobic pace. The goal is to burn fat and lean up. You can drink a cup of plain black coffee or tea before this, but don't consume any calories until you are done. If you can't perform this cardio in the morning, do it after dinner and don't eat anything afterward.

DAY 7

Workout 1: Hot-Cold Contrast

Alternate between a 5-minute cold shower, cold soak, or easy cold-water swim (the water must be 55 degrees or less) and a 10-minute dry sauna or wet sauna session. Cycle between these for as long as possible, preferably for 30 to 45 minutes, which would allow you to perform two or three cycles.

Workout 2: Morning Fasted Fat Burning

Before breakfast, perform 20 to 30 minutes of light cardio: brisk walking, cycling, the elliptical, swimming, hiking, or anything else you can perform while maintaining an easy, conversational, aerobic pace. The goal is to burn fat and lean up. You can drink a cup of plain black coffee or tea before this, but don't consume any calories until you are done. If you can't perform this cardio in the morning, do it after dinner and don't eat anything afterward.

Workout 3: Deep Breathing and Yoga

Engage in deep, nasal belly breathing during a morning yoga routine, which, for this particular day, should ideally last 45 to 60 minutes. Try to do this routine in the sunshine to amplify vitamin D levels. If that isn't an option, use a brightly lit room. Focus on your breath.

The yoga routine you follow is up to you. Whatever routine you perform, you should preferably perform it alone. My top recommendation is Gaia TV and any of their 45-to-60-minute relaxation routines. No power or calorie-blasting yoga! Many of the Rodney Yee DVDs are also good.

BIOHACK YOUR BODY

SCIENCE, GEAR, AND TOOLS FOR BUILDING THE PERFECT HUMAN

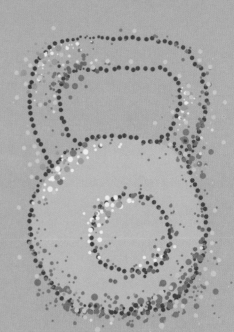

Standing at my basement office desk, I reached for my phone and texted my friend David, who was upstairs at the kitchen table.

"Dude, come downstairs if you want to see my morning writing routine."

Within a minute, David appeared at the open door to the office and immediately stepped back in shock, nearly dropping the French press in his hand.

"What the *hell*?"

I flashed a sheepish grin. I was bare-ass naked in front of my computer keyboard, legs spread wide next to a giant panel of infrared light bulbs that stimulate growth hormone, collagen production, and (hence the nakedness) testosterone and sperm cell production in the testes. A long tube attached to a nasal cannula was blasting my respiratory system with oxidized water for DNA repair. Perched atop my skull was photobiomodulation headgear, designed to enhance blood flow to the brain while reducing inflammation and fixing neural cells. Beneath my feet was a balance-challenging mat patterned after the rice paddy fields in Korea, and attached to both knees were two tiny electrodes to stimulate my muscles as I worked in a standing position—keeping my legs light and free of unsightly varicose veins.

David, one of my clients and a guest at my home for the weekend, raised an eyebrow. I continued to grin. "Nothing you haven't seen before, right, man?" In this case, I was likely wrong.

Admittedly, as a self-experimenting, immersive journalist, guinea pig, and supremely curious adventure-seeker, I realize that my morning writing routine may seem a bit elaborate. But when it comes to sculpting my mind and body into the ultimate human machine, I also sometimes keep things extremely simple, such as when I take a morning-sunshine box breathing walk, spend an afternoon baling hay for the goats, or collect fitness tools simpler than laser lights attached to my balls or an electrical stimulator attached to my skull. This chapter will give you the ultimate blend of ancestral wisdom and modern science to transform your body into a tool that accomplishes any feat you desire.

The fact is, you can drop me just about anywhere on the face of the planet and I'll figure out a way to not just maintain muscle but also build muscle, burn fat, and develop power, strength, stamina, and balance.

Sometimes the tools I use for these objectives are simple—such as an easy-to-use travel kit of just four portable devices—and sometimes these tools are more complex, fringe biohacks that fly under the radar. But from the simple to the complex, every tactic I've discovered to mold the body anytime, anyplace is described in this chapter, which will serve as your ultimate guide to biohacking and building your body using commonsense and easy-to-find tools along with underground and little-known methods, each with plenty of my own highly practical tips from the trenches.

Why We Hit the Gym

Exercise—at least the way most modern gym junkies think of exercise—is not a prevailing characteristic of any of the Blue Zones of longevity, where people live longer than anywhere else on earth. Despite the prevalence of lean, muscular, strong, and fit populations in the Blue Zones, as well as in hunter-gatherer tribes, many indigenous populations, and our ancestors, there's little evidence they enjoy CrossFit boxes, Planet Fitness clubs, fancy health spas, or kettlebell classes.

In fact, the need to hit the gym is largely a fabrication of a postindustrial society in which engines and computers now do much of our manual labor for us, and we humans are now expected to be at a desk or in a largely sedentary environment for eight or more hours each day. The unfortunate consequence of this is that the manual labor our bodies are designed to do no longer needs to get done, and we don't get the all-day-long movement our bodies crave.

To scratch our ancestral itch to move, it only makes sense that at the beginning or end of the day, we'd have a deep-rooted desire to go lace up our running shoes or lift heavy stuff at the gym. Unless we're going out of our way to hack our environment with treadmill workstations, Pomodoro breaks for movement, and brief exercise forays throughout the day, most of us simply don't experience the same natural nudge into movement that people in the Blue Zones have as they collect water from springs, till the fields, walk everywhere, weed the garden, push wheelbarrows, lift rocks, build fences, hunt, and fish. Heck, I remember when I was a painter in college and was up and down ladders the entire day, power-washing walls, hauling heavy paint buckets, and brushing until my shoulders were sore. The last thing I felt like doing at the end of the day was dumbbell curls in front of a mirror at some gym.

So it's only natural that unless you're a construction worker, farmer, gardener, trail builder, or someone else lucky enough to have a relatively physically active job, you're going to want to insert formal, planned exercise sessions into your week. It's also natural that in our relatively coddled, overprotected, safe lives, you'll experience an urge to climb a mountain or slay a dragon, whether those mountains and dragons are marathons, triathlons, obstacle course races, fitness competitions, sporting events, or some other physical challenge. But just don't fool yourself into thinking that it's necessary or natural for optimal health for you to be working on your bench press or training for a marathon, because it isn't. In an ideal scenario, you'd instead be moving all day long at a low intensity, lifting heavy things, sprinting occasionally, and perhaps engaging in a longer stamina-challenging effort once every one to two weeks, not crushing yourself at the gym for forty-five to sixty minutes a day and then staying sedentary the rest of the day.

The gym-based exercise that was once the realm of gymnasts, warriors, bodybuilders, and athletes has now trickled down to the general population. It's not what our bodies were meant for, but in a sedentary society, when it comes to health outcomes, the pros outweigh the cons.

The "Family Reunion with No Gym" Workout

I recently packed up my wife and twin boys and embarked upon our annual family vacation to the tiny, sleepy coastal town of Seaside, Oregon. A somewhat touristy town with far more arcades, candy stores, and ice cream shops than gyms, Seaside wouldn't be my ideal choice for an active, healthy hot spot. But vacationing in Seaside is a long-standing tradition in my wife's family, so I joined in.

As I tend to do for road trips, into the back of the car I threw my kettlebell, my suspension trainer, an elastic band, and a couple of light sliders (think tiny plastic plates the size of dinner plates that can be used for a host of different exercises). With no access to a gym or any other workout equipment, but armed with these four simple and easy-to-transport tools and five basic exercises for each tool, every day I was able to perform an enormous variety of exercises, including the following (you can view any of these exercises at YouTube.com/BenGreenfieldFitness or ExRx.net):

KETTLEBELL

- Swings
- Around the world
- Single-arm clean to overhead press
- Goblet squat
- Bent row

SUSPENSION STRAP

- Pull-ups
- Suspended push-ups with knee-to-chest
- Left and right leg suspended lunges
- Plank rotations

SLIDERS

- Mountain climbers
- Lateral slides
- Pikes
- Bridges
- Crocodile walks

ELASTIC BAND

- Front raises
- Side raises
- Lateral shuffles
- Squat to press
- Kickouts

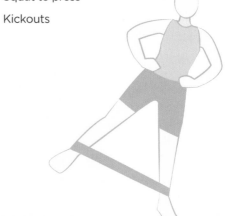

BODY WEIGHT

- Burpees
- Jumping jacks
- Skipping in place
- Sit to stand
- Plank to push-up

As you can imagine, when completed with little to no rest between sets, this workout simulates exactly what I'd get at a highfalutin health club—all performed in the backyard of a beach house.

THE BASICS

Let's begin with the simple and easy-to-use tools that are indispensable to have in your suitcase, car, home office, park, basement, backyard, or anywhere else a "pop-up gym" or minimalist exercise approach is required, including the best choices, workouts, and how-tos.

Kettlebell

One of the best ways to achieve a minimum effective dose of exercise is to toss around a kettlebell. As a matter of fact, a study that appeared in the *Journal of Strength and Conditioning Research* showed that the acute hormonal response to the kettlebell swing exercise (one of the most popular and easy-to-learn kettlebell moves) consisted of an extremely significant rise in growth hormone and testosterone.

A kettlebell is a cast-iron weight that looks like a cannonball with a handle. Originally a tool used by Russian strongmen for training and competition, multicolored, vinyl-coated kettlebells are now a popular fitness device that you can find at many gyms. Kettlebells range from 4 pounds to 175 pounds, but because a kettlebell is shaped differently than a dumbbell, a 4-pound kettlebell can actually feel a bit heavy or awkward. This is because the kettlebell's center of mass is extended farther out from your body, so it can be tougher to handle and maneuver—which is one reason why kettlebells can be so effective for improving your strength, balance, and explosiveness. In most situations, kettlebells are used for increasing grip strength or for performing movements that are designed to build strength and endurance in the lower back, legs, and shoulders. These movements include full-body exercises like the swing, snatch, and the clean and jerk.

I own nearly a dozen kettlebells, littered across my garage, office, and home gym, and nearly every functional weight-training workout I perform uses at least one kettlebell move. Should you want to take your kettlebell skills to the next level, I highly recommend any of the RKC courses offered by Dragon Door and my podcast with Cal Poly strength and conditioning coach Chris Holder, both of which are linked to on BoundlessBook.com/11.

Jump Rope

While many fitness enthusiasts prefer a speed-rope-style jump rope, I'm a bigger fan of a weighted jump rope because it does a better job strengthening the grip and shoulders. When space is limited, you don't have access to a treadmill or good running terrain, or you're doing quick, fast intervals that make it inconvenient to step outside to run or fire up a treadmill, a jump rope is a perfect option. Sure, you could run in place, but the coordination requirements of a jump rope offer a better challenge for your brain. In addition, if you have any type of injury that leaves you unable to unilaterally load one side, as you would when running or jumping rope with alternate legs, jumping rope with both legs is often pain-free and can still train your knees, ankles, and lower leg tendons for the eccentric motion of running.

For an added challenge, you can purchase a short "battle rope," tie an elastic band around your ankles, and do jump rope intervals. This is actually a well-known obstacle challenge in most Spartan stadium races. Incidentally, Muay Thai fighters, some of the best-conditioned athletes in the world, make jumping rope a major part of their training because it combines a full-body workout and endurance training.

Weighted Backpack

On most hunting and hiking retail websites, you can find rugged backpacks designed for packing meat from large animals out of the mountains, or designed for many miles of hard-core rucking with heavy amounts of weight. These same packs can be filled with sandbags, kettlebells, or rocks and used for hiking, uphill treadmill walks, or long rucks through the neighborhood. When my boys were young, I'd take them on hikes, with my "handicap" being 80 to 100 pounds stuffed into my Kifaru Timberline backpack, which sports a biomechanically friendly carbon frame and holds 7,800 cubic inches. I first discovered the muscle, cardio, and grit-training benefits of rucking when I was training for the SEALFit Kokoro, and I still use it as a strategy to amp up the intensity of my walks. Finally, for his hunt training, my friend Joe Rogan uses and recommends the Atlas Trainer, which is a special type of weighted backpack with an attachment option for a standard weight plate.

Weighted Vest

A weighted vest is simply a vest that is either made from a heavy material or equipped with small pockets that can be filled with tiny sandbags, small steel bars, or other weighted objects (these usually accompany your vest order). The purpose of a weighted vest is to add extra weight for bodyweight exercises, walking, distance running, or speed, power, and agility drills. When it comes to performance, research has shown that using this type of extra load during sprinting or speedwork requires your lower-body muscles to generate more force against the ground and can lead to improvements in strength, power, and acceleration during running, as well as increased strength and efficiency during speed, power, and agility drills. It's simple to turn a bodyweight workout into a difficult routine by simply putting on a weighted vest. For example, here's one treadmill routine that I do while wearing my weighted vest:

- Two-minute treadmill run (bicycling in a standing position is another option)
- Twenty weighted vest push-ups
- Twenty weighted vest squats
- Twenty weighted vest "get-ups" (simply lie on your back on the ground, then do a sit-up motion and stand up to your feet)
- Twenty weighted vest reverse lunges

Repeat these five stations as a circuit four to six times through. Because you'll be running, this routine works best with a 10-to-20-pound vest, and if you want an even more advanced version, throw in a round of pull-ups too.

You can also wear a weighted vest during hikes, walks around the neighborhood, at the park, or even when doing stair repeats in a stadium or at a hotel. The sky's the limit—I've even worn my vest through airport security and walked around airports with it on! The useful part about a weighted vest is that no matter where or how you move, it's going to make any aspect of getting from point A to point B just a little bit more difficult. You can add an intense twist to just about any weight-training routine by putting on a weighted vest.

For example, you can try a "5x5" routine while wearing a vest. This routine—five sets of five dead lifts, squats, bench presses, barbell rows, and barbell cleans—gets seriously amplified when it's performed wearing a weighted vest. The main thing you'll notice is that your core, low back, and inspiratory and expiratory muscles are forced to work far harder, which gives you an added calorie burn and challenges your small postural and core muscles.

Medicine Ball

The medicine ball is a simple and versatile way to weave powerful, explosive exercises into your routine—and as you learned in chapter 9, these exercises are essential for slowing aging and gaining compact muscle. Take the example of a medicine ball cannonball toss, in which you drop into a deep squat position with both hands wrapped around the ball, then explode up and toss the ball as high into the air as possible. If you are focusing on the height the ball reaches (if you are trying to hit the ceiling), you are suddenly forced into producing maximum acceleration, full-body extension, and power, with no risk of injury from the eccentric lowering of the weight. The same can be said for some of my other favorite medicine ball exercises, including side tosses, overhead throws, slams, and the classic power squat-to-press move: the medicine ball thruster. If you add 10-, 20-, 30-, and 40-pound medicine balls to your fitness arsenal, the range of power-development, coordination, and functional fitness exercises you can perform is nearly limitless, and if you're training for any type of sport, the addition of medicine ball exercises to your routine is a no-brainer. I'm a fan of the durable, vintage leather medicine balls made by companies such as Champion Sports and Rogue Fitness.

Stability Ball

Also known as the Swiss ball, the giant exercise stability ball seems to have been bastardized of late as a "core-activating chair" for use at a desk. I don't recommend this. Hunched-forward shoulders and a collapsed spine notoriously accompany the use of a ball for a seated position, and you must be hyperaware of your posture if you are sitting on a stability ball. But a stability ball does have a host of beneficial uses. Functional movement guru Paul Chek is a huge fan of the ball, and when he began showing up at Gold's Gym in San Diego, bodybuilders would stand around and make jokes about how ridiculous he looked using it. But they were quite impressed when Paul began performing deep squats on the ball, crunches on the ball with 180-pound dumbbells, and chest-presses on the ball with 110-pound dumbbells (just google "Paul Chek Swiss ball" to see what I mean).

There are a few reasons the stability ball is a beneficial addition to your exercise gear. When properly inflated, it provides a firm but wobbly surface that requires you to react quickly to every tiny movement of the ball caused by a change in your center of gravity. This activates your core and planted leg or arm muscles as stabilizers. At the same time, your body's proprioceptive mechanisms, such as joint mechanoreceptors, spindle cells, your inner ear, and your ocular proprioception, must all stay active, which can improve your sensory perception and spatial awareness. Because of its shape, the ball is also excellent as a stretching tool for the abdominals and spine.

So what do you do if you're not going to sit on the ball while hunched over a keyboard? For starters, try the supine lateral ball roll, an exercise that develops the spinal stabilizers, the foot and ankle complex, hip, pelvis, shoulder girdle, and neck. This is what Paul Chek calls a "Big Bang exercise" because it conditions the body in all planes of motion at once and activates all the weak muscles responsible for stabilizing all body segments involved with the exercise. (For a video demonstration, visit BoundlessBook.com/11.)

Training Mask

Although they are often scoffed at as a gimmicky marketing tactic that makes you look like the villain Bane from *Batman*, training masks actually do work to increase fitness dramatically—just not the way most people think. These masks do not simulate altitude, nor do they actually change the atmospheric pressure you're training in. You need a far more expensive oxygen-scrubbing device designed for intermittent hypoxic training (IHT) or exercise with oxygen therapy (EWOT) in order to truly simulate altitude or to increase or decrease the partial pressure of the oxygen in the air you're breathing. So when you're charging down the treadmill sporting your scary-looking altitude-training mask, you're still breathing air that is approximately 21 percent oxygen, with the same partial oxygen pressure of whatever altitude you happen to be at.

But these masks do make it harder to breathe, and high amounts of carbon dioxide build up in the air that collects in the space of the mask directly in front of your mouth. So these masks can certainly be effective for improving ventilatory capacity and for increasing your mental tolerance and stress resilience, including in situations where you have low oxygen or air availability, but they don't achieve the same physiological adaptations as true hypoxic training.

Training masks have been studied with respect to their effect on respiratory compensation threshold (RCT). RCT is the boundary between high-intensity activity and much higher intensity exertion, when you begin to breathe hard and lactic acid begins to accumulate. Under normal conditions, your body's drive to breathe is based on carbon dioxide levels in the blood. But when RCT is reached, a significant portion of the body's drive to breathe is based on accumulating lactic acid levels. This results in heavier respiration, inspiratory and expiratory muscle fatigue, and an overall inability to sustain high-intensity exercise. In studies, training masks act by increasing RCT, which helps you develop the ability to sustain high-intensity exercise for a longer period of time.

One of my preferred ways to use a training mask is to simulate the "high-oxygen to low-oxygen" environment you'd experience with a spendier EWOT device. I'll warm up on a bicycle or treadmill with the mask off and hung around my neck, then pull it over my face and sprint for thirty to sixty seconds, then pull the mask back down and recover for thirty to sixty seconds, for ten rounds total. On BoundlessBook.com/11, you can find plenty more protocols, including some good diaphragmatic training sessions that you can do while simply resting on your back in a sauna or your living room, along with a discount code for the mask.

PowerLung

Like a training mask, the PowerLung is a small, handheld resistance-training device for the lungs, not an altitude simulator. But the best way to build fitness in your diaphragm and inspiratory and expiratory muscles is—just as with any other muscle in your body—to train them.

I'm often asked why one wouldn't just save some money and breathe through a straw to create this effect. It comes down to the concept of threshold resistance: when you breathe in and out through a PowerLung, you are working against a threshold of resistance that is the same for every breath. You are not breathing through a restricted orifice where the load can be reduced just by changing the way you breathe. The PowerLung has two control dials, one to train your inhale breathing and the other to train your exhale breathing. Both are adjustable to set your level (threshold) of resistance, exactly the way you add weights for strength training. A sample training session you can do with the PowerLung is to simply inhale and exhale through the PowerLung (that's one repetition) for a count of ten seconds, then to recover for 30 seconds to 1 minute, and repeat for ten rounds.

While I'm certain the manufacturers of the device would not encourage this, I tend to do my PowerLung training while driving or stuck in traffic. I find myself in that scenario three to four times a month easily, so I literally get over forty resistance lung-training sessions a year with that approach.

Relaxator

The Relaxator is the final breathwork tool that I'll recommend in this section, particularly because I find it far easier to use hands-free than a PowerLung while on my afternoon walk, and it pairs quite well with the type of breath-hold walks discussed in chapter 3. The Relaxator is a small, no-frills device that you can hang around your neck like a necklace. You then place the mouthpiece in your mouth and, when you exhale, experience an adjustable level of resistance to mouth-based exhalation, while simultaneously being able to breathe through your nose as you normally would. This helps you maintain elevated levels of oxygen and carbon dioxide simultaneously, a health strategy explored in chapter 3.

In addition to making your breathing more rhythmic, slow, and relaxed, the Relaxator also stimulates your diaphragm to work more efficiently, thereby ensuring that the air you inhale reaches the lower part of your lungs. Because you're forced to have a lower respiratory rate while using it, it also activates the parasympathetic nervous system, which comes in handy if you decide to use it while, say, checking email or stuck in traffic. You can also use it while cooking, mowing the lawn, cleaning the garage, or doing any other activity when you want a subtle way to train your breath, without looking like a freak with a training mask on.

Hand Grip Trainer

Grip strength is highly correlated with both full-body strength and, surprisingly, overall longevity. I cannot recommend highly enough that you add a high-quality hand grip trainer, such as the aircraft-grade aluminum Captains of Crush devices, to your briefcase, book bag, or glove compartment. Between a Captains of Crush and a PowerLung stowed in my car or book bag, I can train my lungs and my grip during any road trip or flight. My preferred training method with the Captains of Crush is to squeeze ten times as hard as possible, then hold the last squeeze as long as possible before switching hands, and to repeat for three rounds. Subjectively, it also seems to have a good stress-relieving effect.

Neuro-Grips

Jon Bruney, author of the training book *Neuro-Mass* and my former podcast guest, is known for creating body-blitzing workouts with special combinations of super-slow grinds, isometric holds, and explosive repetitions, in that order. Jon calls these "Neuro-Sets." When performed with proper intensity and in the correct sequence, Neuro-Sets can put your system into neural overdrive and effectively cause your strength to explode. A sample of a Neuro-Set for the upper body would be a set of super-slow push-ups, a push-up hold at the bottom of the push-up for as long as possible, then a final set of explosive push-ups to failure.

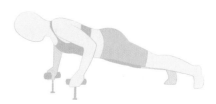

When Jon was seeking a way to intensify exercises like the push-up, he found a suitably primitive device that was up to the challenge: a nail welded to a piece of pipe. Attempting to stabilize the core while performing a push-up with this T-shaped tool proved incredibly challenging. He eventually turned the crude device into a durable, heavy industrial steel set of what he named Neuro-Grips, and he published a training manual to accompany the invention. Normally I can bang out over sixty push-ups without much trouble, but with Neuro-Grips I struggle to perform anything close to twenty reps and can develop a viselike grip in the process. The portability is a nice feature too.

Elastic Bands

In chapter 9, I talked about using elastic bands as my portable gym when I was a bodybuilder on a cycling trip in Italy. Although I've since upgraded to a fancier elastic band system called the X3 bar (which I'll talk about later in this chapter), I still often travel with elastic bands for on-the-go workouts, and they're a good budget-friendly alternative to a fancier system. Problem is, most folks do single-joint movements such as arm curls and side raises with the bands. I instead recommend full-body moves such as these:

- Squat to overhead press
- Side shuffles
- Push-ups
- Torso twists
- Rows

You can easily do those five exercises as a circuit—you'll find video demos at BoundlessBook.com/11.

Suspension Strap

When a pull-up bar is nowhere to be found, there's nothing like a suspension strap to create a pulling and grip-strengthening station. It's also a simple, portable method for balance training, lunges, push-ups, and a nearly unlimited number of challenging exercises. You'll usually find this, elastic bands, slider plates, and Kaatsu devices in the giant 60L backpack I travel with (I usually squeeze it into the overhead compartment on the plane and check zero gear). I prefer a relatively minimalist suspension strap without all the fancy new elastic and pullies in the newer models. The TRX is a good choice.

Slider Plates

Yet another travel-friendly option are slider plates. If you've ever noticed those small discs in the stretching area at the gym and wondered what the heck they are, you're not alone. I originally discovered these no-frills training tools when celebrity trainer Valerie Waters introduced me to her "Valslides" version nearly twelve years ago at a fitness conference. The concept behind these plates is incredibly simple: you place both feet or both hands on the sliders and slide them around in varying directions. They give you the same kind of core workout you'd experience if you were to wear socks on your feet and paper plates under your hands on a wooden floor. Here are a few of the best moves:

- **Knee tuck**: Start in high plank position with both feet on sliders. Pull your knees in to touch your chest. Focus on keeping your core tight, and don't hike your hips up too high. Push your feet back to extend into a high plank. Repeat.

- **Mountain climber**: Start in high plank position with both feet on sliders. Slide your right knee forward to your chest. Push your knee back to return to high plank. Repeat with your left knee.

- **Skater**: Stand with both feet on sliders. Slide your left foot behind your right as far as possible while bending your right leg and touching the fingertips of your right hand to the floor. Pull your left foot back as you return to standing position. Repeat on the other side.

- **Reaching reverse lunge**: Start in a seated position with your knees bent, palms on the ground with fingertips pointing forward, and both feet on sliders. Lift your hips until your knees are at a ninety-degree angle, your arms are straight, and your hips are level, like a tabletop. From here, flex your right ankle so only your right heel rests on the slider. Send your right foot forward, engaging your glutes and hamstrings, then pull back to tabletop. Lower your right foot and flex your left ankle, then send your left foot forward and pull back to tabletop. Repeat.

- **Alligator walks**: Get into a push-up position with a slider under each foot. Walk your hands across the room while keeping your stomach and back tight. For an added challenge, to further strengthen your core, you can do this move with a 25-, 35- or 45-pound weight plate tucked under your toes.

The slider models I like are the original Valslides, the SKLZ Slidez, and Gliding Discs.

Rings

There are a set of gymnastics rings hanging above our family's backyard patio, in the gym, and even above the cold pool (there's nothing quite like a set of ring muscle-ups followed by a drop into ice-cold water). The unique nature of gymnastic rings and the exercises that can be performed with them provide benefits far beyond those of a pull-up bar.

The primary benefit of rings, in addition to their low space requirement and portability, is their inherent instability. Because they independently swing from long straps, the rings move at the slightest touch, forcing you to concentrate every second that you are holding them to keep from swaying and resulting in the significant use of core and stabilizing muscles. Moving your body around rings in a variety of positions requires a surprising amount of upper-body strength and control. Just take a look at the average gymnast's rippling shoulders and biceps to see what I mean.

I recommend using wooden rings. Plastic and metal rings are far more slippery and more difficult to grip properly. The added expense of wood is worth it if you plan on training with the rings for a long time. Both Onnit and Rogue have good models. To get started, simply secure the straps over a bar, through mounted hooks, or from playground monkey bars, and you're set. Once you have your rings, head over to the website gmb.io for some excellent ring-training instructions and a host of gymnastics and functional bodyweight ring exercises.

Hex Bar

Dead lifts and squats are two of the best movements to utilize in a workout routine, primarily because of the significant amount of functional athleticism they produce, as well as the significant hormonal response and neuromuscular response they produce, especially compared to single-joint exercises such as a biceps curl or triceps extension, and even compared to multijoint exercises such as an overhead press, bench press, or lunge. However, both conventional squats and dead lifts performed with a standard barbell are associated with increased risk of back and knee injuries. Enter the hex bar.

Hex bars are modified barbells with open centers that allow you to stand in the middle of the bar while holding handles on each side of the bar. They allow people with back pain or limited range of motion to get all the benefits of a dead lift or squat in a far safer manner. Research has even shown that a hex bar dead lift is not only safer than a standard barbell dead lift, but it's even more effective at building maximum power! I can use my hex bar to lift far more weight with far less risk than with a barbell, and for anyone who wants to maintain or build strength, especially with age, I consider this apparatus to be a crucial addition to a home or garage gym setup.

Blood Flow Restriction (BFR) Straps

In chapter 9, I filled you in on these straps, which are sometimes referred to as Kaatsu training straps, although a true Kaatsu training device is actually a sensor-monitored pneumatic air band that allows a user to set a very precise pressure, whereas a BFR strap is simply a glorified tourniquet. However, the latter are far less expensive and can be faster to put on and use. Both Kaatsu device and BFR bands can be combined with most of the training tools in this chapter and are particularly effective when used with suspension straps, kettlebells, any form of isometric training, and all the cardio machines, such as the rower and the Assault AirBike (just try a Tabata set with BFR straps on your arms and legs).

Underwater Audio Player

If you're anything like me, you can sometimes get a bit bored during a five-minute cold shower, an hour-long paddleboard session, or a lap-swimming workout at the pool—or at least feel as though the experience could be enhanced with a good podcast, audiobook, or music set. Problem is, if you simply carry your phone in a waterproof case, you (a) run a pretty high risk of losing or damaging your phone and (b) are distracted or tempted by the fact that your phone is there should you want to check Facebook or shoot off a quick text message as you rest between swim repeats or wait on your surfboard for the next set. Enter my own personal minimalist, no-WiFi, no-Bluetooth solution: a waterproof underwater audio player, much like the old-school iPod Shuffles that Apple used to make. There are thousands of refurbished waterproofed Shuffles scattered across the internet, and several generic options too. I've listed a few of my favorite options on BoundlessBook.com/11.

THE UPGRADES

Let's move on to more complex or less well-known pieces of exercise equipment that can be added to those listed above to create the ultimate studio or home gym for molding your body. Admittedly, these are slightly spendier upgrades, but they will allow you to get even more out of your training. In a world of "as-seen-on-TV" exercise contraptions, these are the solutions that—of the hundreds I have tried over the past decades—will give you the best bang for your buck during your workout.

Keg

In his book *The Encyclopedia of Underground Strength and Conditioning*, my friend and strength-training coach Zach Even-Esh includes workouts that feature keg carries, keg lifts, keg tosses, and all manner of exercises using an apparatus you're probably more accustomed to drinking beer from. Most breweries, bars, and pubs will cut you a fantastic deal on an empty keg or give you one for free. Simply fill it one-quarter to three-quarters full of water and prepare for one of the best core and full-body workouts you'll ever experience.

Tire

In his book, Zach also teaches tire flips, sledgehammer slams against a tire, tire sled drags, and other brutal workouts that pair perfectly with a keg and sandbag (see below) for the ultimate garage, outdoor, or backyard workout. If you pull a pickup truck around to the back of most tire stores, they'll hook you up with an old, worn tractor tire for free (I recommend calling first to see if they have any available). I own one large tractor tire, a couple of medium-size tires, and even a few smaller ones for my kids and wife.

Sandbag

I made my sandbag in about thirty minutes by purchasing a couple of military duffel bags on Amazon, putting pea gravel into plastic contractor bags, and putting the gravel-filled plastic bags into the duffel bags. (You'll find detailed DIY sandbag instructions on BoundlessBook.com/11, but it's easier to just buy a sandbag from a website such as Rogue Fitness, then fill it with sand or small gravel rocks when it arrives.) In addition to my homemade version, I own two types of sandbags: one with handles that's designed for the same type of exercises you'd do with a barbell, such as cleans or clean and jerks, and a "pancake-style" sandbag more similar to what you'd find in a Spartan Race, which works for exercises such as dead lifts, farmer's walks, throws and tosses, sit-ups, and slams.

Yoga Trapeze

Everyone who comes to my house raises a curious eyebrow when they walk in the front door to see, hanging directly beside the dining room table from the upstairs railing, a bright-purple parachute-like device: a yoga trapeze. Those brave enough to actually attempt hanging from or playing with this device immediately want to own one. The trapeze operates on the concepts of (1) traction and (2) inversion.

Traction refers to any treatment or technique that pulls or lengthens the spine or other joints. Take the spine, for example. A healthy spine has full, firm, and resilient disk tissues that allow for complete range of motion. But after sitting all day in an office or car or after exercising and rotating the spine—combined with years of bad posture, improper footwear, and poorly designed chairs—these disks can bulge, herniate, thin, and become compressed. Your lumbar spine is particularly susceptible; the L4 and L5 vertebrae, at the lower back, are commonly affected trouble areas that can cause radiated pain along the entire spine, as low down as the sacroiliac joint and as high up as the cervical spine and neck.

Inverted positions, such as those assumed in yoga or while hanging upside down from gravity boots or an inversion table, not only provide this traction but also alter the blood flow and the flow of cerebrospinal fluid and can increase capillarization to the brain. Inversion is also a fantastic recovery technique, especially for runners and cyclists.

A yoga trapeze allows for simultaneous inversion and traction and is made from the same material as a parachute. The seams are quad-stitched and rock solid, the hooks are pure steel, and there's no chance that while hanging upside down anything is going to break (unless you happen to weigh over 600 pounds). You can hang a trapeze in a doorway or outside from a beam, bar, or swing set. It is easy to learn how to use, and I personally hang from mine every day for two to five minutes, usually during a quick break from work and to drain my legs after standing at my standing desk for long periods of time. It also works well after you've been on a long road trip or period of airline travel.

Inversion Table

Chapter 12 will teach what you need to know about inversion tables—long, flat tables that can rotate backwards to put your entire body in an upside-down position. Though I'm now a bigger fan of a yoga trapeze, an inversion table can be even easier to use, especially for anyone who can't hoist their body into a yoga trapeze (or strap on a pair of gravity boots). Teeter makes good inversion tables that also include special plugs that allow you to do trigger-point therapy on your low back while hanging.

Rebounder

A recent study conducted by the American Council on Exercise (ACE) showed that, when it comes to heart rate and oxygen expenditure, bouncing on a mini trampoline for less than twenty minutes a day is just as good for you as running, and participants reported that it made them feel better and was a lot more fun than actually running.

In the study, researchers gave a group of twenty-four participants a mini-trampoline workout in the form of a nineteen-minute trampoline exercise video (the video is available online at BenGreenfieldFitness.com/JumpSportWorkout). They then measured the jumpers' heart rates and oxygen expenditure at every minute.

They found that trampolining is a "moderate-to-vigorous intensity" exercise that produces the same physiological benefits as running at six miles per hour, cycling, or playing football, basketball, or ultimate frisbee. But when the participants were asked to rate how they felt during the trampoline workout, they reported that the workout felt far easier than it should have based on their cardiovascular response and calorie burn.

This isn't actually groundbreaking news. Trampoline-based exercise, also known as "rebounding," has quite a colorful history as both a recreational sport and an exercise modality. For example, during World War II, trampolines were used to help increase pilots' spatial awareness and balance abilities. NASA has studied trampoline training for astronauts and found it to be just as effective as running, with no significant differences in maximal heart rate, maximal oxygen uptake, or energy expenditure.

For these reasons, I'm a fan of having a mini trampoline tucked away somewhere in the home or office. You'll find that when you feel like doing absolutely nothing at all, and definitely don't feel like exercising, just two minutes of jumping on a trampoline can give you a burst of energy, and it's a wonderful tool to have on hand for a recovery day too. You don't just have to "bounce." You can do jumping jacks, high-knee running, squats, planks, and plenty more. The best rebounder models are made by JumpSport.

Plyometric Boxes or Bench

Single-leg and double-leg jumping and fast, explosive stepping on a raised surface are efficient ways to create or maintain high-quality muscle fibers and to also boost testosterone. If you're short on space, simply get a bench that can double as a surface for activities such as chest presses or dumbbell rows. If space permits, I recommend having a few plyometric boxes of varying heights. Rogue Fitness and Titan Fitness have good models.

Barbell Rack

A good barbell rack will include an Olympic-style weight-lifting bar, a pull-up bar, plenty of plates (preferably rubber), and sturdy extensions to rack a lift before and after a set. Rogue Fitness has excellent options, and there are several racks that have a small footprint and will even fold up against the wall to take up less space, such as the PRx Performance, originally featured on *Shark Tank*.

Electrical Muscle Stimulator

Flip to chapters 9 and 12 to learn more about electrical muscle stimulation (EMS). I personally own the Compex (a good portable solution for full-body training), a Marc Pro (a good portable solution for recovery, soreness, and injuries) and a NeuFit (not very portable but extremely powerful for full-body training).

X3 Bar

In 2015, my friend John Jaquish authored a research protocol for a London-based hospital to perform a study on human performance and bone. In that study, it was found that individuals could create tremendous forces through the body when exercising using a form of variable resistance, in which a form of training called "isokinetic training" is used to push back against your body just as hard as you push against it. Other studies have shown that this same type of variable resistance training creates muscle gains three times faster than conventional weight training, with double to triple the gains in one-rep max and triple the gains in average power. Variable resistance has also been shown to produce greater anabolic hormone responses and a higher increase in serum testosterone and growth hormone than conventional weight lifting.

Jaquish designed the X3 Bar for isokinetic, variable resistance training, and while using an elastic band–based prototype, he gained 30 pounds of muscle while simultaneously losing body fat. With a series of elastic bands at varying resistances, a small portable bar that simulates an Olympic weight-training bar, and a rugged footplate to stabilize the elastic band, the X3 Bar replicates the same style of training used in these studies, in a small, portable workout system. It allows you to perform any exercise at over 500 pounds of force, without the elastic bands twisting your ankles or applying excessive torsion to your wrists. This system can be used for portable training, low-impact training, or heavy weight lifting without the weights. (For a discount code, visit BoundlessBook.com/11.)

Rowing Machine

Research has shown that the rowing machine is one of best tools in existence for burning calories. A water- or fan-based rowing machine also provides upper-body and lower-body utilization, grip strengthening, and a low-impact training environment, and it can be used for long cardiovascular endurance workouts or high-intensity intervals. I'll often use a 500-meter row to warm up or cool down, or I'll include it throughout a strength-training workout to keep my heart rate boosted during the session. It's also a handy fitness option if you have any ankle, knee, or shoulder injuries that restrict your range of motion. I recommend the Concept2 model.

VersaClimber

While using a VersaClimber is a growing fitness trend now adopted by athlete celebrities such as LeBron James and Peyton Manning, the machine itself is decades old. The first VersaClimber was built by a mechanical engineer in 1981, but as fitness fads came and went over the years, the VersaClimber was mostly forgotten—until recently, when personal trainers and strength coaches started to recognize its extreme efficiency as a training tool.

The seven-foot-tall VersaClimber mimics the natural motion of climbing and consists of a vertical rail with pedals and handles. To use it, you get into an upright position by inserting your feet into the foot straps on the pedals and grabbing the handles. From there, you can adjust handle height, stroke length, and resistance. The longer the stroke length and range of motion you cover with each climbing step, the greater the muscle recruitment, making this a cardiovascular version of variable resistance training. A higher resistance setting allows for a slower-paced strength-building workout, while minimal resistance makes it more cardio focused.

Exercising on the VersaClimber requires a motion of "alternating reciprocal movement," which means when you move one arm up or down, the opposite knee does the same. Performing this motion in an upright position forces your entire body to work at once. Since it's manually powered, you can control your own pace with your movements and go as fast or as slow as you want with little impact. Although it's a big machine, it has a relatively small footprint because it can be tightly stacked against the wall of a gym or garage.

Incline Treadmill

Most treadmills allow for a maximum incline of 15 percent. But an incline treadmill, first introduced to me by famed obstacle course racer Matt Novakovich and his coach, Yancy Culp, allows you to set a maximum incline of 40 percent. This means that you can simulate hiking up just about the steepest mountain you'd ever find, making it a fantastic tool for training uphill without needing to expose your ankles, knees, and hips to the rigors of running back downhill, which can be tough on the joints. Walking at speeds as low as 2.0 mph on an incline of 40 percent can metabolically feel as though you're sprinting on a track. If you're like Matt, you can keep a sandbag, weighted vest, or weighted backpack next to the treadmill for an added challenge. I recommend the NordicTrack model and use it frequently whenever I'm training for a big hike, hunt, or mountainous obstacle race.

TrueForm Treadmill

The TrueForm isn't a treadmill in the traditional sense because there's no motor. Instead, the belt is driven by your own power and curves upward at either end, so that you accelerate when you're closer to the front and decelerate when you back up. On a normal treadmill, the motorized belt cuts out some of your workload by assisting your leg turnover and decreasing the ground reaction forces that would normally require the use of more leg musculature. But the only way to walk or run on a TrueForm is to use your legs to power the belt.

As the name implies, the shape of the treadmill forces you to be true to form. Your core must work harder to stabilize your body on an unstable belt, requiring a strong upright posture, a high cadence without an overstriding heel-strike, and a slight forward lean to maintain your center of gravity for forward momentum. The handrails are lower than on the average treadmill, giving your arms more freedom to pump and assist you. This causes you to burn up to 44 percent more calories compared to walking or running on a regular treadmill.

Currently I use a modified TrueForm with the front dashboard removed as the treadmill for my standing desk. The lack of a motor means it is low in dirty electricity, so I'm not subjected to electrical pollution during a day of work, and unlike other manual treadmills, the speed of the TrueForm allows me to alternate between walking, jogging, or sprinting whenever I want, without pushing any buttons.

Assault AirBike

An upgraded version of the old-school fan bike, with handles for pumping with the arms and pedals for pumping with the legs, an Assault AirBike is a low-impact way to quickly get your heart rate high. The newer models have a built-in computer dashboard that allows you to select, say, a Tabata set (or program in any other interval time and recovery time you desire), and the bike will then beep every time you are to switch from twenty seconds hard to ten seconds easy. My Assault AirBike is an indispensable tool for maintaining cardiovascular endurance even when my body is too beat up to go for a run or do any type of impact training.

Stand-Up Desk

Why the heck would I include a desk as a piece of exercise equipment? Frankly, a standing desk, especially one that you can keep a treadmill or bicycle in front of, allows you to engage in low-level physical activity throughout the day and can make any other workouts you do much shorter (or even optional if your goal is health and not performance). Because treadmills and stand-up desk motors can both produce larger amounts of electrical pollution (more on that in chapter 20), I recommend pairing a manual treadmill or bicycle with a hand-crank or non-motorized stand-up desk that allows you to go from seated to standing with just a few quick cranks. Both LifeSpan and Woodway make a good manual treadmill, but as noted above, I use a modified TrueForm treadmill (with the front dashboard removed). For a stand-up desk, look into models by Varidesk, RebelDesk, Lokus, Human Scale, and Focal Upright. For a done-for-you package, TrekDesk makes a treadmill-and-standing-desk combo. Throw in a few challenging surfaces to stand on, such as a Topo mat, a Kybun mat, or a FluidStance, and you can keep your body in excellent shape during a basic day of desk work.

THE GUILTY PLEASURES

If you like to own nice things and love the concept of better living through science, these fancier, more expensive add-ons will allow you to create the ultimate body-upgrading environment.

Vibration Trainer

In the corner of my living room is a slick black vibration platform called a Power Plate, which I occasionally use for moving lymph in the morning (as an alternative to rebounding), for bodyweight workouts and isometric squat and push-up holds, as a preworkout warm-up, and even as a way to induce a morning bowel movement when I need help "moving things along."

Most vibration platforms are either oscillating or tri-planar. Oscillating platforms have a fulcrum in the center, and the platform rises on one end and lowers on the other. This seesaw motion mimics the motion of walking. Tri-planar platforms rise up and down continuously, imitating the motion of performing tiny jumps over and over again. Tri-planar platforms have a smaller range of motion than oscillating platforms, operate at higher speeds, and are pricier because they are larger and heavier, but they are also more effective at vibrating the entire body rapidly.

A vibration trainer's intensity varies depending on the frequency of vibration, which is measured by the number of oscillations per second expressed in Hertz (Hz). Most research regarding whole-body vibration training has used frequencies between 25 and 40 Hz, so look for a model that can operate at least within this range (most good tri-planar vibration trainers have a frequency between 15 and 60 Hz, while cheaper models operate within a limited frequency range, such as 15 to 30 Hz or 30 to 50 Hz). I recommend the Power Plate, which is a tri-planar platform with a wide frequency range.

Vasper

The Vasper is a fancy training device that can be used for just twenty-one minutes three times per week as a form of high-intensity cardio training. It includes features such as ice sleeves that are wrapped around all your appendages prior to and during training, grounded pads on the pedals that you place your bare feet on to get a grounding effect, and pressurized cuffs to increase blood pressure in arms and legs (similar to Kaatsu training), all in a full-body elliptical-style workout.

Compression on the arm and leg muscles while exercising at a low intensity has been shown to create the physiological effect of high-intensity exercise, even if your intensity isn't quite as high, and also safely compresses the muscle to quickly build up lactic acid, mimicking the physiology of an intense workout that would typically require more extensive time and effort. This high lactic-acid buildup triggers a systemic recovery response, including the natural release of anabolic hormones such as growth hormone and testosterone.

As your body temperature increases while training, blood vessels near the surface of the skin dilate, increasing blood flow to the skin and leaving less blood and oxygen available for the muscles. When there is not enough blood to remove lactic acid from the muscles, physiological fatigue begins to set in. Remaining cool during exercise allows blood oxygen levels to remain high throughout the body, which makes exercising even at higher intensities much more efficient and pleasant. The ice-cold water that circulates through the Vasper's compression sleeves allows for this cooling effect to occur during the exercise session.

Each Vasper protocol that is already built into the software that accompanies the device is a twenty-one-minute interval training session, delivered on a tablet that is fully integrated with the recumbent bicycle-size machine. Each section of the interval training protocol is customizable in duration, intensity, resistance, and speed, and the pressure and cooling can also be modified for ability, comfort level, and performance. There are even heart rate monitors with graphs of power output displayed on the screens to track performance. As you can imagine, the Vasper isn't cheap (around $45,000), but for busy folks—including well-known health, longevity, business, and fitness gurus, like Tony Robbins and Peter Diamandis; research institutions like NASA, Stanford's Sports Medicine Center, and UCSF; and pro teams like the San Jose Sharks and Texas Rangers—this is the ultimate solution to interval training with science.

ARX

Single-set-to-failure training and super-slow training are both part of the training strategies outlined in chapters 10 and 12, and the ARX is a mash-up of both that can be used for extreme strength training or for rehab. In the same way that Vasper "biohacks" cardiovascular interval training, ARX technology "biohacks" strength training with a computer-controlled motorized resistance that is capable of matching any force you produce, giving you a perfect rep with every rep.

Unlike a traditional weight-training machine that requires you to adjust the weight with pins or plates, there is no need to set the resistance while using ARX. Instead, the machine applies opposing resistance in direct proportion to what you are producing at each moment in time throughout an entire rep. The entire effort for that one single set to failure is then measured and displayed by the software in real time.

The ARX Omni allows for over a dozen motions, including the squat, dead lift, pull-down, row, overhead press, and chest press, while the smaller Alpha allows for leg press, chest press, row, calf raise, and torso extension and flexion.

Using the ARX works for any of the super-slow workouts in this book but amplifies their benefits to an entirely new level, especially from an eccentric training standpoint (the strategy outlined by Art De Vany in chapter 9). Like the Vasper, this is one of the spendier devices in this section, but it can be used as little as once per week with significant results for building strength, bone density, and muscle.

PeakFitPro

Because muscle must be overloaded with adequate time under tension, preferably to failure, for a significant adaptive response to occur, anything short of forcing your muscle to work as hard or harder than your previous workout rarely results in an increase in size or strength. In fact, anything less is usually just proof that you are not yet recovered from your last workout, which is why I define workout recovery as the ability to meet or exceed what you were able to do in your last workout. If you don't show up stronger than your previous workout, then what is the point of the new workout? This, along with the ability to produce enormous amounts of force without much joint wear and tear, is why isometric exercises done at a maximal intensity can produce significant gains. Isometric training simply involves pushing against an immovable object while producing large amounts of force, without your joints actually moving. Here's the best example: go to a sturdy wall in your house and use your arms to try to push through it. This should feel like the hardest push-up you've ever attempted in your life because the wall simply won't move.

The PeakFitPro is a static contraction, isometric training machine that allows for up to 5,000 pounds of force (like lifting almost two Toyota Corollas) to be produced during exercises like the squat, dead lift, chest press, pull-down, overhead press, or over thirty additional exercises. It also has a Bluetooth-enabled connection to a phone app to show you if you truly have met or exceeded what you were able to perform in a previous workout.

With traditional weight lifting, if you do a set of ten repetitions before you reach failure, the first nine reps are practically just a warm-up for the last rep, where the real muscle stimulation happens. And those first nine reps can potentially make you weaker for the tenth. With an isometric training machine like this, you can do that last rep first. You simply do one rep of all-out effort for five to ten seconds, creating an immediate and significant muscle-adaptation response. Each exercise is performed at the strongest part of your range of motion, creating maximum stimulation. This position is also the position that is safest for the muscle and joint, so it markedly reduces the chances of injury.

Because this machine is motionless, it's safer than most other exercise machines or free-weight devices—nothing to break or fall or snap or drop. Because you're in the "strong zone" of your range, it's safer for your body, and there are no clanging weights, spinning wheels, fans, or other noisemakers. If you've seen videos of me on the internet struggling against what appears to be an immovable bar attached to a force plate, then I was likely on the PeakFitPro in my basement. This, like many of the other devices in this section, is spendy at $6,495, but you'll find a discount code on BoundlessBook.com/11.

LiveO2

The LiveO2 sits in my office next to a stationary bike and allows me to complete my twice-weekly exercise with oxygen therapy (EWOT) session in just fifteen minutes by simply stepping away from my desk for a quick pedaling session. EWOT is a method of breathing higher levels of oxygen during exercise in order to increase the amount of oxygen in your blood plasma.

Exercise with oxygen was pioneered in the 1960s by a German researcher named Manfred von Ardenne. He wrote a book called *Oxygen Multistep Therapy* that is an extremely thorough reference on oxygen therapy should you want to take a deeper dive.

In the book, von Ardenne describes how stress triggers inflammation—and how inflammation compromises health, a concept I've addressed in previous chapters. He described how plasma hypoxia (low levels of oxygen in the fluid that carries red blood cells) triggers inflammation in the endothelial tissues, which then sets up restriction to blood flow in capillaries.

But, more importantly, he developed a method to quickly and durably fix this problem of hypoxia, specifically by elevating plasma concentrations, increasing oxygen levels to lower capillary inflammation, and restoring circulation.

A substantial body of research has since demonstrated that the administration of oxygen while exercising promotes an expansion of constricted capillaries, which enhances blood perfusion of congested capillary beds. The squamous cells making up the endothelium of capillaries tend to swell when deprived of oxygen, creating a vicious cycle, as this swelling prevents further oxygenation.

Exercise in the presence of high amounts of oxygen opens the arterioles (branches of an artery leading into capillaries), and the oxygenated blood can then reduce any swelling in the capillary endothelium. This creates a positive cycle of lower inflammation and better oxygenation. Repeated administration of EWOT can lead to a lasting reduction of endothelial swelling and an increase in peripheral circulation. It's good for improving performance, strengthening inspiratory muscles, ameliorating asthma, accelerating wound healing, enhancing immune function, decreasing incidence of migraines, and increasing mitochondrial density, among other positive benefits.

The LiveO2 lets you upgrade the effects of EWOT by, with the flip of a switch during your exercise session, alternating back and forth between hypoxia and hyperoxia (this is called "adaptive contrast"). Most EWOT systems take at least one nine-hour workout to deliver therapeutic oxygenation, but with adaptive contrast, you can deliver oxygen flow rates that meet or exceed the levels required and reach a therapeutic result in just fifteen minutes. With adaptive contrast, it is as if you are instantly switching between sea level and elevations of ten thousand feet. These switches make your heart and lungs work harder, so the oxygen does a lot more. I've personally found the results to be enhanced with any blood dilating or blood building supplement, particularly beetroot, cordyceps, echinacea, beta-alanine, and niacin.

Pulse Centers Pulse XL Pro PEMF Table

Chapters 6 and 12 have everything you need to know about pulsed electromagnetic field therapy, a form of "exercise for your cells." I am writing this very chapter while seated on a rocking chair version of the Pulse Centers Pulse XL Pro unit. There is no better way to deliver high-intensity PEMF to your entire body all at once. Originally used by the horse-racing industry, they are now available to consumers.

Infrared Sauna

I'll talk in more detail about infrared saunas in chapter 12. They essentially use light to create heat, which means they can heat your body directly without significantly warming the air around you, and the light waves from the infrared sauna penetrate deep (two to six inches) into your body for a heating effect that allows more activation of your sweat glands than a dry sauna. So an infrared sauna doesn't feel as hot as a dry sauna, but you sweat as much or more.

For years, many folks in the alternative health community have sworn by infrared heat lamps as a source of far-infrared heat, but these lamps can be cumbersome, they can get extremely hot to the touch, and they can be difficult to maintain at a constant temperature.

The temperature inside a typical infrared sauna is adjustable and averages about 100 to 140 degrees Fahrenheit, depending on how long you warm the sauna up before getting in.

Several studies have investigated the use infrared saunas in the treatment of chronic health problems, such as high blood pressure, congestive heart failure, and rheumatoid arthritis, and these studies have indeed found some evidence of benefit. For athletes using a sauna postexercise for thirty minutes, the blood-building benefits can be as powerful as performance-enhancing drugs.

No adverse effects have ever been reported with infrared saunas, and I used infrared therapy with a heating mat called a Biomat for two years before switching to an infrared sauna, without any ill effects.

Choose your sauna carefully. For most people, it's not the slightly lower levels of heat that tend to be the problem with an infrared sauna. Instead, it's the fact that most infrared saunas are concentrated hothouses chock-full of electromagnetic fields, turning what is supposed to be a detoxification and longevity-enhancing experience into the equivalent of hanging out in a microwave or inside a giant WiFi router, leaving you with cell damage, brain fog, and inflammation. In chapter 20, you'll learn plenty more about EMFs and how to mitigate their damage, but for now, the takeaway message is that it can be difficult for a sauna manufacturer to generate infrared light without also generating EMF.

So for my own personal infrared sauna, I chose a model that has a type of heater called a True Wave II, which contains a carbon-based infrared heater with virtually no EMF. It's made by a company called Clearlight using a manufacturing process that allows them to cancel out EMF to levels that are nearly undetectable. All the heaters inside a Clearlight sauna are tested to ensure low and safe levels of EMF, which is uncommon in the sauna industry.

Since I like to move around, exercise, do Bikram yoga, and even occasionally drag an exercise bike or a kettlebell into my sauna, I chose the Sanctuary Y model, which is a combination of a personal hot yoga room and an infrared sauna. You can leave in the two thirty-five-inch benches and have a state-of-the-art full-spectrum infrared sauna for lounging and reading, or you can remove the benches and have your own private hot yoga room with a built-in heated yoga mat floor. (You'll find discount codes at BoundlessBook.com/11.)

THE LAST WORD

So let's say you're overwhelmed by the number of tools in this chapter, but you still want to build the ultimate home gym that incorporates a few key biohacks or upgraded pieces of exercise technology. In other words, you want the minimal effective dose and the 80/20 of everything you've just discovered. The following list is a perfect example of what an ultimate biohacker's gym or home health space would look like if it was designed to be as simple as possible. If you were to walk into my home gym, you would find a setup similar to this:

- Yoga mat
- Bench
- Foam roller and massage ball
- Kettlebells
- A couple of heavy sets of dumbbells
- Weighted vest
- Resistance band or X3 Bar
- Hex bar
- Squat rack with pull-up bar

- Stability ball
- Medicine ball
- Battle rope
- Assault AirBike (or a VersaClimber, or a rowing machine, or a TrueForm Treadmill, or, if budget permits, all four)
- Electrical muscle stimulator (optional)
- Vibration platform (optional)
- Large infrared sauna (optional)

If you wandered out into my garage and backyard, you'd find the icing on the cake: a keg half filled with water, a large tire for flipping, and a pile of sandbags. With this setup, you can do just about any workout on the face of the planet and will have enough exercise variety to last a lifetime. Finally, should you not want to break the budget, rest assured that you can find many of these items on Craigslist or eBay, and you'll find plenty of discount codes on BoundlessBook.com/11.

The fact is, by blending ancestral living with modern technology, you can not only make exercising and molding the body that you desire incredibly fun, but you can also engage in better living through science, using everything that modern science has taught us about efficient exercise to shortcut your way to muscle gain and fat loss and save hours for boundless energy in the process.

You now know how to design the ultimate combination of both simple and complex fitness tools to biohack the body and stay fit in a postindustrial era of airline travel, long car trips, and sedentary, office-based lifestyles.

ONE THING YOU CAN DO THIS WEEK

This week, begin to build your own travel exercise kit. Find some elastic tubing or elastic bands with a handle, a portable foam roller, a jump rope, and a suspension trainer similar to a TRX. Boom. It's that easy. You're now equipped to exercise anytime, anywhere—even in a quiet little seaside town.

For citations for all the research studies mentioned in this chapter and a deeper dive into the topics of this chapter—including links to podcasts, blog posts, recommended tools and supplements, and much more—visit BoundlessBook.com/11.

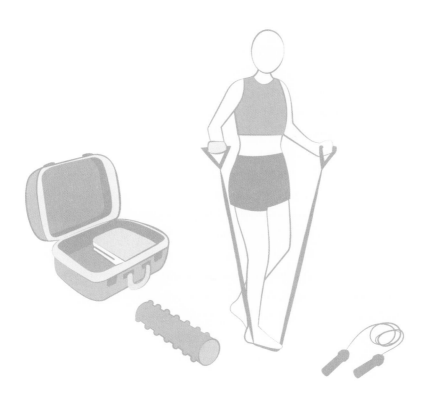

WOLVERINE

A COMPLETE TOOLBOX FOR RECOVERING WITH LIGHTNING SPEED

I was recently splayed out on the bed in a hotel room in Seattle, my entire body throbbing and aching from having just surged across the finish line of a Spartan Super obstacle race—9.8 miles of stumbling through Pacific Northwest rainforest while hoisting sandbags, clambering over logs and rocks, swinging from monkey bars, hauling weighted buckets, crawling through barbed wire, and high-stepping through mud and bogs.

On the hotel room TV was the first movie I'd watched in a long time: *Logan*, from the Marvel Comics X-Men series—which, of course, features the fastest-recovering superhero on the face of the planet. While you certainly can't expect to get punched ten times in the face by a muscle-bound cyborg and have your broken and smashed cheekbones and nose regenerate magically, you certainly can bounce back from many workouts, races, injuries, and surgeries far faster than modern sports medicine and orthopedics would have you believe.

I'll admit it. I used to be pretty old-school when it came to recovery: a postworkout shake, maybe a little stretching or time with the foam roller, and (if things got really bad) an ice massage or a cold bath. Not that there's anything wrong with simplicity. After all, it is easy to get so carried away with new gadgets, toys, and recovery tools that you forget to take time to enjoy a glass of wine while soaking in the sunset at the end of the day.

But I remember when I shared an office with a sports medicine physician named P. Z. Pearce. All day long, marathoners, triathletes, cyclists, and weekend warriors came through the door complaining of aches, pains, and injuries that they had been fighting for weeks, months, and even years. With just a few of the recovery tips I am about to share with you, those folks could have easily saved themselves a lot of pain and frustration, not to mention boatloads of cash on doctor's visits and operations.

So I would be remiss if I didn't equip you with every technique I know to keep your body in pristine shape, especially if you are laying down some serious damage by being more than a weekend warrior.

In this chapter, I will give you the complete download of my favorite potent but often little-known recovery techniques, assembled into one mighty resource that will have you bouncing back from muscle and body damage just like Wolverine.

HOW—AND HOW FAST—DOES YOUR BODY RECOVER?

How fast should you recover from, say, a marathon? Research indicates that the muscle damage from running a marathon can last up to two weeks and that the absence of soreness is not a good indicator of muscular healing. In other words, just because you aren't sore anymore doesn't mean that you are fully healed. Post-marathon muscular soreness fades after a few days, but microscopic damage within the muscle cells lasts for at least a couple weeks.

How about an Ironman? Probably because the non-weight-bearing nature of cycling and swimming allows for faster healing, recovery from an Ironman is not much different than recovery from a marathon and ranges anywhere from eight to nineteen days, depending on the athlete.

A CrossFit Workout of the Day? It appears most folks need at least two to three days of recovery to bounce back from the immune system and nervous system damage that can occur from just one of these hard-core twenty-to-sixty-minute sessions (although, tragically, many Cross-Fitters do back-to-back sessions five to six days a week!). Using heart rate variability testing, I have found that some people bounce back in as little as a day while some take several days, so it can vary quite a bit from person to person.

A hike? Now we're getting more reasonable. It really only takes a day or so to bounce back from a multihour afternoon hike. But even a smattering of the recovery tactics you are about to discover can speed that up and allow you to, say, go for a hard run the day after a hike.

Sure, your body is already a finely tuned self-repairing machine. There are entire branches of medicine built around the fact that the human body has some impressive built-in repair mechanisms that modern medicine seems to have forgotten. You know, of course, that a cut on your finger can turn into a scab and then heal over completely, but all tissues contain similar regenerative processes, and every one of your body's cells and organs has its own regeneration cycle. Intestinal bacteria regenerate within several days, the intestinal wall within a couple weeks, and immune cells within four weeks. Even the liver possesses the capacity to regenerate—25 percent of a liver can fully regenerate within six months! The default state of the body is one of regeneration, and books such as *Bioregulatory Medicine* and the works of Dr. Rudolf Steiner, such as *The Healing Process*, are excellent deep-dive treatises on this concept.

But let's say you don't immediately need to regenerate a lobe of your liver, and you are more interested in bouncing back as fast as possible from a workout, adventure, or stressful day so that you can move on to your next task without feeling like you have bricks tied to your shoes or having a bout of dizziness every time you stand up. In this case, most human performance specialists define recovery as "the ability to meet or exceed performance in a particular activity."

This ability necessitates important physiological functions that can be sped up or enhanced using the strategies in this chapter, including:

- Repletion of creatine phosphate and ATP stores
- Rebuilding of muscle and liver glycogen
- Conversion of lactate into glycogen or removal of blood lactate
- Removal of carbon dioxide via reaction of CO_2 and H_2O to form carbonic acid for subsequent removal via exhalation
- Clearance of acetylcholine and other neurotransmitters from skeletal muscle
- Removal of calcium ions from areas surrounding muscle fibers

- Repayment of oxygen debt postexercise via respiration

- Downregulation of the sympathetic nervous system, blood pressure, heart rate, respiratory rate, and other acute responses to exercise or stress

- Restoration of enzymes that play a crucial role in metabolism, such as phosphofructokinase, a key enzyme in carbohydrate metabolism

Some of these functions, such as the replenishment of ATP and creatine or conversion of lactate into usable fuel, occur during exercise and are referred to as "immediate recovery"; they happen between strides while running or between reps in a set while weight training. Other functions, such as repayment of oxygen debt or removal of carbon dioxide, occur within minutes and are referred to as "short-term recovery": they happen between sets of a weight training session, for example. Full recovery, including restoration of enzymes and stored glycogen, removal of calcium ions, and a nervous system reset, requires more time. These functions occur in the hours and days between workouts or competitions.

Perhaps one of the most important aspects of recovery, and one that is often neglected among hard-charging high achievers, is central nervous system recovery. If you overtax your CNS, then your muscular performance suffers, even after musculoskeletal soreness has subsided. Critical recovery processes related to the CNS include the replenishment of neurotransmitters such as acetylcholine (crucial for CNS function during periods of acute stress) and the removal of chemicals such as ammonia (which is produced by skeletal muscle and is believed to play a role in modulating CNS fatigue).

Then there's the immune system. Exercise increases circulating neutrophil and monocyte counts and reduces circulating lymphocyte counts during recovery. This deployment of white blood cells is an integral part of the physiological stress response to exercise. Given the large changes in the distribution of immune cells among blood and peripheral tissues during and after exercise, it is important to support the restoration of white blood cell counts. Interestingly, of the many nutritional strategies and physical therapies that active individuals turn to for recovery, consuming adequate carbohydrates and getting a lot of deep sleep seem to be the best tactics for supporting immune system recovery.

You are about to discover a comprehensive list of tactics you can use to enhance the healing process, from restoring white and red blood cells to repairing muscle fibers to restoring hormones and neurotransmitters to refilling mineral stores to healing of tiny nerves and blood vessels. Many of these tactics may seem fringe or strange or even extreme, but they all work by a precise biological mechanism.

Take acupuncture, for example. For over five thousand years, Eastern medicine practitioners have used acupuncture to adjust the body's flow of energy (often referred to as chi) to improve health and eliminate disease. While Western medicine practitioners may not agree with traditional explanations of acupuncture's mechanism of action, they have finally come to recognize that acupuncture does indeed work for conditions like depression, chronic pain, allergies, and headaches. An acupuncture procedure involves inserting hair-thin needles into certain points along your meridian, the path through which your energy runs. Needling these points stimulates the body's natural healing mechanisms by (according to Western medicine practitioners) stimulating blood flow, the release of endorphins, and other physiological processes that temporarily relieve pain.

I confess that it may seem odd to include acupuncture as a recovery method, but as a coach and athlete, I have found the occasional acupuncture session to be incredibly useful for everything from healing nagging aches and pains to staving off or speeding up recovery from central nervous system fatigue to addressing full-blown "adrenal fatigue" (whose symptoms, you'll recall from chapter 3, are more likely due to inflammation or overtraining than adrenal dysfunction). You also don't have to duck down back alleys to get treatments in a dank back-alley massage parlor. You can find licensed, well-credentialed acupuncturists operating out of pristine medical clinics throughout the United States through the National Certification Commission for Acupuncture and Oriental Medicine (NCCAOM.org).

But acupuncture is just one example of the recovery methods you should have in your toolbox. Let's delve into twenty-five additional tactics for comic book–level recovery, shall we?

25 RECOVERY-ENHANCING TACTICS

Before we dive into the tactics below, please understand that I realize not everybody has full access to the types of healing strategies and biohacks I'm about to describe just sitting in their basement, as I do in my Batcave in the middle of the forest in Washington State. But it would be fantastic to see more progressively-minded practitioners incorporating these types of therapies and technologies into a traditional physical therapy or sports medicine practice so that they might be available for anybody who wants to heal from an injury or recover more quickly without medications or surgical interventions. For example, consider what organizations such as CognitiveFX and ReviveCenters have done for concussions and traumatic brain injury: they have formulated a multimodal approach that attacks a debilitating condition from multiple angles. Using the information in this chapter, you or your practitioner can do the same for your own injuries and recovery.

1. Stem Cell Therapy

I could probably devote an entire chapter to stem cells alone. Three years ago, *Men's Health* magazine convinced me to inject my penis with stem cells extracted from my back fat for an article on male sexual performance enhancement. After the article went viral, I wrote several follow-up pieces for my website and other publications, stories detailing some edgy procedures like self-administering mannitol (a sugar alcohol) and my stem cells into my bloodstream to enhance neural function (mannitol causes the blood-brain barrier to temporarily become more permeable and allow stem cells into the brain), getting my bone stem cells extracted from my hips and sent overseas to be kept in cold storage, and even undergoing a "full-body stem cell makeover."

The single most important cell for life is actually one type of stem cell: the single-cell fertilized egg, called a zygote, from which all our trillions of cells are formed. The zygote is known as a totipotent cell, which means that it can transform into every other kind of cell. The zygote divides into a cluster of multiple cells known as a blastocyst, which contains pluripotent stem cells—these can turn into almost every other kind of cell. These totipotent and pluripotent stem cells are all embryonic stem cells. The umbilical cord also has embryonic stem cells, but because these are from later stages of fetal development, they are multipotent, which means the types of cells they can develop into are limited.

The Full-Body Stem Cell Makeover

On May 14, 2018, I was completely sedated and underwent a full-body stem cell makeover at a medical clinic in Park City, Utah. The procedure, administered by Dr. Harry Adelson and Dr. Amy Killen, is exactly what it sounds like: the injection of stem cells into literally every joint in the body, along with a special signaling molecule called an "exosome" that carries cell-to-cell messages throughout your entire body.

Mesenchymal stem cells (MSCs) possess a broad range of healing abilities. They are directly responsible for healing damaged tissues after an injury: upon encountering damaged tissue, they release proteins that decrease inflammation, kill invading microbes, and trigger the growth of new connective tissue and blood vessels. In the event of severe damage or cell death, MSCs can turn themselves into healthy versions of damaged or destroyed cells and replace them. Combining them with exosomes "upgrades" MSCs with the ability to travel quickly and efficiently to the areas of the body where the stem cells are needed most, including the brain, joints, and other organs.

Here's how it works: A lab harvests MSCs from placenta. Then, using a process called culture expansion, they expand this stem cell population by hundreds of millions and then they place the cells in a "stressful" culture medium to trick them into thinking that their host is under duress. In preparation for lean times, the MSCs sprout vesicles filled with exosomes. These exosomes are, in fact, the active ingredient of stem cells. One of the reasons our stem cells grow old as we age is that they lose the ability to produce exosomes.

The lab then destroys the MSCs, discards the genetic material, and harvests only the exosomes. At this point, they have the active ingredient of placental stem cells, without the stem cells. They add these exosomes to a person's own stem cells, harvested from bone marrow or fat (or both). Because the membrane of exosomes is identical to the membrane of MSCs, your old stem cells absorb the exosomes into themselves, thereby functionally making them the stem cells of a younger person. This is how adding exosomes to your own stem cells effectively upgrades them.

With a needle nearly a foot long, Dr. Adelson harvested some of the bone marrow from the bones in my hips. My bone marrow was then passed through an ozone machine, which ozonates the bone marrow stem cells to create even more available cells. Then the stem cells were concentrated into bone marrow aspirate concentrate (BMAC), which was supplemented with a large volume of exosomes. Then every major musculoskeletal structure in my body was injected with BMAC and exosomes. This means my entire spine, from the base of my skull to my tailbone, and all major joints (shoulders, elbows, wrists, hands, hips, knees, ankles, feet) were filled to the brim with everything necessary to enhance healing for the rest of my life. Dr. Killen then stepped in and injected the skin of my face, neck, hands, and scalp, along with my penis, with a blend of platelet-rich plasma, exosomes, and stem cells for cosmetic and sexual enhancement.

How does this work? According to the stem cell theory of aging, your tissues age because your body's stem cell populations either fall or cease to function entirely. The full-body stem cell makeover is for people interested in proactively keeping this decline at bay and repopulating the entire musculoskeletal system with turbo-charged stem cells.

As you have probably guessed, the procedure is not inexpensive, but when it comes to recovery and body-upgrading therapies, especially in aging individuals, this one beats out the others in my experience. Old injuries melt away, new injuries heal faster, and the cosmetic and sexual effects are pretty handy too. In chapter 19, I will revisit stem cell therapy in far greater detail.

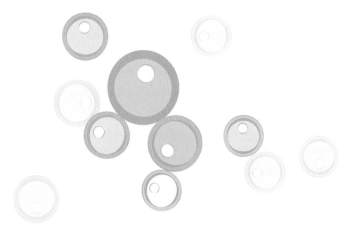

In addition to embryonic stem cells, there are also adult stem cells, which are found throughout the body. Adult stem cells, like umbilical cord stem cells, are multipotent. One kind of adult stem cell that is currently the focus of the majority of stem cell research is the mesenchymal stem cell (MSC), which can differentiate into osteoblasts (bone), chondrocytes (cartilage), and adipocytes (fat). Another important adult stem cell is the hematopoietic stem cell (HSC) which develops into all kinds of blood cells and can be found in bone marrow, peripheral blood, umbilical cords, and the lungs.

Physicians, researchers, and stem cell scientists are now changing the potency of many types of stem cells with different forms of culture expansion or by combining them with signaling molecules like exosomes and very small embryonic-like (VSEL) cells. The chart below gives a quick summary of the types of cells and their potency.

	TOTIPOTENT	PLURIPOTENT	MULTIPOTENT
Cell types capable of generating	Differentiate into any cell type	Differentiate into most cell types	Differentiate into a limited range of cell types
Found in	Early cells of fertilized egg	Inner mass cells of the blastocyst	Many adult tissues (fat, bone, etc.)
Research pros	Easy to isolate and grow	Easy to isolate and grow	Fewer ethical issues, less chance of immune rejection if taken from same patient
Research cons	Ethical issues	Ethical issues, possible tumor formation	Hard to isolate, limited differentiation, scarce

Source: Anna MacDonald, "Cell Potency: Totipotent vs Pluripotent vs Multipotent Stem Cells," Cell Science, Technology Networks, May 29, 2018, www.technologynetworks.com/cell-science/articles/cell-potency-totipotent-vs-pluripotent-vs-multipotent-stem-cells-303218.

Most of the ethical controversy surrounding stem cell research and therapy, especially in the US, surrounds the use of embryonic cells taken directly from fetuses. When a lab wants to harvest embryonic stem cells, scientists wait until the embryo is about three to five days old, when it is a blastocyst containing about a hundred cells, and then harvest the blastocyst and remove the stem cells. The stem cells are then cultured in petri dishes. Another way to harvest embryonic stem cells is via umbilical cord banking, although these cells are only multipotent.

Although adult stem cells are less potent than pluripotent cells, they can still be highly beneficial. For example, HSCs are found in red bone marrow and can differentiate into different blood cells. MSCs are also found in bone marrow and become bone, cartilage, fat, and connective tissue located in bone. Other tissues, like brain, skeletal muscle, skin, and liver, also contain MSCs. New research has indicated that multipotent adult stem cells may be transdifferentiated into other cell types as well. Differentiated adult cells like skin cells could be turned into powerful, body-repairing, embryonic-like stem cells that are capable of becoming almost any of the two hundred cell types in the human body.

Another rising branch of stem cell research focuses on the harvesting of stem cells from amniotic fluid, which is the protective fluid surrounding an unborn baby in the womb. The current protocol for harvesting amniotic fluid during C-section deliveries only adds about ninety seconds to the operation, is completely safe for both the mother and the child, and yields about a liter of amniotic fluid containing MSCs. Although I endorse and am a fan of home births and the avoidance of C-sections whenever possible, amniotic fluid can be an effective alternative to bone, fat, and umbilical cord blood as a source of stem cells.

Stem cell therapy is a powerful recovery method that has flown under the radar for quite some time, but it is now finally becoming mainstream. This is because stem cells' ability to transform into neurons, muscle cells, and several different types of connective tissue leads to rapid joint regeneration and even the reversal of frailty related to aging (much more on that in chapter 19).

In the United States, companies like the US Stem Cell Clinic in Weston, Florida (where I had my fat sucked out to concentrate and store my adipose-derived stem cells), Forever Labs in Berkeley, California (where I had my bone marrow removed to save for future longevity-enhancing injections), and Docere Clinics in Park City, Utah (where I underwent a full-body stem cell makeover) are on the cutting edge of developing injectable stem cell treatments to do everything from regrowing spinal cord cells to eradicating cartilage pain. Clinics such as the Institute of Regenerative Medicine and Orthopedics in Tampa, Florida, inject non-embryonic stem cells into injury sites to stimulate rapid healing or to permanently fix chronic aches and pains. Finally, physicians like Dr. Harry Adelson of Park City, Utah, Dr. Matt Cook of San Jose, California, and Dr. Halland Chen of New York City are now using advanced compounds, such as exosomes and VSELs, to simulate or upgrade the effects of bone- and fat-derived stem cells, often without the time and hassle of harvesting your own stem cells.

How to get started: Read chapter 19 thoroughly. Even one series of stem cell injections into a joint or throughout the body, or delivered intravenously, can have a profound impact on an entire lifetime of recovery, and if you are an active individual with a decent recovery budget, I highly recommend exploring this new frontier of bouncing back faster.

2. Cryotherapy

Cryotherapy, just one form of the broader category of cold thermogenesis, is the treatment of injuries or inflammation via exposure to cold temperatures. While cryotherapy can get extreme (whole-body cryotherapy chambers can plummet to –200 degrees Fahrenheit!), there are much simpler and less expensive ways to engage in cold exposure. I personally favor cold-water immersion because it is easier to do and also triggers the mammalian dive reflex (in which sensory receptors and cranial nerves stimulated by cold water produce a drop in heart rate and a rush of oxygen to the heart and brain). Cold-water immersion also provides hydrostatic pressure from the water, which can be therapeutic, and because of this, in my opinion, it ultimately beats out cryotherapy chambers (although, admittedly, any form of cold-water therapy does require one to get wet and redo hair and makeup).

I personally use some form of cryotherapy nearly every day: cold showers in the morning and evening, a daily dip in the cold pool behind my house. I also have a long history of many swims in frigid lakes, rivers, and seas, which I consider to be a muscular and nervous system reboot. The benefits of cryotherapy include an enhanced immune system, increased cell longevity, reduced levels of inflammatory molecules, and, of course, an incredible tolerance for running outdoors in the cold and performing snow angels in your underwear.

Cryotherapy stimulates the sympathetic branch of the autonomic nervous system by inducing a hormetic stress response. A hormetic stressor, you'll recall, is any light or mild stressor (like exercise) that stimulates a beneficial adaptive response, so you come out stronger than you were before. When you experience cold, the sympathetic nervous system (your "fight-or-flight" nervous system) kicks into gear to preserve your core body temperature. Blood vessels in your extremities constrict, restricting blood flow so that the temperature of your internal organs doesn't drop, your heart rate increases to pump blood where it needs to go, and your lungs breathe powerfully and deeply. The result is a boost to your sympathetically controlled cardiovascular system and an overall improved recovery process.

How to get started: There are many ways to get the benefits of cryotherapy. One way to maximize the effects of cold exposure and heat exposure is to use hot-cold contrast therapy, alternating exposure to hot and cold water or temperatures. Once a week, regardless of my training load or recovery status, I do this hot-cold contrast session: swim, tread water, or move in my AquaFitness pool, which I keep at 55 to 60 degrees Fahrenheit, for eight minutes; soak in my hot tub, which I keep at 104 degrees Fahrenheit, for two minutes; then repeat this cycle for a total of thirty minutes. There are a few ways you can simulate this session:

- take a five-minute shower in which you alternate between twenty seconds of cold water and ten seconds of hot water ten times through
- sit in a sauna for five to ten minutes, then jump into a cold shower for two minutes; repeating for twenty to thirty minutes total
- take a twenty-minute hot magnesium salt bath followed by a five-minute ice-cold shower

The simplest solution? Just take a quick one-to-two-minute cold shower at the beginning and end of each day.

3. Prolotherapy

Like stem cell therapy, prolotherapy is something to consider when you need to bring out the "big guns" because a joint or muscle injury won't go away. Think of prolotherapy as spot welding for an ache or pain. It involves the precise, nonsurgical injection of a natural irritant solution into areas where tendons and ligaments attach to bone and places where cartilage is worn or damaged. When a prolotherapy solution—which can be anything from hyperosmolar dextrose (basically glorified sugar water) to glycerin, lidocaine, or even cod liver oil extract—is injected, it creates a localized, controlled inflammatory response that stimulates the body's own repair mechanisms to heal the damaged tissue. If you have a chronically inflamed joint with built-up scar tissue, prolotherapy can be a good option to reinitiate inflammation and heal the injury for good.

A particularly powerful form of prolotherapy is the injection of platelet-rich plasma (PRP). Platelets, which are small cell fragments, are involved in halting blood flow, antimicrobial defense, cytokine secretion, and tissue-growth-factor production. Using PRP to treat ligament, tendon, and connective-tissue damage is like taking the little particles in your body that are responsible for repairing damaged tissue, concentrating them, and then injecting them into the injured area to accelerate tissue repair and regeneration.

When an inflammatory reaction begins, cytokines mediate a process called chemomodulation. Chemomodulation leads to the growth and strengthening of new connective tissue, increased joint stability, and a reduction in pain and dysfunction. Since cartilage and ligaments have particularly poor circulation compared to tissues like skin and muscle, prolotherapy in these areas results in targeted repair in an area where recovery would normally take much longer to occur.

How to get started: Chapter 19 explains how to self-inject peptides such as BPC-157 and TB-500, which I consider to be a form of prolotherapy. Pain clinics and antiaging clinics also often feature prolotherapy and PRP injections, in many cases combined with more advanced treatments like stem cell and exosome injections.

4. Vibration Therapy

Whole-body vibration (WBV) therapy involves standing or moving on a vibration platform and has been shown not only to increase strength, power, and speed but also to generate hormonal, immunological, and anti-inflammatory responses that can accelerate recovery. Vibration therapy works by triggering reflexive muscle contractions, causing changes in the length of the muscle-tendon complex (a unit of muscles and tendons that work together) and triggering various physiological adaptive responses. Some research has also suggested that the increased gravitational forces experienced during WBV elicit an anabolic hormonal response (testosterone is an example of an anabolic hormone). Vibration therapy also has a side benefit: it can enhance the peristaltic motion of the intestines, making it a great way to induce a morning bowel movement.

Because there is an element of friction when you are standing on a vibration platform, in the early stages of healing, you need to be careful of ankle, knee, or hip injuries that may be irritated by the rubbing of ligaments on bone (such as IT band friction syndrome). I once experimented with vibration for recovery hours after sustaining a knee injury from stepping the wrong way during a trail run, and, unfortunately, the vibration left me reeling in pain for several hours, which probably slowed my recovery. If it hurts, don't do it.

But in the later stages of healing, and for any injured body part not bothered by vibration, a WBV platform can be a handy training and recovery tool to keep in your home gym, garage, or office. You can stand on one for a few minutes in the morning or evening or implement it into your workout routine. The company Power Plate makes a great vibration platform. There are also fantastic handheld devices out there such as the Myobuddy, the Warrior, the Hypervolt, and the Theragun, all of which can achieve similar effects but in a more targeted manner—think of these as vibrating power tools for specific body parts.

How to get started: The best entry-level device, in my opinion, is the Myobuddy, which can be used like a vibrating car buffer for your entire body, including your gut and your head. A close second is the Hypervolt, which is more powerful, has five interchangeable heads in a variety of shapes for different parts of your anatomy, and is relatively quiet compared to other devices—meaning if you have it in your travel bag, you can massage your IT bands while waiting at an airport gate and save yourself from spending serious cash on a formal massage at the airport.

5. Compression

Research suggests that when you wear compression gear during a hard workout, your performance in subsequent workouts may improve, possibly because the increased blood flow resulting from compression helps restore muscle glycogen levels and clear metabolic waste. When you wear compression gear, you may also experience less muscle damage from tissue "bouncing" up and down while you exercise. If you sleep, rest, or travel wearing compression gear, you will find that the improvements in support and blood flow leave you less stiff and sore.

Although I find compression gear a bit annoying and time-consuming to put on for a workout or race, I do wear compression socks or tights while at my standing workstation, I sleep in compression gear after particularly tough workout days, I wear compression gear on airplanes and during long car rides, and nearly every day I take an afternoon nap while wearing a special style of graduated compression boots called NormaTec boots, which combine the following three massage techniques to speed the body's normal recovery process:

- **Pulsing:** Instead of using static compression (squeezing) to transport fluid out of the limbs, pulsing uses dynamic compression, which mimics the muscle pump of the legs and arms, enhancing the movement of fluid and metabolic waste out of the limbs after a workout.

- **Gradients:** Your veins and lymphatic vessels have one-way valves that prevent the backflow of fluid. Via a similar action, a gradient holds pressures to keep your body's fluids from being forced down toward your feet by the pulsing action in the proximal zones of the compression boots. This compression gradient can deliver maximum pressure throughout the entire limb, and the effectiveness of the pulsing action is not diminished near the top of the limb.

- **Distal release:** Because sustained static pressure can be detrimental to the body's normal circulatory flow, sequential pulsing releases the hold pressures once they are no longer needed to prevent backflow. By releasing the hold pressure in each zone as soon as possible, each portion of the limb gains maximum rest time without a significant pause between compression cycles.

In addition to these space-age recovery boots (which have attachments for the arms and torso), I have also experimented with compression shirts made by AlignMed to enhance posture and upper-body blood flow and recovery.

How to get started: Get yourself a decent set of compression socks or tights and wear them during a day of work or for several hours after a tough workout. Look for graduated compression gear, made by companies such as 2XU and Sub Sports. Compression gear also pairs quite well with cold soaks and cryotherapy, as it reduces some of the lymphatic fluid backflow that can occur during long immersion in cold water, making cold thermogenesis more effective.

6. Magnets

Although there is a relative lack of research on the therapeutic use of magnets to help reduce pain or accelerate recovery, there have been some promising studies on their ability to improve nervous tissue regeneration and wound healing. The theory is that magnets increase blood flow, change the migration of calcium ions, alter the pH balance of muscles, and have a positive effect on hormone production and enzyme activity. For example, if a magnetic field is strong enough to attract or repel ions like sodium and chloride in the blood, these ions may eventually encounter the walls of the blood vessels, move more rapidly, and increase tissue temperature or blood flow.

Companies such as Nikken, Promagnet, and Body Glove make thin, light, flexible magnets that you can wrap around your body or apply with adhesive and wear while you are sleeping, exercising, or working, and the company BEMER produces a magnetic mat that you can lie on for full-body therapy. I must admit that aside from occasional experimentation with small adhesive magnets and magnetic wraps for tennis elbow and a sore knee, magnets have not been a huge part of my recovery routine. But many folks swear by slapping them on an injured joint or wrapping sore muscles with a magnetic wrap—and I am not going to argue with as much anecdotal evidence as I have heard.

How to get started: Buy a good magnet and wrap it around the area that is hypoxic or injured. If it's annoying to wear a magnet during physical activity, you can wear it at night while you sleep.

7. HBOT

If you wander into my basement and open a super-secret door at the end of the hallway, you'll discover my cherished, oft-used four-person infrared sauna; a giant float tank equipped with UV, ozone, and hydrogen water; and one of my favorite recovery toys: a soft-shell hyberbaric oxygen therapy chamber. Hyperbaric oxygen therapy (HBOT) involves breathing pure oxygen in a pressurized room or, in this case, a human-sized tube. HBOT has been used in clinical settings to heal wounds, treat carbon monoxide poisoning and smoke inhalation, fix altitude sickness, and even assist with healing from conditions such as Lyme disease, head injuries, stroke, anemia, and dementia. However, HBOT can also be used to maximize performance and recovery. For example, it can facilitate speedier return to activity after a soft-tissue injury or the type of microinjuries and muscle tearing that occur during a hard workout or competition. It can also increase oxygen supply to muscles, increase ATP production, cause new capillary growth and regeneration of nerves, and even mobilize stem cells in a manner very similar to a stem cell infusion.

How to get started: Although HBOT can be supervised by a medical professional your first few times, especially if you're nervous with the slight ear-popping that occurs from pressurizing yourself with oxygen, doing your own HBOT treatment (as I do) is quite simple: you simply flip on an O_2 generator, climb inside the tube, zip it up from the inside, turn the decompression valve, and lie back for sixty to ninety minutes. I've even slept for a full night inside my chamber, and I find that it puts me in a deep sleep in about fifteen minutes flat. For the full antioxidant and anti-inflammatory response, consecutive treatments of up to forty sessions are recommended, but I began to notice better performance and recovery after just two or three sessions, and my "blah" feeling after heavy airline travel disappears within just an hour. The model I use is the Vitaeris 320 by HBOTUSA, and you can find a clinic near you that has one or purchase one for yourself on BoundlessBook.com/12.

8. Deep-Tissue Massage Therapy

I will take a deep dive into deep tissue in chapter 17, but in a nutshell, deep-tissue massage therapy and trigger-point therapy are excellent methods for mobilizing fasciae and removing knots. Having a good foam roller around can save you plenty of money on massage therapy, especially if you are into activities like stretching and yoga. Stretching makes knots in your muscles tighter in the same way that if you tie a knot in a rubber band and pull the ends of the rubber band, the knot gets tighter. Stretching is also often less effective than a deep-tissue massage at restoring the blood flow to a particular muscle. So save your stretching for after your deep-tissue and mobility work with a foam roller, lacrosse ball, tennis ball, or golf ball, as the massaging will release muscle knots and suffuse the tissue with fresh blood and nutrients. Your workout recovery should ideally go in this order: foam rolling, exercise, foam rolling, stretching.

In chapter 9 I talked about Olga Kotelko, who became a track-and-field star in her nineties. Her tip for age-defying muscle was to stay supple. Every night, she gave herself a foam-roller-style massage with an empty wine bottle she kept beside her bed. She understood that you cannot simply beat your body up day in and day out without working into the tissue to massage the fasciae, muscles, and joints. Similarly, I spend ten to fifteen minutes every morning "making love" to a variety of deep-tissue massage tools. Throughout the week, I will hit my lower back, upper shoulders, neck, under armpits, chest, hips, hamstrings, calves, quadriceps, IT bands (the outsides of the thighs), adductors (the insides of the thighs), and even the bottoms of my feet. Once or twice a month, I do a sixty-to-ninety-minute full-body massage or full-body foam-rolling session (there's a great video on my YouTube channel, youtube.com/BenGreenfieldFitness, that walks you through my full routine).

The only problem with a foam roller is that it doesn't fit too well into a carry-on, a suitcase, or a gym bag. This is why it is helpful to have a portable deep-tissue massage device, such as the Muscletrac, Myorope, or Tiger Tail. While it is difficult to get as deep with these sticks as you can when pressing your entire body weight into a foam roller, they do the trick on calves, forearms, the neck, and hips. In a pinch, you can do this type of deep-tissue work with no more equipment than a glass water bottle or wine bottle and a lacrosse ball, although you will be able to go much deeper with tools like ridged rolling balls and foam rollers.

In case you can't get any of these tools at all, there are some tricks you can keep in your back pocket. The corners of dumbbells or kettlebells at the average hotel gym can easily be used to dig into the sides of your sore hips or shoulders. Rocks, the corners of park benches, flagpoles, and anything else with a hard edge or surface can also be used on hips, backs, and the undersides of your knees.

How to get started: Grab a foam roller. Keep it in a highly visible spot in your home or office so you remember to use it. I also recommend picking up the book *Becoming a Supple Leopard* by Kelly Starrett, which you can consider a "cookbook" for all things deep-tissue- and mobility-related.

9. Electrical Muscle Stimulation (EMS)

As you'll recall from chapter 9, EMS causes muscle contractions using electric impulses from an external device. It can be used as a strength training tool, but it can also keep a muscle fit when you are rehabbing from an injury. For example, you could do an EMS strength set for your quads if you have injured your feet and can't do lower-body exercises, or for your pecs if you have injured your shoulders and can't press or do push-ups.

The Marc Pro is an EMS device that uses a specific waveform to gradually and gently grab muscle fibers, which works better for rehabilitation and recovery. This makes it ideal for healing damaged areas of tissue or enhancing recovery, compared with EMS devices that are primarily best for maintaining or building strength, muscle endurance, or power.

The NeuFit is one of the devices that can maintain muscle strength and power with extreme efficacy. It works through something called interferential, microcurrent, galvanic, Russian-stim iontophoresis, which is more compatible with your body's natural electrical wave production. The current also passes through skin and fatty tissue more easily, so it can penetrate much deeper without burning your skin or causing other nasty side effects. Devices like this are also effective at training muscles close to injuries, as they exert no stress aside from the current running through the muscle.

How to get started: I have found that for sore muscles or for sucking inflammation out fast, EMS combined with pressure and ice works well. This treatment is pretty simple: you attach the electrodes to the affected area, place an ice pack over them and secure it with an elastic bandage or kinesio tape, then flip the switch for twenty to thirty minutes. It is crucial to place the electrodes accurately, so make sure that you know your anatomy (most EMS devices come with instructions to make this easier for you).

Near-Infrared vs. Far-Infrared Light

Light can be broken down into wavelengths, and the wavelengths of infrared radiation, also called infrared light, are longer than those of visible light, so it's invisible to the human eye. Infrared light wavelengths extend from 700 nanometers, the red edge of the visible light spectrum, all the way up to 1 mm.

Near-infrared radiation (NIR) exists within the spectrum of natural sunlight. In fact, about half of the total energy of the sun is NIR, which means that our bodies are already naturally adapted to use it for different processes like collagen and elastin stimulation (which tightens skin), combating cancerous cells, and improving circulation. Far-infrared radiation (FIR) has longer wavelengths than NIR, and the benefits of FIR therapy mimic many of the benefits derived from natural sunlight, but without the risk of burns or cancerous effects. FIR can promote blood flow and healthy blood vessel growth and also modulate proper sleep. Both NIR and FIR induce relaxation and detoxification via sweating, and my recommendation is to use a one-two combo of both, preferably along with the visible wavelength of red light so that you get the best of all spectrums.

Keep in mind that the benefits of NIR and FIR exposure are dose-dependent. While moderate exposure to the infrared radiation of the sun throughout the day is beneficial, as is a dose of sauna exposure or the use of PBM devices that simulate or concentrate the conditions of natural sunlight, chronic exposure or doses higher than recommended can lead to skin and cell damage. In addition, certain infrared saunas may expose you to unhealthy levels of electrical pollution (the same type of EMF you'll learn more about in chapter 20), which is especially concerning since these saunas often have FIR emitters all the way around the sauna, meaning you may be bombarded by pollution from all directions. This is why it is important to only use PBM for ten to sixty minutes per day, depending on the power of your chosen device, and to look for an NIR sauna that uses heat lamps or other low-EMF strategies, such as two separate magnetic devices that will cancel each other out, and also has minimal amounts of electrical wiring throughout the walls.

Finally, red light, which occurs at a wavelength of 680 nm, does not penetrate as deep as near infrared or far infrared, but it is more readily absorbed by your skin, leading to increased collagen production and skin health—so if your goal is to minimize scar tissue, address wrinkles, and improve skin tone, you should also include a red-light source in your photobiomodulation protocol.

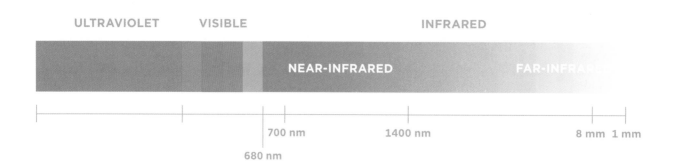

10. Photobiomodulation (PBM)

In chapter 6, I talked about using PBM for cognitive enhancement and a device called the Vielight for cognitive PBM therapy. PBM also can improve physical recovery—at the cellular level, visible red and near-infrared light can stimulate your cells to generate more energy and undergo self-repair. Here's how it works: Each cell contains mitochondria, which produce ATP, your body's primary form of usable energy. A mitochondrial enzyme called cytochrome oxidase-c can accept energy in the form of light for enhanced cellular function. Based on this principle, a kind of photobiomodulation called low-level laser therapy (LLLT), also known as cold laser therapy, uses a particular kind of laser called a light-emitting diode (LED) to reduce pain related to inflammation. It is effective for treating tendinitis, arthritis, and both acute and chronic pain, and it can lower levels of pain-producing chemicals, such as prostaglandins and interleukin, while decreasing bruises, swelling, bleeding, and oxidative stress from free radicals.

Larger PBM devices like the Joovv allow for both full-body treatment and targeted treatment, with similar efficacy to a handheld laser. A device like the Joovv emits red light from mid-600 nm to near-infrared wavelengths in the mid-800 nm range. The benefits of Joovv light therapy include the repair of sun-related skin damage, enhanced muscle recovery and performance, rapid wound healing, the reduction of joint inflammation, improved fertility, and the removal of scars, wrinkles, and stretch marks.

You can also achieve some benefit with a handheld LLLT wand, although I have personally found the Joovv to give better results. If you want to get invisible far-infrared light combined with negative ions, there is a mat called the Biomat that provides a deep heating effect along with healing and recovery-enhancing negative ions, similar to those produced by clean, pure air outside. A daily nap or meditation session on a Biomat can be a great way to recover, and I take an afternoon nap on mine most days.

How to get started: Start small to see how PBM affects you. I recommend getting a Joovv Mini and using it for ten to thirty minutes per day on any spots that need enhanced recovery. This gives you red and near-infrared exposure. If it works well for you, consider a larger Joovv unit, a Vielight (see page 123), a Biomat (which is far infrared, not red and near infrared), or all three.

11. Infrared Sauna

An infrared sauna is considered a type of photobiomodulation because it combines heat and light, but the sauna deserves a category on its own. Infrared light is a source of radiant heat, the same type of heat you get from sunlight or cold-laser therapy. Radiant heat is a form of energy that directly heats objects through a process called conversion, without heating the air around that object. Exposing the body to infrared light has been shown to raise white blood cell counts, enhance immunity, heat tissue, increase blood flow to injured or recovering muscles, and provide a host of additional recovery benefits. The best infrared saunas use infrared heat lamps that produce a combination of near-infrared radiation, which penetrates deeper into the body than far-infrared radiation, resulting in the detoxification benefits of near-infrared light combined with the heat therapy benefits of far-infrared light.

In a typical infrared sauna, ceramic or metallic elements are used to emit energy. Unlike the heat in a regular dry sauna or steam room, this energy penetrates the skin and heats you up from inside as well as outside, so there can be a much more pronounced hyperthermic effect. But one drawback to most infrared saunas is that they can produce a large amount of unhealthy electromagnetic fields (I'll look at that in more detail in chapter 20).

Finally, a treatment that works well in combination with sauna is halotherapy; I have a halotherapy device in my own sauna. Halotherapy involves breathing microcrystalline particles of salt that are infused into a room via a salt generator. It can be wonderful for skin health, pulmonary issues, asthma, coughs, and colds, and it can also cause you to sweat more in your sauna. This can be a handy addition to any sauna setup.

How to get started: Low-EMF infrared sauna brands include Clearlight, SaunaSpace, and Sunlighten. I purchased a large, four-person Clearlight Sanctuary infrared sauna for my basement gym and use it nearly every day for workouts, heat acclimation, building blood volume and new red blood cells, recovery, and detoxification. For a more portable setup, look into the SaunaSpace. Many health clinics and cryotherapy clinics also now offer infrared sauna treatments, although I think it is more convenient to have one at home.

12. Biohacked Water

You no doubt know that water is crucial for hydration, which itself is critical for recovery. But water can now be upgraded using a variety of machines that "structure" water, adding antioxidant-rich hydrogen or even extra molecular-signaling compounds. For example, a company called Eng3 created a device called NanoVi that infuses water with an electromagnetic charge that generates free radicals to subject your body to mild oxidative stress. By charging the water in its humidifier holding tank, then delivering it through a tube to a nasal cannula around your nose or a small pipe you can breathe from while working, the NanoVi creates a signal closely resembling the one given off by free radicals in your body. This stimulates a stronger healing response than free radicals alone would cause, resulting in an improved response to oxidative stress and enhanced cell repair and recovery. It may also enhance protein-folding mechanisms and overall protein repair.

This is important because, as we age, we begin to lose proteostasis, the biogenesis, folding, mobilization, and breaking down of proteins. In all cells, the 100,000 to 250,000 proteins (known collectively as the "proteome") that we need for life can misfold or become misshapen, and the normal 3-D shape of native proteins degrades. Part of proteostasis is refolding or destroying these proteins, but when proteostasis declines, these damaged proteins can accumulate. Indeed, declining proteostasis is now regarded as one of the primary causes of accelerated aging. Misfolded or clumped proteins are significantly implicated in age-related diseases, such as Parkinson's and Alzheimer's, and multiple studies have shown that proteostasis is impaired with age. So anything that can enhance protein-repair mechanisms, such as the NanoVi, not only improves recovery but can also be used as an antiaging tactic.

Then there is hydrogen-rich water, which I drink four to six large glasses of each day. Research suggests that hydrogen (H_2) has potent antioxidative properties, can help control lactic acid levels during exercise, and can even manage postexercise inflammation without blunting your natural adaptive response to a workout (unlike, say, high doses of antioxidants). I have in my home gym an H_2-water generator that is capable of infusing water with extremely high concentrations of H_2. According to Molecular Hydrogen Institute, drinking this water has been shown to boost energy, increase focus, increase immune system strength, enhance performance, elevate mood, eliminate pain, rejuvenate skin, and improve sleep. Because of this wide variety of benefits, I also travel with hydrogen tablets for H_2-enhanced performance on the road and simply drop two to four tablets into a glass of water in the morning and evening.

Interestingly, there is growing interest in using hydrogen-rich water to reduce hydroxyl radicals, a kind of free radical formed in the body from excess iron. Individuals who have either the HFE or SLC40A1 gene variant can absorb too much iron, leading to excess production of hydroxyl radicals and, potentially, unresolved inflammation and poor recovery. Having your doctor run a complete iron panel to see if iron is elevated can be helpful in determining whether this is an issue for you, but keep in mind that if iron is excessively turning into hydroxyl radicals, your iron levels may come back normal or even low. To learn more about this genetic susceptibility, I recommend speaking with Dr. Bob Miller at TOLHealth.com.

How to get started: Admittedly, the NanoVi is a bit expensive (prices range from $5,000 to $14,000, depending on the model you choose), but the convenience of having a cellular-repair device that you can simply have sitting on your desk during a day of work makes it an attractive option for any recovery enthusiast. A hydrogen-rich water generator is convenient but similarly expensive. Grabbing a few bottles of hydrogen-rich water tablets and using them daily is more affordable and can do the trick.

13. Pulsed Electromagnetic Field (PEMF) Therapy

PEMF uses electrical energy to direct a series of magnetic pulses through injured tissue. The electrical signal from each pulse stimulates cellular repair by upregulating a tissue-repair protein called a heat-shock protein and increasing the uptake of oxygen and nutrients into tissue. Studies have shown PEMF to be effective in healing soft-tissue wounds, reducing inflammation and pain, and increasing range of motion. By stimulating ATP production, PEMF can decrease the amount of time it takes to replenish energy stores after a workout. PEMF may also accelerate bone repair, which can come in handy if you have a stress fracture or a broken bone.

There are several smaller, entry-level PEMF devices on the market. For example, I own a small, portable, doughnut-shaped device from EarthPulse, which has options for signals that elicit focus, relaxation, and sleep. Two similar devices are the FlexPulse and ICES M1, both of which I also like, and, finally, there is a small collarbone-worn PEMF device called the SomniResonance SR1. I talked about using these devices for cognitive and sleep enhancement in chapter 6, but they're also useful for recovery: these type of PEMF devices can be held or moved slightly over an area of damaged tissue or healing bone for ten to thirty minutes. Interestingly, the magnetic signal released by a PEMF device is similar to that created by grounding or earthing mats, which professional cycling teams have used for more than a decade during the Tour de France to enhance both sleep and recovery. But unlike these mats, a PEMF device does not need to be plugged into an outlet and grounded, so it exposes you to less electrical pollution.

For spendier, more full-body PEMF treatments, there are two good options. The BioBalance, designed by the same Dr. William Pawluk who developed the FlexPulse, is a mat that you can sleep on all night. For the most powerful PEMF options, Pulse Centers makes a PEMF massage table called the Pulse XL Pro, which can be used for everything from muscle sprains to headaches to sleep induction to noticeable full-body treatments. The Pulse XL Pro generates up to 10 Hz of pulsing power that is safe and completely biologically compatible, so it's more powerful than any other PEMF device on the market (but it's also the price of a small car).

Incidentally, because ultrasonic (ultrasound) waves can penetrate several centimeters into tissue and, like PEMF, increase circulation, oxygen, nutrient delivery, and the removal of waste products from the site of a musculoskeletal injury, you can combine a PEMF unit with ultrasound or have a separate ultrasound unit. For example, I own a sam Sport, a wearable ultrasound unit that delivers 1.3 watts of low-intensity ultrasound energy at a specific frequency that accelerates healing and reduces pain—without the time, hassle, and expense of working with a physical therapist or ultrasound technician. That's an important aspect of many of the recovery modalities in this chapter: the ability to quickly and effectively recover at home without needing to drive to a physical therapist, fancy recovery center, or doctor's office.

How to get started: Begin with an entry-level, portable handheld device like the EarthPulse, FlexPulse, or ICES M1 and see how your body responds to PEMF.

14. Inversion

Hanging upside down like a bat may not seem like a stress-relieving or relaxing activity, but I hang from the inversion table in my garage or the yoga trapeze in my living room for five to ten minutes several times a week, especially after a long day at my standing workstation or several hours sitting in an airplane, and both the traction and the drainage effects are impressive. Heavy, swollen feet and legs almost instantly become lighter, and in addition, inversion has been shown to assist with lymphatic fluid circulation, back pain, blood flow, and spine or hip misalignment from high-impact workouts. Inversion also lengthens the spine, mobilizes the hips, and—in the case of the Pettibon neck traction device that also hangs inside my house—can be used as a chiropractic adjustment tool for the spine and neck.

Of course, you don't have to have an inversion table or yoga trapeze to use inversion. For example, after a long run, you can elevate your legs above your head by lying on your back with your legs propped against a wall—keep your legs elevated for at least one minute for every mile you have run. Other options are yoga inversions like the plow pose, a supported shoulder stand, a supported headstand, or, if you dare, the feathered peacock pose (google any of these inversion poses to see what they look like). Finally, ELDOA, which I'll talk more about in chapter 17, works similarly to inversion as a form of self-imposed decompression and traction for each of your joints.

How to get started: This one is pretty simple, really. Just purchase an inversion table, yoga trapeze, or even a set of gravity boots and keep them in a visible location where you're likely to use inversion on a regular basis. My yoga trapeze and neck traction device hang from my living room balcony, my gravity boots are conveniently located next to the pull-up bar in my home gym, and my inversion table is next to the exercise bike in my garage. I invert for five to ten minutes every single day!

15. Fasting

While the majority of sports nutrition recommendations advise you to shove carbohydrates and protein down your gullet as soon as possible after a workout, there is actually quite a bit of evidence to suggest that fasting, even postworkout, can have a potent recovery effect. When your body enters a fasted state, the process of autophagy is triggered, which is a programmed cellular response that results in cell turnover and recycling. Autophagy is particularly important for nervous system recovery, as the disruption or lack of autophagy has been shown to cause neurodegeneration. Intermittent fasting has been shown to improve motor-skill recovery in rats with spinal cord bruises, the result of autophagy clearing away old neurons to make way for the growth of new neurons. This also improves cognition, muscle function, and movement-pattern recognition.

In a study of cyclists, three weeks of overnight-fasted workouts improved postworkout recovery while maintaining lean muscle mass and performance, as well as keeping body fat low. Another study on endurance athletes suggested that fasted training may more quickly activate muscle protein translation, especially compared with athletes who ate carbohydrates before training, resulting in improved muscle recovery.

Fasting also has benefits for strength athletes. A 2009 study found that subjects who lifted weights in a fasted state had a greater anabolic response to a postworkout meal. In this case, levels of p70S6 kinase, a signaling mechanism for muscle-protein synthesis that acts as an indicator of muscle growth, were twice as high in the fasted group as in the fed group.

Martin Berkhan of the blog LeanGains.com, who is a big proponent of fasting, has a good take on the possible mechanism behind fasted-training adaptations, as does Dr. Jason Fung in his excellent book *The Complete Guide to Fasting*. A simple way to think of it is that when nutrients and calories are concentrated in the body in a fed state, exercise is experienced as less of a stressor than fasted-state training, so there is less need to adapt or compensate to the stressor. A similar phenomenon appears with antioxidant intake, with recent studies showing that ingesting high-dose antioxidants such as vitamins C and E in the presence of exercise may dampen the body's natural response to training, such as free radical formation and satellite cell proliferation. In other words, constantly training in a fed state or eating postworkout may make things too easy for the body.

A word of warning when it comes to fasting: for extremely lean individuals with low stores of essential body fat, people prone to eating disorders, and women who are dealing with adrenal or hormonal imbalances, the risks and stresses of frequent fasting, especially pre- and postworkout, can quickly outweigh any benefits.

In general, women are more susceptible to negative effects from fasting, which makes biological sense from an evolutionary standpoint: women need more calories and nutrients to build up and sustain a reserve that can nourish a growing fetus. Unfortunately, the combination of high levels of physical activity and fasting can rapidly downregulate fertility hormones in women, which has an effect not just on fertility itself but on overall health. Fasting has also been shown to reduce glucose tolerance in women. In addition, the fasting-induced benefits seen in obese women may not apply to leaner women or women in perimenopause. Interestingly, even in obese women, intermittent fasting can result in the loss of lean body mass and muscle, rather than the loss of pure adipose tissue. Finally, it has also been shown that women do not experience the same benefits of fasting-induced autophagy that men do. So proceed with caution, ladies.

How to get started: I fast in two ways: (1) an intermittent, daily overnight fast of twelve to sixteen hours, leaving me with an eight-to-twelve-hour daily compressed eating window, and (2) a weekly or biweekly twenty-four-hour fast from dinnertime to dinnertime. To maintain adequate recovery nutrients during these fasts, I will occasionally "cheat" with low-calorie recovery or energy-enhancing supplements, such as essential amino acids, exogenous ketones, minerals, and/ or bone broth. But any of these are veritable speed bumps compared to a massive postworkout smoothie or preworkout sweet potato.

16. Anti-inflammatory Diet

One huge pet peeve of mine is when someone pulls out all the stops to fix an injury or struggles with constant joint soreness or subpar recovery, all while eating supersized sandwiches on whole-grain bread, living out of the "healthy" bakery case at their favorite coffee shop, eating organic packaged foods laden with vegetable oil, and gulping down several cups of coffee every morning. Glycemic spikes, oxidized oils, and—in excess—acidic beverages like coffee can all aggravate inflammation, so trying to fix an injury without fixing your nutrition is like fighting a fire in your house with water on one side and gasoline on the other.

What makes a food inflammatory? There are at least two dozen factors, including the amounts and proportions of various fatty acids, the amounts of antioxidants and other nutrients, and the food's glycemic impact (its effect on blood sugar levels). But it is not as clear-cut as it might sound because some foods have both inflammation-producing and inflammation-reducing factors. An orange, for example, contains antioxidants that can fight inflammation, but an entire glass of orange juice contains concentrated natural sugars that can have a mild inflammatory effect. Similarly, a nice fatty cut of steak contains enough saturated fats to create inflammation in many people but also contains anti-inflammatory monounsaturated fats.

A resource such as InflammationFactor.com can help you cut through the confusion. Its inflammation factor (IF) rating system allows you to quickly see whether a specific food is going to have an inflammatory or anti-inflammatory effect, and from there you can determine the inflammatory potential of entire meals or recipes. Some convenient anti-inflammatory foods include:

- Pineapple, which is rich in a proteolytic enzyme called bromelain, which produces substances that help fight pain and inflammation
- Blue, red, and purple fruits and vegetables, all of which contain antioxidant flavonoids that limit inflammation, prevent tissue breakdown, improve circulation, and promote a strong collagen matrix
- Ginger, which two studies from the University of Georgia have shown can help fight inflammation and reduce exercise-induced muscle pain in doses of 2 g daily. Just boil several slices of ginger, juice a golf-ball-sized chunk of ginger, or add ginger to a smoothie.

Other foods with high IF ratings include garlic, peppers, parsley, dark leafy greens, onions, salmon, avocados, and apple cider vinegar.

How to get started: Visit InflammationFactor.com, grab their IF rating list for five bucks, then print it and post it someplace you'll often see it for the next few weeks. Familiarize yourself with potentially inflammatory foods that are staples in your diet. Remember, inflammation is natural, and not all inflammation is bad, but when you're trying to pull out all the stops for recovery and your body is already inflamed from, say, a workout or injury, you need to be more cautious. There's a good reason that Tom Brady, a top-ranked NFL quarterback who also has had one of the longest professional sporting careers, doesn't eat tomatoes, potatoes, and eggplants—although one could argue those foods are healthy. He wants every recovery advantage he can get.

17. Vitamin C

Back in the 1940s, physicians began routinely giving their surgical patients 1,000 mg of vitamin C daily for three days before surgery, followed by 100 mg of vitamin C daily during recovery. These doctors reported in the *British Journal of Surgery* that 76 percent of wounds treated this way healed properly, with a three- to sixfold increase in the strength of the wound scar. Russian researchers have shown that surgical patients who take vitamin C are discharged from the hospital one to two days earlier than patients who don't, probably due to vitamin C's crucial role in collagen formation (collagen is the primary component of connective tissue). In fact, when bone broth is combined with vitamin C, exercise-induced collagen synthesis more than doubles.

Vitamin C also works as an antioxidant to limit free-radical damage to tissues and boosts the growth of fibroblast and chondrocyte cells, which produce connective-tissue fibers and cartilage. I don't take a vitamin C supplement unless I am injured, but I do make sure I get an adequate daily dose from fruits, vegetables, and whole-food antioxidant powders.

How to get started: If you are injured, need to speed up recovery, and want to use vitamin C, do not use synthetic vitamin C capsules, which can increase the risk of stroke and blunt the natural satellite-cell proliferation and mitochondrial density induced by exercise. Instead, choose a whole-foods vitamin C source, such as powdered antioxidant supplements like Organifi Red or Green Juice, Life Shotz, the Four Sigmatic rehydration blend, or the Living Fuel SuperBerry powder. A company called American Nutriceuticals also makes a well-absorbed whole-foods vitamin C powder. In addition, many natural-medicine clinics offer high-dose vitamin C IVs, which can be administered on a weekly or monthly basis (if you are an athlete competing in a sanctioned sport, be sure to check into the allowed IV volume).

18. Proteolytic Enzymes

Proteolytic enzymes—such as papain, bromelain, trypsin, and chymotrypsin—promote healing by supporting the production of cytokines, activating immune-system proteins (such as alpha-2-macroglobulins), breaking down soreness-inducing fibrinogen, and slowing the clotting mechanism. This is another tool that, like vitamin C, can help wounds heal faster and help you bounce back more quickly from surgery.

My preferred brand of proteolytic enzymes is Kion Flex, and other good brands are Wobenzym and BiOptimizers.

The best food sources are pineapple, papaya, and red meat, but these are far less potent than targeted supplementation with the actual enzymes, especially because proteolytic enzymes produce the best activity when taken on an empty stomach. This is because proteolytic enzymes taken with food will digest the proteins in the food rather than breaking down the fibrinogen in your body, which is the mechanism by which enzymes modulate blood clotting following tissue damage.

How to get started: Although 100 to 300 mg is a standard dose of enzymes, if I'm injured or have had a very difficult workout day, I take a hefty dose of enzymes—around 800 to 1,000 mg— on an empty stomach prior to bed.

19. Amino Acids

Branched-chain amino acids (BCAAs), such as leucine, isoleucine, and valine, have been a darling of the bodybuilding industry for decades. When used in daily doses (preferably during workouts) of 5 to 10 g per hour, they have been proven to significantly enhance performance, and since BCAAs are the building blocks of neurotransmitters, they are also particularly important for nervous system performance. For neurotransmitter optimization, amino acids are best consumed with vitamin B and minerals, which are the other neurotransmitter precursors. These amino acids also improve physiological markers such as red blood cell count, hemoglobin, hematocrit, serum albumin, and fasting glucose, and they even decrease inflammatory markers like creatine phosphokinase while enhancing the restoration of muscle glycogen. You can find BCAAs in capsule or powder forms.

On the other hand, essential amino acids, or EAAs (also known as whole amino acids), are a far better option than BCAAs because they are a more well-rounded source of amino acids and can keep your body from cannibalizing your own lean muscle tissue during exercise. However, EAAs are relatively pricey, especially if you're popping them during or after every workout. Why are they so much more expensive, and what's the difference between them and other proteins? At the low end of the amino acid spectrum, you will find whey and soy protein powders—only 17 percent of their amino acid content is utilized by the body, with the other 83 percent leaving the body as nitrogen-based waste. Foods like red meat, fish, and poultry fare a bit better, with 32 percent being absorbed and 68 percent being wasted. Eggs are the winners in the food stakes, with 48 percent being utilized and 52 percent being wasted.

Compare those numbers with EAA supplements': a whopping 99 percent of their amino acids are utilized, with only 1 percent wasted. EAAs are also absorbed by the body within twenty-three minutes, compared with several hours for food or powder sources of whole protein (and weight watchers will be happy to know that there is only 0.4 calorie per gram, tablet or capsule). My friend and forty-two-time Ironman triathlete Dr. David Minkoff, a specialist in alternative and antiaging medicine, introduced me to essential amino acids. He swears by them and completely healed a nagging hamstring injury by taking 40 g per day (yes, that is admittedly a boatload of amino acids). He prescribes the same for many of his patients and athletes. The brand I use (and swear by) is Kion Aminos, because of the studied and highly effective amino acid ratios in that particular blend. It is entirely legal to use EAAs in sporting events, and because they have potent fatigue-fighting and recovery-enhancing effects, they are one of my most highly recommended supplements for both performance and recovery.

How to get started: I recommend taking 5 to 10 g of EAAs before a hard workout or race, another 5 to 10 g each hour during the event, and 10 to 40 g per day if you're healing from an injury.

20. Fish Oil

In chapter 4, I explored the cognitive benefits of supplementing with DHA, EPA, and ALA, but the anti-inflammatory properties of these omega-3 fatty acids make them important for physical recovery, too. Omega-3s—found in cold-water fish, algae, and fish oil—can increase muscle protein synthesis and support healthy circulatory and brain function, as well as enhance cognition and mood.

Fish oil supplements generally contain significantly more EPA than DHA (usually at a 2:3 DHA-to-EPA ratio). But mounting research suggests that higher levels of DHA are optimal for recovery, neuronal health, and anti-inflammation, so you should look for a fish oil supplement with a 1:1 DHA-to-EPA ratio. Make sure that it is in a natural triglyceride form and not the cheaper ethyl-ester form, which is not absorbed as well. It should also be packaged with antioxidants, such as astaxanthin and vitamin E, to keep the fatty acids from becoming rancid (and to keep your fish oil from doing more harm than good to your joints).

While the omega-6 fatty acids found in vegetable oils and heated seeds, nuts, and nut butters can produce eicosanoids, which are pro-inflammatory (especially when eaten in the quantity that many endurance athletes tend to eat them), please note that not all omega-6 fatty acids are "bad"—and if you overdose with omega-3 fatty acids while completely eliminating all quality sources of omega-6 (such as flaxseed oil, flax seeds, flaxseed meal, hemp seed oil, hemp seeds, pumpkin seeds, raw sunflower seeds, pine nuts, pistachios, borage oil, evening primrose oil, black currant seed oil, and acai), you can deleteriously affect cardiolipin, which is a critical component of your mitochondrial membranes. For most people, a ratio of 4:1 omega-6 to omega-3 is ideal, although the average American eats a ratio ranging from 12:1 to 25:1! You can test your omega fatty acid ratios from home with high precision using a testing kit like the one from Zinzino.

How to get started: I take 4 to 6 g per day of Living Fuel SuperEssentials fish oil, which contains the ideal DHA-to-EPA ratio. When I am injured or in need of more recovery, I treat myself to 20 to 30 g per day, a "megadose" of fish oil (which many folks in the biohacking community also swear by for cognitive clarity). Other good brands include Pharmax, Barlean's, Carlson, and Green Pastures. Choose wisely, as taking a bad, rancid fish oil is worse for inflammation than not taking any fish oil at all.

Not All Fish Oil Is Created Equal

I am often asked what the healthiest fish oil is. A good general rule is to first look for a fish oil supplement that contains a 1:1 ratio of DHA to EPA, since the additional DHA results in a ratio closer to what you find in many cold-water fish. But this doesn't necessarily mean that more DHA than EPA is a good thing. For example, one study tested the hypothesis that DHA-to-EPA ratios might affect how well the omega-3s are digested and absorbed. The researchers found that a 2:1 DHA-to-EPA ratio reduced the uptake of both omega-3s by 21 to 23 percent, while a 1:2 DHA-to-EPA ratio reduced the uptake by 14 to 18 percent. If you invest in a fish oil supplement, you do not want to lose up to 23 percent of the available omega-3 fatty acids, so it is worth taking the time to look for a supplement that contains an approximate 1:1 ratio. When taken in the right amounts, EPA and DHA work synergistically to affect mood, behavior, and coagulation, as well as brain development, structure, and function.

In addition, it's important to take into consideration whether the fish oil is in ethyl ester (EE) or triglyceride (TG) form. The TG form is best, hands down. This is the form found in nature; in fact, over 98 percent of all fats ingested from any natural food are in TG form. When you take fish oil in EE form, the free fatty acids must be reconverted into TGs before they can enter your bloodstream. This leads to far less absorption, along with a release of ethyl alcohol and subsequent oxidative stress from a release of both free radicals and ethanol, the latter of which must be filtered through the liver in the same way as any other toxin. EEs are also more resistant to hydrolysis by pancreatic lipase than natural TG forms, which further limits their absorption

and utilization. On the other hand, there are virtually no negative side effects from the TG form of fish oils, and nearly all clinical studies demonstrating fish oil benefits are performed with whole-food fish consumption or fish oil supplements in the TG form.

Unfortunately, EE is the prevalent form of fish oil on the market because it is cheaper to produce than the TG form. In fact, the supplements industry created EE because it is easier to work with than TG. The EE form has a much higher boiling point and is easier to process during the molecular distillation protocol used to remove industrial contaminants such as heavy metals and PCBs. Problem is, the process to convert fish oil EE back to the natural TG form is costly, so supplement manufacturers often skip this step. Ideally, they would forgo the option to leave the fatty acids in a free form attached to an ethyl alcohol backbone and instead, re-attach them to a glycerol structure to form a triglyceride molecule. But despite multiple studies showing that of EE, TG, and whole fish, EE is the least bioavailable form of omega-3, supplement manufacturers simply cut corners.

Because I have personally found it to be supportive of cognition, hormones, and joint health, I take a relatively high amount of fish oil, ten to twelve capsules each day of Living Fuel SuperEssentials fish oil, typically with breakfast. It contains both EPA and DHA in their natural TG forms, which results in a 2:3 DHA-to-EPA ratio, but then the manufacturers add additional DHA to achieve the ideal 1:1 ratio. So I am getting both TG and extra DHA, a fish oil win-win scenario.

21. Glucosamine and Chondroitin

Glucosamine is a sugar present in the protective exoskeleton of shellfish, and chondroitin is found naturally in animal tissue, particularly connective tissue like beef cartilage. Glucosamine and chondroitin are also naturally produced by your body. Glucosamine stimulates cartilage production in your joints, while chondroitin helps attract water to the joint, which allows your cartilage to maintain elasticity. Chondroitin may also inhibit the enzyme activity that breaks down cartilage.

How to get started: In addition to regularly consuming shellfish and cartilaginous components of animal meat such as skin, bones (easily made edible in bone broth), and the "gristly bits," I recommend that any aging athlete or exercise enthusiast with joint pain look for a supplement that contains glucosamine sulfate, which is more effective than glucosamine hydrochloride. You need to take at least 1,500 mg per day, usually for at least three months, to notice any improvement in stiffness, pain, or mobility—so stay in this one for the long game. In addition, take 500 to 1,000 mg of chondroitin daily. I personally use Kion Flex for both glucosamine and chondroitin.

What About NSAIDs for Injury and Recovery?

If you are injured or sore, why not simply take non-steroidal anti-inflammatory drugs (NSAIDs), such as ibuprofen? Unfortunately, when you take NSAIDs, you prevent your body from manufacturing prostaglandins, which protect your stomach lining, regulate blood pressure, and bring inflammation to an area that has been injured (yes, pain, redness, swelling, and discomfort are part of inflammation, but that's part of the body's natural repair process).

Because prostaglandins protect the stomach lining, NSAIDs can cause stomach upset, and with long-term habitual use of NSAIDs, there is a risk of stomach bleeding. While many people who exercise pop these pills only every now and again—for example, to reduce pre- or postworkout soreness or to be able to "push through the pain" to complete a competition—even occasional use is not a good idea, and you're going to discover why right now.

A recent study titled "Aggravation of Exercise-Induced Intestinal Injury by Ibuprofen in Athletes" revealed some pretty upsetting information. Nine healthy athletes were studied on four different occasions: (1) taking a standard dose of 400 mg of ibuprofen twice in the hours leading up to a bike workout, (2) taking no ibuprofen before a bike workout, (3) taking 400 mg of ibuprofen twice at rest, and (4) resting without taking ibuprofen.

In each case, researchers measured small-intestinal damage by monitoring intestinal fatty-acid-binding proteins (I-FABPs). They also measured urinary excretion of special sugar probes, which can determine the amount of gastrointestinal permeability—a sign that the gut is becoming leaky.

The researchers found that while both ibuprofen use and working out resulted in increased I-FABP levels, reflecting small-intestinal injury, levels were higher after a workout with ibuprofen than a workout without ibuprofen. Gut permeability also increased, especially after taking ibuprofen and working out, which reflected a loss of gut-barrier integrity. In addition, the amount of intestinal injury from ibuprofen and gut-barrier dysfunction were extremely well correlated. Thus, it is clear that exercise irritates your small intestine slightly, and ibuprofen makes the irritation worse. In fact, the researchers concluded that "NSAID consumption by athletes is not harmless and should be discouraged."

So what about the prevalent practice of taking NSAIDs before a long event like an Ironman or a marathon to "mask the pain"? It turns out that this has been researched, too. One study found that taking 400 mg of ibuprofen four hours before exercise reduced soreness but didn't actually prevent muscle-cell injury, which is cause for concern because it means that by masking pain, ibuprofen may lead to an increased risk of injury.

22. Curcumin

I consume curcumin in some form nearly every day—whether via turmeric root, curries, or curcumin supplements. You may recognize curcumin as the principal compound in turmeric (which happens to be a member of the anti-inflammatory ginger family), and it's a widely recognized herbal anti-inflammatory that has been shown to be as effective at reducing inflammation as injectable cortisone. Curcuminoids are the subparticles that make up curcumin and have been found to be powerful inhibitors of inflammatory compounds called COX-2, without damaging the gut the way ibuprofen does.

Unfortunately, curcumin is notorious for having poor bioavailability. Research suggests that curcumin concentrations in blood plasma, urine, and peripheral tissues are extremely low or nonexistent even when you take a high-dose supplement. This means that, while the curcumin is eliciting fantastic anti-inflammatory action in the gut, it isn't having the same effect elsewhere—so unless all you're trying to do is quell gastric inflammation, you need to read about these three ways to increase curcumin's bioavailability.

The first is to consume black pepper along with turmeric. It doesn't take much black pepper—just one-twentieth of a teaspoon can significantly increase measurable blood levels of curcumin—but a quarter teaspoon of black pepper causes curcumin's bioavailability to increase

Other studies have found that NSAID use during long events, such as a marathon or triathlon, decreases kidney function. This can lead to dangerous issues, including a reduced ability to regulate sodium, electrolytes, and hydration levels. This lack of proper regulation becomes especially dangerous in hot weather, when there is already a lot of stress on the kidneys. The extra stress may create a high risk of long-term kidney damage or kidney failure.

One of the most eye-opening studies on ibuprofen use during exercise was performed during the grueling Western States Endurance Run, a one-hundred-mile ultramarathon. Runners were split into three groups: one that didn't take ibuprofen, one that received 600 mg one day before the race and on race day, and one that took 1,200 mg one day before the race and on race day (having a group taking more ibuprofen allows researchers to see if there is a dose-dependent response). In this study, both of the ibuprofen groups had significantly higher levels of markers for severe muscle damage, including C-reactive protein, plasma cytokine, and macrophage inflammatory protein, with higher levels in the group taking more ibuprofen.

And get this: taking ibuprofen did not affect race time, postworkout soreness, or perceived exertion. This means that ibuprofen did not help at all, and it caused significantly greater inflammation and muscle damage.

NSAID use during training has also been shown to slow down muscle-building processes. The human body responds to muscular exertion by producing prostaglandins. Muscle tissue in injured areas or areas damaged by muscular exertion fills with a particular type of prostaglandin that stimulates stem cells within the muscle to begin multiplying to create new muscle cells. The resulting muscle tissue is stronger than before. NSAIDs block the production of prostaglandins, which means that fewer stem cells become active, fewer new cells are produced, and the muscle tissue exhibits reduced strength and flexibility.

Finally, multiple studies have linked the chronic use of NSAIDs with a higher risk of heart attack and stroke. The mechanisms for cardiovascular damage appear to be mediated through the inhibition of an enzyme known as COX-2, inhibition of the production of a molecule called prostacyclin that relaxes blood vessels and limits platelet clumping, and inhibition of the production of nitric oxide.

So as you can see, the jury is not out when it comes to using NSAIDs. Just don't use them. Period. With so many healthy alternatives, this should be a no-brainer.

by 2,000 percent. The second way is to consume turmeric with a healthy fat source. When consumed with ghee, butter, coconut oil, or olive oil, curcumin bypasses liver processing and is thus less exposed to metabolic enzymes, allowing it to remain in a more absorbable free form. The third way is to heat turmeric. Curcumin becomes far more bioavailable when you heat it in a little warm oil in a sauté pan or sprinkle it into whatever dish you are sautéing.

How to get started: There are a range of highly bioavailable curcumin supplements. The company Thorne produces a supplement called Meriva-SF (Sustained Release), which contains a potent form of curcumin, curcumin phytosome, that has been demonstrated to be twenty-nine times more absorbable than curcumin in whole foods. The curcumin extract is attached to a phospholipid, which allows for higher plasma concentrations of curcumin in a smaller dose.

23. Magnesium

You have probably heard that the magnesium sulfate in Epsom salts baths or float tanks can decrease muscle soreness, enhance relaxation, and displace the calcium ions that can accumulate in muscle tissue during workouts. But concentrated magnesium chloride is even more effective than Epsom salts. Why is pure magnesium so effective for recovery?

As you read this, you have about two ounces of magnesium in your body—mostly in muscle and bone tissue. This mineral is essential for more than three hundred reactions, including nerve and cardiac function, muscle contraction and relaxation, protein formation, and the synthesis of ATP-based energy. A magnesium deficiency can result in muscle cramping, excessive soreness, low muscular force production, disrupted recovery and sleep, immune system depression, and even potentially fatal heart arrhythmias during intense exercise.

Several studies have shown magnesium to be effective for buffering lactic acid, enhancing peak oxygen uptake and total work output, reducing heart rate and carbon dioxide production during hard exercise, and improving cardiovascular efficiency. In addition, supplementing with magnesium can elevate testosterone levels and muscle strength by up to 30 percent, as well as combat calcium buildup from muscle microtearing. While seeds, nuts, grains, and vegetables are good dietary sources of magnesium, active people who eat these foods can still be deficient in magnesium because high activity levels—especially when combined with sweating, which causes mineral loss—deplete it more quickly.

Unfortunately, an oral magnesium supplement may not fully compensate for this deficiency, as oral magnesium in the amount athletes need is not readily absorbed, and magnesium causes diarrhea at high doses. So while the use of oral magnesium (such as magnesium citrate powder) is certainly helpful, a far better way to deliver the required doses is with topical magnesium.

The delivery of drugs transdermally (through the skin) is used to avoid the risk or inconvenience of intravenous therapy, to improve the absorption of a drug by bypassing the gastrointestinal tract, to decrease the metabolism of a drug by the liver, and to provide a more targeted application (for example, in the form of a topical nonsteroidal anti-inflammatory drug patch that's applied directly to the site of injury). This same method can easily be used to deliver high doses of magnesium directly to your muscles pre- or postworkout to enhance performance and recovery. You can magnify this effect by combining it with electrical muscle stimulation.

There are many ways to deliver magnesium transdermally. While Epsom salts provide magnesium sulfate, which can help with postworkout recovery, magnesium chloride is even more effective. You can dissolve 1 to 3 pounds of pure magnesium chloride flakes or crystals in a bath, giving you a dose of about 500 mg for an extremely relaxing and soreness-relieving soak. Alternatively, after a long run or bike ride, you can soak your feet in a magnesium chloride bath for fifteen to twenty minutes. After drying off from my postworkout cold shower, I apply transdermal magnesium lotion to any major muscle groups that I worked that day, rubbing the lotion in for about thirty seconds.

Magnesium chloride is also available as a spray. I use eight to ten shots of the spray or a large dab of the lotion on my shoulders, arms, and legs after a particularly hard workout, often driving it into the tissue with electrical muscle stimulation or a vibration device. In most cases, ten sprays deliver approximately 100 mg of magnesium. Make sure that your skin is dry before applying the spray, and lightly rub the magnesium in after application. Magnesium spray may cause a tingling or slightly annoying burning sensation. This is normal and usually subsides with repeated use.

If you get sports massages, you can give magnesium chloride spray or oil to your massage therapist for use after your session (it likely produces too much friction for your therapist to want to use it during a session). This can assist with the body's natural recovery process and speed up healing from a workout or injury, as well as help prevent future injuries from sore and stiff muscles. If you have a strain or sprain, topical magnesium can also be used to improve circulation or decrease pain. Simply spray the magnesium on any sore area and rub it in.

It is important to keep track of exactly how much magnesium you consume between oral and topical use because anything above 500 to 1,000 mg can cause loose stools or gastrointestinal discomfort. So make sure you keep track of your total magnesium exposure unless you want to spend a lot of time on the toilet.

How to get started: Go to a website like Ancient Minerals (ancient-minerals.com) and grab a bottle of magnesium lotion and a few bags of magnesium bath flakes. Use them regularly during the week. For a heavier dose, google the name of your city and the words "float tank," which will help you find a sensory deprivation chamber in which you can float for one to two hours a few times each month in hundreds of pounds of magnesium chloride at the same temperature as your body.

24. Cannabidiol (CBD)

While THC, the psychoactive chemical found in cannabis, is a restricted substance that is not legal in several states and countries, the compound cannabidiol is—at the time of this writing—perfectly legal in all fifty states, meaning you can take it on a plane to anywhere in the US. CBD is a cannabinoid that composes up to 40 percent of the marijuana plant and is believed by many researchers to be the single most important cannabinoid ever discovered. CBD acts as an antagonist of THC by turning off or turning down anything that would activate the receptors through which THC exerts its effects. CBD itself does not, like THC, attach to receptors associated with addiction, so it is neither addictive nor habit-forming.

CBD also has no psychoactive effects, and there is a growing body of research to support CBD use for recovery. The late Dr. Tod Mikuriya, the former national administrator of the US government's marijuana research programs, stated that no other single drug or substance has as many therapeutic benefits as cannabis. CBD is particularly potent against inflammation, which is one of the leading contributors to conditions like heart disease, cancer, chronic lower respiratory disease, stroke, Alzheimer's, diabetes, and nephritis. CBD is also effective against acute inflammation, which you might encounter, say, after a long day of racing or working out. For example: Cytokines, the signaling proteins synthesized and secreted by immune cells, modulate the initiation and resolution of inflammation. CBD reduces cytokine production by immune cells such as T helper cells TH1 and TH2 (which are the same cells in which overactivity can contribute to autoimmune issues and food intolerances). CBD can also reduce levels of the inflammatory compound interleukin-6.

The problem with CBD is that it is not naturally highly bioavailable because CBD oils, capsules, and powders are not water soluble. Considering that your body is over 60 percent water, you have to find a way to overcome this problem to enjoy the benefits of this cannabinoid. Turmeric plays a significant role here because the isolated curcuminoids (which are the active ingredients of a high-curcumin-containing turmeric plant) mix with the cannabinoids and terpenoids of CBD, causing their bioavailability to explode. When you take CBD with curcumin or turmeric high in curcumin, you can get five to ten times the effects that you otherwise would. Just remember that curcumin itself must be taken alongside black pepper, consumed with a healthy fat source, or heated to get the full effect. Finally, CBD topical lotions can be just as effective as or more effective than oral CBD supplementation for spot-targeting joints.

How to get started: Try the water-soluble CBD capsules from BioCBD, which have been blended with turmeric, or get Thorne's hemp oil, which uses the purest hemp stalk oil possible—certified organic and legal in all fifty states—then blends it with phytocannabinoids (and other active ingredients) from hemp stalk oil, clove, black pepper, hops, and rosemary. It's potent stuff. I recommend just 10 to 20 mg of CBD if you have never used it before, although prior to bed, my personal "sleep cocktail" includes 30 to 50 mg of CBD from either of the sources listed above.

My 1-2-3 Technique for Fast Recovery

I use this three-step recovery process to suck inflammation out of strained and sprained joints and muscles as quickly as possible.

1. **Apply topical magnesium:** You can use any topical anti-inflammatory, including CBD oil, but magnesium chloride seems to work best. I use the Magnetic Clay magnesium oil made by the brand Ancient Minerals because it doesn't contain the heavy metals that most other brands do.

2. **Turn on electrical muscle stimulation:** EMS has the capacity to drive a topical treatment like magnesium deeper into the tissue. After applying the magnesium or another topical anti-inflammatory, place the EMS electrodes in the appropriate sore spots. Remember that it is important to place the electrodes precisely, and be sure to check the instructions that accompany the device you use for information on where to place the electrodes for maximum effectiveness. I use the MarcPro device for recovery, as this waveform is best for avoiding any excess stress to injured muscles.

3. **Place ice over the electrodes:** The cryotherapy from the ice allows you to withstand higher levels of EMS, and this helps drive the topical anti-inflammatory even deeper into your tissue. Once you have the EMS electrodes in place and the device is running, cover the electrodes with an ice pack, even if it's just a ziplock bag of ice (although I prefer the brand Frozen-Peaz). The cold exposure will also reduce inflammation and improve circulation and blood flow once the ice is removed, bringing more nutrients to the injured area and clearing away metabolic and inflammatory debris.

One other factor to consider when using this technique is that icing an injury only reaches its full potency when it is combined with compression. In fact, when you ice an injury without compressing the ice around the sprained or strained area, you can end up with poor lymphatic drainage and backflow of lymph fluid. Because of this, I usually wrap an elastic bandage or other compression wrap tightly around the electrodes and ice. The benefits of compression seem to provide the icing on the cake when combined with magnesium, EMS, and ice.

You can use this 1-2-3 technique two to three times per day for ten to twenty minutes at a time. You will be blown away at how quickly it removes pain and enhances recovery.

25. Sound Healing

Sound healing is the practice of using audio tones and vibrational frequencies to repair damaged tissues and cells within the body. It works on the idea that all matter is vibrating at specific frequencies, and that sickness, disease, depression, and stress cause human beings to vibrate at a lower frequency, while tones that promote healing, happiness, and vitality can produce surprising effects and even allow DNA strands to repair themselves.

You can use sound to improve your mood and switch from a sympathetic ("fight-or-flight") state to a parasympathetic ("rest-and-digest") state, and vice versa. Sound can also help with depression, anxiety, stress, and sleep. But you can also use sound technology to heal you on a cellular level and help with chronic disease. Tibetan singing bowls, tuning forks, drumming therapy, and chanting are all utilized in sound therapy, and many participants experience strong emotions during these therapy sessions (I found myself weeping like a baby at the end of a two-hour session on a sound healing table with a healer named Porangui in Sedona, Arizona). Advocates of sound healing claim that it has the power to heal mental illness, arthritis, and autoimmune disorders, and that it can even shrink cancerous tumors.

My friend and composer Michael Tyrrell has arranged music tracks called Wholetones that are recorded at specific frequencies designed to elicit targeted emotions. I also own and use a Lovetuner, which is a tiny, single-tone flute that plays a tone at the frequency of 528 Hz, which targets the heart chakra. Many videos of tones at 528 Hz frequencies can be found on YouTube, and iTunes also carries works by different artists that explore this harmonic. While you'll usually find me listening to podcasts or audiobooks while working out, driving my car, cleaning, or walking, when I need to boost my mood to the next level and fill myself with positive emotions, I blast Wholetones, energetic techno music, electronic dance tracks, Top 40 hits, or—when my kids are around and ready for one of our prebreakfast or postdinner family dance parties—the Disney channel on Pandora.

How to get started: Here's a practical example of how I personally utilize sound and music in my weekly routine:

- Daily: Occasionally humming (aum chanting) during my morning or afternoon walk
- Daily: Fifteen to twenty minutes of silence, usually while sitting outdoors surrounded by nature sounds
- Daily: My harmonica and Lovetuner are always in my fanny pack for quick practice or sound therapy while traveling.
- Nightly: Guitar or ukulele practice, or family sing-along time
- Weekly: Deep tissue massage while playing Wholetones music tracks
- Weekly: Meditation session in a sauna with earbuds or using full-body surround sound from sauna speakers to play Wholetones or other soundtracks, such as Brain.fm
- Weekly: Deep techno to pump me up before hard workouts or races
- Weekly: Singing or listening to music at church
- Two or three times per week: Chanting, humming, or audible breathing during Kundalini yoga or another yoga session

The Bottom Line

Whew! With this lineup of recovery methods, you have no excuses for not healing your body far more quickly than most folks settle for.

It always surprises me that after getting hurt, many people settle for a once- or twice-weekly visit to the physical therapist, a bit of time on the recumbent bicycle at the gym, some light stretching, and perhaps a cup of ginger tea. But by pulling out all the methods in this chapter, you can, in fact, heal your body far more quickly and rapidly get your musculoskeletal system back to a state that allows you to enjoy life. My home is littered with all the tools and ingredients from this chapter—not only because I live an adventurous life in which I am occasionally strained, sprained, or broken, but also because I want my body to recover from normal day-to-day activities far faster than it normally would, so that I can simply get more out of life!

Finally, should you want to know the best way to identify whether these methods are working, how recovered your body is, and whether your system is fully prepared to handle a rigorous workout or race, check out the sidebar on the Oura "readiness score," which is a simple way to measure how recovered you truly are.

The Best Way to Know Whether You Are Truly Recovered

While attending a biohacking conference in Helsinki, Finland, in 2015, I discovered a small, lonely table in the corner manned by a gentleman who had designed a unique ring for self-quantification. I found the ring—called the Oura—so intriguing that I purchased one from his small start-up company and spent the next year experimenting with the device to track my sleep, physical activity, stress levels, and more. Most importantly, I discovered that the Oura could be placed in airplane mode, disabling the Bluetooth and WiFi signals so commonly emitted by such devices.

Fast-forward to several years later, and the Oura ring has not only taken the world by storm but has also impressively upgraded its tracking capabilities, making it the number one tool I now use to track my readiness to train, using a built-in algorithm called the readiness score.

Ranging from 0 to 100 percent, the readiness score helps you identify the days that are ideal for challenging yourself and the days that are better for taking it easy. The score is affected by a variety of "readiness contributors" that evaluate the balance of your recent and cumulative sleep, physical activity, and recovery. Generally, a readiness score above 85 percent indicates that you are well recovered. A score below 70 percent usually means that an essential readiness contributor has either fallen outside of your normal range or clearly differs from recommended, science-based values.

The following are the most important variables that affect readiness:

- **The previous night's sleep:** How well you sleep has a significant impact on your performance the next day. For a maximum positive contribution to your readiness score, your sleep score needs to be above 85 percent and at the high end of your normal range.

- **Sleep balance:** Sleep balance shows you if your last two weeks of sleep are in line with your needs and is based on a long-term view of your sleep patterns. The ring compares your total time spent asleep in the last two weeks to your long-term sleep history and the amount of sleep recommended for your age. On average, adults need seven to nine hours of sleep per twenty-four hours to stay healthy and maintain peak performance.

- **Previous day:** Yesterday's level of physical activity is one of the primary factors that impacts your readiness score. A contributor bar that reads 100 percent tells you that you've gotten enough rest to balance out your activity and that you've spent a good amount of time performing low-intensity activity. A high amount of inactive time or excess activity causes your readiness score to drop. If your score drops because of intense exercise and high activity burn, you can improve your readiness and fitness by spending time recovering.

THE LAST WORD

If implementing all these recovery tools seems like overkill to you, then you are highly perceptive. After all, you don't need to do everything in this chapter if you have just gone out for a relaxed, sociable Saturday morning bike ride, or even after a typical week of minimalist training or low-level physical activity. But if you are injured, if you are an athlete and have an important competition approaching, if you are truly wiped out from a tough series of workouts, or if you are doing a big deload or rest-and-recovery week after a hard block of training, you should consider pulling out as many stops as possible and geeking out on recovery so that your body is 100 percent repaired from musculoskeletal damage, oxidative damage, chemical damage, or a combination of all three. Consider this chapter to be a cookbook for doing just that.

But maybe your head is spinning from trying to take in vibration platforms and EMS and lasers and proteo-something-or-other. Maybe you want to apply those tools to your own personal recovery plan without spending all your precious time fretting over recovery without enjoying your training or exposing your body to a constant state of underrecovery.

- **Activity balance:** Activity balance determines how your activity over the previous few days impacts your readiness score. A full bar indicates that you've been active but haven't gone all out or trained your absolute hardest, which allows you to recover and restore your energy.

- **Body temperature:** Body temperature is a well-regulated vital parameter. As you sleep, the Oura ring tracks your body temperature variations and compares that night's skin temperature to measures from previous nights. A full contributor bar indicates that your estimated body temperature is within normal variation. When your temperature falls outside of your typical range, your readiness score will fall.

- **Resting heart rate:** Your resting heart rate (RHR) is how many times your heart beats per minute when you are at rest. It's known to be a reliable marker of your state of recovery. By studying your data from active days and recovery days for a couple of weeks, the ring estimates your optimal RHR range, at which point your readiness score becomes more accurate. An RHR slightly below your average means you've recovered well and have good readiness. On the other hand, an unusually high or low RHR means you need to spend some extra time focusing on recovery. Intense training, a big meal right before bed, or an elevated body temperature can elevate your RHR through the night, resulting in a lower readiness score.

- **Recovery index:** Your recovery index tells you how long it takes your RHR to stabilize and reach its lowest point as you sleep. Ideally, you want your RHR to reach its lowest point at least six hours before waking. So if your RHR reaches that point during the first half of the night, it's a sign of excellent recovery. Consuming alcohol or food right before bed, getting sick, and working out late in the day can all elevate your RHR, thus delaying your recovery and causing your readiness score to drop.

- **Heart rate variability (HRV):** HRV is a measurement of the variation in the time interval between heartbeats, which, in an ideal recovery scenario, fluctuates mildly. Both researchers and practitioners consider HRV a good measure of your readiness status, as it can indicate stress and fatigue. Generally speaking, when you're fit, relaxed, and recovered, your HRV is higher. When your body is recovering from stress or strenuous exercise, your HRV is lower. The Oura ring app shows your average HRV (from five-minute measurements taken overnight) and your nightly HRV curve.

Unless you are trying to get yourself into an overreached or slightly overtrained state for the purposes of supercompensating and bouncing back with a higher level of fitness, I highly recommend that you pay attention to your readiness score. When I've ignored it and pushed through, nine times out of ten, it's led to illness and injury.

What would a typical recovery day, week, or month look like if you were uninjured and just trying to maximize the results of your training? What would it look like if you were injured and trying to heal your body as fast as possible? What would it look like if you were overtrained and in a state of chronic fatigue? What would it look like in those last few precious weeks leading up to a competition? What would it look like in the throes of healing your body from something like a Spartan Race or an Ironman or a marathon?

After all, properly programming these recovery techniques can take some serious forethought and scientific application. If you are concerned about how to string all this training and recovery material together into a viable and effective program that doesn't leave you gasping for air during a race because you spent too much time hanging from an inversion table or electrocuting yourself, don't worry. Here's a simple guide to a typical year of optimized recovery. Many of these strategies, such as infrared light or sauna, can be used while doing other productive activities, such as reading, listening to audiobooks, or working.

DAILY			
	Identify inflammatory foods (InflammationFactor.com is a good resource) and avoid them.		Apply full-body photobiomodulation for ten to twenty minutes.
	Fast for 12 to 16 hours.		Drink hydrogen-rich or structured water with minerals added.
	Self-administer foam rolling or deep-tissue work on any tight or sore spots, using books like *Becoming a Supple Leopard* and *Ready to Run* as "cookbook" guides for any areas that need detailed work.		Practice inversion for five to ten minutes.
	Use vibration therapy on any tight or sore spots.		Take 10 to 50 mg of CBD prior to bed.
	Take a quick cold shower or cold plunge every morning and evening.		Take three Kion Flex capsules on an empty stomach sometime during the day.
	Wear compression socks or tights during the day and when traveling.		Take 1 to 20 g of fish oil with one meal each day.

WEEKLY			
	Get a 60-to-90-minute massage.		Take one longer, 20-to-30-minute cold soak or cryotherapy session.
	Have a chiropractic adjustment (I personally swear by a weekly quick adjustment to shoulders, hips, back, and wrists).		Have between two and five 20-to-30-minute infrared sauna sessions.

Apply electrical muscle stimulation one to two times daily for 10 to 30 minutes, preferably combined with ice and topical magnesium or topical CBD.

 Apply pulsed electromagnetic field therapy throughout the day as often as possible. These devices can be worn throughout the day and night.

 Have a sixty-to-ninety-minute HBOT session once or twice a week, especially after periods of heavy workouts or airline travel.

 Take three Kion Flex capsules in the morning and another three in the evening.

 Take 20 to 40 g of Kion Aminos spread throughout the day.

 Adjust your training protocol so you can stay active with less intense activities (e.g., sauna; cold thermogenesis; walking; swimming; non-weight-bearing cardio such as rowing machine, cycling, and elliptical; light weights or bodyweight training combined with blood flow restriction bands).

 Use prolotherapy or stem cell therapy (optional).

 Sleep with magnets on the injured area (optional).

 Take a high-dose vitamin C supplement or get a vitamin C IV (optional).

ONE THING YOU CAN DO THIS WEEK

After your next workout, try one of the simplest recovery techniques in this chapter: inversion. Once you have cooled down from your workout, lie on your back with your feet up against a wall for about five minutes. Not only will you reactivate your "rest-and-digest" parasympathetic nervous system, but you will also recover far faster as blood and metabolic by-products make their way out of your legs. For an added bonus, use the alternate-nostril or box breathing techniques described in chapter 3.

For citations for all the research studies mentioned in this chapter and a deeper dive into the topics of this chapter—including links to podcasts, blog posts, recommended tools and supplements, and much more—visit BoundlessBook.com/12.

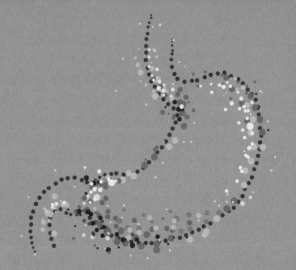

13

CLEAN GUT

HOW TO FIX YOUR GUT, OPTIMIZE DIGESTION, AND MAXIMIZE NUTRIENT ABSORPTION

From marijuana suppositories to coffee enemas to rocket-shaped cocoa butter anti-inflammatory capsules, I have put a lot of strange things up my butt. I have also experimented with just about every detoxification strategy on the face of the planet, from innocent techniques like dry skin brushing and trampolining to more advanced tactics, such as building an entire infrared sauna in my basement, then insulating it, sticking a wine cork in the temperature sensor, jacking up the heat to a level that would cause a Finnish Sauna Society member to spontaneously combust, and sitting in the sauna for hours on end, sweating like a detoxifying pig.

Why do I go through so much trouble? Frankly, it all comes down to attempting to crack the code on fixing the notorious digestive issues that seem to plague even the fittest of folks.

From the digestive glands in your mouth to your esophagus, gallbladder, stomach, small intestine, and colon, there are endless possibilities for what can go wrong in your digestive system. This chapter will focus on the nine primary issues that can create frustrating problems such as constipation, bloating, gas, brain fog, indigestion, leaky gut, irritable bowel syndrome, and a host of other digestive disturbances that can plague even the healthiest of individuals.

After all, boundless energy flows through the entire digestive system, and one of the best ways to avoid disrupting that flow is to have a healthy, flawless gut. This chapter will serve as the last resource you will ever need to unlock the mystery of any gut issue you may have. It explains how the gut breaks and how to fix it, unlocks the surprising truth about detoxification, demystifies food allergies and food intolerances, highlights the serious issue of glyphosate exposure, and even includes a handy guide to healing the gut from occasional bouts of hedonism.

DIGESTIVE SYSTEM 101

You are not alone if you think of your gut as one simple, long, twisting garden hose that extends from your mouth to your butt. Heck, even the classic *Gray's Anatomy*—a go-to manual for every aspiring medical student—describes the gut as "a musculomembranous tube, about thirty feet in length, extending from the mouth to the anus, and lined throughout its entire extent by mucous membrane."

But the gut is far more complex than that description suggests. For example, three-quarters of your immune system resides in your digestive tract. And that entire immune system is protected from the rest of the body by a thin, fragile lining only one cell thick. If that lining is damaged and the barrier that it creates is penetrated, you become allergic to foods you normally would have been able to digest without a problem, you get sick more easily, and your immune system becomes hyperactive, leading to systemic inflammation.

Your gut is also crawling with critters. Five hundred species and three pounds of bacteria in your digestive tract form a giant ecosystem that produces vitamins and other healing compounds and helps you digest food, regulate hormones, and excrete toxins.

Your gut is intimately tied to your brain and mood, too. This is called the brain-gut connection. Jordan Rubin describes this relationship quite well in his book *Patient, Heal Thyself*: "Early in our embryogenesis, a collection of tissue called the 'neural crest' appears and divides during fetal development. One part turns into the central nervous system, and the other migrates to become the enteric nervous system. Both 'thinking machines' form simultaneously and independently of one another until a later stage of development...then the two nervous systems link through a neural cable called the 'vagus nerve,' the longest of all cranial nerves. The vagus nerve 'wanders' from the brain stem through the organs in the neck and thorax and finally terminates in the abdomen. This is your vital brain-gut connection."

This brain-gut connection is why:

- you get butterflies in your stomach before going onstage
- you get nervous or have stomach cramps before a hard workout or race
- antidepressants cause nausea and stomach upset, and stomach upset can, ironically, depress you
- overeating when you are anxious helps your body produce extra feel-good chemicals, often creating a vicious cycle of face-stuffing
- stress makes you want to eat more, and eating more makes you feel stressed
- food intolerances or gut inflammation can cause behavioral issues
- an unhealthy digestive system can make you feel stupid or sluggish

Then there's your liver, which is also part of your digestive system. Your gut has to get rid of all the toxic by-products of digestion by transporting food components to your liver. If the liver, gallbladder, or gut is not functioning properly, toxins accumulate. Your liver destroys old red blood cells; manufactures proteins, blood-clotting agents, and cholesterol; stores glycogen, fats, and proteins; converts fats and proteins to carbohydrates and lactic acid to glucose; transforms galactose (milk sugar) into glucose; extracts ammonia from amino acids; converts ammonia to urea; produces bile; stores fat-soluble vitamins; converts adipose tissue into ketone bodies; and, finally, neutralizes pharmaceuticals and alcohol. The gallbladder, which is sadly absent in an increasing number of populations and is often considered a throwaway organ, stores and concentrates bile and, when not functioning properly, can cause post-meal nausea, bloating, indigestion, fatty stool, constipation, bacterial overgrowth, low thyroid activity, hunger, and blood sugar dys-regulation. (There's an excellent book about healing your gallbladder entitled *Radical Metabolism* by my friend and neighbor Ann Louise Gittleman.)

Just imagine what could happen if any of those important organs broke down. No wonder fixing your gut is at the root of fixing so many health problems.

THE 10 MOST COMMON GUT ISSUES AND HOW TO FIX THEM

While there are many things that can go wrong with the digestive system, most problems—from bloating and constipation to leaky gut, brain fog, and irritable bowel syndrome—can be traced back to ten main issues.

1. Gluten and Gliadin Sensitivities

I have to admit that I was a bit hesitant to begin this section with gluten because these days, everybody and their grandma, their kindergartner, and their dog seems to think they have a gluten intolerance. Sure, gluten intolerance is a legitimate problem and can bring on a host of problems ranging from gut inflammation to autoimmune disease and neurodegeneration. But, as you are about to learn, many people have a completely different problem that they incorrectly attribute to gluten intolerance.

Still, it's important to talk about gluten first so that you can determine if it's a problem for you. Let's begin by taking a look at gliadin, the gut-inflaming substance behind most gluten sensitivities.

Gliadin is a protein molecule found in most (but not all) gluten-containing foods, primarily wheat, rye, barley, kamut, spelt, teff, and couscous, with wheat being the most popular gliadin-containing grain. An inflammatory reaction to gliadin can take place in the small intestine in many people who do not have diagnosed celiac disease or gluten intolerance but who instead have what is called a subclinical sensitivity to gliadin. This is often the case in those of Irish, English, Scottish, Scandinavian, or other Northern and Eastern European ancestries. If you're wondering if your ancestry makes you more susceptible to gliadin sensitivity, you can perform an in-home ancestry test provided by 23andMe and get the results mailed to you, and you can also get a more in-depth and accurate gluten-sensitivity test from Cyrex Laboratories.

If you have a gliadin sensitivity and consume a food containing gliadin, it causes an inflammatory reaction in the gastrointestinal tract that involves heat, redness, swelling, and an interruption in the normal function of the small intestine. The blood vessels in the gut enlarge and become more permeable, which brings more white blood cells and other immune cells to the site of injury. In addition, fluids leak from these blood vessels into the surrounding tissues, bringing even more white blood cells for additional immune activity. A thin filament called fibrin (the same substance involved in blood clotting) also forms at the site of inflammation to aid in the intestinal wall's repair process. Within twelve to fifteen hours after the gliadin-containing meal has hit the gut and the inflammatory response has occurred, immune system activity diminishes, and

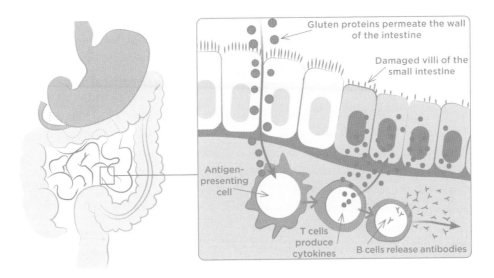

Gluten proteins permeate the wall of the intestine

Damaged villi of the small intestine

Antigen-presenting cell

T cells produce cytokines

B cells release antibodies

the gut is able to begin to slowly heal—assuming that there is no further gliadin exposure. But if you eat more gliadin-containing food, the entire inflammatory response repeats. A vicious cycle sets in and the gut is never allowed to heal before it's hammered with more inflammation.

This is why I am not a fan of a cheat meal of items such as pizza, hamburgers, and breaded and fried foods—you literally never give your gut a chance to fully heal, which generally takes around two weeks after removal of gliadin from the diet (so be patient if you do begin to moderate or remove gliadin!). I personally "cheat" with a tasty grass-fed rib-eye steak, a mess of baked sweet potato fries, brussels sprouts cooked with bacon, a glass of rich, organic red wine, and a bit of dark chocolate with coconut ice cream for dessert. In other words, when I cheat, I cheat with the good stuff.

Constant gliadin-induced inflammatory surges create many problems. First, there may be a loss of nutrient absorption. Your small intestine is lined with tiny, fingerlike projections called villi, which increase the surface area for absorption by up to a thousand times. This means that the absorptive surface area of your small intestine may be roughly the size of a basketball court! These villi allow you to efficiently absorb massive quantities of nutrients from your food. A substance that irritates the lining of the small intestine, like gliadin, can destroy the villi and significantly reduce the total available absorptive area. This not only affects your ability to absorb vital nutrients from food but also leads to indigestion. Typically, this manifests as bloating, tiredness, a hyperactive bowel, and sizable or uncomfortable bowel movements, especially during exercise.

Second, gliadin can increase gut permeability. Your small intestine has a mucosal lining, the same kind of tissue that lines your sinus passages, your lungs, your urinary tract, your mouth, and your throat. This mucous membrane protects your body from infection. Under the inflammatory stress that accompanies repeated gliadin exposure, the mucosal tissue breaks down, and your gut becomes extremely permeable, resulting in leaky gut syndrome. Having leaky gut syndrome is like using a water filter with big holes in it: stuff you don't want to drink gets through the holes and into your water instead of being filtered out. In the case of a leaky gut, undigested food particles, particularly proteins, pass through the intestinal barrier and into the bloodstream, resulting in an immune response in the blood and an enormous amount of stress as your body fights off these foreign particles. Gut permeability already increases as soon as you begin exercising, especially if you are exercising in the heat, and when this combines with the permeability caused by gliadin, the likelihood that you'll get sick, suffer from brain fog, have difficulty sleeping, and experience inadequate energy levels is vastly increased.

Nutrient malabsorption and a leaky gut aren't the only issues brought on by gluten and gliadin. Regular consumption of gluten-containing foods may also cause fat malabsorption and lactose intolerance, even if you weren't prone to them in the first place. Here's what happens with fat absorption: In the tips of your villi are lacteals, which are responsible for breaking down fat into tiny, absorbable droplets. When these lacteals are compromised, as when gliadin destroys villi, you can't properly absorb fat, which is crucial for producing hormones and building cell membranes. You also miss out on the absorption of fat-soluble vitamins, such as vitamins A and E. And yes, this means you may not be getting any benefits from those expensive fish oil pills you pop every day, and you also miss out on many of the benefits of sunlight and photobiomodulation. Fat deficiencies can result in poor blood sugar control, an inability to repair central nervous system damage, poor nerve cell function, low hormone production, and reduced antioxidant levels.

Then there is lactose intolerance. The enzyme lactase normally breaks down lactose in milk into a digestible and absorbable form. But a damaged intestinal wall can't adequately produce lactase, so many people who can normally eat cheese, yogurt, and ice cream can't do so when they consume gluten and gliadin. It is advisable to avoid milk products for several months after going gluten-free (yes, it takes that long for the lining of your digestive tract to heal). On the bright side, many people find that they can comfortably eat ice cream after giving up bread.

Incidentally, even if gluten doesn't bother your stomach, it can still cause brain inflammation and fuzzy thinking, concepts discussed in detail in the books *Why Isn't My Brain Working?*, by Dr. Datis Kharrazian, and *Grain Brain*, by Dr. David Perlmutter.

What can you do about gluten- and gliadin-related gut issues? First, obviously, avoid gluten- and gliadin-containing foods. This can be trickier than it sounds. Many naturally gluten-free foods are treated, processed, and packaged to contain gluten, so it is critical to check labels before loading up on groceries. In addition, some foods that seem like they wouldn't include gluten or gliadin actually do, such as these:

- Canned fruits and vegetables (especially when highly processed, sugary, or dried)
- Uncovered meats in the meat case in the butcher's section at the grocery store (crumbs and other glutinous products often fall in and cross-contaminate the meat)
- Highly processed nuts and seeds, like those found at gas stations and airports
- Chocolate bars that contain wheat or wheat-containing products, especially wafers, and chocolate-coated sweets. Plus, many chocolate bars are produced in facilities that also process other wheat-containing products.
- Nutrition, protein, energy, or weight-loss bars, which often contain wheat or gluten as a binding agent
- Canned soups or prepackaged soup mixes, which often contain gluten as a thickener
- So-called healthy popcorn snacks, which are often coated with not only gluten but also rancid vegetable oils

And then there's cross-reactivity. In some people, foods that do not contain any appreciable amount of gluten are still seen by the immune system as gluten and trigger a similar reaction. This happens because these foods have similar protein structures to gluten and therefore can trigger antigluten antibodies. The foods most often associated with gluten cross-reactivity are these:

- Dairy products (specifically the alpha-casein, beta-casein, casomorphin, butyrophilin, and whey found in dairy)
- Chocolate
- Coffee

- Soy
- Sorghum
- Eggs
- Corn
- Millet
- Oats
- Rice
- Yeast
- Quinoa
- Tapioca

If you do eat glutinous foods, you can take peptidases (often sold as "gluten enzymes") to help break down the gluten. One of my favorite brands is Gluten Guardian—if you break open the capsules and sprinkle it on a slice of bread, it can cause the bread to actually dissolve before your very eyes. To heal a damaged gut lining and reduce gluten-induced gut permeability, you can drink a few cups of an organic bone broth each day (unless you are sensitive to histamines, in which case you may be sensitive to bone broth) and consume marshmallow root supplements, licorice extract, colostrum, L-glutamine, aloe vera juice, chia seeds, probiotics, and digestive enzymes.

Finally, if you want to take the gold-standard test for gluten sensitivity and intolerance, I highly recommend asking your physician to order you a test through Cyrex Laboratories, which has the most thorough gluten-reactivity screening available. Cyrex is the screening method that I recommend for most forms of food allergies and intolerances because so many of the other available tests, such as ALCAT and ELISA, are inaccurate, give a host of false positives, or both.

2. FODMAP Sensitivity

As common as gluten and gliadin sensitivities are, many people with gut distress don't suffer from either of them. This may be especially true if you eat properly prepared, low-gluten or gluten-free grains and fermented foods and still find you have gut issues.

One study found that people with self-reported gluten sensitivities actually had no adverse effects in the gut from eating gluten. In fact, they experienced complete elimination of their gut issues after reducing their consumption of a kind of poorly absorbed, short-chain carbohydrates called fermentable oligosaccharides, disaccharides, monosaccharides, and polyols—more commonly known as FODMAPs. The researchers reported that in all participants, gastrointestinal symptoms consistently and significantly improved during reduced FODMAP intake but significantly worsened when their diets included gluten or whey protein—meaning that combining gluten (even small amounts) with high-FODMAP foods can be a quite problematic one-two combo for many people.

Gluten-induced gut issues are present in a broad spectrum of patients with clinical presentations of irritable bowel syndrome (IBS). But a study published in the journal *Nutrients* found that IBS patients put on a low-FODMAP diet experienced significantly less abdominal pain and bloating than patients who received a high-FODMAP diet, even when gluten was present in the diet.

In other words, it may not be gluten that's upsetting your gut but rather combining gluten-containing foods with FODMAPs, or even FODMAPs all by themselves. How could this happen? Let's back up for a moment and look into what FODMAPs are.

I do indeed eat bread—but it is the mouthwatering, slow-fermented sourdough bread that my wife Jessa makes. The process of fermentation used in sourdough bread not only predigests the gluten but also reduces the glycemic index of the bread, making it far more friendly to your gut and blood sugar levels.

Lest you think that you can go to the grocery store and grab any old sourdough loaf, it is important to note that the fermentation process capable of breaking down gluten is called slow fermentation. Many sourdoughs are short-fermented sourdoughs and are made quickly with chemicals and acids that impart a soured taste without actually allowing natural yeasts and lactic acid bacteria to work through the grain. If you want to experience the full benefits of sourdough, make sure to find a baker who makes slow-fermented sourdough or learn how to make it at home.

This is my wife Jessa's sourdough recipe, in all its tasty, mildly addictive glory. I highly recommend serving it with a pat of grass-fed butter, a drizzle of raw honey or blackstrap molasses, and a sprinkling of coarse salt.

- 1 cup sourdough starter
- 1 cup lukewarm water
- 2 teaspoons salt
- 3 to 4 cups organic all-purpose flour

1. *In a large mixing bowl, combine the starter, water, and salt and mix well. Add 2 cups of the flour and stir until well combined. Allow the mixture to rest for 5 minutes.*

2. *After 5 minutes, add more flour ½ cup at a time, until the dough is sticky but can be handled. Sprinkle the counter with flour, place the dough on the flour, and knead (the dough should feel elastic and easy to knead). Continue to add small amounts of flour at a time while kneading until the dough does not stick to your hands. Knead for 10 to 15 minutes for a high-gluten flour, less for flours with less gluten, like einkorn wheat flour.*

3. *Place the dough in a large mixing bowl and cover it with plastic wrap. Allow the dough to sit for at least 8 hours or overnight at room temperature. The dough should double in size.*

4. *Pop it out of the bowl, knead in about 2 tablespoons of flour, and shape the dough to fit whatever you'll be baking it in, such as a loaf pan. If you are using a loaf pan, grease it now. If you are using a traditional proofing basket, sprinkle it with flour. Place the shaped loaf in the pan or basket and loosely cover it with plastic wrap. Place it on the countertop and let it rise for 2 to 4 hours. You will know it is ready when it is close to or fully doubled in size.*

5. *Preheat the oven to 550°F or the hottest setting (sourdough likes it hot!). If you are using a proofing basket, place a cookie sheet in the oven before preheating. Once the oven is preheated, turn the temperature down to 450°F. If you are using a proofing basket, take the cookie sheet out and gently flip the loaf out of the basket and onto the cookie sheet.*

6. *Place the loaf in the oven and bake for 10 minutes. Turn the temperature down to 350°F and bake for an additional 30 minutes, or until the bread sounds hollow when you knock on it or the internal temperature is 190°F.*

7. *If you are using a loaf pan, remove the pan from the oven and place it on a wire rack to cool. If you are using a cookie sheet, use hot pads to transfer the bread out to a wire rack.*

8. *Allow the bread to cool completely before cutting into it, preferably with a serrated knife to avoid any problematic crumbling.*

TIP: Whole-wheat flour tends to absorb water less quickly, so if you use it, be patient in step 1 and allow the flour mixture to rest for the full 5 minutes. Too little water or too much flour results in a useless brick of dough.

NOTE: A proofing basket is generally made of wicker and is used to produce a rustic, artisan-style bread. It's used during the second ferment of the sourdough, and when you transfer the dough from the basket to the cookie sheet, you will see the spiral design of the basket imprinted on the loaf.

Many of the foods that we commonly eat, even in a healthy diet, are called high-residue foods: when they're digested, these foods leave behind a lot of extra matter, such as lactose, indigestible fiber, and other plant particles, for bacteria to feed on. When bacteria feed and proliferate, fermentation begins, and when there's fermentation in your gut, it causes bloating, cramping, gas, constipation, and diarrhea. What foods tend to ferment more or faster than others? You guessed it: FODMAPs.

FODMAPs often cause symptoms beyond gut-related distress, such as depression, fatigue, headaches, or brain fog (which makes sense, given that whole brain-gut connection you already learned about).

Below is a list of the major high-FODMAP foods. While I am certainly not advocating that you cut these foods out of your diet completely, you may find that when you consume large amounts of them, especially at a single meal or in one day, significant gut issues arise, and that when you eliminate these foods, you can eat gluten-containing foods without a problem. If all of this seems a bit overwhelming, the top two foods to eliminate right away are onions and garlic, the biggest culprits in those with FODMAP sensitivities.

- **Fruit, agave, and honey:** Fructose is a monosaccharide (the M in "FODMAPs") fruit sugar. Fruits that are higher in fructose include melons and tropical fruits such as mangoes, and fruits high in polyols (the P in "FODMAPs"), such as apples, peaches, and pears, also contain high amounts of fructose, as do sweeteners like high-fructose corn syrup, honey, and agave. And of course, fructose is a major ingredient in most sports gels and drinks, so if sports gels make your digestive system go awry, fructose could be the reason.

- **Beans and lentils:** Oligosaccharides are short strands of simple sugars present in all beans and lentils. Maltodextrin, which is found in many sports gels, is also an oligosaccharide, as are isomaltooligosaccharides (IMOs) and other forms of so-called low-carb fiber found in many energy bars. Interestingly, IMOs, despite being marketed as low-carb and appearing in a host of "low-carb" energy bars, along with inulin, are notorious for spiking blood sugar.

- **Wheat, onions, and cabbage:** The culprit in all these is a sugar called fructan, which is found in wheat, onions, scallions, garlic, and cruciferous vegetables such as cabbage and cauliflower. Surprisingly, wheat is even found in many sports bars and energy chews.

- **Dairy:** Lactose, the sugar found in dairy (especially in unfermented forms such as milk, as opposed to yogurt or kefir), is a disaccharide. Large amounts of lactose are found in many postworkout recovery drinks.

- **Sugar alcohols:** Sugar alcohols are also called polyols, which makes them one of the substances FODMAPs are named for. They're also used as sweeteners, especially in sugar-free and so-called health foods, diabetic candy, toothpaste, and chewing gum. Xylitol, maltitol, and sorbitol are examples of sugar alcohols found in many packaged and processed foods. Some sugar alcohols are not as bad as others: xylitol is better tolerated than mannitol, sorbitol, and disaccharide polyols like lactitol, and erythritol's structure and molecular weight keep it from causing the negative reactions seen with other polyols. But sugar alcohols are used as alternative, low-calorie sweeteners because they bypass digestion, and this is known to cause gastrointestinal distress. In most folks, erythritol seems to be the best-tolerated sugar alcohol.

As you may already know from personal experience or pure common sense, eating an entire plate of sautéed onions or a bowl of roasted garlic is probably going to give you gas. Indeed, for most people who have FODMAP issues, onions and garlic tend to be the biggest culprits (although if you are using garlic for its tremendous antimicrobial and antifungal properties, you can take a supplement such as Allimax, which contains high amounts of allicin, the active ingredient in garlic, without causing fermentation issues). You also probably wouldn't mow down a few bowls of beans and lentils or eat a smoothie made with four or five apples and not expect to feel some funky repercussions in your gut. But you can create a nuclear bomb in your gut by consuming 50 to 100 g of fructose and maltodextrin per hour from sports gels during or before a workout or race, downing a wheat-filled energy bar every afternoon at work, or sucking down a lactose-laden postworkout recovery shake or a coffee cup full of heavy creamer in the morning.

While you can get a breath test for FODMAP reactivity similar to that designed for small intestinal bacterial overgrowth (which is discussed later in this chapter and often goes hand in hand with FODMAP issues), a simpler way to assess the situation is to eliminate the major high-FODMAP foods from your diet and observe how you feel—which is basically an "elimination diet" strategy. If you have gas, bloating, indigestion, or other gut problems, I highly suggest that you photocopy the tables on the facing page, stick them on your fridge for easy reference, try a low-FODMAP diet for a week, and see what happens. You may also want to download the Monash University FODMAP Diet app, a handy, relatively inexpensive app that helps you identify foods that are high in FODMAPs.

Finally, if you do eat FODMAPs, you can undo some of the damage with a blend of herbs found in over-the-counter supplements (similar to the way gluten enzymes can assist with gluten sensitivities). One of these supplements, Atrantil, capitalizes on the potency of different plants' polyphenols, which both reduce the effects of some of the bad bacteria and nourish your good bacteria. Atrantil contains three botanicals: peppermint, which relaxes the small intestine and allows the other two to do their work more effectively; quebracho, which soaks up the hydrogen that can fuel uncomfortable methane production and also disrupts the cell walls of methane-producing bacteria; and horse chestnut, which enters the disrupted cells' walls and inhibits the enzyme that allows methane to be produced. After the polyphenols do their work in the small intestine, they move into the colon and are broken down into prebiotics for good bacteria.

3. Insufficient Digestive Enzymes and Low Enzyme Activity

I often see this problem in people who stress their guts by eating large amounts of food, eating in a stressed state, or eating before, during, or after exercise or in a tired, postworkout state. When you consume a meal, an energy bar, or a sports drink, your pancreas and small intestine secrete enzymes that break down proteins, carbohydrates, and fats into absorbable nutrients.

Meat, eggs, and beans, for example, consist of large protein molecules that must be broken down by these enzymes before they can be used to build and repair body tissues. Pepsin, an enzyme found in the digestive juices of the stomach, starts the digestion of protein. Then, in the small intestine, several enzymes secreted by the pancreas and the lining of the intestine complete the breakdown of these protein molecules into even smaller molecules—amino acids. These amino acids can then be absorbed into the blood and carried to all parts of the body.

But there can be problems that keep these enzymes from completely breaking down your food. The amount of food you eat can exceed the capacity of your digestive enzymes, a scenario typical

FOODS SUITABLE ON A LOW-FODMAP DIET

Fruit	• banana • blueberry • boysenberry • cantaloupe	• cranberry • durian • grape • grapefruit	• honeydew melon • kiwifruit • lemon • lime	• mandarin orange • passionfruit • pawpaw • raspberry	• rhubarb • rockmelon • star anise • strawberry • tangelo
Vegetables	• alfalfa • bamboo shoots • bean shoots • bok choy	• carrot • celery • choko • choy sum • endive • ginger	• green beans • lettuce • olives • parsnip • potato • pumpkin	• red capsicum (bell pepper) • silver beet • spinach • squash • swede	• sweet potato • taro • tomato • turnip • yam • zucchini
Herbs	• basil • chili • coriander	• ginger • lemongrass • marjoram	• mint • oregano • parsley	• rosemary • thyme	

Grain Foods	• gluten-free
	  bread or cereal
	  products
		• 100% spelt bread
		• rice
			• oats
			• polenta
				OTHER
				• arrowroot
				• millet
					• psyllium
					• quinoa
					• sorghum
					• tapioca

Milk Products	**MILK**
	• lactose-free
	  milk*
	• oat milk*
		• rice milk*
		• soy milk*
			CHEESES
			• hard cheeses
			• Brie
			• Camembert
				ICE CREAM SUBSTITUTES
				• gelato
				• sorbet
					BUTTER SUBSTITUTE
					• olive oil
					YOGURT
					• lactose-free
					  varieties

Other	**SWEETENERS**
	• sugar**
	  (sucrose)
	• glucose
		• artificial
		  sweeteners not
		  ending in "-ol"
			HONEY SUBSTITUTES
			• golden syrup**
			• maple syrup**
				• molasses
				• treacle	

Check for additives
**Small quantities*

FOODS TO ELIMINATE ON A LOW-FODMAP DIET

Excess Fructose	**FRUIT**
	• apple
	• mango
	• nashi
	• pear
		• canned fruit
		  in natural juice
		• watermelon
			• concentrated fruit
			  sources
			• large servings
			  of fruit
				• dried fruit
				• fruit juice
					SWEETENERS
					• fructose
					• high-fructose
					  corn syrup
					• honey

Lactose	**MILK**
	• milk from cows,
	  goats, or sheep
		• custard ice cream
		• yogurt
			CHEESES
			• soft unripened
			  cheeses
			• cottage
				• cream
				• mascarpone
				• ricotta	

Fructans	**VEGETABLES**
	• artichokes
	• asparagus
	• beetroot
	• broccoli
	• brussels sprouts
	• cabbage
		• eggplant
		• fennel
		• garlic
		• leek
		• okra
		• onions (all)
		• shallots
		• spring onions
			CEREALS
			• wheat and rye in
			  large amounts, e.g.
			  bread, crackers,
			  cookies, couscous,
			  pasta
				FRUIT
				• custard apple
				• persimmon
				• watermelon
					MISCELLANEOUS
					• chicory
					• dandelion
					• inulin
					• pistachio

Galactans	**LEGUMES** • baked beans • chickpeas	• kidney beans	• lentils • soybeans		
Polyols	**FRUIT** • apple • apricot • avocado • blackberry	• cherry • longon • lychee • nashi	• pear • plum • prune • watermelon	**VEGETABLES** • cauliflower • green capsicum (bell pepper) • mushroom • sweet corn	**SWEETENERS** • sorbitol • mannitol • isomalt • maltitol • xylitol

among active, calorie-devouring individuals. Or your pancreas or small intestine can have a genetic inability to produce a certain enzyme, such as lactase. Or perhaps your gut is ravaged from periods of poor eating, gliadin exposure, and the like and is simply unable to produce enough enzymes. Sometimes, enzymatic activity declines because of intense physical activity—so, for example, there may not be enough enzymes to handle that protein shake you slurp down immediately after walking in the door from a hard run. Whatever the case, if your digestive tract can't produce enough enzymes or the enzymes simply aren't working, then nutrients are not completely digested. (Undigested protein is particularly likely to pass through a damaged intestinal wall into the bloodstream and cause inflammation.)

How do you know if you have a digestive enzyme insufficiency? The best way to know is with a stool test, such as a three-day Genova protocol, which involves multiple stool collections that you send to a lab. The lab measures the presence of bacteria, parasites, yeasts, fungi, and other compounds. The lab also measures how well you digest your food and how well your pancreas produces digestive enzymes. Most doctors won't run these tests, and they may not be covered by insurance, but you can oversee the process yourself. The report you get with the test results is pretty self-explanatory.

You can also pay attention to symptoms. Symptoms of digestive enzyme problems include the following:

- Gas and bloating after meals
- Feeling as if you have food sitting in your stomach after you eat
- Feeling full after eating a few bites of food
- Seeing undigested food in your stool
- Frequent and consistent floating stool
- An "oil slick" in the toilet bowl (indicative of undigested fat)

The fixes for digestive enzyme insufficiencies are simple:

- Clean up your diet using some of the strategies you have already learned about, such as avoiding excessive calories, eating when relaxed, and not eating too close to or during exercise, so that your gut can produce adequate digestive enzymes.
- Eat more slowly and mindfully, and avoid rushed, hectic meals. Eating in a relaxed emotional state increases stomach acid production, which aids protein digestion, liberates digestive enzymes for the breakdown of fats, proteins, and sugars, and enhances peristalsis, the wavelike muscle contractions that move food along the digestive tract. My family and I all take one to three deep, slow breaths in through our nose and out through our mouths before every meal, even at restaurants. Try it sometime!
- Engage in intermittent fasts of twelve to sixteen hours daily to give your gut a break. (See page 305 for more on fasting.)
- Jump-start your digestion by taking digestive enzymes (preferably packaged with HCL and bile; Thorne Bio-Gest is a good option) before you eat, and use some of the strategies to reduce glycemic variability from chapter 8.

- If you do need to eat while stressed, in a hurry, or in a postworkout state, try to blend and grind your foods as much as possible so that your digestive system has less work to do. For this reason, I believe every kitchen should be equipped with a good blender, a juicer, a mortar and pestle, and a food processor.

- Fix inflammation. When inflammation is not controlled, the body's ability to make bile is downregulated, but when inflammation is healed, the body's ability to make bile improves. (There's plenty on controlling inflammation in chapters 8 and 12.)

Finally, no discussion of enzymatic issues and nutrient malabsorption would be complete without a nod to your gallbladder. The bile produced by your gallbladder is potent for enhancing digestion of all foods, particularly fat. If your gallbladder is sluggish or not working correctly, even digestive enzymes won't work quite as well. To maximize gallbladder function and health, I recommend ample use of digestifs and bitters before a meal (such as my favorite mix of a little ginger, black pepper, raw honey, and lemon juice), a spoonful of sauerkraut, a digestive enzyme that contains ox bile extract, or a supplement such as Quicksilver Scientific's Dr. Shade's Bitters No. 9. In a pinch, you can even use common cocktail bitters that you would normally add to an alcoholic drink. Mix them in sparkling water or lemon juice. In addition, consider the use of herbal gallbladder-drainage homeopathic remedies, which can be very effective for people with a sluggish gallbladder or the need for increased bile production. A good brand is Pekana.

The book *Radical Metabolism* by Ann Louise Gittleman is an excellent guide for your gallbladder and other digestive issues related to enzyme production or slow digestion, and for even more on bile, listen to the podcast with guest Kelly Halderman, MD, at BetterHealthGuy.com/episode79, in which Dr. Halderman describes bile in detail and recommends specific supplements to help the body make and secrete bile more effectively, including milk thistle, pantothenic acid (vitamin B_5), acetyl-L-carnitine, bitters, phosphatidylcholine, and ox bile.

4. Insufficient Gut Bacteria

A healthy human body has more than 100 trillion microorganisms in its intestines, which is ten times more than the total number of human cells in the body. The metabolic activities performed by gut microflora resemble those of an organ: they train the immune system, attack foreign invaders such as toxins, prevent the growth of harmful pathogenic bacteria in your gut, regulate the development of the intestinal lining, produce vitamins such as biotin and vitamin K, and even produce hormones.

So how do your gut bacteria become imbalanced? In my article "The Art of Using Antibiotics: How to Limit the Damage" (BenGreenfieldFitness.com/anti)—which I highly recommend you read if you have ever been on antibiotics—I explained how pharmaceuticals can deprive your body of precious probiotics. A low-fiber diet can also result in insufficient gut flora. Prebiotics are fiber-based sugars from fruits and vegetables that provide sustenance to probiotics. An inadequate intake of fermented foods rich in good bacteria can also be an issue, especially in a modern Western diet. Unfortunately, most commercial probiotic foods have been pasteurized (which kills the beneficial bacteria), are packaged improperly, or have lots of added sugars to satisfy palates conditioned to sweet foods.

If you do have insufficient levels of gut bacteria, you are likely to experience some serious performance-inhibiting issues, including these:

- The complete absence of gas (yes, you actually stop farting)
- Undigested fiber in your stool, which appears as white or dark specks
- Constipation, with occasional periods of diarrhea or IBS
- Frequent sickness and allergies
- Blood-clotting problems
- Neurological problems and brain fog
- Decreased physical performance

The Crosstalk Between the Gut Microbiota and Mitochondria During Exercise

Your mitochondria play a crucial role in energy generation and the production of reactive oxygen species (ROS) and reactive oxygen nitrogen species (RONS), along with regulation of inflammatory by-products, particularly from endurance exercise. Endurance exercise is beneficial because it can prevent mitochondrial DNA depletion and mutations, promote mitochondrial biogenesis, and increase mitochondrial oxidative and antioxidant capacity.

But chronic stress, particularly from overtraining, can produce inflammation in the gut, which, in turn, causes stress that promotes the movement of toxic lipopolysaccharides from the gut to the bloodstream, as well as the growth of harmful bacteria in the gut. This is why endurance athletes who don't consume the high-carb foods made popular in the marathoning craze of the 1980s and promoted by the Gatorade Sports Science Institute—such as scones, biscotti, processed grains, and sugary drinks, gels, and bars—can still experience gut distress, bloating, constipation, and many other GI issues.

Science is still in the infancy of understanding the bi-directional communication between the gut microbiota and mitochondria, but several studies have shown that gut microbiota molecules, including short-chain fatty acids such as butyrate, are essential for controlling mitochondrial oxidative stress, inflammatory response, and pathogen growth, and also significantly improve metabolism and energy expenditure during exercise.

Furthermore, short-chain fatty acids and their precursors—such as those found in butter, coconut oil, buckwheat, quinoa, millet, amaranth, cultured vegetables, coconut water, kefir, and probiotic beverages—

can induce mitochondrial biogenesis through a variety of mechanisms such as an increase in the activity of PCG-1α (a key regulator of energy metabolism), an increase in redox sensitive energy sensor SIRT1 (a cell-protective and antiaging pathway), and an increase in the enzyme AMPK (crucial for ATP production), all of which suppress inflammatory responses and enhance the beneficial effects of exercise.

Dampening inflammation and oxidative stress during endurance exercise is an ideal approach to restricting the growth of pathogens in the gut as well as the detrimental effects of those pathogens on mitochondrial functions. While treating inflammatory responses with diet is still a challenge, making the right nutritional shifts to tone down oxidative stress can promote the growth of healthy gut bacteria and, thus, protect proper mitochondrial function and gut health during exercise.

But it's not just gut bacteria talking to mitochondria—mitochondria affect gut bacteria, too. Mitochondrial ROS production influences the integrity of your intestinal barrier and mucosal immune responses, which regulate the balance and quality of your gut microbiota. Even mitochondrial DNA mutations can affect the function of gut bacteria, and mutations in mitochondrial genes and oxidative stress can impact your microbiota.

So if you want to perform at your best, you must care for your gut bacteria eating foods rich in healthy short-chain fatty acids, and you must also care for your mitochondria by consuming mineral-rich water and electrolytes, getting enough sunlight and infrared light exposure, grounding, and using pulsed electromagnetic field therapy, cold thermogenesis, and heat therapy.

If you suspect that you have insufficient gut bacteria levels, I recommend the three-day Genova gut-testing kit to test for the presence of bacteria, or even a complete microbiome analysis, which is offered by companies such as Viome and Onegevity. If you discover that you have insufficient bacteria or you have many of the symptoms described above, you have to re-populate your gut with good bacteria and consume adequate amounts of fiber and prebiotics. I recommend the following 1-2-3 combo:

1. **Consume a wide variety of fermented foods,** such as kimchi, sauerkraut, and pickled vegetables, along with yogurts, kefirs, miso, natto, and other foods with naturally occurring good bacteria. This one-two combo provides both good bacteria and the fiber that feeds them. (For a comprehensive guide to finding fermented foods and even preparing your own, see my article "Fermentation: It's What's for Dinner" at BeyondTrainingBook.com/wfxfermentation.) Some people wonder whether prebiotics and fiber can feed the pathogenic bacteria, too, but that's not really the case. While some in-vitro research suggests that certain prebiotics may promote the growth of pathogens like klebsiella, these test-tube experiments do not relate to real-life scenarios in the human gut. The vast majority of evidence demonstrates that prebiotics mainly promote the growth of beneficial bacteria, which, if supplementation with prebiotics is continued, typically outweighs any simultaneous growth of bad bacteria. As good bacteria flourish with prebiotic supplementation and fermented-food intake, the pH of the gut tends to decrease, which is a natural deterrent to the growth of pathogens. When combined with the good bacteria's antipathogenic effects, this helps maintain a healthy balance of good and bad bacteria in your gut.

2. **Consume a full-spectrum probiotic,** such as Seed (my preferred source, as this particular brand seems to be best at populating the gut), Caprobiotics, Thorne Floramend, or VSL-3, along with a soil-based probiotic such as Prescript Assist (which tends to do a decent job surviving the gut to get to where it needs to be but has fewer bacterial strains than Seed). If you have ever been on antibiotics (even if it was years ago!), also take *Saccharomyces boulardii* (Jarrow Formulas and Orthomolecular are good brands). Most of the best probiotic supplements include *Lactobacillus* and *Bifidobacterium*, two of the most-studied strains of gut bacteria. It is a good idea to switch supplement brands every month or two, especially if you are not eating a wide variety of fermented foods. At the time of this writing, the company Seed appears to be developing quite a potent probiotic called a "symbiotic" that can better survive the harsh acidic environment of the stomach and repopulate the gut far more efficiently than other probiotics.

3. **Consume plenty of vegetables and moderate amounts of fiber from other sources,** such as seeds and nuts, to feed the probiotics. If eating salads, smoothies, and plant matter is logistically tough for you, consider a greens powder or greens supplement that is rich in polyphenols, flavonols, and prebiotics and that is derived from organic greens (no exposure to pesticides or herbicides). Good brands include Organifi Green Juice, Living Fuel SuperGreens, Athletic Greens, and EnerPrime.

Prebiotics, Probiotics, Postbiotics, and Modbiotics Decoded

Probiotic is a common term in health and nutrition circles, but prebiotics, postbiotics, and modbiotics tend to fly under the radar. What are they, exactly?

As you probably already know, probiotics are gut-dwelling bacteria: living microorganisms that enjoy a symbiotic relationship with their human host. A prebiotic is a substance that is generally indigestible by humans but nourishes probiotics. Prebiotics include oligosaccharides, arabinogalactans, fructooligosaccharides, and inulin, which are found abundantly in vegetables, grains, and roots. It is important to remember that prebiotics are water-soluble fiber, not insoluble fiber, which is found in foods such as legumes, oats, rice bran, barley, citrus, and potatoes. Insoluble fiber promotes healthy bowel movements and is the fiber that is often recommended for healthy digestion, but it does not selectively fuel growth of beneficial bacteria in the colon in the same way as soluble fiber. However, if you're eating a widely varied whole-foods diet that's rich in plants, tubers, and legumes, you'll get plenty of both forms of fiber.

Postbiotics are exactly what their name suggests: the by-products of probiotics after they have fermented and metabolized prebiotics. Research has shown that postbiotics, which were long thought to be mere metabolic waste, are key factors in maintaining long-term digestive health. In fact, some research suggests that postbiotics may bestow many of the health benefits of healthy probiotic populations—even without the presence of probiotics themselves.

Modbiotics are compounds that influence the growth of gut microbiota through their antibacterial, antifungal, and antiparasitic properties. They can reduce excessive firmicutes (sugar-eating bacteria that drive inflammation, oxidative stress, and metabolic acidosis) and increase gut bacteroidetes (a class of bacteria that are beneficial in the gut but can be harmful when they migrate to other parts of the body).

The interesting fact about naturally occurring modbiotics is that they always occur alongside the sugars that feed firmicutes. So if you eat a natural source of sugars, such as a handful of pomegranate seeds, you get a large dose of modbiotics that would combat the negative effects of harmful sugar-eating bacteria. Modern processed foods high in sugar do not usually contain modbiotics, and neither does the average bottle of so-called superfood juice from the health food store—you need to get modbiotics from whole-food sources.

In summary, to fully capitalize on the power of your gut bacteria, your diet needs to be rich in prebiotic, probiotic, and modbiotic foods. Since postbiotics are the by-products of probiotic metabolism, you do not necessarily need to include postbiotic supplements in your diet, although research does suggest that they can aid in digestion, and a growing number of supplement companies are now selling blends of commonly known by-products of bacterial metabolism, including short-chain fatty acids, antimicrobial peptides (AMPs), B vitamins, vitamin K, amino acids, hydrogen peroxide, and enzymes. Prebiotic foods include raw asparagus, underripe bananas, raw leeks, raw garlic, raw Jerusalem artichoke, raw dandelion greens, and raw or cooked onions. Probiotic foods include yogurt, kefir, coconut kefir, kimchi, kombucha, sauerkraut, natto (fermented soybeans), raw cheese, apple cider vinegar (with the "mother"), and salted gherkin pickles. Make sure that the probiotic foods you consume contain live bacteria cultures and are not pasteurized or heat treated, which kills the bacteria.

To get a good amount of modbiotics, the average diet needs to contain more fruit peels, pulp, fiber, seeds, and skins. Potatoes, lettuce, onions, garlic, ginger, turmeric, tomatoes, green beans, broccoli, coriander, mint, apples, cherries, and pineapple are also good modbiotic sources. Active individuals in particular need to eat a host of whole-food sources of modbiotics so that their digestive systems can keep up with their dietary loads. If you're concerned about lectins or other digestive irritants present in the skins and peels of plants and produce, don't worry: you can generally prepare whole foods to limit the effects of irritants. For example, in the case of a pomegranate, you can dry the skin in a food dehydrator, then pulverize it in a blender or food processor for a modbiotic- and antioxidant-rich powder; and you can juice or blend a mixture of the flesh and the seeds. In the same way that nose-to-tail eating—rather than just eating the muscle meat—has a myriad of benefits, so does eating all parts of a plant, not just the flesh—especially when it comes to the health of your gut.

If this all sounds very complex, the takeaway message is this: eat a diet that includes a wide variety of plant matter, including the outside and the inside of the vegetables, and a moderate amount of natural fruits, along with a diverse array of fermented foods, and you'll be guaranteed to get prebiotics, modbiotics, and probiotics, and your probiotics will have what they need to produce postbiotics.

Finally, if your bacterial insufficiency includes a strange absence of gas accompanied by frequent constipation, which can happen if you have been on some big antibiotic regimens, and you want the shotgun, fix-everything-all-at-once approach, the best solution I have found (if you are not interested in the trendy world of fecal transplants and poop pills) is reinoculating your large intestine with a bacterial strain. There are two options for this: a probiotic enema or the use of a probiotic that can survive the acidic environment of the stomach and effectively "seed" the gut (I prefer the probiotic SEED for this, although an enema is still more effective). Both approaches seed your large intestine with good bacteria without the mess or expense of fecal transplantation or the consumption of someone else's number two. (If you are interested in fecal transplantation, there's a section on it in chapter 19.)

Other strategies that can be helpful to heal the gut after an antibiotic regimen include anything that can be used to heal a leaky gut, particularly colostrum, L-glutamine, John Douillard's "decoction tea" (see page 363 for the recipe), and bone broth.

The Probiotic Enema

As gross or off-putting as it may sound, you can repopulate your good gut bacteria by sticking a tube up your butt and funneling probiotics into your colon—very much like a coffee enema, but with probiotics rather than a cup o' joe. My friend Matt Gallant is a professional poker player and biohacker who has created a recipe for a probiotic enema. It maximizes absorption by minimizing the distance that the probiotics have to travel through the digestive tract, bypassing the acidity of the stomach, and mainlining the bacteria directly into the colon.

For this enema recipe, you will need:

- 1 liter of coconut water
- 5 capsules of Matt's P3-OM Probiotics (for a discount code, visit BoundlessBook.com/13)
- 2 butyric acid (butyrate) capsules (optional, for an even more beneficial effect)
- A large glass jar with a lid, such as a 32-ounce mason jar

If you are too squeamish to give yourself an enema, you can also drink this mixture over two days after it is cultured and refrigerated. (If you decide to drink it, I recommend adding sweeteners, such as pureed fruits like blueberries or strawberries, maple syrup, or liquid stevia.) But as uncomfortable as it may sound, the quickest route is right up the back door.

1. In a large mixing bowl, mix the coconut water and P3-OM capsules with a fork, whisk, or latte frother. (If you're using butyric capsules, break them open and add them to the mixture too.) Pour the whole mixture into the glass jar and put the lid on it.

2. Let the mixture ferment at room temperature for three to six hours, until you see bubbles in the mixture (the warmer the room, the less time you'll need). You can even leave it overnight.

3. Once the whole probiotic bath is cultured and you can see bubbles, keep it refrigerated until you are ready to use it. To administer the enema, you will need an enema tube (you can find the full stainless steel enema kit I use on BoundlessBook.com/13). Administer the mixture, then hang upside down from an inversion table or yoga trapeze, or lay on your back with your legs up against the wall, for about 20 minutes to let the mixture soak in.

5. Too Much Gut Bacteria

Small intestinal bacterial overgrowth (SIBO) tends to fly under the radar, but it can be problematic in people who consume a high-carbohydrate diet (because bacteria in the gut readily feed on sugars and starches) and in people with any of the following:

- Low stomach acid production
- Irritable bowel syndrome
- Celiac or Crohn's disease
- Poor liver function
- A history of multiple courses of antibiotics
- A history of heavy alcohol consumption
- A history of taking oral contraception

SIBO is a chronic bacterial infection of the small intestine. These bacteria normally live in other parts of the gastrointestinal tract, but when they expand into the small intestine, they interfere with healthy digestion and absorption of nutrients and are associated with damage to the lining of the small intestine (leaky gut syndrome). Over time this can lead to deficiencies in the bacteria's favorite nutrients, such as iron and B_{12}, deficiencies that can reduce red blood cell levels. In addition, when damage to the lining of the small intestine prevents foods from being absorbed, these bacteria gobble them up, which creates a vicious cycle of more bacteria growing and damaging the small intestine, more food being available for bacteria, and then even more bacteria growing. After eating your food, these bacteria produce gas, leading to flatulence, abdominal bloating, abdominal pain, and constipation, diarrhea, or both ("constirrhea"). Bacteria also reduce fat absorption by de-conjugating bile, which leads to deficiencies in vitamins A and D and the production of those lovely fatty stools.

Through the damaged lining of the gut, larger, undigested food particles enter the body, and your immune system reacts to them, creating food allergies and sensitivities. Bacteria can also enter the bloodstream and lead to an immune response. This can cause endotoxemia, a condition characterized by chronic fatigue and stress in the liver. Meanwhile, the bacteria secrete acids that, in high amounts, can cause neurological and cognitive symptoms, such as depression and autism.

So how do you know if you have SIBO? The presence of many of the symptoms listed above—nutrient deficiencies, flatulence, bloating, abdominal pain, constipation, diarrhea, food sensitivities—is a good sign. If you have SIBO, you may have a negative reaction to fermented foods, such as kombucha and kefir. You can even get irritable bowel syndrome from consuming probiotics, which often simply aggravate the issue by dumping bacteria on top of excess bacteria. It may seem counterintuitive, but in this case, fermented foods and probiotics could actually aggravate an already bothersome condition.

You can also test for SIBO with a simple at-home breath test that measures the amount of gas produced by bacteria. But even these tests can have high rates of false negatives, meaning the test results come back as negative but you actually do have SIBO—so it can be helpful to simply pay attention to any bloating or gas that occurs when you eat carbohydrate-laden or fermented foods. If that happens, it can be a big clue that you have SIBO.

If you do have SIBO, a combination of lowering your carbohydrate intake, juicing, and doing herbal cleanses can eradicate the issue, as can a special type of diet called an elemental diet. This may be difficult to do when you are in the throes of an intense exercise program, so you will probably need to save it for the off-season—unless you want to take thirty days off to take care of it. There are a variety of SIBO healing programs out there, but here's one basic protocol:

- Eat only nonfermentable carbohydrates, and limit carbohydrate intake in general. (On BoundlessBook.com/13 you'll find an outline of the Specific Carbohydrate Diet, which limits carbs, and a sample meal plan for treating SIBO.)

- If you have a juicer, juice once or twice a day with this recipe: fresh plantain leaves (you can often find them at local ethnic grocery stores—in my town, the Mexican one), one-quarter of a medium-sized cabbage, two small-to-medium-size beets, two carrots, two stalks of celery, and one 1-to-2-inch chunk of ginger.

- Every day, use herbal antibiotics and tinctures such as goldenseal extract, phelloden-dron, coptis, cordyceps, garlic extract, and oil of oregano. People who do not recover after a standard botanical antimicrobial protocol may benefit from the addition of a prokinetic agent such as octreotide or low-dose naltrexone to increase the muscular contractions of the bowel. You will also likely find the supplement Atrantil to be helpful.

- Consider looking into any anatomical issues with your ileocecal valve, which separates the small and large intestines, iliacus muscle (in the pelvis) or psoas muscle (connecting your back and upper thigh), especially any closures or tightness. If the ileocecal valve won't stay fully closed, bacteria can pass through it to relocate from the colon to the small intestine. Here's one way to check: palpate the area about 2 inches to the right of your belly button, or massage it with an iliacus and psoas massage tool like a Pso-Rite. If there's a problem with the ileocecal valve, you'll find that this region is extremely tight and sensitive. (I have some friends who will even use the handle of a kettlebell to mas-sage the area, but that certainly isn't for the faint of heart!)

- Ileocecal valve issues are often correlated to poor vagus nerve tone, so addressing that can be helpful (there are guidelines for stimulating the vagus nerve to improve its func-tion in chapter 2). This is especially important for constipation, since the vagus nerve can modulate bowel movements and slow the heart and breathing so you can relax, es-pecially during bowel movements. If you have a combination of SIBO and constipation, consider supplementation to support the production of the neurotransmitter acetylcho-line, which is needed by the vagus nerve, the brain, and other nerves of the parasympa-thetic nervous system. One such supplement, Parasym Plus, has been successfully used by many people to eliminate constipation issues due to poor vagus nerve function. Inter-estingly, nicotine can act on very similar pathways to support acetycholine production, and some people have even experimented with nicotine patches over the lower right abdomen to stimulate peristalsis or deal with constipation. (This, as well as Parasym Plus, can especially help if your ileocecal valve is closed, but be cautious with nicotine if you have the mast cell activation or histamine issues discussed in chapter 4.)

- Look into the little-known but highly useful peptide LL-37. There's more about peptides in chapter 19, but research on this so-called antimicrobial peptide indicates that it may be highly effective for autoimmune issues and gut-inflammation-related conditions—in-cluding fungal and bacterial overgrowth. The approximate dosage schedule is 100 mcg per week for about six weeks, injected subcutaneously in the abdomen. To learn more about this peptide and how it can be used to eradicate SIBO, I recommend you listen to Super Human Radio, a podcast hosted by my friend Carl Lanore, particularly episodes #2279 and #2289. (Warning: The die-off and Jarisch-Herxheimer reaction to adminis-tration of LL-37 can be uncomfortable and involve flu-like symptoms and diarrhea for up to two weeks. After that, however, many people experience the complete resolution of SIBO symptoms and elimination of bloating and gas in response to carbohydrate intake.)

If you want to learn more about SIBO and how to fix it, check out the comprehensive and helpful website SiboInfo.com, and my friend Dr. Michael Ruscio's website DrRuscio.com, and consider getting a SIBO breath test from DirectLabs. On BoundlessBook.com/13 you'll also find a bonus video and free PDF entitled "The Hidden Killer in Your Gut."

6. Yeast, Fungus, and Parasites

This is nasty stuff to think about, but we humans are constantly surrounded by biological organisms that prefer to use us as their host so that they can feed upon the food that we eat—and I have been shocked at the number of seemingly healthy folks who complain of issues such as insomnia, a raging appetite, or dysregulated mood and who test positive for parasites, yeast, and fungus.

A parasite is a microscopic organism that derives nourishment from its host without benefiting or killing the host. You can have both parasitic fungi and parasitic yeast in your body. Intestinal parasites in particular are quite common and can lead to issues such as abnormal bowel movements, muscle aches and pains, chronic fatigue, insomnia, skin problems, and gut discomfort.

How do you get parasites? They can be contracted in many ways, including from raw meat and fish (had any sushi lately?), polluted water (the open-water swims in many obstacle races and triathlons can be problematic), contaminated fruits and veggies, contact with infected animals and pets, insect bites, and tainted water or food (most commonly, food or water consumed during travel abroad).

Several years ago, within three weeks of returning from a long triathlon training and racing trip to Thailand—which included elephant rides, open-water swims in stagnant, human-made lagoons, liberal consumption of foods cooked in suspect ways, and many insect bites—I had some strange coughing, skin rashes, and seriously smelly poo. I tested with a home poop panel (the three-day Genova gut test that I mentioned earlier) and, sure enough, I had quite a few critters in my gut, particularly yeast, fungus, blastocystis, achromobacter, clostridium, *Pentatrichomonas hominis*, *Chilomastix mesnelli*, and *Helicobacter pylori*. (Note that, as chapter 15 will explain, for overall immunity, your goal should not be to wipe your gut completely clean of foreign invaders, which can modulate your immune system positively. Instead, it's best to specifically address the pathogenic ones.)

Most GI tests will tell you which particular herbal remedies your invaders are sensitive to, and after reviewing my results, I opted to take a high-grade oil of oregano four times per day, use a supplement called mastic gum twice per day, throw down a few capsules of berberine, allicin, and black walnut extract each day, and drink a face-puckering detox beverage once per day. I was good to go with a normally functioning bowel within a month. (Incidentally, if you have other gut issues such as yeast, fungus, food poisoning, or a mild gut bug, that same detox drink can work wonders.) I probably got lucky because, many times, parasitic infections require more serious medication and long-term treatment. It all depends on the type of parasite you have.

How about yeast and fungi? Yeast are microscopic organisms categorized as fungi. The most common culprit for yeast-induced gut issues is *Candida albicans*. It is a normal inhabitant in your body but can wreak havoc if it grows out of control. When that happens, you get chronic fatigue, difficulty losing weight, sugar and carbohydrate cravings, brain fog, and even sensitivities or allergies to foods that were once fine for you to eat. This issue is very similar to SIBO in its consequences, and it even has a similar name: SIFO (small intestine fungal overgrowth). Dr. Mahmoud Ghannoum is a leading SIFO researcher who coined the term *mycobiome* to describe the diverse

I'm not gonna lie: the first time you try this detox juice, it is going to taste absolutely horrible. That's because, unlike the juices found at Whole Foods, it doesn't contain eighteen apples, three bananas, and a pound of other concentrated sugar and fructose sources. The first time I tried it, I had to water it down and chug it so that I wouldn't have to taste the full flavor of the concoction. But between the potent ginger and garlic, the spicy cayenne, and the powerful turmeric, it will knock out just about any major toxins that are floating around in your system. If you must, add stevia to bestow just a bit of sweetness to the brew.

For this detox juice, you will need:

- 1 (1-inch) piece of ginger, chopped
- 3 cloves garlic
- ½ to ¾ cup water
- 1 teaspoon cayenne pepper
- 1 teaspoon turmeric powder
- Juice of 1 lemon
- ⅓ cup apple cider vinegar (see Tip)
- Liquid stevia (optional)

1. *Place the ginger, garlic, and water in a medium-sized saucepan over high heat and bring to a boil. Boil for 10 minutes, then remove from the heat and let cool to room temperature (you can drop a few ice cubes in there).*

2. *Add the rest of the ingredients to the mixture. If you prefer, transfer it to a blender and blend for a minute or two, until smooth.*

3. *Pour it into a glass, slam it, and try not to gag. There's an entertaining video of my first time trying it on BoundlessBook.com/13.*

TIP: Use organic apple cider vinegar with the mother, like Bragg brand.

fungal species that live on and in us humans, and his book *Total Gut Balance: Fix Your Mycobiome Fast for Complete Digestive Wellness* is an excellent treatise on how certain fungi can literally take over your gut and cause a host of digestive issues.

Due to higher levels of estrogen, genetic susceptibility, and natural levels of yeast in the vaginal canal, women (especially those who eat lots of carbs) seem to be most susceptible to candida infection, although men can also grow an overabundance of yeast, particularly when consuming a high-carb diet that includes plenty of processed sugars and alcohol. A low-carb diet combined with a cleansing protocol can eradicate the problem (see the SIBO recommendations above), but often you need an even more comprehensive protocol, including the following:

- Daily consumption of a sludgy but effective drink composed of ½ teaspoon of diatomaceous earth and ½ teaspoon of bentonite clay mixed into 2 cups of water.

- Yeast-eating probiotics such as *Saccharomyces boulardii*, preferably consumed separately from your daily meals

- An antifungal protocol that includes olive leaf extract, grapefruit seed extract, oregano, and other herbs. Mt. Capra's CapraCleanse is my preferred brand, and Mt. Capra also produces CandaCleanse for candida and CapraSite for parasites. (You'll find discounts for these at BoundlessBook.com/13.)

- A diet that restricts sugar, refined carbohydrates, white rice, gluten, dairy, fried foods, fruit, fruit juices, foods made with yeast (such as bread, pasta, and crackers), MSG, vinegar, fermented foods (yes, even sauerkraut, kimchi, kombucha, and yogurt), alcohol, mushrooms, cheese, peanuts, pistachios, and meats from animals that have been exposed to antibiotics
- Evaluation of your personal environment and diet for the presence of mold and myco-toxins (see chapter 4 for more)

So what *can* you eat? Your options include but are not limited to all vegetables (particularly onions and garlic if you do not have FODMAP sensitivities), meats not treated with antibiotics, eggs, gluten-free grains such as quinoa, amaranth, and millet, coconut milk, coconut butter, teas, olive oil, bone broth, nuts, and most beans, provided the beans have been rinsed and soaked. Throughout a candida cleansing protocol, which can take up to thirty days, you can test your progress by using a urine pH strip the first and second time you pee each morning. Look for urine pH values of 6.8 to 7.2 to indicate that your body is recovering from a yeast infection.

Ultimately, I am a fan of a high-quality GI test for a full scan of what exactly is going on inside the gut. This in-home test screens for *H. pylori*, pathogenic bacteria, *Candida albicans*, and fungus, in addition to many types of protozoa and worms, including *Clostridium difficile*, *Giardia lamblia*, *E. coli*, *Blastocystis hominis*, roundworms, *Toxoplasma gondii*, *Trichinella spiralis* (from pork), and tapeworms. In addition, an organic acids test (OATs) is a good urinary panel that can identify candida, 5-Hydroxymethyl-2-furoic, and Furan 2,5-dicarboxylic, all of which can indicate gut fungal issues.

All you have to do is order the test kit, collect a few stool samples when the kit arrives, and send them back to the lab with the included prepaid label. You then receive your test results and recommendations, which may include natural antiparasite herbal formulas, nutritional supplements, and diet or lifestyle changes. Genova Diagnostics offers a GI Effects panel and Diagnostics Solutions produces a GI-MAP DNA Stool Analysis. Both are good, and on BoundlessBook.com/13 you'll find a sample report so you can see what the analysis feedback looks like.

7. Insufficient Stomach Acid

It bugs the heck out of me when I learn that someone with indigestion or heartburn has been prescribed a proton pump inhibitor or some other medication that blocks the production of stomach acid (hydrochloric acid, or HCl). If you're not digesting food properly, the last thing you want to do is further limit your stomach's ability to break down food!

In many cases, the cause of heartburn, gastroesophageal reflux disorder, and the like is, paradoxically, inadequate HCl production, a condition known as hypochlorhydria. Hypochlorhydria is often combined with bacterial overgrowth, a lack of digestive enzymes, and excessive carbohydrate intake. This is a pretty significant issue since HCl sterilizes food in your stomach, reducing your risk of being colonized by harmful microorganisms like parasites or fungi. Stomach acid also plays an important role in the digestion of proteins and the absorption of minerals and vitamins, and it even signals the release of digestive enzymes and bicarbonate from your pancreas.

Insufficient stomach acid can lead to food particles that would normally be digested and absorbed in your upper intestines instead passing into your lower intestines, where they provide fuel for yeast or fungi, promote the overgrowth of pathogens, and cause the poor absorption of vitamins, minerals, and amino acids. They can also pass through a damaged intestinal wall to be attacked by the immune system, leading to food intolerances or allergies.

Low stomach acid levels can be genetic or acquired, and there are a variety of ways to test for it. A gastric acid secretion test is a highly invasive and expensive test that is typically only used by physicians if you have a diagnosed stomach ulcer. The Heidelberg stomach acid test is considered the gold-standard test for stomach acid and precisely measures the stomach's ability to produce acid. You can also diagnose low stomach acid levels from routine complete blood counts and comprehensive metabolic panels if you know what they are looking for. When you get the test results, the numbers to pay attention to are chloride, which should be less than 100, and CO_2, which should be greater than 27. You can also simply pay attention to your symptoms.

You can also do a simple at-home baking soda test. Simply mix ¼ teaspoon of baking soda into ½ to ¾ cup of cold water. Drink the baking soda solution before eating or drinking anything else, then time how long it takes for you to burp or belch. If you don't burp within five minutes of drinking the solution, then you aren't producing enough stomach acid.

However, in most cases, if you have heartburn after a meal (especially a protein-containing meal), your HCl is probably low. So what can you do about insufficient stomach acid? A combination of the following protocols can be very effective:

- Add crushed raw garlic to your diet. It contains the natural antimicrobial allicin, which can help reduce levels of harmful bacteria and fungi, such as candida. You can also purchase allicin in supplement form; the brand Allimax is quite good.

- If you eat grains, legumes, seeds, and nuts, soak, sprout, or ferment them to improve their digestibility.

- Increase your fiber intake and encourage healthy bowel movements by adding a daily handful of dried prunes or ground flax or chia seeds to your diet.

- Consume two to three tablespoons of extra-virgin coconut oil a day. The antiviral, antibacterial, and antifungal properties of the medium-chain fatty acids and triglycerides in coconut oil have been researched since the 1960s. Microorganisms that can be inactivated by coconut oil include bacteria, yeast, fungi, and viruses. If you're not a fan of coconut oil, you can use monolaurin capsules or powders, since monolaurin is one of the more effective antimicrobial components of coconut oil.

- Avoid refined carbohydrates. These include white bread, pasta, cookies, cakes, crackers, and so on. Also avoid soda, alcohol, wheat and gluten, peanuts, shellfish, excessive caffeine, artificial sweeteners like aspartame and sucralose, nitrites (which are found in processed meats like hot dogs, lunch meats, and bacon), MSG, hydrogenated and partially hydrogenated oils, which are found in most processed foods, deep-fried foods, fast food, junk food, and nightshade vegetables such as tomatoes, eggplants, potatoes, and peppers of all kinds and colors.

- Eat smaller, more frequent meals instead of fewer large, heavy meals, not because snacking a lot will magically boost your metabolism, but because it may be easier for you to digest small meals until you have fixed your HCl problem.

- Do not eat right before bed, and maintain an upright position for about forty-five minutes after eating to allow for easier digestion. If gastric reflux becomes a serious issue at night and you've tried everything else, consider using a zero gravity bed or zero gravity sleeping position, lying on your back with a pillow tucked under the knees and your head and shoulders elevated.

- Do not drink ice water before, during, or after meals, as this can reduce HCl production.

The following supplementation protocol can enhance the gut-healing effects of the above strategies:

- Take half a capsule of HCl with pepsin immediately before eating. If you experience no burning or indigestion, the next day take one tablet the same way. If you still have no burning or indigestion, the next day take two tablets the same way. Continue until you experience burning, then back off.

- Consume one to two servings of organic bitters or a bitters supplement immediately before a meal. If you drink cocktails, consider something like a Ben & Gitters, which, aside from being named after yours truly, is a wonderful digestif consisting of a shot of gin on the rocks splashed with two to four dashes of bitters such as angostura.

- Consume a tablespoon of a fermented vegetable, such as sauerkraut or kimchi, before a meal.

- Consume 1 to 2 cups of bone broth, a large 8-to-12-ounce glass of chia seed slurry (see page 305), or 1 to 2 g of L-glutamine each day.

If you want to read more about the issues with heartburn medications and the methods you can implement to restore proper HCl production and heal gastroesophageal reflux disorder (GERD), I highly recommend the heartburn and GERD section of Chris Kresser's website (chriskresser.com/heartburn/). Physician Dr. Carolyn Dean also discusses this concept in detail in her post on my website, "Why Kill Your Stomach Acid?" (BenGreenfieldFitness.com/article/digestion-articles/why-kill-your-stomach-acid/).

8. Other Food Intolerances or Sensitivities

Let's say Joe and Jane both have problems eating fruit or, for that matter, anything that contains fructose. They both get horrible bloating and gas from fruit, especially concentrated fruit sources such as dried fruit. But they don't have the same underlying problem. Joe's sensitivity is related to the type of the digestive enzyme deficiencies you read about earlier in this chapter, but Jane's is due to something else: fructose intolerance. Unlike Joe, Jane suffers from impaired fructose absorption due to a deficiency of fructose carriers in the small intestine, which are responsible for carrying fructose across the gut barrier and into the bloodstream.

The terms *food intolerance* and *food sensitivity* are widely used to refer to a variety of unpleasant responses to specific foods or compounds that don't reach the level of an allergy, which involves a serious and immediate immune response. While you have already learned about gluten intolerance, a combination of the following six factors can also create other food intolerances:

- A lack of the chemicals or enzymes necessary to digest a certain food

- Malabsorption, which is an inability of the digestive system to absorb specific nutrients

- A negative reaction to a normal amount of a substance, usually some type of pharmacological compound, like a food additive, preservative, or coloring

- An immune antibody response to food that is less serious than a full-blown food allergy (for example, gluten intolerance)

- A toxin present in food from either contamination or mold (for example, aflatoxin from peanuts or coffee)

- A psychological reaction to a food associated with a past experience, such as being unable to eat chili without feeling nauseated because of that time you ate chili on a road trip and got carsick

Lactose and gluten are the substances most commonly associated with food intolerances, and they have sparked entire industries of lactose-free and gluten-free foods. But there are also lesser-known intolerances to food additives, preservatives, artificial colors and flavors, fructose, and foods that contain high levels of salicylate, such as many fruits, juices, vegetables, spices, herbs, nuts, teas, wines, and coffees.

If you experience gas, bloating, frequent bathroom trips, or cramping after a meal, you likely have an intolerance to one or several compounds in those foods. While moderate indigestion is normal from high-carbohydrate and high-calorie intakes, especially during a long workout or race, it is not normal to have excessive mucus, coughing, itching, rashes, sinus inflammation, or headaches, which dozens of my clients have reported after a big workout or race. These are all potential signs of food intolerance.

The good news is that by accurately identifying specific intolerances, adjusting dietary intake, and choosing the right training and racing fuels, food intolerances can become a nonissue. Unfortunately, testing for food intolerances is confusing, to say the least. Options include breath testing, skin pinpricks, stomach gastroscopy, intestinal biopsy, stool analysis, skin sample analysis, electrical current testing, muscle testing, and more—and there is a lot of controversy in the medical and nutrition communities about which test is best. Results go all the way from questionable to downright useless.

If you suspect a specific intolerance, that hunch can help you choose the proper test. Fructose intolerance is best identified by a breath test, which measures undigested fructose levels through hydrogen levels in the breath, whereas lactose intolerance is better measured by analyzing the blood sugar response to lactose consumption. Meanwhile, an IgG and IgA test (not to be confused with an IgE test, which identifies a true food allergy) can measure immunoglobulin levels for specific protein-based food intolerances, such as those to chicken or eggs.

However, I think that Cyrex Labs food sensitivity tests are the most accurate tests and don't supply you with a long list of false positives—I'll discuss the reasons why in detail in chapter 16.

For a simpler solution than a lab test, keep a record of everything you eat for a few weeks and a list of any symptoms that develop in response to specific foods. Doing so can help you narrow down the list of foods that may be causing you problems. The next step is a food-elimination diet, in which you avoid suspected triggers.

In my opinion, the most accurate, gold-standard method for determining food sensitivities—aside from Cyrex tests—is to do an elimination diet. This consists of eliminating all of the foods that are suspected as possible allergens for seven to ten days and then adding them back, one at a time, every two to three days. Try to keep the foods you eliminate as pure as possible, meaning that if you are testing for a dairy allergy, you could test with cottage cheese, sour cream, or milk, but not ice cream, because ice cream contains sugar and other ingredients that might skew the results. If no reaction occurs within forty-eight to seventy-two hours, you can move on to the next food group. But if there is a reaction, you should wait for two to three days to clear your intestines and then try the next food. When testing foods, it is important to eat quite a bit of the chosen food to provoke a reaction. This is because small amounts may not cause a noticeable reaction, so you miss out on important information.

What do you do if you discover that you do indeed have a food intolerance? The nature of the food intolerance will determine the steps you take to address it. For example, since a gluten intolerance is related to an immune system response, you would need to switch to a gluten-free diet or use a dipeptidyl peptidase supplement prior to consuming any gluten. The same can be said for a fructose intolerance, which requires you to eliminate fructose and sucrose (which contains fructose and glucose) from your diet. In other cases, eliminating the food entirely isn't necessary. For example, if you are lactose intolerant (as I am), taking a lactase enzyme pill immediately before eating any dairy, or eating only raw, unpasteurized dairy, in which the natural lactase enzymes are fully intact and active, may do the trick.

Since having several food intolerances is quite common, you may also need to adopt a diet that is free of the usual food culprits, especially if you are an active exercise enthusiast who chows down on thousands of calories a day. If you want an extremely clean autoimmune diet that eliminates just about every possible food-sensitivity trigger, check out the four-week autoimmune diet on BenGreenfieldFitness.com/diet or follow the guidelines in *The Autoimmune Paleo Cookbook*, which is one of the better and tastier autoimmune diets out there. You'll also find a few other options in chapter 21.

9. Food Allergies

A true food allergy is usually a much bigger deal than a food intolerance. A food allergy is often accompanied by serious, and sometimes even fatal, symptoms. It occurs when the body's immune system mistakenly identifies a protein—such as the proteins in shellfish or peanuts—as harmful. Some proteins or fragments of proteins are resistant to digestion and are tagged by the antibody immunoglobulin E (IgE). These tags fool your immune system into thinking that the protein is an invader, and your immune system triggers an allergic reaction to defend the body. So unlike food sensitivities, which can arise from several different causes, allergic reactions to foods are characterized by elevated allergen-specific antibody levels in your blood.

These allergic responses can range from mild to severe and include hives, a severe drop in blood pressure, dermatitis and other skin reactions, gastrointestinal and/or respiratory distress, anaphylactic shock, and even life-threatening anaphylactic reactions in which the throat swells and closes, requiring immediate emergency action.

Unlike food intolerances, you usually know for sure when you have a food allergy because the response is readily identifiable and highly uncomfortable or severe. You can get IgE tests online from companies like DirectLabs. But if you suspect that you have a food allergy, don't mess around: consult with a licensed medical care provider who specializes in allergy treatments.

If you decide to take an alternative route, you can look into Nambudripad's Allergy Elimination Techniques (NAET) or sublingual immunotherapy, in which small drops of the substance you are allergic to are placed under your tongue in increasingly greater doses. An alternative medical or homeopathic practitioner can walk you through either of these methods. I personally used this strategy with small amounts of peanut powder to successfully cure one of my twin boys of a peanut allergy he developed early in life.

10. Mold and Mycotoxin Exposure

In many cases, I've discovered that the type of mold and mycotoxin exposure discussed in chapter 4 can further aggravate gut issues. Mold toxins have a direct inflammatory effect on the stomach and intestinal lining and can cause gastric pain, heartburn, diarrhea, and constipation. The intestinal inflammation they create also weakens the tight junctions in the lining of the gut, allowing the entry of foreign proteins to which the immune system can make antibodies, causing food allergies and autoimmune disease. This disruption of the gut microbiome causes a further inflammatory response, including the production of inflammatory cytokines that can cross the blood-brain barrier and create inflammation in brain tissues, most notably the vagus nerve and nervous system. This then further interferes with intestinal motility and adds to the inflammatory damage of the intestinal lining. So, as you can imagine, the vicious cycle created by mold (and, similarly, Lyme disease), dictates that you should revisit chapter 4 if you are having gut issues so that you can learn how to rule out mold and mycotoxin exposure as the potential culprit.

The Bottom Line

Perhaps your head was spinning as you read through the nine gut issues just described and thought, "I have that! No, wait—I have *that*!" Don't worry. It's quite typical for gut issues to be multifactorial. In fact, people often carry a cocktail of bacterial imbalances, food intolerances or allergies, a leaky gut, and a toxic liver.

The best way to begin figuring out what is going on in your gut is to (1) test your gut, (2) alter your diet and use targeted nutritional supplements based on your test results, and (3) manage stress as much as possible during this process, since stress can significantly exacerbate gut issues.

If you want to learn more about the gut, I highly recommend the following resources:

- *Clean Gut: The Breakthrough Plan for Eliminating the Root Cause of Disease and Revolutionizing Your Health*, by Alejandro Junger, MD
- *A New IBS Solution: Bacteria—The Missing Link in Treating Irritable Bowel Syndrome*, by Mark Pimentel, MD
- *Gut and Psychology Syndrome: Natural Treatment for Autism, Dyspraxia, ADD, Dyslexia, ADHD, Depression, Schizophrenia*, by Natasha Campbell-McBride
- *Healthy Gut, Healthy You*, by Dr. Michael Ruscio
- *Radical Metabolism*, by Ann Louise Gittleman
- Dr. Allison Siebecker's website, SIBOInfo.com

Finally, you'll learn more about my favorite diets and clean-eating options in chapter 21. Now that you have learned how to fix your gut, it is time to discover the truth about detox and the best way to clean up the rest of your body, too.

DETOXIFICATION 101

Think of detoxification, or detox, as spring cleaning for your body. Heavy metals, toxins, pesticides, and other compounds that your body is unable to metabolize can accumulate in your tissues, cells, and digestive tract. This may not occur to the extent that some of the more extreme folks would have you believe (no, there is not twenty years' worth of rotting meat simply hanging out in your colon in a giant meat brick), but you may indeed have amassed enough toxins to affect the way your metabolism and brain and other organ systems function. And there are certainly different natural compounds that can aid your body's natural processes in removing these toxins.

But recently, I read an article in the *Guardian* with the headline, "You Can't Detox Your Body. It's a Myth. So How Do You Get Healthy?" In the article, author Dara Mohammadi said, "Detoxing—the idea that you can flush your system of impurities and leave your organs squeaky clean and raring to go—is a scam. It's a pseudo-medical concept designed to sell you things."

Is this true? Is detoxing a scam?

To answer this question, it is important to first understand what toxins are. No matter how cleanly or toxin-free you live your life, just about everyone has some toxic buildup somewhere in their body. When the Centers for Disease Control and Prevention (CDC) published the most recent *Fourth National Report on Human Exposure to Environmental Chemicals* in 2009, it revealed some pretty shocking results. On average, the CDC's report found 212 chemicals in people's blood or urine, 75 of which had never before been measured in the US population. These chemicals included the following:

- Acrylamide, which is formed at high temperatures when foods are fried or baked and is also a by-product of cigarette smoke
- Arsenic, which is found in many home-building products
- Environmental phenols, which include bisphenol A (found in plastics, food packaging, and epoxy resins) and triclosan (used as an antibacterial agent in personal care products such as toothpaste and hand soap)
- Perchlorate, which is used in airplane fuel, explosives, and fireworks
- Perfluorinated compounds, which are used to create nonstick cookware
- Polybrominated diphenyl ethers, which are found in fire retardants in products like mattresses
- Volatile organic compounds (VOCs), which are found in paints, air fresheners, cleaning products, cosmetics, upholstery fabrics, carpets, dry-cleaned clothing, wood preservatives, and paint strippers

These chemicals, especially in combination, can create a dangerous toxic load in the body, accumulating in blood, urine, and tissues. While detox organs such as the liver and kidneys can process much of this toxic burden, exposure to these chemicals can potentially cause medical problems if the liver and kidneys are not functioning well or are overburdened by a poor diet, or if other important detox pathways are not working properly, most notably the Nrf2 pathway, which turns on over two hundred genes, many of which are related to detoxification.

While the kidneys are indeed an important filtration mechanism for removing waste and excess water from the body, the liver has the most crucial job when it comes to detoxification. In addition to filtering toxins out of your blood, your liver uses a four-phase process to eliminate chemicals and toxins.

In phase 0, a fat-soluble compound that needs to be removed from the body or undergo detoxification—such as a xenobiotic, toxic compound, or synthetic drug—is transported into a liver cell. During phase 1, detoxification officially begins as these fat-soluble toxins are broken down into smaller fragments. Then, in phase 2, the fragments are bound to other molecules, such as glutathione or a methyl group, creating new nontoxic, water-soluble molecules that can be excreted in bile, urine, sweat, or stool. Finally, in phase 3, these water-soluble molecules are transported out of the liver cells and into the bloodstream, to eventually be excreted. But for this entire liver detoxification pathway to work efficiently, your body must have adequate nutrients, particularly those that support phases 1 and 2. There are specific nutrients that support both pathways.

Phase 1 supportive nutrients

- B vitamins, specifically B_2, B_3, B_6, B_{12}, and B_9 (folic acid)
- Flavonoids, which are found in fruits and vegetables
- Vitamins A, C, and E, which are found in carrots, oranges, wheat germ, and almonds
- Glutathione, which is found in avocados, watermelon, asparagus, walnuts, and other fresh fruits and veggies
- Phospholipids, which are found in eggs, lean meats, organ meats, fish, and soybeans
- N-acetylcysteine, cysteine, and methionine, which are found in many high-protein foods such as eggs, meat, fish, seeds, and nuts
- Branched-chain amino acids, which are found in animal protein sources such as dairy products, red meat, and eggs

Phase 2 supportive nutrients

- Indole-3-carbinol, which is found in cabbage, broccoli, and brussels sprouts
- Limonene, which is found in oranges, tangerines, caraway seeds, and dill seeds
- Glutathione (see the phase 1 list)
- Fish oil from fatty cold-water fish like salmon, herring, and sardines
- Amino acids (protein)

Now let's look into whether supporting these detoxification pathways with specific compounds actually works.

The Evidence for Detoxification

The *Guardian* article mentioned earlier included a quote from Edzard Ernst, a professor of complementary medicine at Exeter University, who said, "There are two types of detox: one is respectable and the other isn't." The respectable one, the article explained, treats people who are addicted to drugs in order to save their lives. "The other," said Ernst, "is the word being hijacked by entrepreneurs, quacks, and charlatans to sell a bogus treatment that allegedly detoxifies your body of toxins you're supposed to have accumulated."

The article went on to explain that when it comes to "detoxifying" dietary supplements, smoothies, and shampoos, not one manufacturer can define what it means by "detox" or name the toxins that these products are supposed to remove. But just because a manufacturer of, say, spirulina powder can't say how it works doesn't mean that there is no evidence of its power to eliminate toxins.

For example, cyanobacteria are a type of bacteria found in spirulina that act as accumulators (also known as "biosorbents") of heavy minerals, meaning they can effectively bind to large minerals and metals. They do this via a process called ion-exchange binding and can significantly reduce heavy-metal toxicity in tissue. In fact, 100 mcg (a tiny amount) of spirulina hexane extract has been shown to remove over 85 percent of arsenic found in tissue. At a dose of 250 to 500 mg per kilogram of body weight (about 20 to 40 g for a 170-pound individual), spirulina has been shown to prevent metal toxicity in pregnant rats' offspring when the mothers were given fluoride. Spirulina has also been shown to reduce lead accumulation in brain tissue, protect against cadmium buildup, and attenuate mercury accumulation in the testes.

Granted, spirulina is one of the few substances that has a large body of evidence to support its detoxifying activity, but other compounds such as dandelion extract, ginseng, and zinc have also been clinically proven to reduce heavy-metal buildup. And while heavy metals are only one form of the toxins that can accumulate in your tissues, there is no doubt science has proven that these toxins can indeed be removed via certain natural compounds. So while the *Guardian* article guffaws at the idea of superfoods like spirulina, the evidence suggests that there is more to the story.

Take milk thistle extract, another popular detox supplement. While the *Guardian* article would have you believe that there is no value whatsoever in consuming this type of nutrient, studies show that milk thistle protects and promotes the growth of liver cells, fights oxidative stress, and blocks toxins from entering cells. Silymarins, plant compounds extracted from the seeds of milk thistle, have antioxidant properties several times greater than those of vitamins C and E. In fact, silybin has been shown to be especially effective in promoting liver health. Milk thistle also helps prevent the depletion of glutathione, which is necessary for phase 2 liver detoxification.

We can look to farming for another example of detoxification. Glyphosate, the active ingredient in herbicides used on crops around the world, has been shown to cause gut and genetic damage as it builds up in the bodies of animals. So some farmers use activated charcoal and humic acid (a claylike substance extracted from soil) to detox their cattle after the animals have been exposed to glyphosate chemicals while feeding.

As you can see from these examples, to claim that detox supplements and diets simply do not work is a gross oversimplification. While there is no evidence for the efficacy of the cayenne pepper, lemon, and maple syrup cleanse your coworker has been bragging about, evidence of other nutrients' detoxing capacities does indeed exist.

But what about colon cleanses? The *Guardian* article's author, Dara Mohammadi, wrote, "Proponents will tell you that mischievous plaques of impacted poo can lurk in your colon for months or years and pump disease-causing toxins back into your system. Pay them a small fee, though, and they'll insert a hose up your bottom and wash them all away." She also went on to say, "Some colon-cleansing tablets contain a polymerising agent that turns your faeces into something like a plastic, so that when a massive rubbery poo snake slithers into your toilet you can stare back at it and feel vindicated in your purchase."

When you think about it, the idea that toxins might somehow be reabsorbed by your body as they sit in your colon makes some sense. After all, rectal suppositories are used to rapidly administer drugs. If drugs can enter your bloodstream from your colon, it is certainly possible that toxins could enter that way, too. But your colon is equipped with several mechanisms to keep toxins from building up. For example, bacteria naturally present in the colon can detoxify food waste. Mucous membranes in the colon can keep toxic compounds from reentering the blood and settling in your tissues. The colon also sheds old cells about every three days, preventing a buildup of harmful material and even allowing for the expulsion of parasites.

I suspect that if colon cleansing, colonic hydrotherapy, or enemas have any effect in making you feel like you have more energy or have been "cleansed," it more likely has to do with an activation of reflexes in your gut that cause your nervous system to relax and increase the peristaltic movement of food through your digestive tract. These protocols may also increase the production of bile by the liver or the release of bile by the gallbladder, which can indeed improve digestion, and they may have a mild laxative effect and relieve constipation. This could potentially make you feel better by allowing you to better break down or absorb nutrients from your food or even to pass some feces that had built up over the previous few days, but this is one point on which I completely agree with the *Guardian*. There is no evidence that waste can sit inside you for years, slowly rotting and leaking toxins into your body.

Glyphosate is the active ingredient in many commercial, agricultural, and residential herbicides, causing it to have a significant presence in many modern crops and produce, including wheat and many other grains, vegetables, and anything using these types of foods as ingredients, such as the pasta or salad at your favorite restaurant. A host of scientific research has implicated glyphosate exposure in various systemic disorders: it suppresses the biosynthesis of cytochrome P450 enzymes and amino acids by gut microbes, directly damages DNA, disrupts glycine homeostasis, inhibits succinate dehydrogenase, affects the chelation of minerals such as manganese, changes natural biological compounds to more carcinogenic molecules, and disrupts fructose metabolism, all of which significantly impact metabolism and lower immune function.

Glyphosate works synergistically with other factors, which means that problems such as exposure to other toxins, insufficient sun exposure, and deficiencies in nutrients like sulfur and zinc can all aggravate glyphosate's effects. In other words, eating a diet rich in glyphosate and poor in nutrients and minerals while spending a lot of sedentary time indoors is one of the worst things you can do for your gut.

Glyphosate exposure can affect the gut microbiota by damaging or killing bacteria, which, in turn, can affect behavioral expression and lead to anxiety and depression. Research performed by Stephanie Seneff at MIT links glyphosate's suppression of proper gut bacteria function to many modern diseases, including autoimmunity, cancer, and Alzheimer's. In fact, research has shown that glyphosate is ten times more potent than gluten in its ability to degrade the tight junctions between cells in the intestinal wall, meaning that glyphosate can "poke holes" in the gut lining. The tight junctions between cells in the gut lining is what allows certain particles, like tiny digested food particles, into the bloodstream while keeping out other particles, like large undigested protein molecules. As you have already learned, when unwanted particles get through the gut membrane and into the bloodstream, they can lead to food intolerances, food allergies, and systemic inflammatory responses.

There is a simple solution to preventing this type of gut damage. The company Biomic Sciences, owned and operated by my friend and brilliant physician Dr. Zach Bush, has demonstrated that the liquid supplement RESTORE, which contains the active ingredient lignite, can increase and strengthen tight junctions and also protect against everyday exposure to pesticides and herbicides. Both clinical experience and cell-culture studies have shown that RESTORE creates a gut environment in which twenty thousand to thirty thousand different strains of gut bacteria can thrive and protect the entire GI tract against agricultural herbicides, antibiotics, GMOs, gluten, and foodborne toxins.

In addition to minimizing our exposure to glyphosate and other gut irritants by choosing organic, non-GMO foods, my family also prevents potential damage to our guts by taking a single shot of RESTORE before any plant- or grain-containing meal. (You'll find a discount code for RESTORE, as well as a link to my podcast with Dr. Bush, at BoundlessBook.com/13.)

Aiding Your Body's Natural Detox Through Diet

Your body has its own powerful methods of detoxing and can activate these methods without fancy diets or detox spa visits. For example, your liver prevents pathogens from passing into your bloodstream, processes environmental toxins for safe removal, and helps rid your body of excess nitrogen that builds up from the breakdown of proteins and amino acids. Your kidneys filter blood, remove excess water, pass urea (a toxin that builds up as a by-product of protein breakdown), and send this all out of your body via your urine. So if you eat foods that support your liver and kidneys and avoid foods that stress them, you are already detoxing every day. This is why I am a fan of using strategies like herbal blends and colonic cleanses only sparingly—such as if you test for extremely elevated liver enzymes or heavy metals, or you're suffering a significant bout of constipation—and using natural detox habits all year long.

For example, a natural detox habit for your liver would be to avoid high amounts of omega-6 polyunsaturated fats from processed and packaged foods, such as canola oil and french fries. Instead, eat healthy fats from fish, meat, seeds, and nuts, along with plenty of plant matter and minerals. You should also avoid high amounts of fructose and sugar, limit alcohol intake, consume plenty of egg yolks (rich in choline, which your liver uses to process fats), and eat organic liver or use dessicated liver powder a few times a month. Additionally, you can simply pay attention to the kinds of soaps, shampoos, and household cleaners you use. Many contain toxins that can tax your liver over time (more about that in chapter 20).

For your kidneys, you can limit your intake of high-fructose corn syrup, drink plenty of water along with a full spectrum of minerals, limit alcohol intake, and—if you are predisposed to renal issues—limit protein intake to no more than 200 g per day.

As the *Guardian* article notes, many popular detox and cleansing diets probably seem beneficial because of the foods they eliminate and not because of any magical ingredients. In other words, all that lemon juice, cayenne pepper, maple syrup, and fancy water is probably not doing as much as you think when it comes to cleansing and detoxifying your body. But eliminating processed fats, high-fructose corn syrup, alcohol, candy, soda, conventionally raised and processed meat, and snack foods while on a detox diet can indeed give your liver and kidneys a chance to step up and perform their normal duties instead of dealing with toxins from your food.

Healthy Detoxing Protocols

Simply adjusting what you eat can support your body's detox, and you can fix your gut with the methods in this chapter. But if you have been exposed to overprocessed and refined foods, chemical additives, antibiotics, pharmaceuticals, pesticides, herbicides, chlorinated water, artificial sweeteners, or anything else that might be considered remotely "unnatural," you should think about performing a more thorough detox protocol.

For example, have you consumed lots of diet soda at some point in your life, eaten much non-organic or non-farm-raised meat, traveled extensively, chomped on fruits and vegetables without washing them, been sick and taken pharmaceuticals, engaged in a few nights of excessive drinking, been exposed to secondhand smoke, or inhaled the fumes of household cleaning supplies? I don't know about you, but my answer to many of those items is "Yes!" So I perform a more thorough detox of my body once a year—typically in the winter, when I am more often indoors, I am exercising and traveling less, and I have more time for a bout of intensive self-care. After I perform these more complete detoxes, I feel reborn and rebooted in a way, with less brain fog, gut distress, fatigue, joint pain, and other symptoms of toxic buildup.

The idea behind doing a complete detox or cleanse is to use herbal or medicinal compounds to induce peristalsis (the contraction of gastrointestinal muscles that propel contents through the digestive tract) and a rapid, thorough clearing of waste from your colon. Other herbal compounds can enhance the ability of the liver to bind and excrete toxins. By also restricting calories and doing light exercise and other activities to strengthen lymph fluid circulation, sweating, and fat loss, you can accelerate the rate at which your body metabolizes fat tissue. Since your body stores many toxins in fat, this can increase the rate of detoxification.

In a nutshell, you clean out your digestive tract, remove toxins from your body, and accelerate fat burning. What's not to love? Believe it or not, you don't need to sequester yourself in some exclusive spa on a mountaintop or spend the entire day on or near the toilet to do a detox like this. I do a yearly detox at home while living my regular life—you'll find my protocol on page 304.

I perform this program every year, typically in January, and do it for one to three months. (I'll also vouch for two other safe and structured detox programs, listed on page 310.) Many of the elements of my yearly protocol—from the hot and cold therapy to the coffee enema to the dry skin brushing—can be introduced throughout the year as daily or monthly habits, so you naturally detox all year long rather than living a toxic lifestyle and waiting until January for one giant, very uncomfortable detox. Once you systematize these practices, they become easy and effortless and can flow quite nicely into the type of daily routine you will discover in chapter 21.

Because you will be moving a higher amount of compounds through your digestive tract during a protocol like this and experiencing increased peristalsis and bile production, you can expect to spend an extra fifteen to twenty minutes or so on the toilet in the morning and possibly again in the late afternoon or early evening, depending on how many toxins you need to eliminate. Incidentally, this is where a Squatty Potty device—or any squatting position that raises your knees above hip level and helps to relax your pelvic ligaments—can come in quite handy. (You'll find an article I wrote about why I recommend this type squatting position for defecation on BoundlessBook.com/13.)

An important note for those who have been exposed to the type of mold issues discussed in chapter 4: mold can significantly compromise your body's ability to detoxify, meaning that mycotoxins from mold have literally poisoned the very systems needed to remove these toxins, including the liver, GI tract, kidneys, and lymphatic system. If you've been exposed to mold or mycotoxins, please revisit that section in chapter 4 to better understand how to clean up your system—or at least test for these issues—prior to a detox protocol.

As you embark on a detox protocol, be sure to never discount the power of wild plant intake, which is also a longevity strategy discussed in chapter 19. Phytochemicals in plants have unique properties that support detoxification pathways. For example, perhaps your mother or grandmother encouraged you to eat your broccoli. There is now a solid scientific explanation for why it is so good for you: Broccoli contains a phytochemical called sulforaphane that stimulates the protein Nrf2. Nrf2 is the master controller in your body for making, utilizing, and recycling glutathione, an antioxidant that's necessary to help remove toxins!

Turmeric also supports Nrf2 and has been shown to downregulate mammalian target of rapamycin (mTOR) signaling pathways. This is important because overstimulation of the anabolic and growth-promoting mTOR pathway contributes to inflammation and impaired detoxification.

Another common plant that has been used for centuries is milk thistle, which turns out to support Nrf2 and the production of glutathione. Here's another example: when the enzyme nitric oxide synthase (NOS) is not functioning optimally, a free radical is produced rather than the beneficial nitric oxide. One of the cofactors needed to make nitric oxide is called BH4, and royal jelly, which is the food fed to queen bees and bee larvae, is a naturally occurring source of BH4. In addition, if NOS is not working properly to make nitric oxide, certain nutrient-dense foods and herbs, such as green coffee beans, beet root, and hawthorn berries, can also provide necessary support. There are even phytochemicals that appear to help "scavenge" the excess free radicals produced when nitric oxide pathways aren't working properly, including those from echinacea, garlic, rosemary, and witch hazel. (For more on NOS pathways, I recommend a test from StrateGene or a visit to the website of Dr. Bob Miller at TOLHealth.com.)

Finally, no discussion of detoxing would be complete without a foray into fasting, which allows the body to engage in its own cellular cleanup protocol. While there are entire books on fasting (Dr. Jason Fung's *The Complete Guide to Fasting* is one of the best) and websites devoted to dozens of different fasting protocols and religious and traditional fasting techniques, my own fasting protocol is quite simple:

My Full-Body Detox Protocol

This is what my annual full-body detox protocol typically looks like. If I'm home for a long enough stretch (without traveling), I'll stick to this protocol for up to four weeks, but if it's the first time that you're doing it or you need a deep "spring cleaning" for your body, I recommend following it for three months. It is okay to continue your normal workout routine during this time, although you may find that for the first several days or even the first couple of weeks, you are a bit more fatigued than usual and may need to primarily get your movement in with yoga, sauna, swimming, hiking, or easier bodyweight workouts.

Daily Diet Guidelines

- Avoid frequent snacking; shoot for two or three meals per day with just one to two snacks, maximum.

- Avoid any foods that have been heavily cooked or exposed to high heat.

- Avoid baked goods.

- Avoid soy, wheat, legumes, and dairy unless fermented, soaked, or sprouted.

- Avoid high intake of heavy foods like cheeses and nut butters.

- Avoid extremely spicy foods.

- Avoid white sugar, simple starches, high alcohol intake, high caffeine intake, and frequent recreational drug use.

- Include fermented foods such as kimchi, sauerkraut, natto, kefir, and kombucha, as long as they do not have added sugars.

- Include a wide variety of bitters and digestifs, such as ginger, lemon, lime, and dandelion.

Teas and Broths: Drink several cups of any of the following each day, preferably spread throughout the day:

- Pau d'arco tea, preferably blended with a tablespoon of soy lecithin or sunflower lecithin and a teaspoon of turmeric powder. You can add stevia for flavor.

- Organic bone broth. I prefer Kettle & Fire beef or chicken broth. You can also find instructions for making your own bone broth on BoundlessBook.com/13.

- Decoction tea. You'll find more information and the recipe on page 363. Read John Douillard's book *Body, Mind, and Sport* for more on the science behind this tea.

- Fresh celery juice

Hot and Cold Therapy: Stay in a dry sauna, steam sauna, or infrared sauna for ten to thirty minutes, at least long enough to begin sweating and preferably long enough that you begin to get uncomfortably hot. You can kill two birds with one stone and do any of the day's other activities in the sauna. You can also read or simply sit and breathe—staying still in a sauna can increase parasympathetic nervous system activity and enhance detoxification. Just stay away from your phone, WiFi, Bluetooth, and other emitters of electromagnetic fields. Another good sauna activity is breathwork: resisted breathwork, restricted breathwork, holotropic breathwork, breath holds, or any of the other breathwork tactics in chapter 3. Follow this sauna session with a two-to-five-minute cold shower, soak in a cold bath, dip in a cold pool, or any other cold thermogenesis activity.

Dry Skin Brushing: Either in the sauna or after a shower, perform a full-body dry skin brush for two to five minutes. You can find dry skin brushes, as well as full instructions for how to use them, on BoundlessBook.com/13.

Rebounding: At any point during the day (I prefer first thing in the morning to get the lymph fluid circulating), jump on a rebounding trampoline for five to fifteen minutes. I recommend any of the JumpSport model trampolines. It is okay to alternate between single- and double-leg bouncing. A vibration platform or tai chi full-body shaking are also good options.

Oil Pulling: This practice involves simply swishing oil in your mouth for five minutes (not twenty minutes) each morning. You can find full instructions on how to do this on BoundlessBook.com/13. Be sure to spit the oil out instead of swallowing it when you're finished. For oil, I prefer The Dirt brand oil-pulling oil or extra-virgin coconut oil.

Intermittent Fasting (daily): After dinner, wait for a minimum of twelve hours (and up to sixteen hours) before your next meal. The closer you can get to sixteen hours, the better.

Meditation (two to five times per week): Meditate for fifteen to sixty minutes. This can include yoga, prayer, transcendental meditation, mindfulness meditation, box breathing, underwater swimming, nature sit spots, or the use of a meditation app such as Headspace, Calm, Oak, or Sam Harris's meditation app. You do not need to do the same form of meditation each Sunday.

24-Hour Fast (once a week): At either breakfast, lunch, or dinner on Saturday, begin a twenty-four-hour fast until breakfast, lunch, or dinner on Sunday. During this fast, you can consume a maximum of 2 cups of each of the teas listed above, as well as bone broths and celery juice. You can also drink good, clean water liberally, and, especially if you are an athlete concerned about energy levels or muscle maintenance, you can use any or all of the following:

- Up to 30 g of essential amino acids, split into several 5-to-10-gram portions

- Two or three shots of trace liquid minerals, or sea salt and lemon juice in water

- Two or three handfuls of EnergyBits organic spirulina or chlorella. Swallow them whole or chew them. (You'll find a discount code on BoundlessBook.com/13.)

- One to two servings of exogenous ketones, such as HVMN, KetoneAid, PerfectKeto, KetoForce, or Ancient Nutrition. (You'll find discount codes on BoundlessBook.com/13.)

- Chia seed slurry: Fill a 16-to-20-ounce glass mason jar with 2 to 4 tablespoons of chia seeds. Fill the rest of the jar with water, place the lid on the jar, and refrigerate overnight. Try not to consume more than 4 tablespoons of chia seeds in the course of twenty-four hours (1 tablespoon is about 60 calories). You can add stevia, lemon juice, or sea salt to this chia seed slurry.

- Any low-calorie or no-calorie beverage, such as Pellegrino or Gerolsteiner with stevia, Bragg's apple cider vinegar drinks, coconut kefir, Zevia, or any of the teas listed above

When you break your fast, begin with a light, easy-to-digest meal. One of the best, most comprehensive guides to fasting and what you can and cannot consume before, during, and after a fast is *The Complete Guide to Fasting* by Dr. Jason Fung with Jimmy Moore.

Coffee Enema (one to two times per week): Since an enema is something you don't want to make a mistake with, you can find full instructions for how to do this on BoundlessBook.com/13. After you have used a stainless steel enema kit and tube to add 20 to 40 ounces of organic black coffee to your colon, lie on your left side for twenty minutes. If you have trouble retaining the enema, add a tablespoon of blackstrap molasses.

- Perform a twelve-to-sixteen-hour intermittent fast each day. For example, if you finish dinner at 8 p.m., you do not eat again until at least 8 a.m. the following day. Water and noncaloric coffee or tea are fine. Most of the benefits of fasting come not from overall caloric restriction but rather from going relatively long periods of time without food. Unless you are attempting to lose a significant amount of weight, it is fine to eat as many calories as you normally would. You simply move all those calories into what is called a compressed eating window.

- Perform a twenty-four-hour fast two to four times per month, in which you do not eat from dinner on one day until dinner the next day. In my case, I consume only water between dinner on Saturday and dinner on Sunday.

- Perform a three-to-five-day fast once per year, preferably during a period when you can devote this time to meditation, yoga, and a vision quest or journey of self-discovery, such as a camping trip or nature immersion experience. Trust me, it pays to be far away from your refrigerator and pantry during this time.

To further understand how fasting encourages detox and a self-programmed cellular turnover called autophagy, I recommend you check out my friend Naomi Whittel's book *Glow 15* and Dr. Bryan Walsh's detox educational program at MetabolicFitnessPro.com, along with chapter 19.

HOW TO NEVER GET A HANGOVER AGAIN

No discussion of clean eating or detoxing would be complete without some tips on how to never get a hangover again, or at least how to mitigate the effects of alcohol or a hefty bout of hedonism. After all, we healthy, active folks like to get our party on every now and again, right?

Most people think that hangovers are the result of dehydration. But even if you have followed the sage advice to drink a glass of water for each alcoholic beverage consumed, you can still wake up feeling less than stellar. Preventing a hangover is way more complicated than simply chasing your beer or margarita or glass of wine with a pitcher of water (or coconut water or Gatorade or Pedialyte).

This is because dehydration is just one factor in a hangover. Your pituitary gland normally produces antidiuretic hormone (ADH), which increases your blood pressure by causing your body to retain water. When you drink alcohol, your pituitary gland churns out less ADH, so you stop retaining so much water, which is one reason the bathroom line is so long at parties. But as soon as your buzz begins to wear off, ADH production increases once again, which causes a rebound of fluid retention, swollen hands and feet, a puffy face, and a headache as blood pressure rises.

At the same time, your kidneys pump out more of the enzyme renin and the hormone aldosterone. This promotes the secretion of vasopressin, which increases blood pressure by inducing sodium retention and potassium loss. This is why people with heart problems are most prone to a heart attack when they have a hangover: the cardiovascular system goes into electrolyte-roller-coaster hyperdrive trying to retain fluids.

And that's not all. Cortisol works with aldosterone to balance electrolyte levels, so when you are hungover, your body pumps out more cortisol. This not only contributes to even more fluid retention but also raises blood sugar levels by converting amino acids into glucose in your liver, a process known as gluconeogenesis. As blood sugar levels rise, the pancreas produces more insulin, resulting in abnormal stress on both the pancreas and the liver. These elevated levels of cortisol can also cause catabolism (decreased protein availability in skeletal muscles) as well as a redistribution of body fat from your legs and arms to your belly. Oh yes, there's still more.

As you drink and force your body to metabolize alcohol, your liver converts ethanol into acetaldehyde and acetate, which causes increased production of tiny blood vessel constrictors called thromboxanes. Thromboxanes also cause blood platelets to stick together and form clots and decrease levels of natural killer cells, which are crucial to the immune system. This surge in thromboxane creates symptoms very similar to those of a viral infection, including nausea, headache, and diarrhea.

Finally, most alcoholic beverages contain congeners, which significantly contribute to hangover symptoms. Congeners, which are found in high concentrations in dark-colored liquors like brandy, wine, dark tequila, and whiskey, contain free radicals and positively charged molecules that can significantly disrupt your acid-alkaline (pH) balance and increase your body's need to step up antioxidant activity to scavenge all those free radicals. As your body goes into fight-or-flight mode to help you handle all these congeners, you get gastrointestinal issues, nausea, headaches, sweatiness, clamminess, and/or chills.

So what can you do about this cluster of reactions that can occur once you foray into the realm of two or more alcoholic drinks? Here are my best practices for a bout of higher-than-normal alcohol intake (or any other outburst of hedonism, toxic excess, or partying).

1 to 3 days before the party

- Log as much sleep as possible. Research has shown this helps to mitigate the effects of later sleep loss.

- Limit your intake of vegetable oil and omega-6 fatty acids and emphasize monounsaturated fatty acids (MUFAs) and saturated fatty acids (SFAs). Animal studies have confirmed that high amounts of omega-6 fatty acids from polyunsaturated fatty acids (PUFAs) increase liver damage in response to alcohol intake, while more stable fats like cocoa butter and coconut oil protect against it. If you do eat omega-6s, try to make sure they come from whole foods, such as nuts, seeds, and eggs.

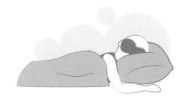

The day of the party

- Work out. Strength training or HIIT prior to heavy eating or drinking can improve glycemic response to carbohydrate-laden foods or drinks. Exercise also increases antioxidant activity and reduces alcohol-induced liver damage.

- Eat several egg yolks or a serving of liver. Your liver will be burning through its choline stores so it can mitigate the damage of drinking, and this will top off those stores. Choline supplementation or doubling your normal dose of fish oil can also work well.

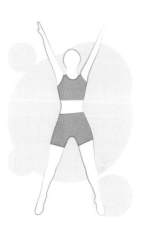

1 hour before the party

- Eat a spoonful each of extra-virgin avocado oil, extra-virgin olive oil, and red palm oil. The polyphenols in olive oil and avocado oil and the vitamin E in red palm oil can protect against alcohol-induced oxidative stress, and the monounsaturated and saturated fats in all three protect the liver. In a pinch or in a hurry, just choose one.

- Eat a light meal. Although a liver that is emptied of glycogen stores does allow you to convert the fructose in cocktails and wines into liver glycogen, which might make you consider a complete liver-glycogen-emptying fast before partying, if you plan to drink heavily, you want some food in your stomach to slow the absorption of the alcohol, but not so much food that you're overloaded with calories from both the meal and the booze. If you do not eat, you risk flooding your body with too much ethanol too fast, and the subsequent conversion into acetaldehyde can overwhelm your antioxidant defenses. Preferably, this meal should include plenty of polyphenol-rich plants and spices, including turmeric powder, ginger, berries, and beets, since anything pungent or colorful is fantastic for alcohol metabolism. Another way to get in herb or plant matter is to take 1 to 2 g of curcumin or a spoonful or two of Dr. Thomas Cowan's potent vegetable powders. Examples of good light meals include a fresh salad topped with fish, beets, and nuts; a mess of scrambled eggs, turmeric powder, and kale served up in a corn tortilla or nori wrap; and a few small handfuls of nuts, dried ginger, dark chocolate, and berries (not only does the cocoa fat in chocolate protect against ethanol-induced liver damage, but the cocoa polyphenols can increase your antioxidant capacity). Make sure you salt these types of light meals with a good mineral-rich salt.

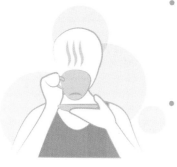

- Take 500 to 600 mg of N-acetylcysteine (NAC) and 1 g of vitamin C. NAC is a precursor to glutathione, the antioxidant responsible for metabolizing alcohol. Hospitals give NAC megadoses to treat Tylenol-based and alcohol-based liver poisoning. Vitamin C helps NAC supply glutathione, an essential antioxidant.

- Take 300 to 400 mg of magnesium. Alcohol depletes magnesium and can also cause constipation, and this helps with both. You may want to save this tactic for after the party if you find the magnesium gives you loose stool, which is common, or use a time-release magnesium formula such as Jigsaw MagSRT.

- Mix a few spoonfuls of collagen powder into a smoothie or drink of your choice (such as green tea—see below) or drink a cup of organic bone broth. The glycine in collagen and gelatin reduces lipid peroxidation and antioxidant depletion in the liver. Adding vitamin C with a supplement or a squeeze of lemon can increase glycine absorption.

- Drink a cup or two of green tea or matcha. Green tea contains polyphenols that protect against ethanol-induced oxidative stress, and the caffeine and L-theanine in the tea can give you a stable, slow release of energy for a night of fun. You can certainly double up and make yourself a green tea cocktail that includes the oils, vitamin C, and collagen powder as well, which is far more effective than forking over ten bucks for an overpriced detox juice or anti-hangover supplement.

During the party

- Drink only the highest-quality alcohol available and avoid high-fructose corn syrup, added sugars, and other nasty ingredients. (For the healthiest alcohol choices and my favorite cocktail mixes, visit BoundlessBook.com/13.) A few particularly good choices are gin or vodka mixed into sparkling water with bitters or a splash of fresh juice; organic or biodynamic wine; or a noncaloric soda such as Zevia mixed with wine and ice for a sparkling cooler.

  - Unless you are drinking the super-fancy, expensive stuff, dilute wine and other spirits with sparkling mineral water to improve hydration. If people ask why you're bastardizing the wine with water, inform them that you are making yourself a fancy French sparkler.

  - Add a pinch of salt or one effervescent electrolyte tablet to each glass of water you consume (ideally from a glass bottle, such as Pellegrino or Gerolsteiner).

  - Stay active to ensure you metabolize snacks and alcohol better. My own trick? I perform forty air squats every time I use the restroom at a long alcohol-fueled dinner or party, and I try to walk the room or dance as much as possible.

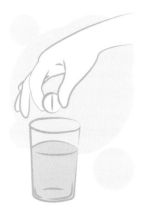

Before bed

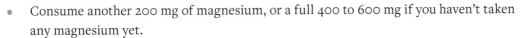

- Mix ½ teaspoon of sea salt, the juice from 1 lime or lemon, 1 tablespoon of blackstrap molasses, and 1½ cups of water (preferably mineral water or, despite the extra sugar content, coconut water, as long as you have been careful not to have too much sugar at the party). Ideally, drink this thirty to forty-five minutes before bed to give yourself enough time to pee before you fall asleep. A second, easier option is to drink sea salt mixed with water, or suck down a sachet of QuintEssential Hypertonic Elixir, which tastes more or less like seawater but works fantastically. You can also include up to 1500 mg of any vitamin C supplement with this water.

- Consume another 200 mg of magnesium, or a full 400 to 600 mg if you haven't taken any magnesium yet.

- Take four capsules of activated charcoal to sop up any toxins in the gut. Contrary to popular belief, charcoal does not absorb alcohol, but it does absorb toxins, so this step is only truly necessary if you're unsure of the purity of the compounds you've been consuming, or if you have gas and bloating from excess sugars or strange party foods.

- Take 3 to 10 mg of melatonin. Alcohol reduces melatonin secretion, which can contribute to annoying early awakenings when all you want to do is sleep in.

In the morning

- Drink the same pre-bed drink from the night before.

- Take four more capsules of activated charcoal or drink a large mason jar of 16 to 32 ounces of charcoal lemonade (Four Sigmatic makes a tasty one).

- Consume a breakfast that includes eggs so that you can get more choline and/or consume a handful of desiccated liver capsules, or, better yet—although you'll be hard-pressed to find pâté at Denny's or a pancake house—eat a serving of organ meat.

- Exercise lightly (e.g., take a walk in the sunshine) or sit in a sauna. Do anything that gets you sweating (infrared sauna therapy is best due to the added detox effect). Afterward, take a cold plunge or a cold shower, or take a five-minute shower in which you alternate between twenty seconds of cold water and ten seconds of hot water.

- If you're truly hungover, try my ultimate hangover cure: combine all of the following ingredients in a blender until smooth.

- 1 cup coconut water

- ½ avocado

- Juice of ½ lemon

- 1 (1-to-2-inch) piece of ginger, peeled and chopped

- 2 large egg yolks

- 1 heaping teaspoon chlorella

- Pinch of sea salt

  For added efficacy, include 2 to 3 tablespoons frozen broccoli sprouts, a handful of dandelion greens, and 200 to 300 mg of ginseng, which can accelerate the clearance of acetaldehyde.

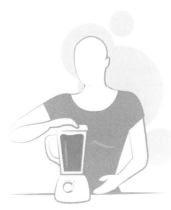

Finally, if you can't get into the sunshine because you're, say, stuck in a maze of Vegas casinos or don't have the energy to leave your hotel room, to jump-start your circadian rhythm, you can utilize the HumanCharger, the ReTimer, or similar blue-light-producing devices in the morning (or, if you need to stay awake and phase-shift your circadian rhythm forward, before the actual party) and use the ultra-sexy blue-light-blocking glasses at night as much as possible. I often refer to these as "birth-control for your head," but several manufacturers—including Ambr, Ra, and Felix Gray—do now make some relatively attractive options. (See chapter 7 on sleep for more details on light-blocking and light-producing strategies.)

Finally, I should mention that I don't endorse drunkenness. I personally drink about one serving of alcohol each night, and—I suspect because I am never tempted to cheat on the weekends after abstaining every weekday—haven't been drunk in over six years. But I also understand that having occasional bouts of partying tends to be a societal norm, and I decided I wanted to equip you with all the tools you need to combat the damage and keep a night or weekend of partying from destroying your productivity and happiness for days on end.

Avoiding Dangerous Done-for-You Detoxes

Sure, every single day you can consume certain foods and supplements—from cruciferous vegetables to chlorella—and engage in certain lifestyle activities—from fasting and rebounding to spending time in a sauna—that help your liver, your lymph, and the rest of your detox organs perform their jobs better.

But when you find yourself mowing down a shopping-cart-sized blender full of cilantro, chomping through an enormous mug of chlorella or charcoal each day, or jumping on the latest diet or juicing craze, detox gets a bit more complex and downright dangerous. As you learned in chapter 4, my friend Dr. Dan Pompa gave himself mad hatter's disease by detoxing the wrong way—specifically by mobilizing toxins and metals from fat tissue and other storage areas into his body. He experienced the disturbing and often permanent side effects that can occur if these compounds are simply deposited into other tissues, like the brain and central nervous system, rather than excreted.

At a recent mastermind meeting of functional medicine physicians whom I consider to be some of the world's leading experts in detoxification, including Dr. Dan Pompa, Dr. Chris Shade, and Dr. Joseph Mercola, the consensus on detox was this: the willy-nilly, daily consumption of compounds reported to detox your body, especially in the excessive amounts found in most daily detox supplements, is likely risky. Ironically, many popular compounds used in this type of approach, including carrots, celery, and curcumin, can inhibit detox pathways when consumed in very high amounts in the absence of a systematized detox program. On the other hand, a detox system that is planned and programmed to guide your body through specific detox pathways in a precise order is a far more intelligent and less risky approach.

For such a detox program to be effective, the following three principles must be in place:

- **Toxin mobilization:** engaging in activities that involve lipolysis (breakdown of fat cells, which store toxins), including sauna exposure, caloric restriction, fasting, exercise, and rebounding

- **Detox:** stimulating and supporting all major detox pathways with both foods and supplements, such as mung beans, cruciferous vegetables, milk thistle extract, N-acetylcysteine, glutathione, vitamin C, and green tea polyphenols

- **Excretion:** binding and removing the toxins with high-fiber foods, common binders such as charcoal and chlorella, advanced binders such as clinoptilolite fragments and clay, and activities such as exercise, sweating, and enemas

There are only three programs that satisfy these criteria and that I endorse as effective and safe detox programs overseen by intelligent, well-informed medical professionals. The first is Dr. Bryan Walsh's Walsh Detoxification Program, which primarily uses real food and lifestyle strategies and takes ten days. The second is Dr. Chris Shade's Detox Qube, a four-week program that must be overseen by a medical practitioner. The final program is Dr. Dan Pompa's True Cellular Detox, which is my annual strategy and is detailed on page 304. It is three months long, includes all my personal biohacks and strategies that I worked on with Pompa, and is followed by daily use of Dr. Pompa's Cytodetox supplement. (For more information about each of these programs, see BoundlessBook.com/13.)

Supplementing with Glutathione

I'll admit it: I personally self-administer a glutathione injection into my right butt cheek once a week and mainline glutathione into my bloodstream via a push IV once a week. Glutathione acts as an antioxidant, helps cells repair themselves, keeps mucus fluid, helps prevent asthma, enhances liver detox pathways, and much more, and ever since I discovered its wonders over three years ago, I've been working intensively to keep my levels elevated, especially because my genetic testing revealed that I produce lower-than-normal amounts. Your body naturally produces glutathione every day, but extra doses—which are very well absorbed via the bloodstream as opposed to the gut—can specifically help facilitate phase 2 liver detoxification. In simple terms, adding higher amounts of absorbable glutathione allows for more garbage trucks to come pick up the trash that is overflowing on the liver's curb.

Injections and IVs deliver far more absorbable glutathione in less time compared to many glutathione-containing supplements (especially if the glutathione is combined with phosphatidylcholine, which a good medical practitioner will often do). This is because when administered orally, much of the glutathione can be broken down and oxidized before it can be absorbed. But this doesn't mean you have to rush out to grab a handful of needles, a diagram of the appropriate butt-cheek injection location, or a nurse practitioner to shove an IV needle into a vein on your forearm. Because I have very low levels of endogenous glutathione production, I go out of my way to take these added steps, but oral glutathione supplementation combined with the consumption of glutathione-rich foods can also get you plenty of this crucial antioxidant. Research has demonstrated that lab animals absorb orally consumed glutathione intact, and that glutathione can cross intestinal cells in humans. And contrary to what many nutritionists preach, significant amounts of orally administered glutathione can be absorbed intact if the glutathione is in liposomal form and is administered sublingually (under the tongue).

Research has shown that taking glutathione sublingually results in better absorption than taking an encapsulated supplement. Liposomal glutathione administered sublingually can be very effective. Liposomes are small, fat-like droplets that are very similar to the membranes that encase your own cells. These membranes protect the contents of the liposomes from the process of digestion, so by taking glutathione that has been packaged into liposomes, you may be able to increase your absorption of orally administered glutathione. Liposomal oral glutathione seems to be taken up particularly well by the kidneys, heart, brain, lungs, skin, and small intestine.

People with insulin resistance, diabetes, chronic inflammation, or infection can't produce sufficient glutathione on their own, so glutathione supplements, IVs, or injections may be the best option for them. An effective glutathione supplemental dose is between 250 and 1,000 mg daily. For oral administration, I prefer a sublingual, liposomal form, such as Quicksilver Scientific or Almsbio glutathione; the latter also contains several mitochondria-supporting compounds, such as PQQ and CoQ10. You can also improve your body's own glutathione synthesis by supplementing with glutathione precursors or compounds that enhance glutathione recycling.

Your body produces glutathione from three amino acids: cysteine, glutamate, and glycine. The most important of these when it comes to supplements is cysteine, as your body has more trouble creating it. Since cysteine degrades easily, it is best to supplement with N-acetylcysteine (NAC), which is broken down into a readily available form of cysteine. PharmaNAC is a very powerful supplemental form of cysteine, and also quite handy for hangovers and liver detox protocols. For glutathione recycling, particularly via raising glutathione levels inside cells, R-lipoic acid and resveratrol are both effective.

If you want to include glutathione-supporting foods in your diet, you need to start eating sulfur-rich compounds. The foods with the highest sulfur content are beef, fish, poultry, broccoli, brussels sprouts, cauliflower, kale, watercress, mustard greens, garlic, shallots, and onions. Other ways to support glutathione production include consuming whey protein, which has a cysteine precursor for glutathione; turmeric powder or curcumin, which both increase glutathione and glutathione enzyme levels; and organ meats, avocado, spinach, and okra, all of which are naturally rich in glutathione.

Another very good method to deliver large amounts of highly absorbable glutathione into your system very quickly is via a suppository (yep, up the butt) or a nebulizing intranasal spray. For either of these methods, I recommend my friend Dr. John Lieurance's glutathione products; you'll find a link to his website on BoundlessBook.com/13. He also sells high-dose melatonin and CBD suppositories that are very effective for sleep, even in people who notice nothing at all from traditional oral administration.

THE LAST WORD

Congratulations! You have now learned everything you need to know about what to do when your digestive tract gets off track, how to hit the reboot button, how to detox your body, and much more.

As you no doubt now realize, the gut is quite complex, and there are plenty of resources that had to be omitted from this chapter simply for lack of space. You can find these in complete detail on BoundlessBook.com/13.

Finally, you are going to find that detoxing your body goes hand in hand with detoxing your home and workplace. Chapter 20 has everything you need to know about how to fully detox the air, light, water, and electricity in the important areas of your life. I also suggest paying close attention to chapter 15, which has plenty more about the immune system, which also goes hand in hand with gut optimization.

ONE THING YOU CAN DO THIS WEEK

Here is a simple strategy to help your digestive system that you can begin immediately: every time you eat a meal, chew each bite of food twenty-five times. Yes, twenty-five. Your mouth, like your stomach, is full of digestive enzymes, such as salivary alpha-amylase, so by taking your time and chewing, you are giving those enzymes a chance to do their job. You're also allowing optimum time for your gallbladder to release bile into your stomach. Chewing thoroughly can also activate hormones like cholecystekinin that will make you feel fuller faster, stimulate hydrochloric acid to begin breaking down proteins, and even stimulate your parasympathetic nervous system so that you're not eating in a stressed, fight-or-flight state.

> For citations for all the research studies mentioned in this chapter and a deeper dive into the topics of this chapter—including links to podcasts, blog posts, recommended tools and supplements, and much more—visit BoundlessBook.com/13.

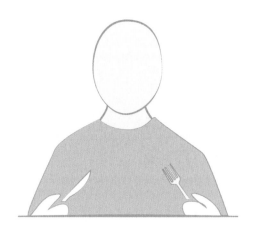

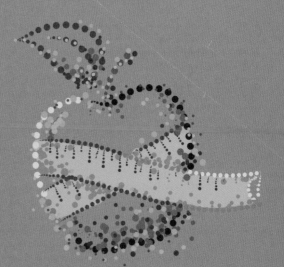

14

F&*K DIETS

HOW TO CUSTOMIZE YOUR NUTRITION TO YOU

I shook my head at the baffling reading on the blood glucose monitor: 140. *140?* That's the blood glucose level of a diabetic who just chugged a giant Coke—not the level I'd expected for myself after consuming a handful of roasted macadamia nuts (without a chocolate coating).

Could the numbers be lying? An equipment malfunction, perhaps? I fumbled with my finger, squeezed out another drop of blood, and tested again. 10, 9, 8 … The screen counted down and finally displayed my new reading: 142. Damn. Even higher.

What the hell? *Nuts* are not supposed to spike one's blood sugar. That's the realm of cookies, bananas, and soda, not friggin' *nuts.* Considering I'd tested my genes and discovered a higher-than-normal risk of type 2 diabetes, and I was patting myself on the back for having consumed a high-fat, low-carbohydrate diet for the past three years, this blood sugar value in response to nuts was even more alarming.

So I picked up the phone and called Grace, my poop doctor, who not only happens to specialize in just about any issue pertaining to the gut, diet, and food reactions but also possesses the results of my food allergy, food intolerance, and digestive inflammation tests and has a microbiome printout of every tiny shred of bacteria in my inner tubes.

"Oh, that's easy!" she exclaimed after I filled her in. "You don't tolerate oxalates. Oxalates are in nuts, so you produce the stress hormone cortisol when you eat nuts."

I nodded. Of course. Contrary to popular belief, your blood sugar can massively spike not just when you eat something sugary but also when you eat something "stressful," such as something you are allergic to or can't digest properly—in my case, the innocent macadamia nut. This happens because stress causes cortisol to send a message to my liver to break down stored carbohydrates and dump them into my blood so that I can run from the lion and live to fight another day. Problem is, I was dealing with a nut, not a lion, and didn't need the boost of blood sugar to fuel a speedy retreat. As a result, my blood sugar shot through the roof, causing rampant inflammation and blood vessel damage.

I hung up the phone and sighed. Thank you very much, biochemical individuality. I should have known. After all, one of the prized books on my shelf is a 1998 gem by Roger Williams entitled (you guessed it) *Biochemical Individuality*. The back cover sums up its argument nicely: "There is no such thing as the average person—we are all genetically and biologically unique. But when sperm meets egg, our characteristics are not locked in stone. Bad genes do not cause disease by themselves—nutrition and environment can alter the outcome."

The book, recommended to me at a health conference by Dr. Jeffrey Bland, a man deemed the "father of functional medicine," explains the fascinating diversity that exists from human to human, including surprising variations in everything from the shapes of our hearts and livers to the rate at which we excrete fatty acids and amino acids, our natural enzyme production levels, how well we digest certain foods, and a host of other elements.

For example, even though they're found in just about every multivitamin on the face of the planet, some people don't actually need to supplement with any ascorbic acid (vitamin C), vitamin A, or a form of vitamin B called riboflavin. Why? They harbor intestinal bacteria that produce ample amounts of each of these vitamins. But the only way to know if you possess that bacteria is to do the type of simple, at-home poop testing you will read about later in this chapter.

Take vitamin D as another example. There are well-authenticated cases of "vitamin D–resistant" people. These folks produce heart-damaging amounts of calcium and phosphorus deposits in their blood vessels when they consume the FDA's current recommendations for this vitamin (about 20 mcg per day). That should be a big warning sign to anyone popping vitamin D like candy, especially given the health media's infatuation with this so-called cure-all vitamin. At the same time, many people—especially those with darker skin tones, which can limit the amount of vitamin D they produce from sunlight—can develop serious health issues, such as osteoporosis and hormone deficiencies, when they don't supplement vitamin D.

But despite the enormous amount of biochemical individuality that exists from person to person, there are still a plethora of diet books published each year (particularly close to swimsuit season and New Year's) that promise to be the ultimate solution for everything from losing body fat to banishing acne to beating cravings and building muscle—when in fact the same ketogenic diet that helped your neighbor shed 20 pounds can result in rampant inflammation, brain fog, and oxidized cholesterol for you.

Roger Williams put it quite elegantly:

Genetic influences are far better understood now … for major nutrition-related problems such as alcoholism, heart disease, diabetes, hypertension, and cancer. Yet we seem frustratingly slow to integrate this knowledge into clinical practice and common knowledge. Most clinicians still treat and write about these problems as if inborn differences are unimportant. Professional and lay authors still recommend restrictive diets they assume are best for nearly everyone. They debate heatedly about which one of the conflicting diets is "right"—high-carbohydrate, low-carbohydrate, vegetarian, high-protein, etc. When will we automatically consider that all these diets likely have merit, but only for some individuals?

Get that? For dramatic emphasis, allow me to repeat what Williams says at the end of that paragraph: "All these diets likely have merit, but only for some individuals."

So f&*k diets. Diets suck, which is why I have never written a diet book and also why I think most diet books are silly marketing ploys (and the primary way for authors to prey upon our desire to find the holy grail of dieting; they make oodles of money by publishing a diet book and then a few months later publish a cookbook to grab even more cash).

Most diets apply a one-size-fits-all approach that paints an entire population with a broad nutritional brush without considering genetics; personal health history; nutrient, vitamin, and mineral deficiencies that need to be addressed; and, as you have just learned, biochemical individuality. To optimize the flow of energy through your body, doesn't it seem logical to account for the type of gas you put in the tank? You don't want to pump unleaded fuel into a diesel engine. A diet that works for one person leaves another person completely stripped of the ability to tap into their life force because it causes food intolerances, brain fog, bloating, and other chronic food-related problems.

In this chapter, you're going to discover what happens when diets such as keto, carnivore, vegan, and others go wrong, exactly how you can determine your own biochemical individuality, and how to know what way of eating is perfect for you.

THE KETOGENIC DIET

Let's start with a look at why a popular diet that many people swear by can be the wrong choice for some. The ketogenic diet is an extremely high-fat, low-carb diet that's championed by fat-lovers as the perfect way to lose weight, enhance cognition, and increase endurance. And for many people, the diet does indeed work for these goals.

I personally followed a strict ketogenic diet for years while competing in Ironman triathlons, and I even participated in a fascinating high-fat-diet experiment called the FASTER Study (an acronym for "fat-adapted substrate use in trained elite runners"). In this experiment, I and eighteen other elite endurance athletes followed a strict 90 percent fat-based diet for twelve months, then appeared at a University of Connecticut lab to subject ourselves to a series of blood, urine, and stool measurements followed by a brutal three-hour treadmill run, along with a painful biopsy of muscle tissue from the quadriceps and fat tissue from the ass cheeks (imagine a miniature guillotine shoved into your flanks to cut out tissue samples). The results of that experiment (which you can read more about on BoundlessBook.com/14) completely rewrote exercise physiology textbooks by revealing that long-term adherence to a high-fat diet nearly doubles the human body's fat-burning capacity, both at rest and during exercise, without harming performance. I still occasionally use a high-fat, very-low-carb ketotic diet—and even supplement with exogenous ketones, which are a drinkable strategy to very quickly put yourself into ketosis—as a brain-boosting strategy on mentally difficult days.

But when I do fitness and nutrition consulting for people who are following a ketogenic diet, I have witnessed concerningly high levels of LDL cholesterol (skyrocketing over 400 mg/dL), along with rampant inflammation and inflated triglyceride levels (which can be a risk factor for heart disease and liver problems). These metrics are often accompanied by issues such as anxiety, joint pain, gastrointestinal discomfort, general malaise or fatigue, and poor physical performance. How can some people thrive on keto while others struggle? It comes down to how an individual's body processes fat.

When Fat Metabolism Goes Wrong: Why Keto Isn't Right for Everyone

Fact is, many people have problems metabolizing and utilizing fat that aren't related to clinical conditions or missing nutrients but are instead the result of variations in the genes that encode for fat metabolism. If you have one of the following four genetic factors, you may not respond well to a high-fat or ketogenic diet. Indeed, you may not benefit from a constant state of ketosis at all—especially one achieved not by fasting and sugar restriction but by high fat intake—and you may instead perform better on a low-fat diet or a primarily Mediterranean-style diet high in monounsaturated fats like olive oil.

FAMILIAL HYPERCHOLESTEROLEMIA

One relatively common condition affecting fat metabolism is familial hypercholesterolemia (FH), which affects up to 10 percent of the world's population. People with this condition tend to experience a metabolic firestorm in response to a high-fat diet because their cholesterol and inflammatory biomarkers increase dramatically in response to foods like coconut oil, butter, fatty fish, red meat, and eggs. This condition is also associated with chest pain during physical activity, fatty deposits around the elbows, knees, and butt, cholesterol levels high enough to be a true cardiovascular risk factor, and cholesterol deposits around the eyelids.

While a very high LDL cholesterol (typically above 300 mg/dL) is a sign you may have FH, you can more precisely determine your status by getting a genetic test through a company such as 23andMe, then looking for risk markers such as these: (1) a TT polymorphism (genetic variation) on the CETP gene; (2) an AT polymorphism on the PCSK9 gene; or (3) an AA or AG polymorphism on the APOB gene. (If polymorphisms and genetic terminology are new to you, visit BoundlessBook.com/14 for a helpful guide on how to analyze your 23andMe raw results.)

When I presented this conundrum of people with FH on a ketogenic diet to my friend Chris Masterjohn, one of the brightest guys I know when it comes to nutrition geekery, he explained to me that the best way to deal with FH is to "take the one gene for the LDL receptor responsible for contributing to this condition and try to bring it up to the expression level that would be found in someone without FH." Chris went on to explain that from a scientific standpoint, this can be accomplished by maximizing the biological activity of thyroid hormone and suppressing the activity of a gene called PCSK9, both of which can be achieved by increasing insulin signaling through, for example, frequent physical movement, the use of insulin-sensitizing herbs and spices, and moderation of processed sugar and starches.

POOR ALPHA-LINOLENIC ACID CONVERSION

Alpha-linolenic acid (ALA) is a short-chain omega-3 fatty acid found primarily in plant-based foods, such as flax seeds, walnuts, and other seeds and nuts. ALA is an essential fatty acid because, like essential amino acids, it cannot be produced in the body, so it must be obtained through food. Plant sources of ALA are popular among vegetarian- and vegan-diet enthusiasts because once in the body, ALA can be converted into DHA and EPA, critical fatty acids that enhance cognition and brain health and help stabilize a state of ketosis and that are found primarily in animal foods (especially fatty fish).

But research suggests that only 2 to 10 percent of all ALA consumed is actually converted into DHA or EPA. In addition, the expression of ALA-converting genes, known as FADS, can vary widely. One variant of the FADS gene increases conversion, while another reduces conversion—so people with one variant are less able to convert ALA to DHA and EPA than those with another variant.

The FADS variant that improves ALA conversion is most common in African, Indian, Pakistani, Bangladeshi, and Sri Lankan populations. It is moderately common in European populations (although there is also variation across European populations; the conversion-increasing variant is most common in southern Europe) and least common in Native Americans and indigenous Arctic populations. This variation is likely due to the relative availability of plant sources of omega-3s and genetic adaptations to that availability: The more an ancestral population relied on plant sources of fatty acids, the more the population adapted to convert ALA into usable DHA and EPA. Conversely, the more a population consumed DHA and EPA directly from animal and fish sources, the more the conversion-increasing variant was replaced by the conversion-decreasing variant.

So if you have, say, African or Southern Asian ancestry, you likely carry the conversion-increasing variant of the FADS gene and don't need to consume as much DHA and EPA from animal or fish sources. It is important to note that this doesn't mean you don't need to consume animal or fish sources at all, simply that you don't need as much of them as people of other ancestral heritages do.

If you have far northern European, Iberian, Native American, or indigenous Arctic ancestry, you most likely can't effectively convert ALA into usable DHA and EPA. Those of British and Northern European ancestry may have more effective conversion rates, but the conversion-increasing variant is not as common as in Tuscan and southern European populations. If your genetic heritage comes from these groups, you need to get your DHA and EPA directly from meat and fish.

UPREGULATED ELONGATION OF OMEGA-6 FATTY ACIDS

Omega-6 fatty acids are, like omega-3s, polyunsaturated fatty acids, and they are found most commonly in poultry, eggs, grains, seeds, nuts, and most vegetable oils. Omega-6s are precursors to molecules called eicosanoids, which, when derived from omega-6s, can be pro-inflammatory, especially when omega-6s are consumed in excess. Eicosanoids derived from omega-3 fatty acids, on the other hand, are anti-inflammatory, but humans cannot efficiently convert omega-6s into omega-3s, so a high intake of omega-6 fatty acids without a proportionally high intake of omega-3s can lead to rampant cellular inflammation and weight gain.

But even if you do consume adequate omega-3 fatty acids (a balanced ratio of omega-3s to omega-6s is 1:1), you may not be able to handle omega-6s as well as other people. The process of converting omega-6s into inflammatory compounds is called elongation. The expression of the gene responsible for elongation varies from person to person, and some people have upregulated elongation, which results in more inflammatory compounds. If you have upregulated elongation, a significant amount of the linoleic acid (an omega-6 fatty acid) you consume in food like seeds and nuts will be converted into arachidonic acid, a precursor to inflammatory compounds. To avoid that inflammation, you will need to avoid common ketogenic fat sources high in linoleic acid, such as poultry, eggs, and nut butters, or, if you do consume them, you'll need to increase your intake of omega-3 fatty acids from fatty cold-water fish like tuna, mackerel, herring, and sardines. You can determine the status of your omega-6 elongation with an omega-3 and omega-6 fatty acid index test, which tells you whether you have excess inflammatory arachidonic acid levels. These indexes are offered by companies such as WellnessFX and Quest Diagnostics.

THE THRIFTY GENE HYPOTHESIS: FTO AND PPAR VARIANTS

The geneticist James Neel proposed the thrifty gene hypothesis in 1962 in an attempt to explain why certain populations are more susceptible to type 2 diabetes; it has also been used to explain why humans tend to accumulate body fat. The hypothesis claims that in the past, "thrifty genes" allowed some people to quickly build fat reserves in times of plenty as a buffer against food scarcity in leaner times. As food became overabundant in the modern era in developed nations, these genes continued to allow people to build fat reserves, even though times of food scarcity were less common. In addition, the calorie-dense foods responsible for triggering the thrifty genes (think about dishes high in both sugar and fat, such as butter with potatoes, ice cream, and eggs with waffles) are consumed in much higher quantities today than they were in the past.

Granted, the thrifty gene hypothesis has received much criticism over the last few decades, and even Neel himself found some evidence that suggested the hypothesis might not be accurate. But there are indeed certain genes that cause some people to gain fat more easily than others, especially in response to high-fat foods. The most common nutrients associated with genetic obesity are fatty acids, and the two most notorious genes responsible for storing these fatty acids are the FTO and PPAR gamma genes.

The FTO gene (which codes a protein associated with fat mass and obesity) is responsible for regulating body fat and overall weight. Research suggests that the FTO gene is the primary genetic factor associated with weight gain and that diet is the primary environmental factor that triggers the FTO gene. A high saturated-fat intake is particularly associated with FTO-induced weight gain, so if you carry either one or two copies of the FTO rs9939609 polymorphism, you will likely do better on a diet low in saturated fat, particularly from dairy, butter, coconut oil, and fatty beef, lamb, and pork.

The PPAR (peroxisome proliferator-activated receptor) gene is also associated with weight gain following a high fat intake. The PPAR gamma polymorphism is responsible for regulating fatty acid storage, the uptake of fatty acids, and the growth of new fat cells. A variant of the PPAR gamma gene has shown significant increases in weight in response to dietary fat and mono-unsaturated fatty acid intake, suggesting that the PPAR gamma gene is one of the primary genes responsible for causing weight gain. Polyunsaturated fatty acids, such as the omega-6 arachidonic acid, also activate PPAR gamma, so if you have PPAR gamma (instead of, say, PPAR alpha), you will probably achieve greater dietary success by limiting your intake of fats.

You can find out if you possess either the FTO rs9939609 polymorphism or the PPAR gamma gene by taking a 23andMe genetic test at home and then searching for these gene variants in your raw results. There is a growing body of websites, such as DNAFit, MyHeritage, StrateGene, and Genetic Genie, that can make digging through this data a bit easier. (BoundlessBook.com/14 also has a guide to analyzing your 23andMe raw results, and you can also visit BenGreenfieldFitness.com/rawdata for a quick list.)

So if you have one of these genetic factors and can't thrive on keto, what should you eat? Much to the chagrin of ketogenic zealots, it all comes down to (drumroll please) eating a low-fat, fiber-rich, high-carbohydrate diet and replacing saturated fat with polyunsaturated fat. The best approach is to follow a diet similar to an ancestral protocol common among the inhabitants of the island Kitava, who happen to possess the FH gene but do not experience heart disease. This diet is rich in fiber-dense carbohydrates, such as coconut meat, starchy tubers, and fresh fruit (notably, none of these are processed, refined carbohydrates).

How to Do Keto the Right Way

When you think about it, it may seem strange that some people don't do well on keto. After all, our ancestors were often in a state of ketosis, as are many hunter-gatherer tribes today; so are many people in Blue Zones—parts of the world where people tend to live longer than average. But they all achieve ketosis via natural habits such as frequent fasting, low intake of processed sugary or starchy foods, high plant intake, and "drowning" real, whole foods with healthy fats such as extra-virgin olive oil. This stands in stark contrast to the modern, somewhat bastardized version of ketosis, often called "dirty keto," which involves buying ketone supplements that cost $15 a serving, eating ungodly amounts of butter, coconut oil, and other saturated fats, eating surprisingly sparse amounts of actual, real food, and spending many precious minutes each day hunched over a ketone monitor in a form of endless self-quantification.

As long as you don't have one of the genetic factors listed earlier, a ketogenic diet can indeed be an effective method for enhancing focus, boosting physical and mental energy, and improving physical performance. But even if you respond well to a carbohydrate-restricted or fat-rich diet, it is easy to make mistakes that may prevent you from entering a state of ketosis, cause you to accumulate nutrient deficits, and give you low, sluggish energy (particularly during workouts) on a strict ketogenic diet.

In particular, two main issues often arise on a ketogenic diet. The first problem, stemming from a tendency to focus on animal foods and avoid plant foods, is the loss of key nutrients, such as phytochemicals, antioxidants, fiber, and plant-based vitamins. For example, the phytochemicals contained in kale, spinach, blueberries, raspberries, collard greens, Swiss chard, and sweet potatoes are responsible for a phenomenon called xenohormesis. Recall from chapter 3 that hormesis is a phenomenon in which exposure to low doses of compounds that could be toxic or lethal in higher doses results in a beneficial effect, such as improved health, muscle growth, or longevity. Eliminating plants from your diet because they're carbohydrate-based, as many do on keto, means eliminating these phytochemicals and the benefits they bring.

These same plants are also sources of antioxidants that are crucial for neutralizing free radicals, which can cause a host of physiological and neurological problems, including neuro-degeneration and damage to muscle tissue. Vegetables and fruits are some of the densest sources of a full spectrum of antioxidants you can consume. They also—unlike butter, coconut oil, and hefty cuts of fat-streaked meat—include fiber. Fiber is important for satiety, maintaining healthy digestive function, and feeding robust populations of beneficial gut bacteria (although it's worth noting that, paradoxically, in people with compromised guts, fiber can increase issues such as gas, bloating, and constipation). Finally, plants are potent sources of a wide range of vitamins, minerals, and micronutrients, including vitamin A, vitamin C, B vitamins, calcium, potassium, and iron. While some vegetables, particularly starchy tubers like sweet potatoes and white potatoes and sweet fruits like bananas and apples, are too high in carbohydrates to be strictly keto-friendly, most vegetables, such as dark leafy greens and cruciferous vegetables, are keto-friendly and can be consumed in relatively high quantities.

Of course, one wrench thrown into this equation is the potential for other hormetic stressors—such as exercise, cold thermogenesis, sauna, sunlight radiation, and even the heterocylic amines and other charred compounds formed during the cooking of meat—may allow for adequate hormesis even in the absence of high plant intake, a theory proposed by my podcast guest Dr. Paul Saladino in our carnivore diet episode. However, there is very little long-term research comparing the hormetic effects of a plant-based diet to those of a carnivore diet.

The second problem that can accompany a low-carb, ketogenic diet is a cluster of symptoms known collectively as the "keto flu," also known as carbohydrate withdrawal. Keto flu can manifest as any or all of the following symptoms:

Brain fog	Irritability
Headaches	Muscle soreness
Chills	Nausea
Sore throat	Poor focus
Confusion	Stomach pains
Dizziness	Sugar cravings
Insomnia	

Keto flu typically begins twenty-four to forty-eight hours into a ketogenic diet and can last anywhere from a few days to several weeks. The flu is caused by three changes that can occur as your body shifts from glucose metabolism to fatty acid metabolism. First, as you cut out carbohydrates, your insulin levels drop. This signals your kidneys to flush sodium out of your body, which can result in losing up to 10 pounds of water weight in just a few days. The accompanying loss of muscle glycogen and minerals, along with low insulin levels, can cause dizziness, nausea, headaches, muscle cramping, diarrhea, and constipation.

Second, there are diet-induced changes to thyroid hormones. The hormones T3 and T4 are produced by the thyroid gland and regulate body temperature, metabolism, and heart rate. Thyroid function relies heavily upon adequate carbohydrate intake, so as you cut back on carbohydrates, levels of T3 and T4 may fall, resulting in brain fog and fatigue.

Third, at the same time as your T3 and T4 hormone levels fall, your cortisol levels can rise. This is because extreme carbohydrate restriction signals to your body that glucose is a precious commodity, and your body responds by attempting to increase glucose levels via increased levels of stress hormones like cortisol. This can result in irritability and insomnia.

So how can you beat these nutritional deficiencies and carbohydrate withdrawal symptoms? The following are seven tactics for getting the most out of a low-carb, ketogenic diet without experiencing significant reductions in physical or cognitive performance.

1. CONSUME VEGGIES AND TAKE SUPPLEMENTS.

Most vegetables are keto-friendly. There is no reason you can't liberally consume kale, collard greens, brussels sprouts, and Swiss chard and moderately consume low-glycemic-index fruits such as blueberries, raspberries, and blackberries. You can also supplement the phytochemicals, antioxidants, and fiber you get from these whole-foods sources via prebiotics, probiotics, and antioxidants like GSH (glutathione) and turmeric extract (curcumin), along with a quality multi-vitamin. Interestingly, microgreens, which are the shoots of leafy greens such as arugula, Swiss chard, and mustard picked just after the first leaves have developed, can help modulate cholesterol levels and lower inflammation. Microgreens are very simple to grow at home in a sunny window or under an LED grow light.

In addition to eating more vegetables and microgreens, you should also consider consuming the following supplements:

- Choline, which helps your liver process fat and prevents nonalcoholic fatty liver disease
- Magnesium, which improves bone health, immune system function, and nerve and muscle function. It also helps minimize muscle cramps, dizziness, and fatigue.
- Potassium, which is necessary for proper cellular function. It also minimizes cramps, constipation, and muscle weakness.
- Sodium, which, as mentioned above, is dumped by your kidneys as insulin levels drop. If you are performing heavy training sessions, you need to maintain sodium levels because you lose a lot of sodium through sweat. Sodium also reduces fatigue, headaches, and thirst.
- Creatine, which will allow you to perform high-volume, high-intensity workouts without relying on high levels of muscle glycogen (since these stores will be depleted as you restrict carbohydrate intake). This is known as a carbohydrate-sparing effect.

2. CONSUME MORE FATS, ESPECIALLY MCT OIL.

Consuming more of the right types of fat may accelerate your adaptation to a ketogenic diet. MCT (medium-chain triglyceride) oil, which is derived from coconut oil, is particularly potent. Most fatty acids must travel through your lymphatic system to your heart, muscles, and adipose tissue before entering the liver to be metabolized. But MCT oil goes straight to the liver to be immediately metabolized into energy, and just adding MCT oil to your diet may allow you to avoid the keto flu altogether. You can also add coconut oil to your morning coffee and eat more foods rich in healthy fats, such as grass-fed beef, fatty cold-water fish, and eggs. Extra-virgin olive oil, coconut oil, and MCT oil can also be drizzled liberally on almost any dish. Just remember to include plants, too, as these can eliminate the potential for a high intake of oils (particularly saturated fats) to become inflammatory.

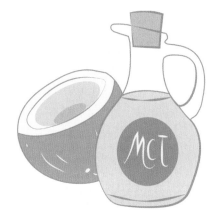

Is It Healthy to Put Fat in Your Coffee?

You are no doubt familiar with the current craze of dumping butter, coconut oil, MCT oil, or ghee into what your grandparents would have consumed as a no-frills, plain ole cup of coffee.

There is definitely something to this trendy practice. When blended with fats, cognitively enhancing cholesterols found in the mighty coffee bean, including cafestol and kahweol, can cross the blood-brain barrier, increasing coffee's cognitive benefits and extending the mental boost to a level beyond that which caffeine can provide. In addition, adding fats to coffee can keep you satiated for long periods of time, boost ketone production if you use MCT or coconut oil, provide anti-inflammatory effects and feed beneficial bacteria in the gut if you use butter, and even provide a slight elevation in metabolic rate if you use MCT oil (due to the thermogenic effect of combining caffeine and MCT oil).

So I am certainly a fan of blending fat into your coffee. But you also can't consume oodles of saturated fat in large doses without taking some steps to mitigate the potential damage. For example, the long-chain fatty acids found in coconut oil can cause a rise in inflammatory T cells that, if left unchecked, can lead to and exacerbate autoimmune diseases or gut discomfort. The short-chain fatty acids found in vegetables can reverse this damage, so if you do add concentrated amounts of fat to your coffee, make sure to consume several servings of vegetables throughout the day, especially antioxidant-rich greens, herbs, and spices. In other words, don't have fatty coffee for breakfast, sardines and an avocado for lunch, and a rib-eye steak and mashed potatoes for dinner and expect your cholesterol, inflammation, and other biomarkers to respond favorably. A better scenario would be a fatty coffee for breakfast, a giant salad for lunch, and boatloads of roasted vegetables with dinner.

Keep in mind, too, that you are often drinking many, many calories in a fatty coffee beverage—remember, fat has twice as many calories as protein or carbohydrates—so it counts as a full meal and isn't best consumed along with, say, a big plate of bacon and eggs, assuming you care about the size of your waistline. And finally, if intermittent fasting is your thing, be aware that a cup of high-calorie fatty coffee will definitely take you out of a fasted state, although because it is unlikely to spike glucose or insulin levels, it is one of the better choices for staying "semi-fasted."

Now don't get me wrong: there's nothing wrong with a big black cup o' joe, but occasionally it's fun to spin the brain's dials with inventive deliciousness. So here are three of my favorite fatty coffee recipes to get your creative wheels churning: two hot, for those chilly fall or winter days or when you crave the comfort of a hot brew, and one cold, for a pre- or postworkout pick-me-up or a cognition-enhancing treat on a warm summer day. Pro tip: For all these recipes, I pretty much only use a smaller NutriBullet blender. A big countertop blender is unnecessary, unwieldy, and leaves too much of your coffee goodness stuck to the sides of the blender jar.

COFFEE-CACAO SIPPER

Prepare yourself for an intense chocolate experience with a hint of java. The Ceylon cinnamon helps control blood sugar, and though the collagen is optional, I recommend it for active individuals. The cardamom or rosemary is also optional but will enhance the coffee's antioxidant properties.

- 12 to 16 ounces brewed coffee, hot
- 1 scoop unflavored collagen peptides (optional)
- 2 tablespoons cacao powder
- 1 tablespoon almond or other nut butter
- 1 tablespoon coconut butter or coconut manna
- 1 teaspoon Ceylon cinnamon
- Drop of butterscotch toffee–flavored or vanilla-flavored liquid stevia
- Pinch of cardamom or dried ground rosemary (optional)

Place the ingredients in a blender and blend for 1 minute, until smooth and oh-so-frothy. Oh, and be careful when you open the lid: this stuff can get a bit fizzy under pressure. Just ask my wife, who has—perhaps more than once—had to help me clean a coffee explosion off the kitchen walls.

CRUNCHY COFFEE FROSTY

This drink is like a milkshake-coffee combo with a bit of a superfood crunch at the end. I'll occasionally break off a few chunks of a nice, very dark chocolate bar and stir that in instead of the cacao nibs.

- 8 to 12 ounces brewed coffee, chilled
- 4 ounces full-fat coconut milk or coconut cream
- 2 tablespoons cacao powder
- 1 teaspoon ground Ceylon cinnamon
- Drop of butterscotch toffee–flavored or vanilla-flavored liquid stevia
- Cacao nibs, for topping
- Unsweetened coconut flakes, for topping

Place all the ingredients except the toppings in a blender and puree until smooth, adding water and ice to achieve your desired texture. After blending, top with or stir in the cacao nibs and unsweetened coconut flakes.

GHEE-COCONUT-CACAO COFFEE

This wonderful morning brew keeps me satiated for hours, and the cacao offers a nice boost of dopamine too. I occasionally use two packets of Four Sigmatic mushroom extract instead of coffee.

- 8 ounces brewed coffee, hot
- 2 tablespoons cacao tea (I recommend the MiCacao brand, which is a delicious mix of cacao shells and nibs)
- 1 tablespoon coconut butter or coconut manna
- 1 tablespoon ghee (optional, but if you don't use it, I'd double up on the coconut butter or coconut manna)
- Drop of butterscotch toffee–flavored or vanilla-flavored liquid stevia (I prefer Omica Organics)

Place the ingredients in a blender and blend for 60 to 90 seconds, until well combined and smooth.

3. IMPLEMENT A CYCLIC KETOGENIC APPROACH.

Unless you're using a ketogenic diet to treat a health condition such as epilepsy or Alzheimer's, you don't necessarily need to stay in ketosis indefinitely. Occasional and even regular dips into ketosis via strategies like fasting, occasional carbohydrate refeeds, and carb cycling are sufficient for providing the benefits of a ketogenic diet without requiring you to eliminate carbs for months at a time. While you can, especially if you aren't a hard-charging athlete, certainly remain in a state of ketosis for years at a time without experiencing any adverse effects (assuming you eat a healthy ketogenic diet that includes plant foods), you can also get the same benefits from brief, frequent forays into ketosis.

For example, you can consume all of your carbohydrates at the end of the day, especially if you have a hard exercise session in the late afternoon or early evening. This exercise session ensures you are highly sensitive to glucose, so that the glucose you do eat is stored as muscle glycogen. If you fast for twelve to sixteen hours after this meal, you will still be able to enjoy the fat-burning and brain-boosting benefits of ketosis without depleting your energy. Many of my athletic clients perform evening carb refeeds of up to 200 g of carbohydrates every day and spend most of their time in ketosis. Most of my other clients perform at least a weekly carb refeed, typically on their most physically active day of the week to reduce any excess glucose response.

The Carnivore Diet

The carnivore diet falls into the same general category as the ketogenic diet because it is a very-low-carbohydrate protocol that can potentially set you up for many of the same deficits or issues people experience when going keto. The difference between a carnivore diet and a ketogenic diet is that although a carnivore diet can (and should) be ketogenic, it is higher in protein and lower in (or devoid of) many of the common staples of a ketogenic diet, such as butter, coconut oil, seeds, nuts, and plant-based oils.

On a strict carnivore diet, one eats meat (preferably nose-to-tail), fish, water, and little else, although some variations allow for animal-derived foods such as butter, dairy, and eggs. So breakfast might be a cut of wild salmon, lunch a large rib eye, and dinner a serving of a rack of lamb.

However, if you eat exclusively meat, you can disrupt your microbiome, particularly because the notable lack of fiber can cause a shortage of short-chain fatty acids (SCFAs), which your gut bacteria use as fuel to maintain the integrity of the intestinal wall. Research has shown that an all-meat diet can lead to SCFA deficits. But an interesting study found that cheetahs are able to ferment collagen from bones and cartilage into SCFAs; humans on a carnivore diet who consume bone broth, bone marrow, and other cartilaginous sources, such as many of the newer bone broth powders with added cartilage, may be able to do the same.

In addition, many of the benefits of fiber are attributable to its fermentation by bacteria that produce SCFAs, especially one called butyrate, in the colon. However, it turns out that SCFAs have metabolic properties that are very similar to those of a ketone called beta-hydroxybutyrate (BHB). In the presence of low carbohydrate intake, the liver's production of BHB may reduce or eliminate the need for butyrate, which is produced from a higher-fiber diet. This can be especially good news for people who experience gas, bloating, or other gastrointestinal distress from a high consumption of seeds, nuts, grains, or vegetables (particularly roughage and raw veggies).

Therefore, a well-formulated ketogenic or low-carbohydrate carnivore diet may provide many of the benefits of fiber, without a high carbohydrate intake or the unpleasant side effects that some people experience from high fiber intake. In other words, if you are in nutritional ketosis from a ketogenic diet or a low-carb carnivore diet, it may not be necessary to consume a lot of fiber to achieve the health effects attributed to fiber.

Since red meat is quite high in the amino acids cysteine, tryptophan, and methionine, which can be pro-cancer and pro-aging in excess, anyone on the carnivore diet should prioritize getting adequate glycine, proline, and hydroxyproline, all of which can balance out the other amino acids and also support a strong gut lining. This is another good reason to consume bone broth, collagen, glycine, essential amino acids, and organ meats, which are high in these particular amino acids.

Finally, because it includes so little (or no) plant matter, the carnivore diet tends to be low in vitamins C and E, and, if dairy is not included, also vitamin K_2 and calcium. If a carnivore diet doesn't include organ meats, it also becomes low in vitamin A, folate, manganese, and magnesium, which are crucial compounds for normal, healthy metabolic function.

In reality, it is very rare to find a long-lived, healthy population that subsists entirely on meat, especially muscle meat. For example, several Asian, Latin American, and African tribal cultures that are often thought of as carnivorous actually consume the intestines of ruminant animals like goats, sheep, deer, and cows, which contain high amounts of the vegetables and fiber those animals consumed—a literal stomach salad! These include dishes such as the Spanish zarajos, the Filipino dinuguan, the Korean gopchang, and the Latin American chinchulines.

Many argue that some ancestral populations were carnivorous. While it's true that many of our ancestors thrived on large quantities of animal products, every single one of the commonly cited carnivorous groups also took significant advantage of plant foods. For example, as my friend Chris Kresser notes in his excellent write-up on the carnivore diet:

- *The nomads of Mongolia ate plenty of meat and dairy products, but consumed wild onions and garlic, tubers and roots, seeds, and berries.*

- *Gaucho Brazilians consumed mostly beef, but also supplemented their diet with yerba mate, a tea rich in vitamins, minerals, and phytonutrients.*

- *The Maasai, Rendille, and Samburu tribes of East Africa primarily consumed meat, milk, and blood, but also occasionally consumed herbs and tree barks. Women and older men in these communities consumed ample amounts of fruit, tubers, and honey.*

- *The Russian Arctic Chukotka thrived on fish, caribou, and marine animals but always paired these animal foods with local roots, leafy greens, berries, or seaweed.*
- *The Sioux of South Dakota ate large amounts of buffalo, but also consumed wild fruit, nuts, and seeds that they came across as they hunted the buffalo herds.*
- *The Canadian Inuit subsisted primarily on walrus, whale meat, seal, and fish, but also foraged wild berries, lichens, and sea vegetables and even fermented many of these plant foods as a preservation method.*

Granted, one could argue that many of these populations turned to these plants only in the absence of animal foods, and that they—and modern humans—could thrive on eating fish and animals nose-to-tail in the absence of such plant matter. However, this may not be sustainable for the planet, accessible for many people, or enjoyable (since it would require getting rid of a rich, tasty, and satisfying tradition of consuming plant compounds such as coffee, red wine, sourdough bread, sweet potato fries, beet salad with goat cheese, and all of your other favorite foods that are plant derived).

Finally, researcher Richard Wrangham presents good evidence that the relatively large brain and small gut of the human didn't happen from eating more meat (which the carnivore diet enthusiasts propose) but from eating tubers and root vegetables.

All things considered, if I were to eat a carnivore diet, I would not only eat organ meats, bone marrow, and bone broth, but I would also add:

- small amounts of root vegetables and tubers, along with pureed, mashed, or canned pumpkin and sweet potato purees, preferably skipping the skin of these compounds and any excess fiber
- homemade fermented yogurt made from coconut milk and the *L. reuteri* probiotic (see chapter 15 for a recipe)
- raw, organic honey as a sweetener
- small, antioxidant-rich, low-sugar berries, such as blueberries, lingonberries, bilberries, and blackberries
- bitter, tannin-rich teas and organic coffee
- organic dried insects such as crickets, grasshoppers, caterpillars, and ants (which have extremely high nutritional value and can be purchased from websites such as BenGreenfieldFitness.com/edibleinsects)

- seeds and nuts, if tolerated by the gut and prepared via the ancestral practices of soaking, fermenting, or sprouting
- nutrient-dense vegetable powders that offer plenty of phytonutrients without excess roughage and fiber, such as Dr. Thomas Cowan's heirloom vegetable powders
- twelve-to-sixteen-hour daily intermittent fasting to ensure that mTOR pathways aren't excessively activated
- consumption of my friend Dr. Joseph Mercola's "autophagy tea" before my nightly fast, to limit mTOR activation and increase autophagy (1 teaspoon pau d'arco powdered tea, ½ teaspoon hydroxycitrate and garcinia (HCA/garcinia powder), ½ teaspoon quercetin powder, ½ teaspoon glycine powder, ½ teaspoon chamomile powder)

For a deep dive into the ins and outs and dos and don'ts of a properly structured nose-to-tail carnivore diet, including its sustainability, ethics, and my own approach to this diet, please listen to my interview with Dr. Paul Saladino at BenGreenfieldFitness.com/carnivore.

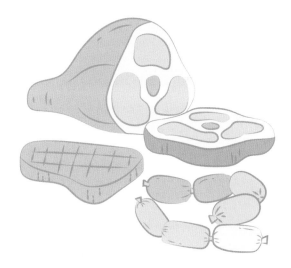

4. GET GOOD SLEEP.

Sleep helps to regulate cortisol levels, which rise as thyroid hormones levels drop in response to carbohydrate restriction. As you sleep, levels of the fat-burning hormones leptin and adiponectin rise, which further stabilizes appetite and improves your adaptation to a fat-based diet. Review chapter 7 for recommendations on optimizing your sleep.

5. PERFORM LIGHT EXERCISE FOR A FEW DAYS.

Hard exercise elevates cortisol levels, which are already elevated from the process of adapting to a ketogenic diet. Since excessively elevated cortisol levels can signal insulin to shovel the food you eat into fat cells (which is the opposite of what you want to achieve with a ketogenic diet), until you adapt to burning fat, perform lighter exercise sessions. Do some yoga, hit the sauna, go for a swim or paddleboard session, or embark on an easy sunshine walk or hike. Incidentally, if you perform this activity in a fasted state before eating breakfast, it will boost your fat-burning capacities even more and make your shift into ketosis go more smoothly.

While you don't want to overdo any hard exercise sessions, lifting heavy weights can help prevent loss of muscle on a high-fat, lower-protein ketogenic diet. Lifting weights will send signals to your muscles to enter an anabolic, muscle-building state without taking you out of ketosis. Ideally, these initial weight-lifting sessions should be short and intense rather than high-rep or high-volume.

6. TAKE ACTIVATED CHARCOAL.

Adipose tissue can act as a storage depot for toxins like molds, BPA, and pesticides. As you burn stored body fat while on a ketogenic diet, these toxins can be released back into your bloodstream and, if left alone, can be reabsorbed into more-sensitive tissues like the brain and other vital organs. Consuming activated charcoal, which binds to toxins, will help your body flush these toxins out. (Chapter 13 also describes other effective methods for truly detoxing your body as you burn fat.)

7. TAKE EXOGENOUS KETONE SUPPLEMENTS.

By definition, the goal of a ketogenic diet is to get your body to generate ketones, molecules produced during fat-burning that your body uses for fuel. But you can also mainline exogenous ketones into your body with the use of supplements, such as ketone salts and ketone esters. They can help reduce fatigue and boost energy by quickly raising ketone levels in your blood. While exogenous ketones aren't a replacement for a true state of nutritional ketosis, they can help you get through the keto flu during the first few days or weeks of a carbohydrate-restricted diet.

A PLANT-BASED DIET

Heavy consumption of animal products, such as the steaks, burgers, chicken, giant slabs of fish, and massive omelets that often characterize a Western diet, can certainly be detrimental to the environment and, particularly when it comes to high intake of meat, may even be detrimental to your health or longevity. For example, people who are overmethylators may not be able to consume as much red meat due to meat's high content of methyl groups (I'll explore this in more detail in chapter 19). Several observational studies suggest that eating a lot of red meat may increase the risk of diabetes, heart disease, certain types of cancer, and premature death. Admittedly, observational studies cannot prove causality, and scientists are still not entirely sure if high red meat intake itself is harmful or if other factors related to high red meat intake are responsible, such as an overall lower-quality diet, low consumption of fruits and vegetables, or high intake of heavily processed meats or fast food. Nevertheless, certain components of red meat, especially those found in processed or overcooked meat, are indeed linked to adverse health effects. While researchers have hypothesized that eating plenty of herbs, spices, fruits, and vegetables may partially offset the harmful effects of high red meat intake, this doesn't justify a 16-ounce rib-eye steak every night for dinner just so long as you have a side of kale.

One controversial study reported that a diet too rich in meat, eggs, milk, and cheese could be as bad for you as smoking. High intake of dietary animal protein in people under sixty-five was linked to a fourfold increase in risk of death from cancer or diabetes and nearly double the risk of dying from any cause over an eighteen-year period. These negative effects were almost eliminated when the protein came from plant sources, such as legumes and whole grains. Based on results from studies such as this, Valter Longo, a fasting and nutrition researcher and director of the Longevity Institute at the University of Southern California, advises that people should restrict themselves to no more than 0.8 g of protein a day for every kilogram of body weight.

Finally, a dominant characteristic of many Blue Zones residents and ancestral hunter-gatherer tribes is that during certain parts of the year, meat or excess protein is restricted, similar to the "Meatless Monday" habit many diet-conscious health enthusiasts have adopted.

So should you not eat meat and instead adopt a plant-based diet? While eating only plants may seem like an effective option, there are several problems that accompany a diet devoid of meat. First, it is just as easy to eat poorly on a plant-based diet as it is on an omnivorous diet. Vegetarians can gorge themselves on ice cream, Twinkies, Taco Bell, Domino's pizza, and McDonald's milkshakes all day long. Even vegans can stuff their faces with crap like fast-food french fries, potato chips, and highly processed "meat" products made with soy and wheat and still technically be eating a plant-based diet. Second, certain nutrients can only be acquired via the consumption of animal products, including these:

- Creatine, which increases muscular power output and enhances cognitive function
- Vitamin B_{12}, which maintains healthy myelin sheaths to protect your neurons
- DHA, which is vital for proper cognitive development and cell membrane function
- Carnosine, which enhances antioxidant activity in the brain to protect it against oxidative damage
- Taurine, which plays a role in preventing heart disease

If you are a vegetarian, you are likely missing out on at least one of these critical nutrients, and if you eat the types of junk foods listed above, not only are you creating nutritional deficiencies in your diet, but you are filling those gaps with inflammatory compounds like rancid vegetable oils and excessive levels of sugar.

But let's say you already eat a healthy vegetarian diet, with an emphasis on real, whole foods. What should you do to make sure you're getting all the nutrients your body needs? Here are my top ten suggestions.

Try to Include Eggs and Dairy

While eggs and dairy will certainly break a strict vegan diet, they can fill in plenty of nutritional gaps without requiring you to eat meat. Eggs provide long-chain omega-3 fatty acids, including ALA. The best eggs are pastured eggs or eggs from chickens on a diet designed to boost levels of omega-3s. Eggs also provide the most bioavailable food-based protein on the face of the planet. Our bodies absorb and use 50 percent of the protein from eggs, the highest proportion of all food-based protein sources. Eggs contain high levels of choline, which is necessary for the proper metabolism of fat in the liver, as well as vitamin B_{12} and retinol, a form of vitamin A that our bodies use far more readily than plant-based vitamin A.

Assuming you don't have a dairy intolerance, dairy is a potent source of healthy fatty acids, minerals like calcium, and highly bioavailable proteins like whey and casein. If you do have a sensitivity to milk, try consuming fermented dairy products, such as yogurt, kefir, and hard aged cheeses like Pecorino Romano, gouda, and Parmigiano-Reggiano. The fermentation process breaks down lactose and also adds probiotics and creates new nutrients like vitamin K_2, which shuttles calcium into your teeth and bones. Vitamin K_2 is critical for a healthy heart and skeletal system and is notoriously absent in a plant-based diet. Especially if you are forgoing dairy, I highly recommend supplementing with about 100 to 200 mcg of vitamin K_2 per day, along with generous amounts of natto (which goes well with avocado, sea salt, and extra-virgin olive oil for a nice breakfast).

Take Taurine, Creatine, and Carnosine

These micronutrients are found only in meat and animal foods. Taurine is an amino acid that fights free radicals and protects your vision and is crucial for brain development, healthy blood pressure, and blood glucose stability. Your body can synthesize taurine from a combination of other amino acids, but this can be difficult for vegan athletes to pull off in adequate volume. There are vegan taurine sources out there, such as NOW Foods Vegan Taurine Powder (trust me, it's a much healthier alternative to Red Bull), and I recommend using 1 g per day.

Creatine plays a crucial role in the production of ATP, the molecule that supplies energy to all the cells in your body. Naturally produced in the body from other amino acids, creatine is also found in meats, eggs, and fish and is commonly deficient in active people, the elderly, and people who eat a primarily plant-based diet. With increases in exercise or muscle damage, your physiological need for creatine is increased. Research suggests that creatine supplementation can increase your muscles' work capacity and power output while enhancing your lean body mass and physical endurance. Outside of the athletic population, creatine has been shown to reduce muscle breakdown and even to support cognitive function, especially in the elderly. Because creatine stores high-energy phosphate groups in the form of phosphocreatine, it releases energy to aid cellular function during stress. This effect causes strength increases after creatine supplementation and can also benefit the brain, bones, muscles, and liver. I recommend 5 g per day, preferably in one to three doses and mixed into warm water or another warm liquid to maximize absorption.

Carnosine is made of two amino acids, histidine and alanine. Most carnosine research has shown its potential as an antiglycation agent and athletic performance aid. A carnosine deficiency can lead to premature aging, impaired mental health, decreased muscle tone, and vulnerability to certain diseases, such as cancer and diabetes. Like creatine and taurine, carnosine is not produced by plants. Instead, it's synthesized in animal tissue, particularly brain and muscle. In fact, one study demonstrated that vegetarians have less than 50 percent of the amount of carnosine in their muscle tissue that omnivores do. The limiting factor in carnosine production is the amino acid beta-alanine, and while you can supplement with carnosine, beta-alanine supplements have also been shown to increase muscle levels of carnosine on their own.

Take Niacin and Thiamine

Niacin, otherwise known as vitamin B_3, is notoriously lacking in plant-based diets. Severe niacin deficiency can cause dermatitis, dementia, diarrhea, and death (a cluster of effects known as the "4 Ds" of the disease pellagra). Thiamine, or vitamin B_1, is necessary for proper neuronal function and even digestion. The most effective vegetarian sources of niacin and thiamin are peanuts and sunflower seeds, but to get enough of these nutrients from these sources, you would need to consume quantities that can lead to other health problems, such as reduced absorption of iron, zinc, and calcium due to high levels of phytic acid. Alternatively, you can eat mushrooms to get your daily niacin. For example, two cups of grilled portobello mushrooms provides over 75 percent of your daily niacin requirement.

Consume Algae

While eggs contain high levels of long-chain omega-3 fatty acids like ALA, there are vegan forms of omega-3, such as algae in the form of spirulina and chlorella, that provide some EPA and DHA. These fatty acids are critical for neuronal growth, cellular function, and cognitive development.

Take Iodine

Plant-based diets are particularly lacking in iodine. The best natural and vegetarian sources are sea vegetables, such as nori, kelp, kombu, and dulse. In a pinch, you can also consume a daily dose of liquid iodine such as Lugol's (aim for 400 to 1,200 mcg).

Properly Prepare Grains, Legumes, and Nuts

Fermentation and soaking or sprouting can make grains, legumes, and nuts more digestible and their nutrients more bioavailable. See BoundlessBook.com/19 for instructions.

Maximize Iron Absorption

Iron found in plants is less bioavailable than the iron in meat. You can improve iron absorption by consuming vitamin C. Combine foods such as Swiss chard, spinach, beet greens, lentils, beans, and quinoa with foods like tomatoes, bell peppers, lemon juice, strawberries, oranges, papaya, kiwis, pineapple, and grapefruit. You should also moderate coffee and tea consumption with iron-rich foods since both of these beverages reduce iron absorption.

Take Vitamin D

Cholecalciferol, or vitamin D_3, is essential for bone health. Although vitamin D is found in plants in the form of vitamin D_2, it is nowhere near as potent as vitamin D_3, which is the form found in fish and dairy products. Intake of vitamin D on a plant-based diet is often below the recommended range, and this inadequate intake can reduce bone mineral density, depress immune system function, and cause higher levels of inflammation. If you want to keep your bones and teeth strong and give yourself adequate hormone and steroid precursors, I recommend 35 IU of vitamin D_3 per pound of body weight per day. This could be tough if you are a strict vegan, because most supplemental vitamin D_3 is derived from wool, and most vegan versions contain vitamin D_2, the less potent form. Garden of Life is one of the few vegan D_3 brands out there.

Take Vitamin B$_{12}$

Vitamin B_{12} is vital for cell division, metabolism, and maintenance of the nervous system. Vegans have been shown to be significantly deficient in vitamin B_{12}. This can cause weakness, numbness, and an increase in an amino acid called homocysteine that can increase the risk of heart disease, dementia, and Alzheimer's. B_{12} deficiency can also cause peripheral neuropathy and cognitive impairment, eventually leading to Alzheimer's, dementia, and Parkinson's. I recommend a sublingual liposomal vitamin B_{12} spray for fast absorption of this vitamin.

Be Careful with Soy

In addition to often being genetically modified, unfermented soy contains digestive irritants and digestive enzyme inhibitors like lectins, phytates, and protease inhibitors. Sure, most of these problematic compounds can be rendered harmless by fermenting soy and consuming it in forms such as miso, natto, and tempeh, but it's best to avoid processed foods and unfermented forms of soy, such as edamame, soy milk, and tofu. Soy also contains high levels of compounds called goitrogens that prevent your thyroid from using iodine correctly. Consuming a lot of soy could lead to hypothyroidism. Finally, soy contains plant estrogens in the form of isoflavones, which can raise estrogen levels and reduce testosterone levels. Women with estrogen dominance and men and women with testosterone deficiencies certainly shouldn't eat soy.

It is certainly possible to thrive on a plant-based diet. You just need to be careful to fill in the gaps and pay far greater attention to proper food preparation and combinations so that you unlock and consume the vitamins, minerals, and nutrients that are notoriously lacking in a modern plant-based diet.

In addition to those listed above, several other nutrients, from zinc to selenium to glycine, are also often absent in a plant-based diet, but the guidelines above address most of the major compounds that research has shown to be lacking in a plant-based diet.

THERE'S NO ONE-SIZE-FITS-ALL DIET

Even outside a specific diet like keto, which doesn't work for people who have certain genetic factors, examples of individual, idiosyncratic reactions to foods abound. At the beginning of this chapter, I described my own reaction to the oxalates in nuts and explained how some people don't benefit from supplementing with vitamin C, vitamin A, or riboflavin—and for some people, supplementing with vitamin D can be actively dangerous.

Another example is sulfur. Foods rich in sulfur—including garlic, cruciferous vegetables (such as kale, broccoli, and cauliflower), and egg yolks—are often touted as some of the healthiest compounds you can eat, and it's true that sulfur is important to detoxification, gut-lining integrity, lowered risk of cancer, and oxidation reduction. But unfortunately, some people may actually be "over-sulfured," a concept explored in the book *The Wildatarian Diet* by Teri Cochrane, and this is further aggravated by the nearly inescapable presence of the chemical glyphosate on foods. Typically, sulfur reactions are due to a variation in CBS—not the TV channel but a gene family that provides instructions for the enzyme cystathionine beta-synthase, which plays an important role in the breakdown and metabolism of sulfur. Some telltale signs of sulfur sensitivity include deleterious reactions to garlic, eggs, wine, and dried fruits that have sulfites added to them, along with joint pain, inflammatory bowel disease (Crohn's disease and ulcerative colitis), irritable bowel syndrome, and neurotransmitter imbalances. As you can imagine, this is a serious issue, especially considering that several popular dietary plans encourage us to consume as many sulfur-containing foods as possible, and that juicing and blending with sulfur-rich vegetables such as kale and cabbage is quite common and encouraged. In other words, while the dietary advice to eat more sulfur may be fine for many people, those with genetic vulnerabilities in sulfur metabolism can be harmed by this dietary practice. (For more on sulfur sensitivities, look up the works of Dr. Greg Nigh at ImmersionHealthPDX.com and Heidi Turner at FoodLogic.org.)

Or consider glutathione. Many medical practitioners do not realize that glutathione levels are carefully monitored and regulated by the body. When glutathione is consumed, the body's feedback systems sense that it has plenty of glutathione on board, so it can stop making glutathione through the process of methylation. This means people who have a genetic susceptibility for poor methylation, which can be tested for, can unwittingly turn off their ability to methylate, which is counterproductive!

Another example of biochemical individuality (and one big reason why, despite the prevalence of diet books, we have failed so miserably to control the obesity pandemic) is the wild variation in blood sugar responses to foods like cookies, bananas, sushi, and whole-grain bread. The latest research on this phenomenon, detailed in nitty-gritty specifics in Paleo icon Robb Wolf's book *Wired to Eat*, suggests that the capacity to extract energy from food differs dramatically from person to person because the interactions between one's genes, microbiome, diet, environment, and lifestyle are extremely complex. This also suggests that common measurements of the sugar content of foods, such as the glycemic index, may be less useful than individualized measurements of blood sugar responses to different foods.

One recent six-month European study, called "Food4Me," investigated 1,500 participants in seven European countries. The participants were randomly divided into two groups: one was given personalized dietary advice based on genetic data, and one was told to follow standard dietary prescriptions, such as eating lots of fruits and vegetables (I have always been confused about why pineapples and pears are lumped together with collard greens and kale), lean meats (I run away from lean meat because I have never once field-dressed an animal and found meat devoid of fat), and whole grains (which can spike your blood sugar more than a Snickers bar). The participants in the personalized diet group fared far better in terms of important longevity blood biomarkers and weight than those in the one-size-fits-all diet group.

Coffee is another perfect example of why we need customized diets. Current guidelines advise consuming no more than four or five cups of coffee per day. This is fine for the subset of the population who are genetically fast caffeine metabolizers, but for many people who have a particular variant of a gene called CYP1A2, having more than two cups of coffee per day vastly increases the risk of a heart attack and hypertension.

Scientists are slowly beginning to tease out all these connections and have now linked at least thirty-eight different genes to nutrient metabolism. Roger Williams wasn't aware of these genes when he wrote *Biochemical Individuality* (although he hypothesized about genetic influence on the propensity to thrive on specific diets), but they are now known to hinder or help the absorption and metabolism of different nutrients. These genes include MTHFR (folate metabolism), FTO (body weight and fat composition), TCF7L2 (blood sugar regulation), APOE ε4 (cholesterol), and FADS1 (fatty acid metabolism). This means that your genetic makeup, microbiota, health history, and living environment all play a role in determining whether you should consume more or less choline, vitamin C, fatty acids, starches, caffeine, and folate.

From the failures of a high-fat diet to individual blood sugar responses to carbohydrates and genetic variations in the need for major vitamins, minerals, and nutrients, the importance of dietary customization is enormous.

The million-dollar question is, how can you customize your diet?

HOW TO CUSTOMIZE YOUR DIET

We live in a magical modern era in which the same kind of self-quantification and lab testing that highfalutin CEOs would have paid tens of thousands of dollars for at fancy longevity institutes decades ago is now available for the general population at a fraction of the cost. Let's take a look at some of the best methods for figuring out how much carbohydrate, fat, and protein you should eat, which supplements you should and should not take, and how many calories you should consume.

Blood Testing

A good blood test can locate holes in your diet that need to be filled by measuring health markers, such as blood sugar response to certain foods, mineral status, thyroid status, cholesterol status, red and white blood cell levels, vitamin B levels, acidity, alkalinity, and vitamin D status (vitamin D can be quite toxic if your levels are adequate and you are simply taking it because you heard you should). Some blood tests can even determine food allergies and intolerances, although most of these are inaccurate and will give you an exhaustive "false positive" list of foods you shouldn't eat.

For blood tests, I recommend the Longevity Panel, which can be purchased from the direct-to-consumer blood-testing company WellnessFX. For this test, you will need to drive to the nearest lab to give blood, but WellnessFX is currently developing a state-of-the-art microneedle that will allow you to test painlessly in the comfort of your own home. For food allergies, a company called

Cyrex offers the gold standard in testing. After a simple blood test, rather than sending you a dizzying and frustrating laundry list of hundreds of foods to avoid (which is what you get from most popular food allergy tests), Cyrex will send you a list of just a few proven foods to which you are guaranteed to be allergic.

Stool Testing

Your blood won't necessarily tell you what's going on in your gut, but a stool panel allows you to determine the presence or absence of certain types of bacteria, yeast, fungi, parasites, and digestive inflammation, all of which can then be used to determine whether you need to take certain probiotics or cleansing compounds, or whether you should avoid fermentable substances such as simple sugars, starches, and FODMAPs (review chapter 13 for information on FODMAPs).

This type of test is pretty important because poor digestion and nutritional malabsorption can lead to immune dysfunction, nutritional insufficiencies, various chronic diseases, food allergies, and other toxicities. For years, the gold standard test was a complicated home stool panel in which you pooped into the equivalent of a hot dog tray for three days, but the company Viome now gives you the same details with just a speck of your stool, making complicated, uncomfortable poop testing a thing of the past. A Genova Diagnostics GI Effects or Diagnostics Health GI MAP stool panel, in which you collect stool at home and then send it off to the lab, can also give you plenty of insight into your gut. Although these tests will not reveal the same microbiome details as a test such as Viome's, they do reveal bacteria, parasites, viruses, normal flora, fungi, and antibiotic-resistant bacterial genes, along with immunologic markers for GI health and function, including SIgA, elastase, calprotectin, and anti-gliadin markers, all of which allow you to see whether your gut is balanced, inflamed, or in need of a healing protocol. Finally, at the time of this writing, the company Thorne is taking things to the next level with an at-home stool test that promises to be the most thorough on the market. It will give you a glimpse of everything going on inside your gut, including your microbiome.

MICROBIOME STOOL TESTING

Viome offers a complete gut microbiome analysis that provides a snapshot of every living organism in your gut. Born at the prestigious Los Alamos National Lab and originating from technology designed for national security, the Viome test uses a small stool sample to create a complete sequencing of the gut microbiome. By analyzing the genes that your microbes express, Viome can identify which metabolites they produce and the role of those metabolites in your body's ecosystem. Viome then recommends specific probiotics and foods so you can fine-tune the function of your gut microbiome to minimize the growth of harmful microbes and maximize the growth of beneficial ones. This test is still controversial, as it is somewhat unclear whether the bacteria in your large intestine reflect the biome of your small intestine, and whether you can simply toss probiotics into your gut to replace what you appear to be deficient in. But Viome seems to be constantly expanding its ability to give you gut insight based on the samples you send in, so in my opinion, it is worth completing this test if you can afford it (although you will still get plenty of good data from Viome's more basic stool panel).

Saliva Testing

You can test your DNA via a simple and inexpensive at-home saliva collection. This is an excellent way to determine not only what your ancestors traditionally ate but also how your genes affect everything from your antioxidant needs to your blood sugar response to whether you're sensitive to lactose or gluten, and much more. While 23andMe primarily delivers ancestry data along with a few health insights, you can grab your raw genetic data from their website and then upload the results to a more in-depth and extremely affordable service such as MyHeritage, StrateGene, or Genetic Genie to take a deeper dive into your health-related genetic results. You can also go to BenGreenfieldFitness.com and listen to my podcast interviews with the physicians at companies such as Thorne, Tree of Life, and Youtrients, which, for a slightly higher price, test for a far larger number of genetic variables called SNPs. Practitioners like Dr. Ben Lynch at StrateGene, Dr. Bob Miller at Tree of Life, and Dr. Mansoor Mohammed at the DNA Company in Ontario, Canada, can help you make even more sense of the data and allow you to personalize your diet based on your genes in a very precise manner.

Urine Testing

A urine test called an "organic amino acids evaluation" is optional but can be helpful for identifying small nutritional deficiencies that can add up and become detrimental over time. (For example, a slight drop in uric acid excretion over ten years can mean getting or not getting painful gout in your older years.) These nutritional deficiencies can cause a variety of chronic health conditions, and if you struggle with poor sleep, less-than-stellar workouts, brain fog, appetite cravings, sore joints, or any other mysterious problems, this profile can help uncover issues with micronutrients and other small components that a basic blood test won't reveal. You can determine your levels of organic acids, fatty acids, amino acids, vitamins, minerals, and antioxidants via an in-home urinalysis and blood-drop test, then use that information to prevent the types of problems mentioned above. I am also a fan of the DUTCH urine test, which can give you an accurate analysis of testosterone, estrogen, cortisol, melatonin, DHEA, and other hormones.

Exercise Testing

A resting metabolic rate test determines the amount of energy (in calories) your body uses while at rest. This measurement is calculated by analyzing the amount of oxygen your body uses and the amount of carbon dioxide your body produces. Almost all the energy your body produces is created through aerobic (oxygen-utilizing) metabolism: oxygen is combined with carbohydrates and fats to make ATP (cellular energy) in your body's tissues, and carbon dioxide is produced as a metabolic by-product. An exercise metabolic test can tell the same kind of data relevant to exercise: for example, how many calories you burn at any given heart rate. Armed with both sets of information, you can figure out precisely how many calories you need to eat to maintain a healthy weight and perform at peak capacity. I recommend you google the name of your city with the phrase "metabolic testing." Many universities, health clubs, and medical institutions offer these tests to the general public.

The Testing Protocol I Recommend

This may seem like a dizzying array of tests, but it isn't that much once you systematize them. For example, I recommend everyone do the following protocol:

- Blood test once yearly
- Gut test once yearly
- Microbiome test once yearly
- Urine test if you have symptoms the other tests can't identify
- Metabolic test once in your lifetime (or when your body composition or fitness dramatically changes)
- DNA test once in your lifetime

Yes, your total cost for this entire range of tests may be higher than for a typical fifteen-minute visit to your overworked doctor. But these costs pale in comparison to what you will shell out for medical care and insurance during your lifetime if you accumulate nutritional deficiencies; chronic diseases, such as obesity, cancer, diabetes, Alzheimer's, dementia, or colitis; constipation; and the host of other nasties that can manifest in the human body when the fuel you give it isn't tailored to your biochemical individuality. In addition (perhaps this is my inner propeller-hat-donning nerd talking), it's pretty cool to keep your finger on the pulse of everything going on inside your body, provided you resist the temptation to become obsessive-compulsive by adding a microgram scale to the kitchen counter for weighing every last shred of Parmesan cheese.

I will take a much deeper dive into the world of self-quantification in chapter 16, and in chapter 21, I'll introduce many of the diets that I endorse (along with sample dishes for breakfast, lunch, dinner, and snacks) and explain how to decide, based on your lab tests, which diet is perfect for you.

YOUR DIET AND YOUR ENVIRONMENT

No discussion of diet would be complete without mentioning the impact your dietary choices have on the environment. Harvesting and preparation techniques, treatment of animals, food processing, pesticide use, the harvesting and shipping scalability of different foods (like tree nuts and eggs), and growing methods all significantly impact the local and global environment, which, in turn, impacts the quality of the food we eat. Indeed, experts suggest that, in America, food production and consumption practices have a greater effect on our well-being than any other human activity.

Contrary to popular belief, healthy food isn't simply synonymous with high-quality, nutrient-dense food. Instead, an ideal healthy diet needs to be part of a sustainable production and consumption system that benefits not only human health but also the natural resources involved, the ecosystem in which the food is produced, and the food sources themselves. With a finite amount of land, water, and resources, along with a growing population and a deteriorating food system modeled around mass production, the need to produce and consume food in a more sustainable way has never been more pressing. If we accept the status quo, we will likely remain in an ecological overshoot until the earth can no longer handle it.

One of the most useful concepts I discovered while researching this issue came from Christian Peters, a nutrition professor at Tufts University. According to Peters, an ethical synergy occurs when a dietary decision benefits both our health and the environment. An ethical dilemma occurs when a dietary decision benefits personal health but is detrimental for the environment. For example, consuming more legumes is an ethical synergy: it would likely improve our health and allow us to be more efficient with land and resources. Consuming fewer processed sugars is also an ethical synergy because it would likely improve health and reduce unnecessary land use. On the other hand, consuming more fish and fish oil is an ethical dilemma: it could potentially improve health, but it would have a negative impact on fish populations and the environment, especially if the fish and fish oil are not sourced sustainably, which most are not. Increasing meat consumption is also an ethical dilemma: it could potentially improve health (in certain people), but it also means using resources more inefficiently, especially in a myopic era in which we do things like eat only muscle meat rather than the entire animal, as our ancestors used to, or stay closed-minded to alternative protein sources such as algae or insects.

These concepts of ethical synergy and ethical dilemmas got me thinking more about why people make certain food choices. I believe there is a powerful factor that we are currently not harnessing to its full potential, especially in the US: how our food choices affect the greater good.

One of the most common problems I hear from my coaching clients is that they lack the motivation each day to make the right nutritional choices. I think this is because, in the nutrition world, we often emphasize our self-interest a little too much, which blinds us to the rest of the world.

Consider all the actions we do with the greater good in mind. We donate blood; we volunteer; we bring meals to people who've recently lost a loved one. We don't do these things for money or celebrity status, and we often don't have to resort to white-knuckled willpower. We do them because these behaviors align with the people we want to be and make us feel more hopeful, grateful, needed, and inspired. And all of this points to the powerful notion that when a cause is bigger than ourselves, we are more likely to stick with it in the long term.

As a nutrition professional, I am often tempted to look at food through a lens that considers only nutrients and calories. While these are indeed important, I challenge you (and myself!) to broaden this perspective to include the environment as well. You can achieve this by implementing the following strategies.

1. Identify Your Minimum Effective Dose of Animal Products.

In other words, don't eat more animal foods than you need. To best help the environment, your optimal intake of animal foods is likely around 10 percent or less of your total daily calories. Focus on eating more tubers, root vegetables, legumes, whole grains, and seeds. While they're nutrient-dense, tree nuts and eggs can pack more of an environment-harming punch (especially when they aren't organically grown tree nuts and pasture-raised eggs), so consume only moderate amounts of these. Don't forget alternative protein sources, particularly insects, and vegetarian strategies such as combining lentils and rice to get all nine essential amino acids.

2. Minimize Food Waste.

Use leftovers, plan meals, compost your food scraps, freeze and dehydrate foods, learn to can and/or ferment food, give food scraps to livestock or pets, make trips to your local homeless shelter or soup kitchen to donate extra food, and buy visually unappealing fruits and veggies (which are higher in nutrients anyway). Minimize your intake of processed foods, which cause metabolic food waste due to their relative lack of nutrients. Case in point: I'm writing this just after Thanksgiving. Rather than scrapping all the turkey bones, turkey liver, and turkey heart, I used the bones to make a giant vat of bone broth with black pepper, turmeric, salt, and saffron, and then dredged the organ meats in coconut flour and butter and fried them in olive oil. Remember that there is a creative and tasty way to eat just about anything.

3. Eat a Variety of Foods.

Try new foods regularly. For example, when you go out to eat, try to order dishes with strange or unfamiliar ingredients. Eating a variety of foods enhances your likelihood of selecting a nutritionally adequate diet and also increases the likelihood that you won't deplete one single food source (just imagine what would happen to the world's spinach crops if everyone suddenly decided the only dark leafy green they were going to eat in their lunchtime salad was spinach). Hunter-gatherer tribes and people in many longevity hotspots around the world eat 130 to 150 different plant varieties and foods throughout the year; most Westernized diets include only a paltry 30 different plant species.

Getting Started

BoundlessBook.com/14 has links to plenty of websites that contain more information and practical tips for implementing these and other environmentally friendly sustainability practices. Here are a few to get you started:

- Monterey Bay Aquarium Seafood Watch (SeafoodWatch.org), which can help you make more sustainable seafood choices
- Water Footprint Calculator (WaterCalculator.org), which can help you learn more about how much water your household uses
- The Cornucopia Institute's Organic Dairy Scorecard (cornucopia.org/scorecard/dairy/), which ranks dairy brands by sustainability
- The Cornucopia Institute's Organic Egg Scorecard (cornucopia.org/scorecard/eggs/), which ranks egg brands by sustainability
- BuyingPoultry.com, which rates poultry products by how the animals are treated
- EatWild.com, which has a directory of local farms and ranches selling grass-fed, humanely raised meat, eggs, and dairy
- LocalHarvest.com, which helps you find local farms and farmers markets
- BetterWorldShopper.org, a database that tracks companies in a range of areas, including the environment and animal protection
- CarboTax.org, which asks you a series of questions to help you compare your climate impact to that of the average American
- The Global Footprint Network's ecological footprint calculator (footprintcalculator.org/signup), which asks you a series of questions to help you identify your environmental footprint

- Consumer Reports' Greener Choices initiative (GreenerChoices.org), which provides information on products' environmental impact
- The Climatarian Challenge app (LessMeatLessHeat.org/app), which gives you a budget of "carbon points," calculates the carbon footprint of your meals, and subtracts the appropriate number of points from your budget—the goal is to get through a month on just the budgeted points

WHAT ABOUT KIDS?

Feeding kids can be a daunting task. After all, they are not just miniature adults. Their blood-brain barriers are far more permeable than those of adults, they lay down new bone on a daily basis, their cells are rapidly dividing, and their metabolisms are rampant. But kids do have the same cellular metabolism mechanics as adults and require the same set of nutrients that adults do, including the following.

Calcium

Kids produce new bone tissue on a daily basis. In fact, minimizing the effects of age-related bone loss begins during childhood and particularly puberty, when bone tissue undergoes massive spikes in growth. Kids from four to eight years old need 1,000 mg of calcium per day, and kids from nine to thirteen years old need 1,300 mg per day. It is crucial that calcium be accompanied by adequate levels of vitamin D and vitamin K.

The source of calcium is also important. I personally was raised on a half to full gallon of processed, homogenized, pasteurized 2 percent cow's milk each day, and I suffered gastric distress regularly as a child and adolescent. In raising my own children, I have realized that kids (and adults) digest organic raw dairy, goat's milk, camel's milk, and A2 dairy (dairy that doesn't have A1 protein, which some people are sensitive to) far more easily than commercial cow's milk, and without risk of gut damage unless a true food allergy is present. The best sources of calcium are sardines with the bones, hard cheeses like cheddar and pecorino, raw milk, full-fat fermented dairy products like yogurt and kefir, and dark leafy greens like collard greens, kale, and Swiss chard.

Iodine

Iodine is an essential nutrient (meaning it is not produced by the body; it must be ingested from an outside source) and is necessary for proper thyroid hormone production. Thyroid hormone regulates growth factors, such as growth hormone, that contribute to cognitive and physical growth. Iodine deficiencies are associated with stunted height as well as lower IQ scores. Kids from four to eight years old need 90 mcg per day, while kids from nine to thirteen years old need 120 mcg per day. The best sources are seaweed (kombu, kelp, and nori have the highest content) and milk. For example, my children often strike off to school with sardines, anchovies, mackerel, or herring wrapped in nori.

Iron

Iron supports neurological development and blood cell formation. Kids from four to eight years old need 10 mg per day, while kids nine to thirteen years old (for girls, prior to menarche) only need 8 mg per day. The best sources are red meat, organ meats such as chicken liver, and shellfish (especially clams, if your kid has a taste for shellfish). Meat is a better source than plants because the iron bound to heme—the non-protein part of hemoglobin and the molecule that carries oxygen in the blood—is more bioavailable than iron that is not bound to heme. Iron from non-meat sources, such as spinach, lentils, beans, and cashews, should be combined with high sources of vitamin C, such as citrus fruits and dark leafy greens, to improve the bioavailability of the iron. For example, another frequent lunchbox item for our children is thinly sliced chunks of steak; organic elk, bison, buffalo, or beef jerky; braunschweiger; pemmican; or headcheese; along with kiwis, orange slices, and steamed greens.

Zinc

Zinc supports physical growth and immune system development. Research suggests that 5 to 6 mg of supplemental zinc per day can reverse delayed growth in kids. Other research suggests that zinc supplementation in zinc-deficient kids under the age of five can reduce diarrheal infections and pneumonia. Kids from four to eight years old need 5 mg per day, while kids from nine to thirteen years old need 8 mg per day. The best sources are red meat (particularly lamb), oysters, crab, and lobster.

Vitamin A

Severe vitamin A deficiency can cause night blindness and permanent blindness and mild deficiency increases the risk of upper respiratory tract infection, while adequate amounts can enhance eye health, bone health, and balanced hormones. Kids from four to eight years old need 400 mcg per day, while kids from nine to twelve years old need 600 mcg per day. The best sources are liver, cod liver oil, eggs, full-fat dairy, sweet potatoes, kale, spinach, and carrots. A mess of scrambled eggs with cheese, sweet potatoes, and kale is a typical breakfast for our kids, and dinners include roasted carrots, yams, or steamed greens.

Vitamin B$_{12}$

Vitamin B$_{12}$ is critical for the growth and maintenance of myelin sheaths, the protective coats that encase your neurons' axons. If these sheaths deteriorate or you don't consume sufficient vitamin B$_{12}$, the result is cognitive decline or poor cognitive development. The B$_{12}$ requirement for kids from four to eight years old is 1.2 mcg per day, while for kids from nine to thirteen years old, it's 1.8 mcg per day. The only sources of vitamin B$_{12}$ are animal products like red meat, poultry, fish, and shellfish, so if you are raising a plant-based eater, they will definitely need to supplement with B$_{12}$.

Vitamin C

Vitamin C supports collagen formation, connective tissue health, recovery from injury, and immune system function. Kids from four to eight years old need 25 mg per day, while kids from nine to thirteen years old need 45 mg per day. The best sources are fruits and vegetables, such as oranges, lemons, limes, kale, broccoli, brussels sprouts, and cauliflower. Whole foods are, of course, far superior to concentrated juices.

Vitamin D

In the absence of frequent exposure to unfiltered sunlight, vitamin D must be obtained through diet. Kids of all ages need 15 mcg per day. Along with the mighty mushroom, the best dietary sources are meat, fish, eggs, and cod liver oil. Research suggests that animal-based sources of vitamin D are about five times more effective than the supplemental form vitamin D_3. My own children eat meat and mushrooms, but they also supplement with vitamin D because their genetic testing revealed that, in response to sunlight, they naturally produce lower amounts of vitamin D than most people do.

Vitamin K_2

Vitamin K_2 is responsible for the proper absorption of calcium and for shuttling calcium into your teeth and bones. Effective doses for adults tend to range between 50 and 200 mcg per day, and since vitamin K_2 is very safe to consume, it is fine for kids to consume the low end of that range. The best sources are natto (a Japanese fermented soybean dish), egg yolks, grass-fed butter (particularly Green Pastures X-Factor Butter Oil), cream, ghee, liver, gouda cheese, kefir, sauerkraut, and emu oil. (Emu oil contains over fifty times more vitamin K_2 than chicken liver or cheese, four times more than duck fat, twenty-five times more than cream and butter, and ten times more than ghee and egg yolks. Walkabout Australian Emu Oil is a good brand.)

Choline

Choline assists the liver with processing fat and toxins and acts as a precursor to the neurotransmitter acetylcholine, making choline a critical part of enhancing memory formation and skill acquisition. Kids from four to eight years old need 250 mg per day, while kids from nine to thirteen years old need 375 mg per day. The best sources are egg yolks and liver. (Getting the impression yet that your child should be eating eggs and organ meats?)

EPA and DHA

Omega-3 fatty acids are crucial for brain development. EPA and DHA in particular are responsible for improving memory, mood, neuronal health, and learning. Research suggests that 250 to 500 mg of combined EPA and DHA can be especially beneficial. In addition to a high-quality fish oil (my children take Living Fuel SuperEssentials Omega), the best sources are cold-water fatty fish like salmon, mackerel, and herring, as well as salmon roe (which kids love on rice crackers). (Check out chapter 4 again for more information and tips on EPA and DHA consumption.)

Saturated Fat

Your and your child's cells are encased by membranes, and each of these membranes is composed of saturated fat, which is a more stable fatty acid that's less prone to oxidation. Saturated fats are also responsible for shuttling proteins between cells, stimulating the release of neurotransmitters, and forming memories. Saturated fat is found in dairy products like butter, ghee, full-fat milk, and cheese, and in fatty cuts of beef, pork, and lamb. It is important to remember that cell membranes also depend on other fats, particularly oleic acid, which is found in high quantities in extra-virgin olive oil. Many of the plants, tubers, eggs, and other foods recommended in this section can be dipped, drowned, dosed, and soaked in a good olive oil.

Cholesterol

Cholesterol is necessary for the production of steroid hormones, such as estrogens and progesterone, and vitamin D. While the liver naturally produces cholesterol, consuming dietary sources of cholesterol like egg yolks and shrimp allows your kids to also consume other beneficial nutrients, such as choline, omega-3 fatty acids, and protein.

Prebiotics and Probiotics

By producing postbiotics, probiotics provide kids with vitamins and nutrients and make existing nutrients more bioavailable. They also support healthy digestive processes and even secrete mood-stabilizing neurotransmitters like serotonin. Probiotics can be found in fermented, "living" foods like raw dairy, natto, kimchi, sauerkraut, and kefir.

Prebiotics in the form of soluble and insoluble dietary fiber allow beneficial gut bacteria to thrive and promote healthy bowel movements. Prebiotics are found in high quantities in jicama (Mexican yam), Jerusalem artichoke, garlic, onions, leeks, underripe bananas, and dandelion greens.

Dealing with Picky Eaters

I realize that at this point you may be wondering how the heck you are going to get your kid to eat sardines, liver, and natto. I got lucky. From the time our kids were very young, my wife and I would often "mommy bird" our food, chewing—or cutting with knife and fork—into tiny, edible bits the same natural whole foods that we consumed and spitting it onto our children's plates. So our kids grew up with palates accustomed to real food. In addition, we never created kids' versions of dinner while the adults ate the grown-up food. If the adults were eating bacon, onions, liver, and brussels sprouts for dinner, the kids had no other options: there was no separate macaroni and cheese or frozen pizza for them to eat so they could avoid the real, wholesome food. If they didn't want to eat what we were having, that was their choice, and they could go to bed with growling stomachs. It was always the same at restaurants, and now my kids turn down the kids' menu of chicken wings, breaded vegetables, sliders, and mini pizzas and instead opt for a nice cut of fish or steak with roasted vegetables from the adult menu. (Admittedly, this comes back to bite us when the restaurant check arrives.)

Of course, I realize that you may not have gotten so lucky as to start your kids at such an early age, and I know that kids can be picky eaters, so any diet plan for children should be enhanced with some practical tips to overcome this obstacle.

- Encourage your kids to take at least five bites of a dish before deciding they don't like it. If you have multiple kids, make it a competition to see who can eat the most of the dish.
- Egg yolks can be added to everything from spaghetti sauce to mac and cheese without changing the flavor.
- When they contain the right ingredients (like kale, green bananas, egg yolks, kefir, Brazil nuts, cod liver oil, and frozen fruit), smoothies are an excellent way to provide essential nutrients in dessert form.
- Smoothie leftovers can be made into ice pops.
- Instead of cooking rice in water, cook it in bone broth, add some trace minerals such as a pinch of salt, and throw in some kelp granules for added iodine.
- Although they're nutrient-void on their own, rice crackers are great vehicles for tuna salad, liver pâté, cheese, and hummus.
- Fish sauce made from fermented fish is full of glutamate, which can help picky kids develop a taste for the umami flavor of many novel foods. We began including fish sauce in our children's dishes at an early age, and as a result, they developed an Asian-like palate and appreciation for this flavor, which is seldom found in Western diets.
- Sticking scallops or steak on toothpicks or skewers instantly makes them fun to eat.
- Bribing kids with small prizes for eating healthy food can work temporarily.

Supporting the symmetry, growth, and beauty of children via nutritional strategies is a topic I will explore in detail in chapter 17, but in the meantime, here is one last tip: kids require a lot of energy, so don't limit (or let them limit) their caloric intake unless there is a valid medical reason.

THE LAST WORD

Allow me to finish with one important consideration: your diet can fluctuate and change as your body and your gut transform. For example, many people who have digestive issues, bathroom troubles, or other health complaints need to initially fix their gut, heal their digestive tract, or detox with an extremely clean and restrictive diet that eliminates common problem foods such as dairy, grains, nightshades, and red meat—even the healthy, organic, natural versions of these foods (the Autoimmune Paleo diet, or AIP, is perhaps my favorite such diet). But once the gut is healed, these foods can gradually be reintroduced and enjoyed, and, in my case, macadamia nut face-stuffing can ensue once more.

Finally, for books that are packed with recipes and diets and are not trendy diet rags written to make a quick buck but are instead thorough reads appropriate for customizing both plant-based and omnivorous diets, I recommend all of the following:

- *The Plant Paradox: The Hidden Dangers in "Healthy" Foods That Cause Disease and Weight Gain*, by Dr. Stephen Gundry
- *Returning to an Ancestral Diet*, by Dr. Michael Smith
- *Perfect Health Diet: Regain Health and Lose Weight by Eating the Way You Were Meant to Eat*, by Paul Jaminet
- *The Wahls Protocol: A Radical New Way to Treat All Chronic Autoimmune Conditions Using Paleo Principles*, by Terry Wahls
- *Deep Nutrition: Why Your Genes Need Traditional Food*, by Dr. Cate Shanahan

ONE THING YOU CAN DO THIS WEEK

Order a genetic test. It's so simple and affordable these days to have a genetic test kit delivered to your home from a company such as 23andMe, drip a bit of saliva into a tube, and within just a couple of weeks get a report that allows you to see your ancestry and identify genetic variables that will affect your diet. You can also go to BenGreenfieldFitness.com/rawdata to see a host of websites that allow you to import your genetic data and find out plenty more about how you should eat, supplement, exercise, and much more. Practitioners like Dr. Ben Lynch at StrateGene, Dr. Bob Miller at Tree of Life, and Dr. Mansoor Mohammed with the DNA Company can help you make even more sense of the data and personalize your diet based on your genes in a very precise manner. So what are you waiting for? Go forth and salivate.

For citations for all the research studies mentioned in this chapter and a deeper dive into the topics of this chapter—including links to podcasts, blog posts, recommended tools and supplements, and much more—visit BoundlessBook.com/14.

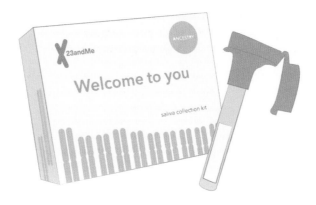

15

NEVER GET SICK

HOW TO BUILD AN UNSTOPPABLE IMMUNE SYSTEM

I watched from the porch as my tiny twin boys toddled across the goat pen in our backyard, cooing and laughing as our dwarf goats dished out gentle head butts and high-pitched bleats. My eyes narrowed as I observed Terran, the younger of my twins by a solid nine seconds, gingerly place his hand in a pile of steaming goat dung, then smear it across his lips and cheeks. Ten years ago, I would have broken into a Tom Cruise sprint across the lawn to save him from certain intestinal death, but now I simply smiled: a proud papa confident that his children would grow up with unstoppable immune systems. Heck, this same proud papa now throws open his refrigerator every two weeks to drink pig whipworms and rat tapeworms.

See, in my bouts with intestinal invaders—from parasites contracted during a triathlon in the jungles of Thailand, to a series of nasty Vietnamese gut bugs that left me bedridden for weeks, to flesh-eating MRSA from barbed wire wounds sustained in a Spartan Race—I have had to fight uphill battles against immune system assailants and have picked up some handy tips along the way. The key takeaway? The more bacteria to which you are exposed (within reason, of course), the stronger your immune system becomes. Hence my nonchalant reaction to my children's interacting with goat fecal bacteria.

You no doubt already have an intimate relationship with your immune system. You probably care about it, or at least think about it with some frequency. You regularly wash your hands, take vitamin C, and eat plenty of fruits and vegetables. But somehow you find yourself sniffling, coughing, and sneezing more frequently than you would like, even when it's not flu season. For hard-charging high achievers, this issue often strikes in the middle of an important work project, a family vacation, a bout of travel, or a crucial block of workouts or training sessions.

Just think of a few of the ho-hum, standard, old-school pieces of advice for kicking a cold:

- Take oodles of vitamin C and zinc.
- Get plenty of bed rest and don't exercise.
- Avoid exposure to cold temperatures.
- Use antibiotics or a handy-dandy Z-Pak to fight off viruses.

The problem is, most of these strategies simply don't work and may wind up weakening the immune system even further. For example, some supplements can help, but you need to take a high-enough dose in a form that you can absorb when you're sick. Exercise can actually facilitate the detox process, while staying sedentary will keep lymph fluid stagnant, and antibiotics will wipe out the good bacteria in the gut that support the healthy environment our body needs to heal.

The immune system just isn't as simple as it seems, so in this chapter, you will discover the inner workings of human immunity and little-known in-the-trenches methods to strengthen your immune system and bounce back from sickness fast, including how to channel the power of your emotions, beliefs, and thoughts to heal your body.

Immunity Tips from the Experts

Over the years, I have collected a host of immunity tips from several physicians who specialize in outside-the-box thinking. Here are a few of my favorites that aren't addressed elsewhere in this chapter.

"For travel, I would go with colloidal silver spray for topical antimicrobial activity, and DHEA, 20 mg for women and 50 mg for men, to boost immune function the day before and the day of travel. Science identifies DHEA as an immune modulator, but the dose is just a personal guess (and a touch of expectation/placebo)."

—Justin Mager, MD

"At the first sign of a viral infection (fever, chills, body aches, runny nose), I advise . . . a dose of Oscillococcinum, a homeopathic remedy. Although Oscillo doesn't prevent the flu or colds from occurring, clinical studies have shown that it reduces [the duration] of illness."

—Yasmin Nibbe, MD, FAAP

"I have recommended many natural remedies for colds and flu and tried most for myself. Aside from being healthier to prevent these infections, the most effective single remedy is simply sitting in the sun to provide the body with a 'shot' of vitamin D. Even in most winter locations, fifteen to twenty minutes of sun exposure to as much skin as possible will work wonders to ward off illness."

—Phil Maffetone, PhD

"One incredibly powerful means of preventing colds is the use of colloidal silver gel as an antibacterial immune defense barrier."

—Jeff Spencer

"For shoring up your immune function during cold and flu season, here's rule #1: do not overeat. In fact, if you feel you have been exposed to a bug or feel something coming on, then light fasting is an excellent idea. Digestion takes more energy than just about any other daily human activity. Placing an excessive burden on your digestive processes diverts energy and resources that might otherwise be devoted to better quality immune function...Avoiding sugar and starch in particular is critical."

—Nora Gedgaudas

"Oral or transdermal sodium bicarbonate, oral iodine, and oral or transdermal magnesium, along with selenium, would be number one. A Biomat is essential too—especially if you get the flu."

—Mark Sircus, OMD, DM

"Fever is part of the body's normal response to infection...Hippocrates knew this when he said, 'Give me a fever and I can cure any disease.' Suppressing the fever may interfere with healing and prolong the infection . . . A technique called 'wet sock hydrotherapy' (google it) can support the immune system and dramatically decrease healing time."

—Toby Hallowitz, ND

IMMUNITY 101

The complex immune system has six components:

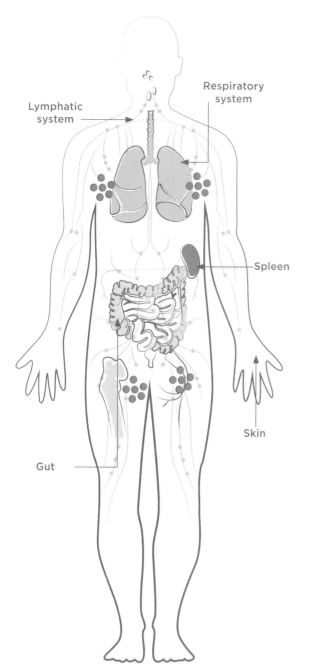

- The lymphatic (lymph) system, which is a network of organs, nodes, vessels, and tissues that transport lymph fluid throughout the body. Lymph fluid contains infection-fighting white blood cells, and the organs and nodes are where toxins, waste, and other unwanted debris are filtered.

- The respiratory system, which consists of a series of organs, including the mouth, lungs, pharynx, larynx, and trachea, that take in oxygen and expel carbon dioxide. Airways are covered in a mucus layer that traps pathogens and other particles before they can reach the lungs. Tiny hairlike, muscular projections called cilia propel the mucus layer.

- The skin, which is the human body's largest organ and serves as a barrier to the external environment. The skin's immune system contains an estimated twenty billion T cells (a type of white blood cell), which control skin microbes and educate the immune system as a whole.

- Lymphocytes, small white blood cells that seek out and destroy pathogens and orchestrate an immune response. The two types of lymphocytes are B cells, which make antibodies that attack bacteria and other toxins, and T cells, which help destroy infected or cancerous cells. Killer T cells are a subgroup of T cells that kill cells that are infected with pathogens or are otherwise damaged. Helper T cells determine which immune responses the body has to a particular pathogen.

- The spleen, which stores white blood cells and platelets, filters blood, and recycles old red blood cells. It also helps fight certain kinds of bacteria.

- The gut, which harbors many different kinds of bacteria and other organisms that make up what's called the gut microbiome. Good bacteria help control harmful colonies of bad bacteria, fight pathogens by producing antimicrobial substances, and affect the pH of the gut environment to provide a chemical barrier against harmful microbes. Gut flora also regulate inflammation and activate immune functions. As a matter of fact, 60 percent of the immune system is found in the gut-associated lymphoid tissue (GALT), which is located just outside the intestinal lining. In addition, the intestines are lined with immune cells called mast cells, which coordinate the immune system's and nervous system's responses to toxins and infectious agents.

Little-Known Diet Strategies to Hack Your Killer Cells

Natural killer (NK) cells are a type of lymphocyte and are critical to the immune system. They are produced in your bone marrow, lymph nodes, spleen, tonsils, and thymus gland and then enter into the circulation to control tumor formation, microbial infection, and tissue damage. People lacking adequate NK cells have been shown to experience more frequent viral infections, including herpes and HIV, and to die prematurely from cancers.

Circulating NK cells remain in a resting, inactive state until they are activated by inflammatory cytokines and invade any tissues that possess pathogen-infected cells. The NK cells then secrete cytokines such as interferons and TNF-alpha and release a membrane-disrupting protein called perforin, which causes the death of the target cell.

But more NK cells are not better, and your goal should be to modulate normal, natural activity of NK cells, not to increase the number NK cells. For example, in a state of rampant inflammation or excess abdominal fat, the number and activity of NK cells is increased, which can result in insulin resistance, pancreatic damage, exacerbation of autoimmune issues such as asthma, and miscarriages in pregnant women. On the other hand, impairment of and deficits in NK cells are associated with cancer, viral infections, multiple sclerosis, rheumatoid arthritis, lupus, and advanced aging.

Research-proven ways to modulate the normal activity of NK cells include many of the same antiaging strategies and compounds you will learn more about in chapter 19, including these:

- Exercise
- Massage
- Curcumin
- Zinc
- Selenium
- Astaxanthin
- Melatonin
- Astragalus
- Spirulina
- Eleuthero
- Blueberry
- Echinacea
- Thymus peptides (particularly epithalon)

When I interviewed nutritionist Jonathan Clinthorne on my podcast, he also highlighted a few other little-known, research-proven methods for increasing NK cell activity, including these:

- Avoiding the synthetic forms of folic acid often found in B vitamins, multivitamins, and folic acid–fortified foods such as cereals and packaged/processed foods. Always use the natural form of folate called 5-methyltetrahydrofolate.

- Regular consumption of aged garlic extract (approximately 2.5 g daily), especially during cold and flu season or intense periods of exercise or travel stress

- Avoiding frequent oscillations in calorie intake—both too few and too many calories have been found to suppress NK cell function. This is not to say that intermittent fasting or alternate daily fasting suppresses killer cells, but rather that long-term calorie deprivation or frequent excess calorie intake should be avoided.

Finally, although it is not available in the US, nor is it FDA approved, several overseas clinics are offering a type of immune system upgrade via NK cell infusions. Originally developed for cancer patients, this protocol involves obtaining billions of white blood cells from your body, washing them, sterilizing them, growing them, combining them with cytokines to speed up the process of cell expansion, and finally infusing them back into your body. For this protocol, look up practitioners such as Dr. Matt Cook, who offers this protocol in Mexico City, or Dr. Rafael Gonzales and Dr. Eduardo Ulloa at the World Stem Cell Clinic in Cancun.

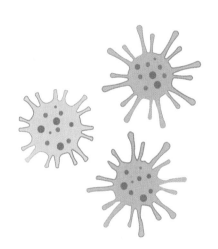

The immune system can also be divided into two distinct but complementary systems: the cell-mediated (also called innate) immune system and the adaptive (also called humoral) immune system. Innate immunity is your body's first line of defense and protects you from a range of pathogens via the following:

- Physical and chemical barriers, such as the skin, the mucosal epithelium, and gastric and respiratory chemicals
- Blood proteins
- Immune cells, such as natural killer cells, macrophages, heterophils, thrombocytes, eosinophils, and basophils. These protector cells engage in phagocytosis (devouring other cells) to eliminate invaders.

When the cell-mediated immune system is overwhelmed by invaders, your adaptive immune system kicks into high gear. This is the part of your immune system that allows you to encounter different bacteria and foreign invaders throughout your life and become more resilient as a result. It acts by learning to recognize specific features of a given pathogen—such as chicken pox—then eliminating the pathogen, and then creating a memory of the pathogen so that the next time you encounter it, you don't get sick. The primary cells of your adaptive immune system are lymphocytes.

To make things just a bit more complex, the adaptive immune system can also be broken down into adaptive humoral immunity and adaptive cell-mediated immunity. Adaptive humoral immunity is the primary line of defense that eliminates extracellular pathogens (invaders acting outside of your cells) and their toxins and involves the activity of antibodies in your blood, which are responsible for identifying pathogens. These antibodies are produced in different parts of your body, such as the gastrointestinal and respiratory tracts. On the other hand, adaptive cell-mediated immunity involves the activity of T cells to eliminate intracellular pathogens (invaders inside your individual cells) that antibodies can't reach. Both T cells and antibodies protect you by identifying and remembering certain features of each pathogen and recognizing the pathogen when you encounter it in the future, so that you adapt and develop a stronger overall immune system. The most important way you can support proper cell-mediated immunity is by not deactivating your natural immune system response with vaccinations and antibiotics but instead by allowing the natural immune response to take its course and letting the body simply be equipped to heal itself.

Taking these multiple components of the immune system into account, creating unstoppable immunity begins with moving lymph fluid throughout the body, keeping the respiratory system ready, limiting pathogens passing through the skin, keeping white blood cells elevated, strengthening the spleen, and repairing and maintaining proper gut health. You can fortify these defenses every day with various strategies while also ensuring you limit the amount of antibiotic-resistant and pathogenic invaders you come into contact with and simultaneously exposing yourself to the "good germs"—all strategies you will discover in this chapter.

The Importance of Letting Your Body Heal Itself

By Dr. Thomas Cowan

Over the years many patients have asked me how to take care of their immune systems. My response is always that—in contrast to what we generally believe—we don't have an immune system. Rather, we have two distinct immune systems. Only when these two immune systems are working together harmoniously do we have the possibility of being in robust health. The way to understand the functioning of our two immune systems is to examine what happens when we encounter a simple viral infection.

Take chicken pox, for example. When we are first exposed to the virus that causes chicken pox, we have no immunity against it, so it enters through our respiratory tract and infects thousands or perhaps millions of cells. These infected cells are distorted and dysfunctional and must be eliminated from the body. The elimination of these infected cells is the job of our first immune system, the cell-mediated immune system, otherwise known as the innate immune system. This system relies upon nonspecific defense mechanisms that activate either immediately or soon after a toxic or bacterial attack begins in your body. The nonspecific defense mechanisms include chemical defenses in the blood, immune cells like white blood cells, and even physical barriers, like your skin. The job of the cell-mediated immune system is to target infected cells, digest them, and eliminate them through the various elimination channels of the bowels, lungs, nasal passages, skin, etc. The crucial point here is that what we generally call being "sick," such as having a fever, mucus, cough, or rash, is actually the working of the cell-mediated immune response. A virus or toxin only stimulates the activity of this crucial innate immune response.

I know that this is so because you can infect someone with a virus, then inhibit the activity of their cell-mediated response and innate immune system, and they will never show any signs of sickness! They could die of the infection, but there will be no fever, no mucus, no outward signs of being sick. On the other hand, we can use various chemical stimulators of the cell-mediated response, with no infection needed, and we will show all the signs we typically associate with being sick. Fascinating, eh? This cell-mediated response is crucial to our health. It is how we detoxify, it is how we clear diseased cells and tissues from our bodies, and it is how we eliminate unwanted toxins and microorganisms from our bodies. Without a robust cell-mediated response, we are like a house that is unable to take out its garbage: over time we become more and more toxic.

The cell-mediated response usually lasts seven to ten days, after which we are restored to good health. But the body in its wisdom has realized it would be no good to keep going through the same illness over and over in our lives, so it has developed a second immune system, called the humoral or antibody-based immune response. The humoral immune system recognizes a certain unique protein associated with a particular virus or any other foreign assailant (called the antigen) and makes antibodies to that specific antigen. As a result of the antibody production, from that time on we are able to clear the infection from our bodies without ever having to involve the innate immune cell-mediated response. Since the humoral response has no outward symptoms, we will never again get "sick" in response to infection from that same microorganism. When these two systems—the innate and humoral immune systems—work together as they are meant to, your immune system is almost 100 percent foolproof, and it is extremely rare for a person to suffer the same viral disease more than once in their lives.

Up until the twentieth century, prior to the era of vaccinations, it never happened that we made a humoral response without at least some prior innate immune cell-mediated activity. Remember: in a normal immune response, we first have to clear the infection and only then can our immune system remember what happened. Vaccines changed all that because the theory behind vaccines is that we can develop immunity to a microorganism even if we bypass the cell-mediated response. Vaccines are essentially engineered to create minimal or no cell-mediated response and to only stimulate an antibody response.

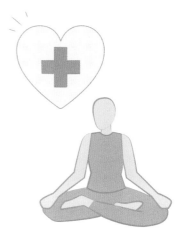

There are many problems with this unnatural approach. The first is that toxic chemicals, like aluminum, must be used to stimulate an antibody response in the absence of cell-mediated activity. Second, the immunity from this antibody approach is never lifelong, as proven by the continual need for booster shots. Third, and most crucially, a strategy of downplaying the cell-mediated immune system in favor of repeated stimulation of antibodies is guaranteed to produce a nation of people who suffer from chronic autoimmune disease and cancer. Autoimmune disease is defined as the state in which a person has developed excessive antibodies to their own tissues and includes conditions such as low thyroid, celiac disease or gluten sensitivities, acne and eczema, inflammation, joint pain, and much more. Conventional medicine says we don't know the etiology of this excessive antibody activity, but many studies have proven that repeated vaccination leads directly to this high-antibody disease state. Sure, there are other ways to develop autoimmune diseases, but vaccinations certainly are not helping.

And then there's cancer. The case of cancer being related to a suppressed cell-mediated response was dramatically demonstrated by a sarcoma (a virulent type of bone cancer) specialist named William Coley in the early part of the twentieth century. Coley was able to cure thousands of cancer patients simply by injecting them with a bacterial toxin that stimulated a high fever response. Fever is the quintessential sign of an activated cell-mediated immune response, and intensely stimulating fever for about a month is a powerful enough

therapeutic maneuver to cure even some end-stage cancer patients. There can be no better demonstration of the value and power of our cell-mediated immune system, and the body's innate ability to heal itself through built-in immune system mechanisms, than the story of Coley's toxins.

We are in a dangerous time in the history of medicine. We are the first medical system in the entire long history of human beings that has waged war on our cell-mediated immune system. A system that ignores the healing power of fever and acute illness is a medical system that will produce a nation of chronically sick people. It is far past time to reevaluate how we do medicine and how we care for our vital two-part immune system.

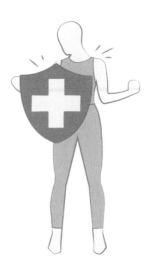

HOW TO BUILD AN UNSTOPPABLE IMMUNE SYSTEM

Now that you're armed with a basic road map to the immune system and an understanding of why dealing with illness is far more complex than simply popping pills and getting some rest, I'm going to equip you with fourteen of my favorite proven strategies for building an unstoppable immune system.

1. Lymph Flow

Your lymph system is one of two major circulatory systems in your body. Its primary role is to transport immune cells and dead cellular debris through the body to where they can be removed or recycled. While most members of the allopathic medical research community have focused on investigating the vascular system or developing pharmaceutical drugs and antibiotics for the immune system, the health of the lymph system seems to be given far more attention by the holistic and ancestral medicine community.

Think of the lymph system like the drains in your home: when there is a clog in any of the pipes, you experience odors and flooding, along with the accumulation of particles such as hair and food that then become a breeding ground for bacteria. In the same way that you must be careful what goes down the drain and also maintain your pipes in order to avoid a clog, you must do the same for your lymph system.

A congested lymph system can lead to the accumulation of waste, debris, dead blood cells, pathogens, toxins, and cancer cells, along with the inadequate flow of crucial compounds such as white blood cells and fat-soluble vitamins. Since, unlike the cardiovascular system, the lymph system does not have a heart to pump its fluids, the flow of lymph fluid depends on the motions of the muscles and joints during physical activity. In addition to engaging in low-level physical activity throughout the day and occasional vigorous exercise sessions, the best ways to ensure that your drains don't get clogged include the following:

- **Rebounding and vibration:** While anyone visiting my house, including the guy who mows the lawn and the woman who delivers the mail, may think I'm a complete freak of nature, in the spring and summer I sneak outside each morning and bounce up and down on my mini trampoline for ten minutes. During the colder months, I perform a similar activity on a vibration platform in my living room. When I travel, I simply perform full-body qigong shaking when I wake in the morning. (For a video of this shaking technique, visit BoundlessBook.com/15.)

  The g-forces generated during rebounding, the vibration that occurs when standing on a vibrating platform, and the motion of the muscles and joints during whole-body shaking all increase lymph flow and lymph fluid drainage and filtration via the six hundred to seven hundred lymph nodes spread throughout your body.

- **Chiropractic care:** According to chiropractic medicine, when something is obstructing the organs and structures in the upper part of the chest—such as a problem with the spine or rib cage—it can prevent the lymph system from properly collecting and removing toxins. This makes sense because the rib cage actually operates as a major pump for lymph fluid. A chiropractor can help correct any anatomical displacements to improve lymph flow. Adjusting the torso and thoracic region can also improve oxygen delivery to cells.

- **Sweating:** Perspiration is one of the primary mechanisms by which your body eliminates toxins. Although exercise can, of course, cause perspiration, infrared saunas are also an excellent method of circulating lymph flow via sweat.

- **Dry skin brushing:** Dry skin brushing involves gently moving a coarse brush along the skin in the direction of the heart. This is a perfect activity when you're in an infrared sauna, and I keep a simple, affordable brush on the floor of my sauna at all times.

- **Hydration:** Just as your blood needs water, so does your lymph fluid. I make it a habit to consume at least half my body weight in pounds in ounces of water per day (so, at 170 pounds, I drink at least 85 ounces of water, or about 2.5 liters). I usually drink purified and mineral-rich water and add the occasional squeeze of lemon or shot of apple cider vinegar. Along with the decoction tea on page 363, my friend John Douillard recommends a lymph rehydrating technique that involves sipping warm water every fifteen minutes throughout the day for two consecutive weeks, which stimulates lymph flow, relieves lymph congestion, and improves a sluggish immune system.

Panchakarma: Ayurvedic Detox

Stephen Cabral, the author of the book *The Rain Barrel Effect* and a former podcast guest of mine, is the man who first introduced me to Panchakarma, an ancient Ayurvedic detoxification ritual.

Panchakarma is a Sanskrit word that means "five actions" or "five treatments." The protocols used in traditional Panchakarma are:

- Vamana (emesis—an induction of vomiting by drinking an herbal solution)
- Virechana (purgation—similar to an herbal colonic)
- Niroohavasti (an enema using an herbal decoction)
- Nasya (infusion of medicine through nostrils)
- Anuvasanavasti (an oil enema)

While the protocols above may sound like a trip to a medieval torture chamber, there are other, gentler cleansing methods included in modern Panchakarma:

- Shirodhara (gently pouring a warm mixture of herbs and oil over the forehead)

- Garshana (dry skin brushing with either a wool or silk glove.
- Swedana (an herbal steam bath, during which the head and the heart are kept cool while the rest of the body is heated)
- Udvartana (an herbal paste lymph massage)
- Shiro-Abhyanga-Nasya (a combination of a deep head, neck, and shoulder massage and facial lymph massage, followed by inhalation of therapeutic aromatic steam, and a nasal and sinus "nasya" cleanse with herbal nasal drops)
- Pinda Swedana (a massage treatment using rice cooked in milk and herbs)

There are many suggested benefits of Panchakarma, including enhanced detoxification, improved digestion, and better skin health, but increased immunity is one of the more studied effects.

- **Massage:** Foam rolling, deep tissue therapy, and massage all improve the flow and drainage of lymph. I often get my massage on top of a Biomat or PEMF mat to enhance the flow even more. Herbal lymphatic drainage can also be very effective, especially for those with chronic illnesses.

- **Loose clothing:** Tight-fitting garments can place unnecessary restriction on lymph vessels—especially underwire bras, since lymph nodes are highly concentrated around the chest region to drain fluid from the breasts, arms, and chest. This goes for men too: guys I highly respect, such as wellness pioneer Paul Chek and Finnish health icon Veli-Jussi Jalkanen, both wear very loose fitting clothing nearly reminiscent of medieval tunics and cloaks or Scottish kilts. At least go boxers, not briefs, fellas.

Herbal Lymphatic Drainage

A major part of the lymphatic system is the interstitium, which is a network of connective tissue that surrounds nearly every organ system in the body, particularly the digestive and respiratory systems and under the skin.

Although it was previously thought to be simply dense connective tissue, researchers have now discovered that the interstitium consists of a series of interconnected fluid-filled sacs, and, along with being the primary source of lymph fluid, is a major fluid compartment for the entire body. Addressing this component of the lymphatic system is critical for many important lymph functions, including immune system tasks, the delivery of triglycerides as fuel for between-meals energy, picking up and processing proteins and fats that are too large to enter the bloodstream, draining waste from every tissue in the body, including the heart and digestive system, and draining nearly 3 pounds of plaque and other toxins from the brain each year.

My friend John Douillard at the LifeSpa clinic in Boulder, Colorado, is an Ayurvedic physician who specializes in lymph fluid circulation and detoxification, and he recommends several herbs to boost and detoxify the lymphatic system:

- Red root: This herb helps decongest lymphatic vessels and offset the age-related development of fibrous tissue. Red root cleans out the intestinal lymphatic ducts that direct protein and fat into the blood. This can help reduce swelling in the limbs, heaviness after big meals, and postprandial "food comas."

- Ocotillo stem: Native tribes of the southwestern US have traditionally used this compound to boost lymphatic detoxification processes.

- Stillingia root: Stillingia, or queen's root, aids in decongesting lymphatic vessels and mucous membranes. It also boosts the lymphatic system's detox capacities.

- Astragalus: This plant is particularly helpful for cleaning out the skin-associated lymphatic tissue, as well as supporting the lymphatic system as a whole. It also helps calm an overreactive immune system, since a congested or toxin-laden lymphatic system can cause hypersensitivity and overstimulate the sympathetic nervous system.

- Ginger root: In Ayurvedic medicine, ginger is known as the "universal spice." In addition to cleaning and boosting the lymphatic system, it also clears metabolites from the kidney's collecting ducts.

Although you can purchase many of the herbs above from websites such as Mountain Rose Herbs or Amazon, LifeSpa also sells "done-for-you" herbal cleansing products (you'll find links to them at BoundlessBook.com/15). You can also look into the homeopathic lymphatic drainage tinctures made by the company Pekana, which aid in the detoxification and drainage of the lymphatic system and the major organs of elimination, including the liver and kidneys.

Here's a quick summary of the best practices for lymph flow:

- Engage in low-level physical activity throughout the day and occasional bouts of vigorous exercise.
- Stay well hydrated with pure water.
- Practice whole-body shaking or rebounding on a trampoline or vibration platform every day.
- Use a sauna (preferably infrared) one to five times per week, and dry skin brush for at least one of those sauna sessions.
- Visit a chiropractic doctor two to four times a month.
- Get a full-body massage two to four times a month or regularly make love to your foam roller.
- Consider a Panchakarma treatment once per year.

2. Thieves Oil

There's this old tale of four thieves. During the fourteenth century, when the bubonic plague was running rampant through Europe and Asia, these four thieves became notorious for robbing dead bodies of all their possessions—yet the thieves miraculously never contracted the highly infectious plague. According to lore, after they were caught and charged, the court magistrate offered them a deal: in exchange for a reduced sentence, they could share their secret to immunity from the plague. The thieves took the deal and told of a blend of medicinal herbs they consumed each day, specifically cloves, lemon, cinnamon, eucalyptus, and rosemary. Hundreds of years later, this blend of aromatic herbs was proven to be a potent way to kill airborne bacteria, enhance the activity of white blood cells, and increase lymph fluid circulation.

Whether or not the story is true, the "four thieves" remedy was developed into an herbal formulation in Europe between 1413 and 1722. Because of its touted protective benefits, herbalists have passed along its recipe for hundreds of years, and it typically involves a combination of various herbs and spices, most often cinnamon, eucalyptus, rosemary, cloves, and lemon.

Several variations of this formulation have been passed down through the years. Thomas Jefferson is said to have fancied a version that consisted of vinegar spiked with lavender, rosemary, sage, wormwood, rue, mint, and garlic to keep his presidential body infection-free. In contrast, the *Scientific American Cyclopedia of Preparations* gives this formula:

> 4 oz dried rosemary tops
> 4 oz dried sage
> 2 oz dried lavender
> 5 oz fresh rue
> 1 oz camphor dissolved in vinegar
> ¼ oz sliced garlic
> 1 oz bruised cloves
> 1 gallon strongly distilled wine vinegar
>
> Digest for 7 or 8 days, with occasional agitation: pour off liquor: press out the remainder, and filter the mixed liquids.

Even with the variation in ingredients, there are multiple research-proven benefits of thieves oil. For example, multiple research studies have shown that allicin, a compound released when a garlic clove is crushed, smashed, or chopped, can boost immunity against viruses, and that aged garlic extract can reduce the severity of colds and flus by enhancing the function of immune cells. Following are more of the proven benefits of thieves oil.

CLEANING THE AIR OF MICROBES AND MOLDS VIA DIFFUSION

An experiment was done to see if the aerosol use of essential oils could alleviate some of the microbial causes of sick-building syndrome, a cluster of symptoms such as chronic fatigue, frequent headaches, and illnesses, all traceable to exposure to a polluted or moldy indoor environment. The researchers used a blend of clove, lemon, cinnamon bark, Eucalyptus radiata, and rosemary and found that this blend did inhibit certain microbes. The researchers concluded that "thieves [oil] can significantly reduce the number of aerosol-borne bacteria and may have application in treating air for enclosed environments and preventing transmission of aerosol-borne bacterial pathogens."

A follow-up field study also found that diffusing this same blend of essential oils decreased airborne black mold. Mold management will be addressed in greater detail in chapter 20, but it's quite an important consideration for the immune system because mold can significantly contribute to the development of a hyperactive immune system, an issue discussed in detail in Dr. Neil Nathan's excellent book *Toxic*.

RESPIRATORY SUPPORT

One key ingredient in thieves oil, eucalyptus oil, is well known for its respiratory support when inhaled or taken orally. One article in *Alternative Medicine Review* states: "Application by either vapor inhalation or oral route provides benefit for both purulent and non-purulent respiratory problems, such as bronchitis, asthma, and chronic obstructive pulmonary disease (COPD). There is a long history of folk usage with a good safety record. More recently, the biochemical details behind these effects have been clarified. Although other plant oils may be more microbiologically active, the safety of moderate doses of EO and its broad-spectrum antimicrobial action make it an attractive alternative to pharmaceuticals."

In another study, *Eucalyptus globulus* was tested for cytotoxicity and antibacterial activity against common pathogens linked to respiratory infections. The study demonstrated that the pathogens, including influenza, pneumonia, *Staphylococcus, Klebsiella,* and adenovirus, were highly susceptible to eucalyptus oil. Cinnamon bark oil has also been shown to inhibit gram-positive and gram-negative bacteria associated with various infections and to be toxic to various fungi related to respiratory tract infections.

ANTIMICROBIAL ACTIVITY

Probably one of the most famous uses of thieves oil, besides its aromatic applications, is to eliminate microbes. The antimicrobial effects of essential oils are vast. The *Journal of Biological Chemistry* explains that cyclic hydrocarbons found in essential oils, including aromatics, terpenes, and alicyclic compounds, likely have a direct toxicity effect on the cell membranes of certain bacterial species.

One study tested the antimicrobial activity of the essential oils from clove and rosemary. The authors reported that after testing clove and rosemary essential oils against *Staphylococcus epidermidis*, *Escherichia coli*, and *Candida albicans*, they found that "both essential oils possessed significant antimicrobial effects against all microorganisms tested."

An in vitro study that tested twenty-one selected essential oils against six bacterial species (*Escherichia coli*, *Klebsiella pneumoniae*, *Pseudomonas aeruginosa*, *Proteus vulgaris*, *Bacillus subtilis*, and *Staphylococcus aureus*) found that nineteen of the oils showed antibacterial activity against one or more strains of the microbes tested. They reported: "Cinnamon, clove, geranium, lemon, lime, orange and rosemary oils exhibited significant inhibitory effect. Cinnamon oil showed promising inhibitory activity even at low concentration, whereas aniseed, eucalyptus and camphor oils were least active against the tested bacteria. In general, *B. subtilis* was the most susceptible. On the other hand, *K. pneumoniae* exhibited a low degree of sensitivity."

MICROBIOME SUPPORT

The oils in the thieves blend have been shown in many studies to prevent microbial infections of the gut when ingested, and there is evidence that any disturbance of the microbiome or "killing off" of good bacteria is unlikely due to the immune-modulating effects of the oils. A 2012 article provided support that essential oils can work synergistically with probiotics to have complementary antimicrobial effects with practically no side effects.

I first fell in love with thieves oil when I used it topically to successfully kill the flesh-eating bacteria (MRSA) that I contracted while swimming in dirty water with open wounds during a triathlon. Here are just a few suggestions I have for the use of thieves:

- Apply a few drops to open cuts and wounds to prevent infection and promote healing.
- Mix with a tablespoon of water, gargle, and swallow for a sore throat.
- Put a drop on your thumb and apply to the roof of your mouth for a headache.
- Breathe in the vapors when you have lung congestion.
- Put a few drops in any oil-pulling oil to maintain healthy teeth and reduce cavities.
- Apply a drop or two to gums and teeth for pain relief from toothaches. Mix one or two drops with a tablespoon of raw honey for cough relief.
- Use it in an essential oil nebulizing diffuser and breathe it in for sinus headaches.
- Buy a FLO Pen and vape thieves (or any other essential oil, such as oregano oil, peppermint oil, or lavender oil) just as you would with a vape pen. The FLO essential oil pens are an effective way to breathe in oil compounds without the use of a vaporizer or diffuser.

3. Echinacea

Echinacea is, like thieves, an incredibly versatile immune-supporting compound. It has been shown in research to relieve upper respiratory symptoms such as inflammation, whooping cough, and the common cold, and a fascinating meta-analysis from the University of Connecticut showed that echinacea, when taken during cold and flu season, could cut the likelihood of getting a common cold by over half and also reduce the duration of the common cold by almost one and a half days!

But the benefits of echinacea go far beyond coughs and colds. For example, like a regular sauna practice, intake of echinacea increases the expression of heat shock proteins and also boosts white cell counts. Heat shock proteins are typically induced when cells are exposed to environmental stressors, such as heat, inflammation, and oxidative stress. They play a role in the assembly and transport of newly synthesized protein within cells and also remove denatured proteins, so they're important for preventing cell damage and repairing cells after injury. They are also important in antigen presentation and the activation of lymphocytes and macrophages. Antigen presentation is especially important after a viral infection, as it signals to the body that an antigen is "foreign" and "non-self." It has been proposed that heat shock proteins are part of the body's adaptive immune response because their circulation in the bloodstream signals danger to the host.

Echinacea also boosts the immune system by stimulating phagocytosis, the process by which white blood cells and lymphocytes attack invading organisms such as parasites and bacteria. Echinacea also stimulates the production of T cells and macrophages in the bloodstream while enhancing the concentration of interferon, interleukin, immunoglobulin, and other natural immune compounds in the blood.

Echinacea intake also protects red blood cells against oxidative damage. The membranes of the red blood cells contain high concentrations of polyunsaturated fatty acids that are highly susceptible and sensitive to free radicals, but echinacea can act as a free radical scavenger (although, whether you use antioxidants or any other method to quench free radicals or reactive oxygen species, there is a law of diminishing returns—see the sidebar below).

Are Antioxidants Actually Bad for You?

You have no doubt heard that free radicals can damage cells and that reactive oxygen species (ROS) should be ruthlessly mitigated with antioxidants. But the fact is that some amount of free radicals and ROS are necessary for a number of cellular pathways involved in cellular growth, survival, and proliferation, and in metabolism and blood vessel formation. It's certainly true that, for example, cancer cells generate higher levels of ROS that are essential for that cancer to grow, and this is likely why cancer cells express elevated levels of a large number of cellular antioxidants, to protect against oxidative or stress-induced cell death.

If ROS were only toxic, antioxidants would be great, but since ROS can help with immune function, antioxidants may blunt adaptive immunity. In fact, in the case of sepsis, which is a systemic infection accompanied by significant amounts of inflammation and autoimmunity, antioxidants have been shown to make the situation worse. And in trials, high doses of antioxidant vitamin E do not show a benefit for cancer and in fact show possible harm.

In addition, activation of the innate immune system requires ROS signaling. This signaling is necessary for surveillance receptors of the immune system and the release of protective pro-inflammatory cytokines, which then cause an appropriate immune response.

Decreasing ROS levels too much has been shown to inhibit activation of proper immune responses, eventually leading to immunosuppression. At the same time, excessively elevated ROS levels can contribute to autoimmunity by increasing the release of proinflammatory cytokines and proliferation of too many adaptive immune cells.

Finally, if you consume high doses of antioxidants after exercise, they can turn off the beneficial genetic transcription response to exercise, which can limit the number of mitochondria you can produce.

So what's the takeaway message? Consume antioxidants, but not too many of them, and be especially careful consuming antioxidants before, during, and after exercise—particularly antioxidants in concentrated supplement forms. In addition, while taking antioxidants when you're sick is good, this doesn't necessarily mean that more antioxidants are better. Unfortunately, research has yet to show what the magic amount of antioxidants is to support a balanced ROS seesaw, but my general rule is to take small amounts each day, eat a moderate amount of wild plants and other whole-food antioxidant sources, and then to allow my body to create its own antioxidants via normal signaling pathways.

Echinacea is also a proven performance-enhancing aid, particularly for aerobic and endurance athletes and athletes competing at high altitudes (for similar reasons, it is quite good for altitude sickness). This is because echinacea has been shown to stimulate macrophage activity, which can result in an increase in prostaglandin E2 (PGE2) secretion. PGE2 is a protein that stimulates the production of serum erythropoietin (EPO). EPO, which you may recognize as a banned performance-enhancing drug in its exogenous form, is a hormone that is secreted by the kidneys to stimulate stem cells in bone marrow to develop into red blood cells. In addition, PGE2 has been shown to stimulate the release of granulocyte-macrophage colony-stimulating factor (GM-CSF) from smooth muscle cells, which causes it to act as a growth factor for new red blood cells.

Currently, the primary form of echinacea that I use, particularly to load with for about two weeks leading up to any competition or adventure I have at high altitudes, is a blend from Biotropic Labs that combines echinacea with other blood-building compounds such as beetroot, chlorella, desiccated liver extract, blue-green algae, cordyceps, and several other compounds that support both red blood cell production, exercise performance, and immunity. (You'll find discount codes on BoundlessBook.com/15.)

Finally, echinacea appears to work best as an immune booster when taken in the early stages of a cold or upper respiratory tract infection because it can shorten the duration of both colds and flus. Effective doses range from 900 to 1,500 mg per day split into three doses.

4. Zinc

During cold and flu season, if you see me mumbling with a mouthful of what appears to be a breath mint, it is more likely a zinc lozenge, and it is one of the four to six zinc lozenges that I dissolve in my mouth each day if I have been exposed to sickness.

Zinc is hands down one of the best, if not the best, immune-hacking supplements. If you read the medical literature, this is one modality that has been shown to work over and over again.

Zinc is a micronutrient found in many foods, like meat, cheese, and especially seafood, particularly oysters. If you're wondering just how important this micronutrient is, since 1963, scientists have learned of over three hundred enzymes and over one thousand transcription factors that require zinc for proper function. And, not only does zinc modulate cell-mediated immunity, but it also has antioxidant and anti-inflammatory properties that can provide a potent cure for the common cold. But I wouldn't suggest simply running out to your local drugstore and grabbing a bottle of any old zinc. The type and the dose matter significantly.

While zinc itself is essential for immune function, zinc lozenges, which are best if you're trying to stave off or shorten a cold, appear to work through a different mechanism entirely. When you pop a zinc lozenge into your mouth, it begins to release ionic zinc, which is the key to its antiviral activity. Dissolving a lozenge slowly in the mouth provides a steady release of free ions into the pharyngeal region in the nasal cavity, which can have a greater effect on reducing respiratory and nasal symptoms associated with sickness than taking a zinc capsule or tablet. In fact, studies have shown that zinc lozenges can decrease the duration of a cold by five to seven days (if you think about how long a cold usually lasts, that's almost getting rid of the cold!).

But you must make sure you are consuming the correct type of high-dose zinc lozenge. First, make sure it doesn't contain any additives that would prevent proper dissolution and ionization. I also suggest avoiding any lozenges that contain citric acid, as this commonly added compound can bind tightly to zinc ions, preventing them from being released. Instead, look for a form of zinc called zinc acetate, which is twice as effective as zinc gluconate. Avoid effervescent lozenges, which also can reduce the production of ionic zinc.

Finally, for zinc to actually do its job, you need to start taking it right away—at the first sign of symptoms, when you feel you have been exposed to sickness. That's because it works by interfering with a virus's replication. So you essentially have only two or three days before it's too late to use zinc. After you're already sick, zinc can't do much to help your sniffles.

In summary, here's my recommended protocol for using zinc:

- As soon as you realize that you have cold symptoms, pop a zinc acetate lozenge (a good brand is Life Extension).
- Let it dissolve in your mouth for twenty to thirty minutes.
- Pop a new lozenge every two to three hours until your symptoms are gone.

5. Elderberry

One of the highlights of my year is when the old elderberry tree in the forest behind our house comes into full production and creates oodles of elderberries, which my wife collects, ferments, and turns into a dark, dense, immune-boosting elderberry wine. Elderberry teas, tinctures, and supplements are all excellent options to have on hand in your medicinal pantry and combine quite well with many of the other compounds discussed in this chapter.

The anthocyanins in elderberry have been shown known to have potent immunostimulant effects. In fact, a 2016 study showed that elderberry supplementation can vastly reduce the duration and symptoms of colds in air travelers. Another study found that when the elderberry extract is used within the first forty-eight hours of the onset of flu symptoms, it shortens the duration of symptoms by an average of four days.

Because of its sweet, tart, and refreshing taste, elderberry juice is an excellent alternative to elderberry wine, especially if you don't have time to make the wine. Good brands include River Hills, Biotta, Biona, and Wyldewood Cellars—all of which have a tart and tannic flavor, with a mild sweetness. An elderberry tincture is another good option. Effective doses of elderberry extract range from 600 to 900 mg per day. As a word of caution, the elderberry plant is poisonous aside from the berries, so should you choose to prepare an elderberry treatment yourself, be sure to use only the berries and to prepare them properly via a process such as fermentation.

6. Colostrum

Ever since I discovered the potent ability of colostrum to keep the gut lining from becoming permeable during workouts and races in hot weather, which can result in gut distress and endotoxemia, I have been a fan of using this supplement. Turns out, it's also beneficial whenever I'm exposed to any type of immune system assailant.

Colostrum, the first secretion of the mammary glands in both humans and animals, serves as a form of passive immunity, transferring antibodies from mother to infant. Colostrum provides a substantial dose of antibodies such as IgA, IgG, and IgM, all of which help to fight pathogens in the intestinal tract. The growth factors in colostrum stimulate the gut to patch up the gaps in the intestinal lining that lead to leaky gut (and then to autoimmune disorders). In fact, infants have greater intestinal permeability at birth, but their gut lining quickly becomes less permeable due to the intake of colostrum from their mother's breast milk. Later in life, excess inflammation and damage from toxin exposure, glyphosate, processed foods, rancid vegetable oils, and other assailants can cause the gut to become permeable again. Research shows that colostrum can restore a leaky gut lining to normal permeability levels, and also shows that athletes who pop colostrum prior to exercising in hot weather can completely banish the gastric distress that so notoriously accompanies exercise in the heat.

Because of its ability to repair a leaky gut, colostrum is fantastic for controlling the rampant, full-body inflammation and overactivity of the immune system that so often comes with leaky gut. As a matter of fact, one of the best protocols for managing autoimmune conditions, as outlined by my friend and physician Dr. Thomas Cowan in his book *Vaccines, Autoimmunity, and the Changing Nature of Childhood Illness*, is this:

- Follow the GAPS diet (see GAPSDiet.com).
- Take low-dose naltrexone, one of the most underrated medications for modulating immune system issues (see *The LDN Book* by Linda Elsegood for details).
- Take the liquid supplement RESTORE, whose active ingredient, lignite, can improve gut permeability (see chapter 13 for more details).
- Take a colostrum supplement to repair the gut lining.
- Take glandular extracts (such organ meats, liver capsules, and thyroid glandular), which help to modulate the immune system.

Colostrum is also fantastic for building muscle, as it is a potent growth hormone precursor and enhances levels of insulin-like growth factor 1—compounds that many bodybuilders inject with a needle but that you can easily get with a natural colostrum supplement. I get my colostrum from an organic goat farm in western Washington, and this is the same colostrum you can find at GetKion.com. Effective doses range from 20 to 60 g per day.

7. Bone Broth

I often consume the equivalent of a full cup of bone broth in my morning Wendy's Frosty–like smoothie (see the recipe below). But I triple or quadruple my bone broth consumption anytime I want to boost the health of my immune system, such as during cold and flu season, when there's

My Perfect Wendy's Frosty–esque Morning Smoothie

- 8 to 12 ounces bone broth, or 1 cup frozen bone broth (such as Kettle and Fire)
- Large handful of ice
- 2 teaspoons ground Ceylon cinnamon
- 1 drop Omica Organic vanilla stevia
- 2 scoops of a good protein powder (I prefer Organifi, Thorne, Ancient Nutrition, or Living Fuel brands)
- Juice of ½ lemon (this enhances collagen absorption from the bone broth)

For topping (optional):

- Coarse sea salt
- Fermented cacao nibs
- Spirulina
- Unsweetened coconut flakes

Blend for 3 minutes on high (this is key for proper consistency—a long blend time!). Top with coarse sea salt, fermented cacao nibs, spirulina bits, and unsweetened coconut flakes, if desired.

nearly always a pot of bone broth on the stove with other immune-supporting goodies thrown in, such as chaga mushroom extract, a bit of the decoction tea on page 363, or a dropperful of oregano oil.

There is a reason why native peoples have been consuming bone broths for thousands of years, why your grandmother's chicken soup always seemed to cure what ailed you, and why there's a South American proverb that claims "bone broth raises the dead." Whether bone broth is as magical a healing aid as it is touted to be remains to be proven by robust research, but nonetheless, there are numerous health benefits to simply drinking liquid that has been simmering with the marrow and joint bones of beef, chicken, lamb, and even fish for twenty-four to forty-eight hours.

Bone broth contains substances that are vital to the innate immune system, such as the amino acids arginine (which is critical for immune system and liver function), glutamine (which assists with cellular metabolism), and glycine (which aids in glutathione production and improves sleep quality). The marrow in bone broth contains lipids called alkylglycerols that are crucial for the production of white blood cells. These same alkylglycerols also appear in colostrum and have been shown to control the growth of cancer cells. According to research by Dr. Matthias Rath, the collagen in bone broth may also prevent cancer tumor metastasis, and the gelatin in bone broth is beneficial for autoimmune diseases related to a leaky gut. The glycosoaminoglycans found in bone broth can similarly help to restore a healthy intestinal lining. The chondroitin sulfate in bone broth, has both anti-inflammatory and immunoregulatory effects.

Be sure to proceed with caution if you purchased packaged bone broth, as not all bone broth is created equal. Almost every company selling bone broth online—even the ones using grass-fed and organic ingredients—are simply freezing their broth and shipping it with lots of dry ice and harmful Styrofoam containers. Furthermore, many do not even list bones on the ingredients label. If bones aren't on the label, the broth won't contain nutrients from bone marrow, such as collagen, immune-boosting alkylglycerols, or omega-3 essential fatty acids.

I personally prefer Kettle and Fire bone broth. They maintain strict standards to deliver bone broth made from the bones of cattle that are humanely raised, with no antibiotics or hormones, 100 percent grass-fed and grass-finished.

For a particularly nourishing morning breakfast, I recommend you experiment with my friend Dr. Thomas Cowan's healing broth recipe. The following is adapted from his excellent book *Cancer and the New Biology of Water*:

- Heat a generous amount of grass-fed ghee in a saucepan over medium heat, then add 1 to 2 tablespoons of turmeric powder and stir until it dissolves.
- Add 3 to 7 different vegetables of choice (sprouts such as alfalfa sprouts and mung bean sprouts are particularly good) and sauté until the vegetables are soft.
- Next, add 1 to 2 cups of bone broth. Turn the heat down to low and simmer for 1 to 2 minutes, then stir in a generous portion of powdered vegetable extract.
- Finally, ladle the broth into a bowl and add 1 tablespoon each of naturally fermented miso and natto.

For that recipe, I cannot recommend highly enough the ashitaba, burdock, and three-fold blend of powdered vegetable extract from Dr. Cowan's website, which is linked to on BoundlessBook.com/15.

Finally, please note that those with histamine sensitivities or mast cell issues may need to proceed with caution when it comes to bone broth and fermented foods—pay close attention to any symptoms you experience after eating them.

8. Fermented Foods

If you open my refrigerator, you will immediately see that the entire top shelf is chock-full of mason jars packed with fermented vegetables—from sauerkraut to pickles to kimchi and beyond—along with plenty of homemade coconut yogurt, kefir, natto, miso, and more.

My typical lunchtime salad and my side dish at dinner include a heaping tablespoon of sauerkraut or kimchi, a dollop of yogurt, a fermented pickle, a teaspoon of miso, and an occasional glass of my wife's wonderful homemade kombucha. When I began incorporating these types of fermented foods and probiotics into my diet, my frequent seasonal colds suddenly dwindled. I was getting sick once a year rather than once a month. By supporting my gut bacteria, I was drastically improving my immune system.

It is estimated that three-quarters of your immune system resides in your gut. Indeed, immunity begins with the bacteria in our digestive tract, as these creatures play vital roles in nutrient absorption, mucosal barrier function, support of gut lymphoid tissue, and immune function.

For example, take lactic acid bacteria, also known as *Lactobacillus paracasei*, which is found in naturally fermented foods like sauerkraut and yogurt. It produces the enzyme lactocepin, which is able to destroy immune system messengers called chemokines. In a healthy gut, chemokines guide white blood cells to an infection, but in individuals with inflammatory bowel disease, they can exacerbate an autoimmune response. Consuming sources of lactic acid bacteria can thus reduce autoimmune symptoms.

Another strain of bacteria, the probiotic bifidobacteria, secretes gamma-aminobutyric acid. Macrophages, which are immune cells that engulf bacteria and virus-infested cells, contain butyric acid receptors that, when activated by the acid, can reduce the production of inflammatory compounds. The cell walls of bifidobacteria also contain a dipeptide that activates the synthesis of lymphocytes, which are immune cells that produce antibodies and are responsible for acquired immunity. Scientists have also examined the effect of kefir, which is probiotic-rich fermented milk, on the immune systems of rats. The rats were given kefir daily for twenty-eight days and then injected with a cholera toxin. The rats that had been eating a daily dose of kefir exhibited significantly higher antibodies to the toxin than the control group.

To get more details on supporting natural, healthy gut flora, revisit chapter 13. In addition, I highly recommend combining a high intake of a wide variety of fermented foods with daily use of the supplement RESTORE, also mentioned in chapter 13. Over the last sixty years, there has been a steady loss of biodiversity in our gut membrane's bacterial ecosystem, and a large part of this is due to factory farming, processed foods, and widespread antibiotic use. This loss of biodiversity has left our gut membrane walls vulnerable. But the most potent of the common causes of the damage to the gut wall in our diet is glyphosate—an ingredient in weed killers—because it triggers the activation of a protein called zonulin. Zonulin is produced in the gut, where it opens the tight junctions between cells in the intestinal lining, then circulates systemically and can open the blood-brain barrier, kidney tubule systems, and blood vessel walls.

RESTORE is a liquid supplement that delivers bacterial metabolites to promote a healthy firewall of tight junctions in the gut wall and blood-brain barrier, and it rapidly increases production of the enzymes that break down zonulin. Although I always buy organic, because of the widespread prevalence of glyphosate toxins, even in organic food, I take RESTORE several times per day. (For discount codes, see BoundlessBook.com/15.)

9. Decoction Tea

If I ever get a bout of gut issues, one of the first things I do is make myself a big ole cup of my friend John Douillard's decoction tea, which contains slippery elm bark, marshmallow root, and licorice root (you'll find the recipe at the bottom of this page). The combination of these herbs softens and soothes mucous membranes all the way from the throat to the stomach to the small and large intestines, flushes the lymph system, and allows good bacteria to multiply while providing adaptogen-like effects that protect these bacteria from stress and environmental irritants.

To understand why this particular tea works so well, it's important to understand that the environment of the intestinal tract that supports beneficial microbes is very delicate. For intestinal villi to function well, they cannot be too dry or too wet (excessive mucus production, for example, will hamper their function). John Douillard has been using his decoction tea in his Ayurvedic health practice for almost thirty years to correct both dry and overly damp mucous membranes. When these herbs are cooked down into a concentrated tea, the soluble fiber from the roots and barks are released. This fiber is naturally slimy and soothes dried-out intestinal mucosae. The fiber also feeds beneficial intestinal microbes as a natural prebiotic. This is a critical part of the tea's restoration effect: it creates an environment that allows healthy microbes to proliferate while restoring the function and environment for the intestinal villi and gut mucosa, so nutrients can be digested and assimilated optimally. Think of this tea as coating your entire digestive tract with a mucilaginous, microbe-boosting layer. When this happens, new intestinal skin can grow, a healthy intestinal environment can be restored, and microbes can repopulate.

The first ingredient in the tea—licorice—is a classic Ayurvedic herb that's used as a natural lubricant for the intestinal and respiratory airways. Licorice lubricates and coats mucous membranes and, as an adaptogen, protects them from stress and environmental irritants and pollens. In addition, glycyrrhizin, found in licorice root, can inhibit the replication of influenza virus while also reducing virus-associated inflammation.

The next ingredient, slippery elm bark, has long been used in Ayurvedic medicine for digestive and intestinal concerns because of its lubricating and gut-defending properties. It has also been shown to support healthy antioxidant activity in the intestinal tract.

Finally, the chopped marshmallow root is perhaps the most slippery of the three herbs in this formula. It has been shown to support the health of the stomach lining and to protect the intestinal tract from irritants, such as the toxic form of carrageenan found in many packaged foods. It has even been approved in Europe for clinical use to improve the integrity of the gastric, oral, and pharyngeal mucosae.

The key to the success of this tea is to consume it every day for a month or two, 1 tablespoon every two hours, apart from a meal. You must also use chopped, not ground, herbs (if you use ground herbs, you will basically make a muddy tea, and it won't work).

Here's how to make the tea: Boil 1 to 2 tablespoons each of organic chopped licorice root, organic marshmallow root, and organic slippery elm bark in a pot filled with 2 quarts of water. If you can let it simmer overnight, uncovered, until about 2 cups of water remain, it's even better, but if not, that's okay. Strain the mixture, save the liquid, and discard the herbs. This should make 2 cups to sip on throughout the day.

DIY Antiaging Yogurt

by Dr. William Davis

Note from Ben: I first discovered the wonders of home-made yogurt from my friend and cardiologist Dr. William Davis, author of Undoctored. *He was kind enough to share the secrets behind this powerful and delicious creamy treat.*

I've been discussing this idea of making yogurt by starting with a specific strain of Lactobacillus reuteri ATCC PTA 6475, based on the detailed studies conducted at MIT and elsewhere, both experimental animal and human, that have suggested dramatic effects. Those effects include:

- Complete shutdown of appetite, an "anorexigenic" effect, that can be used to facilitate intermittent fasting or break a weight-loss plateau

- An increase in metabolic rate, which also contributes to weight loss

- A dramatic increase in skin thickness and skin collagen, along with acceleration of skin healing, a surrogate for overall youthfulness and health. I'm a big fan of dietary collagen, such as those in collagen hydrolysates, bone broths/soups, slow-cooking meats, the skin on chicken and fish, etc. This *L. reuteri* strategy amplifies this effect considerably.

- Increased oxytocin. A doubling of oxytocin levels was observed in mice. This effect is responsible for the extravagant skin benefits, reduced insulin resistance, dramatic increases in testosterone in males, increased estrogen in females (magnitude unclear), and thicker and more plentiful hair (though the consistency of this effect is not yet clear). Other studies have demonstrated substantial weight loss, especially from visceral fat, along with increased muscle mass and increased bone density.

Put all these effects together—reduced appetite, increased skin health, increased bone density, fat loss, muscle gain, etc.—and you have one of the most powerful antiaging, youth-preserving strategies I have ever come across.

Because the most robust data were generated using the ATCC PTA 6475 strain of *L. reuteri* (and, to a lesser extent, the DSM 17938 strain), I have been confining my efforts to this strain. Other *L. reuteri* strains may mimic these effects, but we don't know that for certain, as the studies have not been performed. Strain specificity can be a crucial factor. After all, all of us have several strains of *E. coli* in our intestines that live quietly and don't bother anyone. But get exposed to selected strains of *E. coli* from contaminated produce, and you develop life-threatening diarrhea that can be fatal, especially in children. Same species (*E. coli*), different strains—strain specificity can be a critical factor.

So we start with *L. reuteri* ATCC PTA 6475 provided by the Swedish company BioGaia, which has somehow locked this species up with patents. Their product is called Gastrus and combines the ATCC PTA 6475 strain with the DSM 17938 strain. Problem: there are only 100 million CFUs (live organisms) per tablet. I have not observed any substantial health benefits by ingesting the tablets.

However, the counts can be increased with fermentation in the presence of prebiotic fibers, so I have been amplifying bacterial counts by making yogurt. Just as ingesting prebiotic fibers increases bacterial counts in your intestines, so it goes in yogurt as well.

This yogurt is thick and delicious, and given its extraordinary thickness of the end-product, it is likely that trillions of CFUs are present, sufficient to convert the soupy liquid of your starting coconut milk to rich yogurt that's thick enough to stand up on a plate. People who consume ½ cup per day of this preparation are reporting the effects listed above.

There are probably many ways to make this yogurt and yield the bacterial counts you desire. But this is how I did it.

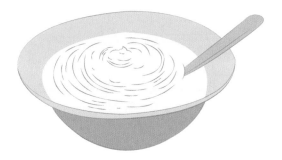

- 1 quart organic half-and-half, cream, whole milk, canned full-fat coconut milk, goat's milk or cream, or sheep's milk or cream (see Note)
- 1 tablespoon inulin or another prebiotic, such as sucrose, glucose, or potato starch
- 10 tablets BioGaia Gastrus, crushed

1. *In a large glass or ceramic bowl, combine 2 tablespoons of the half-and-half with the inulin and crushed probiotic tablets. Mix thoroughly and make sure the inulin and sugar are dissolved. Then add the remaining half-and-half and stir to combine well.*

2. *Turn the oven to 300°F for about 60 to 90 seconds, just until a desert-hot temperature is reached. Place the yogurt in the oven and turn the oven off.*

3. *After 4 to 6 hours, turn the oven back to 300°F for 60 to 90 seconds and then turn it off again. The goal is to keep the temperature at 100°F for around 24 hours; this method isn't precise, but it works fine when using dairy for fermentation.*

Note: If you use coconut milk, you will need to add 1 tablespoon sugar because there is no lactose to ferment in coconut milk. Don't worry, the sugar is fermented to lactic acid, so there's little sugar in the yogurt. Just as the cucumbers you grow in your garden were fertilized with cow manure but ripe cucumbers contain no cow manure, so the final fermented yogurt should contain little to no sugar.

In addition, fermenting coconut milk is much fussier than fermenting dairy, and you'll need to have more precise control over the temperature. It's best to use a yogurt maker, Instant Pot, sous vide device, rice cooker, or any other device that allows you to maintain a constant temperature. (I used a yogurt maker with good results.) Any of these devices can also be used to make this yogurt with dairy.

To make more batches, reserve a few tablespoons from the original batch and use it in place of crushed tablets, since your yogurt should contain plentiful microbes. The first batch tends to be a bit thinner with curdles, but subsequent batches tend to be thicker and smoother.

There are some uncertainties:

- Is there a reduction in bacterial counts or contamination by air organisms when you make yogurt from prior batches? Some people have "re-seeded" their yogurt by adding a few more crushed tablets of probiotic after several rounds of yogurt-making.
- We've arrived at the dose of ½ cup by trial and error, as judged by the anorexigenic effect that results when oxytocin levels increase. But is that the ideal dose? Don't know yet.
- Can we improve on taste, texture, and bacterial counts by altering fermentation temperature, choice of prebiotic, or other conditions?

Despite the uncertainties, I am witnessing some dramatic changes in the people trying this yogurt.

Note from Ben: I have been able to achieve a perfect texture and taste by stirring in 4 heaping tablespoons of organic Great Lakes unflavored beef gelatin and 4 dropperfuls of Omica Organics vanilla stevia to the mix, then refrigerating it for one day after fermentation. For a step-by-step audio demonstration of the yogurt-making process we use, go to my children's podcast at GoGreenfields.com and listen to the coconut yogurt episode.

10. Vitamin C

Although vitamin C is often celebrated as a powerful antioxidant, the benefit of vitamin C for the immune system is, at first glance, less than stellar. For example, several studies have shown that vitamin C supplementation has little or no effect on colds. Most of these studies involved supplementation at small doses or supplementation after the onset of colds. But other studies do indeed show benefit from larger doses and from taking vitamin C prior to the onset of illness. Some newer studies confirm that 1,000 mg per day of the right type of vitamin C can shorten the duration and mitigate the severity of colds while also preventing colds from developing, especially in people with low vitamin C levels.

In addition, many of the negative studies done on vitamin C look at a form known as ascorbic acid. Ascorbic acid is actually a synthetic form of vitamin C that is typically made from genetically modified corn, and it lacks the beneficial bioflavonoids present in whole-food forms of vitamin C. Also, keep in mind that approximately 80 percent of the world's vitamin C supplements come from China, where the manufacturing and quality controls aren't as stringent as in the United States. There is even some concern that the vitamin C we consume so much of in supplement form and that is often used as an additive in processed food is tainted with impurities such as heavy metals.

But contrary to popular belief, there is little difference between the various forms of vitamin C as far as bioavailability is concerned. According to the Linus Pauling Institute, natural and synthetic vitamin C are chemically identical and have the same effect on vitamin C levels in the blood. The same can be said for powders, tablets, capsules, liquids, and food forms of vitamin C. So your primary concern should be the purity and quality of a vitamin C supplement, not its bioavailability.

To find a good-quality vitamin C product, look for an all-organic food-based supplement or a USP-grade vitamin C, produced in a GMP-certified facility (GMP stands for "good manufacturing practices," and supplements produced at a GMP-certified will be higher-quality and safer). A few good products that fit these criteria include Whole Foods Market Food-Sourced Vitamin C, American Nutraceuticals Vitality C, and OrthoMolecular Buffered C Capsules.

If you take more than 500 mg at a time in an oral form, you'll likely experience stomach upset. But you may not get any extra benefit from a dose higher than 500 mg in any case. Dr. Mark Levine, chief of molecular and clinical nutrition at the National Institutes of Health and author of a research project proposing increasing the recommended daily amount of vitamin C, said: "At 100 milligrams all the tissues are saturated, at 200 milligrams, the blood plasma is saturated, but at 500 milligrams dose, then absorption levels appear complete, and rate of absorption begins to decrease." Dr. Andrew Weil, an alternative medicine physician, reduced his recommended dosage of vitamin C, from 2,000 to 6,000 mg divided into three doses a day to only 200 to 500 mg divided into two doses per day. He made this change after he examined two studies that showed lower levels of ascorbic acid more than adequately saturate the body's tissues and are sufficient to protect against cancer, heart disease, and other chronic illnesses. And a review of clinical trials published in the Journal of the American Medical Association concluded that 200 mg a day is the maximum humans can absorb when taken orally. But aside from the potential stomach upset, you don't need to worry if you do take higher doses because vitamin C is water soluble, and anything not used by the body quickly passes out. Ultimately, based on all this evidence, I suggest taking 200 to 500 mg oral vitamin C during cold and flu season.

Of course, the best, most natural sources of vitamin C have a single thing in common: they are all plant foods! Although most mammals can produce vitamin C in the liver, humans (and, oddly enough, guinea pigs) cannot, but plants provide a rich, highly bioavailable source of vitamin C. All citrus fruits, including orange, grapefruit, lime, and lemon, are excellent sources of vitamin C. Many non-citrus fruits are also rich in vitamin C, including papayas, strawberries, pineapples, kiwis, cantaloupes, and raspberries. Green leafy vegetables such as Swiss chard and cruciferous vegetables such as broccoli and cauliflower are also excellent sources, as is parsley, which provides over half of the recommended daily amount of vitamin C!

Finally, should you want to take things to the next level for vitamin C, then you can do as I do and get a quarterly high-dose vitamin C injection. Every few months, I visit the clinic of Dr. Jason West in Pocatello, Idaho, where I receive a variety of high-end medical treatments, including a nervous system reboot of my gut via procaine injections, chiropractic adjustments, live red blood cell analysis, and a ninety-minute-long 100-gram (yes, that's 100,000 mg!) vitamin C IV. An intravenous vitamin C protocol involves the slow infusion of vitamin C at doses on the order of 0.1 to 1.0 g ascorbate per kilogram of body weight. Of course, it would be absolutely impossible to consume this amount of vitamin C orally without severe gastric upset, but high plasma ascorbate concentrations can be safely achieved with IV infusions. In the past decade, the popularity of this tactic has exploded among functional medicine practitioners. It can be used to combat infections, treat rheumatoid arthritis, enhance collagen synthesis, and manage autoimmune diseases, and it has generated the most interest for its potential use in adjunctive cancer care.

11. Oregano Oil

When I was sixteen years old, my father suddenly began smelling like a giant Italian pizza. See, dear Dad had read a book by Dr. Cass Ingram called *The Cure Is in the Cupboard*, in which he discovered a potent herb that he used to heal a fungal infection of his foot. From that point on, I would hear him drone on and on about the wonders of oregano—which is considered to be the healing "hyssop" alluded to in ancient scriptures—at the dinner table, and I slowly became well versed in something called "oil of oregano." I later added it to my travel kit and immune system protocol as an absolute must-have—I use it all the time, from dripping it into my mouth before airplane travel to sprinkling it on my feet after using the shower at a health club or gym to cleaning external wounds, scrapes, and cuts with it.

Dr. Ingram in his book claims that wild oregano oil (unlike the standard thyme-based oregano oil found in most grocery stores) can help to reverse digestive complaints; boost the immune system; cleanse the body of fungi, yeasts, bacteria, and viruses; and protect against common illnesses.

So what makes oregano oil so special? Oregano (*Origanum vulgare*) is an herb that is a member of the mint family and has been valued for over 2,500 years in folk medicine for treating colds, indigestion, and upset stomachs. PubMed, a database of published medical and life sciences literature, lists almost two hundred studies on the beneficial properties of oregano oil and over eight hundred studies showing the benefits of carvacrol, one of the primary ingredients of oregano, for bacterial infections, fungal infections, parasites, viruses, inflammation, allergies, tumors, indigestion, candida, small intestine bacterial overgrowth, and even to reduce side effects from medications and drugs.

Carvacrol and thymol provide oregano's antiseptic and antioxidant properties. In addition, the terpenes in oregano, pinene and terpinene, contribute to its antiseptic, antiviral, anti-inflammatory, and anesthetic properties. Two long-chain alcohols, linalool and borneol, provide additional antiseptic and antiviral qualities. Finally, the esters linalyl acetate and geranyl acetate act as antifungal agents. It is the combination of these components working together that makes oregano such a potent protector of the immune system.

Good uses for oregano oil include these:

- Using it on skin to kill fungal infections or remove warts
- Applying several drops to wounds or infections (including MRSA and staph) externally
- Consuming one or two dropperfuls per day during cold and flu season, or when traveling (if the taste is too overwhelming, dilute in water with a bit of stevia)
- Adding tea tree oil and lavender to it, then placing several dropperfuls in a spray bottle filled with water to kill household mold
- Using a few drops on your toothbrush in addition to your toothpaste or when you can't find your toothpaste

I recommend that if you add oregano oil to your immune system arsenal, you look for oregano oil that contains a natural carvacrol level of over 80 percent. The fake stuff at the grocery store or on a bulk supplement website typically consists of thymol or is harvested from thyme, which doesn't give you the same potent effect as an oil high in carvacrol. Finally, should you purchase the 100 percent pure version of oregano, be cautious. It is extremely caustic and can burn the skin or the mouth, so you must mix it into a carrier oil that both dilutes it and maintains its bioavailability (almond is a good carrier oil).

12. Mushrooms

Mushrooms are a nutritional powerhouse, providing B vitamins, minerals, fiber, protein, antioxidants, and beta-glucans and other bioactive molecules that fight harmful bacteria, viruses, and toxins. Many mushrooms are also immunomodulators that stimulate the immune system's defense mechanisms.

For example, one study found that daily consumption of 5 to 10 g of shiitake mushrooms for four weeks significantly improved immunity and lowered inflammation. Shiitake mushrooms also exert antitumor activity and, when used in conjunction with chemotherapy, have been shown to prolong survival time, restore immunological parameters, and improve quality of life. The American College of Nutrition has found that shiitake mushrooms can improve the efficiency of the immune system, improve gut immunity, and decrease inflammation, and lab tests on human cell lines show that shiitake mushrooms can prevent malignant tumor growth by signaling tumor cells to burst in a process called apoptosis. Lastly, shiitake mushrooms have potent antimicrobial properties, making them effective natural antibiotics. Amazingly, one study showed that shiitake only killed disease-causing microbes, leaving beneficial bacteria unharmed (in contrast, prescription antibiotics kill off both beneficial and bad bacteria in your body).

Maitake mushrooms are also powerful immunomodulators that stimulate the immune system's defense reaction through enhanced cytokine production, phagocytosis, and NK cell activity. Cordyceps, which is a fungus that lives on certain caterpillars in the high mountain regions of China, also exhibits potent antitumor effects and immunomodulating effects. Studies have shown that cordyceps can help improve the body's innate immune function, and it's so effective in modulating immunity (which involves both improving an immune reaction to an invader or tumor and reducing an immune overreaction like asthma) that it has even shown benefits in studies on people with severe asthma. Evidence also suggests that cordyceps can help autoimmune issues and decrease the number of harmful bacteria in the gut.

The turkey tail mushroom contains bioactive compounds called beta-glucans, which can stimulate the immune system by enhancing macrophage and natural killer cell function. Studies also suggest that beta-glucans can help the immune system slow the growth of tumors and protect the body from the effects of cancer-causing compounds. Turkey tail also contains a high number of prebiotics, which feed the good bacteria in your gut and support immunity.

Another little known but highly effective mushroom is the tremella, which is rich in vitamin D and fiber, and contains specific compounds that protect the liver. Research suggests that tremella mushrooms can help the body fight infections, and in ancestral medicine, it has long been used as an immune tonic.

Finally, there's one of the most powerful mushrooms for immune systems, the "king of medicinal mushrooms": chaga. Chaga has an abundance of beta-glucans, and research has also shown that it activates immune cells responsible for combating cancer growth. Chaga increases the production of immune cells IL-6 and lymphocyte, which can help increase the ability to fight pathogens. Other compounds in chaga help the immune system to differentiate between the body's cells and foreign cells. Chaga reduces immune hypersensitivity and even reduces the risk of cardiac shock from severe allergic reactions. Chaga also has antiviral properties and can help fight off viral infections—it may even reduce the ability of HIV to replicate and prevent herpes and Epstein-Barr viruses from infecting new cells and replicating.

Most of these mushrooms help to regulate cell-mediated and adaptive immunity the process of modulation—both potentiating and suppressing the immune system similar to the way that an adaptogen can modulate endocrine and hormonal balance.

My favorite way to get a daily dose of immune-boosting mushrooms is to take Four Sigmatic's 10 Mushroom Blend, which includes a hefty dose of vitamin C (from rosehips), along with chaga, reishi, cordyceps, lion's mane, shiitake, maitake and a few other choice immune-boosting mushrooms. You can easily put a teaspoon of this into your morning cup of coffee or tea, especially during cold and flu season.

13. Bee Products

When it comes to creating compounds that support the immune system, bees are definitely a valuable resource. You're no doubt familiar with honey, but there are also three other immune-supporting bee products: bee pollen, royal jelly, and propolis.

Real raw honey stands in stark contrast to the fake, pesticide- and herbicide-laden, nutrient-poor honey you find in the average plastic honey bear at the grocery store. Raw honey has so many enzymes that it's the only food in the world that never goes bad, and it's full of minerals and antioxidants. In addition, honey contains minor amounts of the same type of bioactive components found in antioxidant-rich fruits and vegetables, including phenolic acid, flavonoids, α-tocopherol, ascorbic acid, proteins, and carotenoids.

Honey also has potent antiviral properties and can speed recovery from viral infections. Manuka honey, a type of honey produced by bees that feed on the nectar of the tea tree, inhibits flu virus replication and has been shown to be more effective than the active ingredients in popular cough medicines at improving both cough and sleep quality in individuals with upper respiratory infections. Methylglyoxal (MGO) is the primary anti-flu component of manuka honey. When selecting manuka honey, look for the MGO label on the jar and choose a brand with an MGO content of 83 or above (the higher the MGO rating, the higher the level of antiviral activity of the honey).

Bee pollen is one of the most nutrient-dense foods found in nature. It's packed full of vitamins and minerals, and it has nearly a full spectrum of essential nutrients. Pollen is the colostrum of the insect world—it contains more protein per gram than any other animal-based food, as well as free-forming amino acids. Research suggests that bee pollen has potent antifungal, antiviral, anti-inflammatory, antimicrobial, anticancer, liver-protecting, and local analgesic properties.

Royal jelly, secreted by glands in the heads of nurse bees, is the exclusive food of queen bees, who live about forty times longer than worker bees. Cleopatra used royal jelly on her skin regularly because of its regenerative and healing effects. Research suggests that nutrient-dense royal jelly may also support nerve health, mental acuity, and memory and protect against nerve damage because of its high acetylcholine content. It's certainly a superfood. It contains proteins, fatty acids, polyphenols, adenosine monophosphate, and hormones like testosterone, estradiol, progesterone, and prolactin.

Finally, there's propolis, which is the most potent of the immune-supporting compounds we can borrow from the bees. Propolis, taken from the Greek words for defense (pro) and city or community (polis), is known commonly as "bee glue" and is literally the immune protection for the beehive. Bees use propolis to seal holes and cracks in the beehive; it hardens the walls and even makes the inside of the hive aseptic. Studies on humans have shown that it has several applications in treating a host of diseases because of its antiseptic, antibacterial, antioxidant, anti-inflammatory, antifungal, antiulcer, antimycotic, anticancer, and immunomodulatory properties. It contains over three hundred natural compounds that have been shown to help immunity, and there's evidence that humans have been using propolis to support health since 300 BC.

In my pantry you'll find the royal jelly, propolis, bee pollen, and raw honey from Beekeeper's Natural, the bee-based superfood elixir from Gosha's Organics, and the drinkable blend of royal jelly, propolis, bee pollen, and wasp extract from Vespa (which is also a fantastic, ketogenic-friendly fuel for endurance athletes).

14. Germs

Don't be afraid to get dirty.

Did you eat your own boogers when you were a kid? If so, you're not alone—it turns out that we may actually be hardwired to eat our own boogers. Studies have shown that a kid's snot harbors bacteria that, when eaten, help strengthen the body's immune system. Don't worry, that doesn't mean that you need to harvest your or your kid's boogers and consume them as dietary staples, but it does highlight the fact that we need to allow our bodies to be exposed to germs and to get dirty.

I must admit, when my shiny new twin baby boys were brought onto the planet nearly eleven years ago, I certainly had my doubts about the value of letting their soft and innocent bodies roll, crawl, and toddle among the dirt and doggy-doo. But since then—and especially after learning what I'm about to share with you—I have become extremely lax about germs, and my boys now clamber up and down farm animals near our house and elephants in third-world countries, wallow like hogs in every mud puddle they find, and eat fistfuls of olives with faces and hands still stained from exploring every corner of the garage and backyard. Turns out, it's good for them.

THE HYGIENE HYPOTHESIS

Although the idea that exposure to certain infections may decrease the risk of allergies is not new, Dr. David Strachan was one of the first to formally propose it as the "hygiene hypothesis" in scientific literature, in an 1989 article in the British Medical Journal. In the paper, Strachan pointed out that hay fever and eczema were less common in children from larger families, and that children from larger families were probably exposed to more germs through their siblings. Since then, epidemiological studies have confirmed the protective effects of large family size, as well as of growing up on a farm.

Then, in a 2003 article in a journal of immunology, Dr. Graham Rook proposed the "old friends" hypothesis, arguing that we have become so dependent on microbes that coevolved with mammalian immune systems that our immune systems can neither develop or function properly without them. These microbes include species that inhabit our skin, gut, and respiratory tract; species that inhabit the domesticated animals and pets we live with; and even organisms such as symbiotic bacteria, viruses, and parasites or worms that establish chronic infections that we can actually tolerate and that help us develop specific immunoregulatory responses.

Finally, in the past several years, the "microbial diversity" hypothesis has emerged. This idea holds that the health and diversity of the bacterial species in our gut mucosae is a key factor for strengthening the immune systems: more-diverse microbiomes are better for our health than those with a limited number of bacterial species. This may relate to the hygiene hypothesis. Dr. Rook compared the embryonic immune system to a computer that contains many programs but little data. During gestation and childhood, the immune system builds a "database" of organisms that allows it to identify and respond to harmful agents in the internal or external environment. This microbial diversity hypothesis is why I recommend vaginal delivery of babies, which exposes newborns to the variety of bacterial species in the vaginal canal.

Each of these hypotheses is based on the general concept of upregulation of the body's T cells in response to infectious agents and appears to be well supported by epidemiological data. Many studies have proven that autoimmune diseases are much less common in developing countries than in industrialized countries and that people who emigrate from developing countries to industrialized countries develop immunological disorders such as asthma and disorders only upon spending a certain amount of time there.

Sure, not all germs are created equal, and there are definitely some situations in which you should protect your kids. For example, if MRSA (a staph infection), rabies, measles, rotavirus, anthrax, or Ebola is sweeping through your city, it's a good idea to keep the kids indoors and not send them out to sweat and blow snot with the other kids. But these situations are few and far between. By and large, exposure to a wide range of germs will help your kids develop strong immune systems and help them avoid allergies and autoimmune problems.

BOOSTING YOUR CHILD'S IMMUNE SYSTEM

One of the best ways to jump-start the immune system with beneficial flora is to be born via vaginal delivery—even Mom's fecal matter can be a boon. But there are also plenty of other ways to get dirty and boost your immune system. Here are ten that children can highly benefit from—and although these are aimed at kids, you'll find that implementing them helps your immune system, too.

1. Let your children touch and taste things.

Although your natural reaction may be to slap that handful of leaves, patch of dirty grass, clump of mud, or slightly discolored snowball out of your child's exploring hands, resist the urge! The

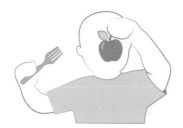

same goes for their propensity to gnaw on shopping cart handles, lick random windows, and chew on the seat belts in the car. Allow your children to experiment touching, handling, and even tasting the natural world around them. My kids kiss our dog on the lips. When they were infants, I often saw them lick the floor of the public bathroom at coffee shops, crawl through airports with their noses to the ground, and even rip their diapers off and eat their own poop. This may disgust you and make your parenting, caretaking heart want to leap forward with an antibacterial wipe, but frankly, the pros outweigh the cons when it comes to your kids' noses and mouths getting down and dirty with nature.

2. Don't be a bottle boiler.

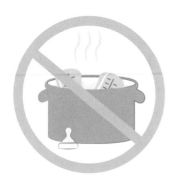

Sure, just like other dishes, bottles (and pacifiers) should be cleaned of fluid and food residue every now and again via boiling or washing, but you don't need to nuke the pacifier every time it touches the carpet or boil the bottle nipple after the dog sniffs it. Your children can (and should) eat and drink from slightly germ-tainted surfaces every now and again.

3. Avoid antibacterial soaps.

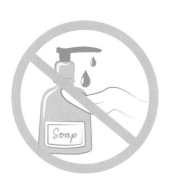

When I used to pick my kids up from childcare at the YMCA, I would sometimes get strange looks from the other parents because I went out of my way to remind my kids not to use the antibacterial hand soap. That stuff can actually can hurt your kids. By constantly using antibacterial soaps and hand sanitizers, we may be not only inhibiting immune development in our children but also creating "superbugs," bacteria that are resistant to pharmaceutical and natural antibiotics. So stick to good old soap and water, and even with these compounds, avoid excessive hand washing.

4. Avoid antibiotics.

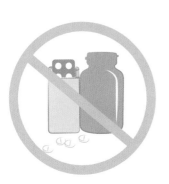

Don't rush out and grab a Z-Pak or an antiviral medication when they get the flu or are knocked down by a nasty bug. This can create the same kind of drug-resistant bacteria that antibacterial soaps do. However, if your child is seriously down for the count with the flu, you may need to be worried about secondary infections such as pneumonia, bronchitis, or sinusitis. In this case, I recommend you look into natural ways to boost white blood cell count or introduce natural antiviral or antibacterial substances, many of which I describe in this chapter, such as thieves oil, oregano oil, echinacea, mushrooms, and elderberry tinctures.

5. Visit farms and have pets.

You don't need to fly to Asia and play with monkeys and elephants to expose your children to beneficial worms and germs. Instead, go on the occasional field trip to your local farm to pet the sheep or feed the horses. And pets count! Cats, dogs, gerbils, guinea pigs, and even fish can expose children to a variety of bacteria and other living organisms they might not otherwise encounter. In a modern era of virtual pets and GigaPets, consider being the parent who instead builds a backyard chicken coop or visits the pet store for the occasional birthday gift.

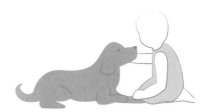

6. Increase your kids' time with other kids.

For the first several years of school, we homeschooled our twin boys, but we also made sure to put them in gymnastics and jujitsu, where they were able to tumble around on slightly dirty floors or mats surrounded by other children. We also went out of our way to ensure they frequently visited the gym's childcare facilities; participated in basketball, tennis, and soccer; went to music camps and ski school; and engaged in a variety of other extracurricular activities—all of which exposed our young children to other kids' sniffles, skin, and sweat.

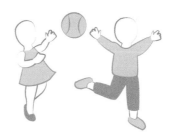

7. Eat a variety of cultured foods.

For years I have told my wife that she needs to write a cookbook called *Dirty Kitchen*, alluding to the amount of lactofermentation and bacterial cultures she uses during food prep (good idea, eh?). I love this title because it refers to the wide variety of bacteria in foods such as natto, kimchi, kefir, pickles, yogurts, sauerkraut, rakfisk, poi, kombucha, and even chocolate. Earlier in this chapter, I explained the importance of fermentation for the immune system, and there's no reason that children shouldn't be exposed to these same foods early in life. Remember that variety is important, and simply feeding your child the same probiotic pill day after day is probably not going to be adequate stimulus for their immune system.

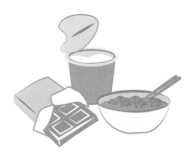

8. Encourage your kids to play outside.

I wish this tip could go without saying, but the sad truth is that a great percentage of children spend more time indoors on Wii, PlayStation, and Xbox than they do outdoors getting dirty. On any nice afternoon, we kick our kids out into the backyard to explore, and since they were tiny toddlers, they've always returned with dirt under their fingernails (or possibly animal dung), mud around their noses and mouths, and weeds and wild grasses lodged in their clothes. These

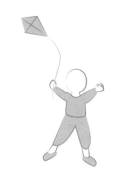

are all immune system boosters that far outweigh the inconvenience of having to wash dirty children. Of course, our kids have learned first-hand the ravages of itchy poison ivy, the sharp stings of a hornet nest, and the pain of road rash from tricycle tricks and bike crashes, but the pros outweigh the cons, and it's okay to take pride in a dirty, cut-up kid sitting down to dinner at the dining room table.

9. Don't make your kids bathe or shower every day.

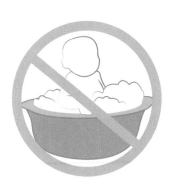

In our post-Victorian, cleanliness-obsessed culture, it can be tempting to give our children a daily warm bath, followed of course by a perfect hairdo and a color-coordinated outfit from the Gap. But sometimes it's okay to let the dirt ferment on your child. On many a summer day, our boys go two or three days getting dirty and playing outside without a bar of soap in sight—and while they get a bit stinky and stained, this is a fabulous stimulus for their immune system. Let those soil-based organisms thrive on your child's skin! If "no soap showers" are just not your thing, then you may be interested in AOBiome, a biotech start-up that has created a spray that contains billions of cultivated bacteria commonly found in dirt and untreated water—so now you can basically pay for an expensive skin cosmetic to get the same thing you would get from rolling around in your lawn.

10. Don't do excessive loads of laundry.

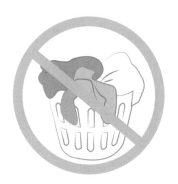

Germs, dirt, and bacteria thrive on clothing. Prior to reading the other parts of this chapter, you might have been tempted to take this as a sign to do a daily load of laundry. While you shouldn't necessarily send your child to sports, school, or social events smelling or looking like a pigpen, it's okay to give clothes a few good wears before laundering—in the same way that you don't need to be constantly boiling bottles and pacifiers. Most of the time, it's okay for kids to smell just a little bit like ... kids.

While this list of ways to get you or your kids dirty is by no means comprehensive, hopefully it gets your wheels turning about exposing your children to (gasp!) pathogenic organisms—including bacteria, worms, parasites, germs, fungus, viruses, and even other sick kids and dirty animals. This may be one of the best favors you can do for your family, and if you have kids, you will probably be giving them an advantage later in life, especially compared to children who grew up in a bubble. Your own immune system will benefit quite a bit too—and you'll have one less reason to be grossed out when your little one sneezes in your face, coughs at the table, or tracks a trail of dirt into the house!

THE POWER OF THE MIND

So far this chapter has focused on the body—all the ways that you can boost your physiological immune system. But the mind plays a powerful role in physical well-being, too.

There are over 150,000 different proteins that make up your body. The shape of each protein can change as a result of electromagnetic fields, and when it changes shape from one configuration to another, the protein molecule moves, as do all the other protein molecules surrounding it, which cooperate in functional assemblies called pathways. Respiratory pathways, digestive pathways, and muscle contraction pathways are all examples of assemblies of proteins whose coordinated movements produce specific biological functions.

Studies have shown that this change in the shape of proteins can change the expression of genes. Electromagnetic fields are generated by thoughts and emotions, and since proteins are altered by electromagnetic fields, this means that genes can be turned on and off by those same fields. That's right: you can control gene activity by focusing on your beliefs.

Beliefs, true or false, positive or negative, creative or destructive, influence the very cells of your body. This means that DNA does not control your biology by itself, and that information can be transmitted throughout your body, to other people's bodies, and even to your descendants in ways other than through the base sequence of DNA. It means that that harnessing the power of your mind can be just as effective or even more effective than pharmaceuticals, supplements, and biohacks, and that your perception of your environment significantly affects your health.

So is it true that a sunny outlook means fewer colds and less heart disease, that hope can somehow protect against hypertension, diabetes, and respiratory tract infections, and that happier people live longer? It turns out that the biology of emotion—and what it may teach us about helping people to live longer—has been studied at prestigious institutions such as Harvard. Laura Kubzansky of the Harvard School of Public Health is at the forefront of such research. In a 2007 study that followed more than six thousand men and women aged twenty-five to seventy-four for twenty years, she found that emotional vitality—a sense of enthusiasm, hopefulness, engagement in life, and ability to face life's stresses with emotional balance—significantly reduces the risk of coronary heart disease, even when accounting for healthy behaviors such as not smoking and regular exercise.

A Story of Emotions and Cancer

I first realized the power of emotions and stress to affect disease when I traveled to Israel for a tour of the country's collection of health spas, fitness centers, healing retreats, and wellness facilities. In northern Galilee, I visited the home of a former professional basketball player, Doron Sheffer.

Doron had been an amazing athlete. He was an achiever. A hard-charger. As a guard for the dominant college basketball team at the University of Connecticut, he averaged five assists and thirteen points per game, hit 40 percent of his three-point attempts, and led the team to a brilliant 89-13 record. He then became the first Israeli ever drafted by the NBA in 1996, but he instead signed a lucrative contract with an Israeli professional basketball team, which he then led to four consecutive national championships.

But then Doron got testicular cancer. When I sat down with him in his backyard garden looking over the beautiful hills of Amirim, eating a meal of organic figs, goji berries, and sweet local almonds, he described how the tremendous pressure, pent-up emotions, and stress in the life of a hard-charging professional athlete eventually built up inside him and culminated in disease.

As a matter of fact, scientists at Yale University have discovered that the conditions for developing cancer can be significantly affected by your emotional environment, including everyday work and family stress. In this case, Western medicine is catching up to the traditional Chinese medical view of cancer, which has long held that emotions are a major contributing factor. For example, researcher Sun Binyan wrote in his book *Cancer Treatment and Prevention*, "According to our understanding of the tumor patient, most have suppression of the emotions. They tend to hold in their anger. Although some patients have good results after treatment, emotional stimulation may cause them to decline again and then the previous treatment would have been in vain. Some people have a severe phobia about cancer. Before they know the real disease, they have a lot of suspicion. Once they know they have the cancer, their whole spirit breaks down. This kind of spiritual state is very bad for the treatment." And in the book *Prevention and Treatment of Carcinoma in Traditional Chinese Medicine*, author and researcher Jia Kun gives ten recommendations for cancer prevention. In addition to having a good environment and personal hygiene, getting proper amounts of physical activity and rest, having good eating habits, and avoiding smoking, he states that "emotional changes, such as worry, fear, hesitation, anger, irritation, and nervousness, should be prevented. Mental exhaustion is harmful and life should be enriched with entertainment."

Western research supports the idea that depression can impair immune system function, which can contribute to the development of cancer, since the immune system normally attacks and destroys cancerous cells. For example, it has been shown that tumor-relevant lymphocyte subpopulations, also known as natural killer cells (NK cells), which can attack cancer cells, have receptors for various neuropeptide proteins, including those released during stress. This means that NK cell activity can be influenced by emotions. The level of NK cell activity has been shown in research to be a good predictor of breast cancer outcome, and a loss of NK activity in cancer patients has been shown to be correlated with an increase in the patient's stress levels, lack of social support, and fatigue or depression.

Another recent report analyzed the findings of close to a hundred studies that demonstrate how the sympathetic nervous system (SNS), the fight-or-flight portion of the nervous system, can encourage cancer metastasis. During acute stress, the SNS is activated, but soon as the stressful event has passed, the body returns to homeostasis within about an hour. But under chronic stress, the SNS is turned on virtually all the time, and in this chronically stressed state, adrenaline and noradrenaline can alter genetic expression. This genetic alteration can lead to a number of pro-cancer processes, including activation of inflammatory responses, inhibition of immune responses and programmed cancer cell death, reduction in the cytotoxic function of NK cells, inhibition of DNA repair, stimulation of cancer cell angiogenesis, and activation of epithelial-mesenchymal transition, which is one of the ways new cancer stem cells are created.

One researcher, Dr. Harold Burr, measured the energy fields of mice and noted which mice later developed cancer. After taking more than ten thousand measurements, he found that the electromagnetic signature of cancer appeared in the mouse's energy field before there was any detectable cellular malignancy! Burr also looked at a group of healthy women who did not have a diagnosis of uterine cancer. The women who had an electromagnetic signature for uterine cancer—even though they were apparently healthy—went on to develop cancer later. Cancer was showing up in the field of energy before it showed up in the physical cells.

Burr's body of work demonstrates the wisdom of an ancient saying in traditional Chinese medicine: *The mind controls the qi, and the blood follows the qi.* The ancient sages were referring to life energy, and by "blood" they meant the body. Energy influences matter! Perhaps this is why research has shown tumors shrinking to less than half their original size within just a few hours of an emotional therapy session that elicited positive emotions, why studies have shown the DNA in lab-grown cancer cells to disintegrate when positive emotions were directed toward those cells by Chinese traditional medical practitioners, and why practicing mindfulness meditation for just three months has been shown to have an antiaging effect on telomeres.

Now here's the deal: I'm a hard-charging guy focused on personal and professional excellence in everything I do. But I truly believe that unless you are able to relax, breathe, de-stress, and simply stop and smell the roses, you're going to eventually develops a chronic-stress-related disease that forces your fast-forward life into slow motion. So you have to put on the brakes on before your body does, perhaps with the flu, perhaps with back pain, or perhaps with cancer. Make sense?

This is exactly what Doron figured out, and his new aura of peace and calm spoke strongly to me. He defied conventional medicine and naturally healed his body of cancer, and his approach to life is now refreshing, relaxed, and incredibly peaceful. When I visited Doron at his home and private health resort in the mountains of northern Israel, I was surrounded by a laid-back community of aromatherapists and massage therapists that featured herb gardens, spas, a health food shop, an organic olive oil shop, art galleries, restaurants, and wellness bed-and-breakfasts. These mountains were where Doron slipped away from chronic stress, reinvigorated his body, and underwent his own spiritual cleanse to win his battle against testicular cancer.

Holistic Healing Strategies

The ultimate question is this: How can you slow down before your body forces you to slow down? How can you stop the constant barrage of emails, text messages, and phone calls, the stress of overexercising, eating to train and training to eat, going to bed late, 24-7 self-quantified biohacking, trying to have everything, getting up early, and still somehow managing to squeeze in some semblance of quality in your friend and family relationships?

Now that you understand how your thoughts, stressors, emotions, and beliefs affect your biology, it's time to identify the techniques and tools that can help you to use your body as your own pharmacy and heal yourself from the inside out.

QIGONG

Literally translated as "life energy cultivation," qigong is a system of coordinated body postures and movements, breathing, and meditation used in traditional Chinese culture to promote health and spirituality. According to Taoist, Buddhist, and Confucian philosophy, qigong allows access to higher realms of awareness and awakens your true nature. Qigong typically coordinates slow, flowing movements with deep, rhythmic breathing and a calm, meditative state of mind. My favorite qigong master is Robert Peng, who is quite good at distilling this ancient Chinese practice so that even my eight-year-old twin boys were able to learn qigong along with me over the course of an eight-week program.

ACUPUNCTURE

While many folks think acupuncture is something you seek out when you have tendinitis, knee pain, or some other musculoskeletal injury, it is actually effective not only for treating pain but also for increasing the amount of qi—life force energy—flowing through specific meridians in the body. The spiritual elements of acupuncture that often conflict with Western beliefs and modern medicine have been abandoned by many acupuncture therapists in favor of simply tapping needles into acupuncture points. But in traditional Chinese medicine, illness and imbalanced emotions are perceived as a disharmony or imbalance in qi, and acupuncture therapy is designed around the pattern of disharmony.

My own acupuncturist in Spokane, Washington, works out of the office of a physical therapist in a modern medical clinic but still practices traditional acupuncture and examines things like the color and shape of my tongue, the strength of my pulse, the quality of my breathing, the sound of the voice, and (sorry, dude) even the smell of my breath. So you don't have to hop on a plane to Hong Kong to get acupuncture done right, even if you are seeking it out—as I am—for emotional balance and to achieve a higher level of consciousness, rather than to simply fix an injury (though it works for that too).

Some studies suggest that acupuncture causes a series of events within the central nervous system that results in the release of adenosine, and that this may deactivate the fight-or-flight sympathetic nervous system. This may make acupuncture a way to use neurochemicals to cause an electromagnetic change in your body.

ELECTRIC ACUPUNCTURE

An NES scanner is a frequency-based device that can be used to identify specific aches, pains, health disorders, and emotions—you can think of it as an electrical form of acupuncture. When I first began to use an NES scanner, I placed my right hand on a computer mouse–shaped object that mapped my body's energy field. I then plugged the scanner into my computer. Once the scan was completed, in a few seconds, the software returned a graphical representation of any distortions in the body's information, as well as recommendations for therapy to stimulate the body's healing response and correct the noted distortions.

The skin indicates what's going on underneath it and has a magnetic quality, so wherever there is a blockage in energy flow or some other problem, the skin in that area becomes more magnetic or sticky, which the scanner detects. You then stimulate that area a handheld biofeedback device called the miHealth, which comes with the NES scanner. As you treat the area, the body's magnetic quality begins to change as it heals, and the scanner detects that change.

Here's another way of looking at this: Cells have an electrical potential. Sick, tired, and malfunctioning cells have a low electrical potential, and this is what surfaces as magnetic or sticky quality on the skin. By putting energy back into the problem area, this system can apparently raise the electrical potential of those cells, restoring them over time to their normal, optimal functioning. This also stimulates the nervous system, sending a signal to the brain to direct resources to that part of the body as part of the natural healing response.

While this may seem like a modern bastardization of traditional acupuncture, I consider it to be one of the more potent biohacks I own for identifying issues with my vibrational frequency and electromagnetic field and then fixing those issues with a targeted medical device.

TAPPING (EFT)

Tapping, also known as emotional freedom technique or EFT, is also somewhat similar to acupuncture. Acupuncture heals by stimulating the body's meridians and energy flow, but surprisingly, you can also stimulate these meridian points by tapping on them with your fingertips—no needles or trip to the acupuncturist required. Tapping has been shown to provide relief from chronic pain, emotional problems, disorders, addictions, phobias, posttraumatic stress disorder, and chronic diseases. For example, research done at Harvard Medical School during the last decade found that the brain's stress and fear responses, which are controlled by an almond-shaped part of your brain called the amygdala, can be downregulated by stimulating the meridian points.

Although these studies focused on acupuncture and used needles, follow-up double-blind research revealed that stimulating the points through pressure, as in tapping, gives rise to a similar response. Other studies have shown tapping to reduce cortisol by up to 50 percent!

Here's how tapping works: First, identify a problem on which you want to focus. It can be general anxiety, or it can be a specific situation or issue that causes you to feel anxious. Then compose a setup statement acknowledging the problem you want to deal with, such as "I feel very anxious right now." You then follow this statement with an affirmation of deeply and completely accepting yourself. For example:

- "Even though I feel this anxiety, I deeply and completely accept myself."
- "Even though I'm anxious about my interview, I deeply and completely accept myself."
- "Even though I'm feeling this anxiety about this relationship, I deeply and completely accept myself."
- "Even though I'm having trouble sleeping, I deeply and completely accept myself."

Then you begin tapping five to seven times in each of these locations, in order: on the outer edge of the hand, the eyebrows, the side of the eyes, under the eyes, under the nose, under the chin, under the collarbone, under the arm, and on top of the head. You then finish with a deep breath to clear the emotional dirt away.

If you include EFT, acupuncture, and other energy healing methods, there are over one thousand studies showing that energy healing is effective for an astounding number of health conditions. (You can find a list of these studies on the National Institute for Integrative Healthcare website, niih.org.)

MINDFULNESS MEDITATION

If I offered you a pill that could increase your levels of stem cells, lengthen your telomeres, dissolve beta-amyloid plaques in your brain, improve your memory and attention, boost serotonin, repair DNA, regulate inflammation, increase the strength of the immune system, repair skin, bone, cartilage, and muscle cells, increase growth hormone levels, and enhance the neural connections in your brain, would you would take it? Fact is, such a priceless pill is free and backed by research. It's called mindfulness meditation.

From holotropic breathwork to transcendental meditation to two-hour-long chanting sessions, I've toyed around with just about every form of meditation that exists (save for the notorious ten-day silent meditation retreat known as Vipassana, which is on the bucket list), and I can tell you without a doubt that mindfulness meditation couldn't be simpler: you take a seat in a comfortable place, pay attention to your breath, and when your attention wanders, you return it to your breath. Heck, even my boys—who are currently ten years old—perform a style of this meditation for fifteen to twenty minutes one to two times per week. Most often, they do it outdoors in a traditional Native American–style sit spot, during which they mindfully observe with their eyes, ears, nose, and mouth the world around them, or inside our sauna, during which they focus their attention on a candle or an hourglass, both of which are fantastic tools to keep the mind from excessively wandering during meditation. The steps for mindfulness meditation are simple:

1. Take a seat on the floor, the ground, a chair, a meditation cushion, a park bench, or anything else on which you can sit comfortably for five to forty-five minutes.

2. Straighten your upper body so that your head and shoulders comfortably rest on top of your vertebrae.

3. Let your hands drop onto the tops of your legs and lightly rest on your thighs.

4. Drop your chin a little and let your gaze fall gently downward. It helps to gently rest the tongue against the roof of the mouth. Your eyes can be open or closed.

5. If possible, breathe through your nose. Bring your attention to your breath and feel your breath (some say to follow your breath) as it goes in and out.

6. Most likely, your attention will leave your breath and wander. Don't worry. There's no need to try hard to stop this from happening. When you notice your mind wandering, don't judge yourself or think you're failing. Instead, just gently return your attention to the breath.

7. Before making any physical adjustments, such scratching an itch, pause for just a moment. Then, with intention, shift at a moment you choose. This creates space between what you experience and what you choose to do.

8. When you're ready, gently lift your gaze (if your eyes are closed, you can now open them). Take a relaxed, focused moment and notice any sounds in the environment, how your body feels, any thoughts and emotions you have. After you've paused, simply move on and continue with your day.

That's it. It's that easy. One final note: I've found that the box breathing described in chapter 3 (four-count in, four-count hold, four-count out, four-count hold) is incredibly effective during this style of meditation. Two other very impressive forms of guided mindfulness meditation that I have found to be highly beneficial are Dawson Church's EcoMeditation (available for free online) and Emily Fletcher's Ziva Technique.

VISUALIZATION

In the book *Getting Well Again: A Step-by-Step Self-Help Guide to Overcoming Cancer for Patients and Their Families*, radiation oncologist Dr. O. Carl Simonton and his wife Stephanie Matthews-Simonton, a trained psychologist, document how people can influence the disease process of cancer through healing their emotions. They provide example after example of how visualization prolongs life and improves quality of life in cancer patients, and in some cases aids in healing cancer altogether. Research backs this up: a host of studies connect visualization (often referred to as guided imagery) with improved mood and quality of life in cancer patients. But visualization doesn't just work for chronic diseases. It can also serve as a quick way to transform yourself out of stress and to a higher level of energy vibration, which is literally the frequency at which cells oscillate within the human body.

Visualization involves creating a detailed mental image of an attractive or peaceful environment and is often paired with physical relaxation techniques such as progressive muscle relaxation, which involves tightening then relaxing every muscle in your body, one by one. When visualization is paired with physical relaxation techniques like this, the aim is to associate the sensations of relaxation with the peaceful visual image so that future practice sessions with visualization will quickly bring back the physical sensations of relaxation. My collegiate tennis coach often used this strategy with us young, nervous players: as we lay on the floor of the tennis court, we would progressively relax our bodies while visualizing fluid serves and flawless ground strokes. Later, during match play, we could achieve the same level of relaxation without stopping to lie down on the court and do the actual physical relaxation technique (which could possibly have annoyed our opponents, I would imagine).

Of course, the beauty of visualization is that it and requires nothing more than your imagination and concentration. Here's a simple step-by-step guide:

1. Find a quiet and calm space and make yourself comfortable.

2. Take a few slow and deep breaths to center and calm yourself.

3. Close your eyes.

4. Imagine yourself in a beautiful place where everything is as you would ideally like it, such as a beach, a mountaintop, a peaceful meadow, or a forest.

5. Imagine yourself becoming calm and relaxed—smiling and feeling full of joy.

6. Focus on the sensory details of your scene to make it more vivid. For example, if you imagine the beach, spend time imagining the warmth of the sun on your skin, the smell of the ocean, seaweed, and salt spray, and the sound of the waves, wind, and seagulls.

7. Remain within your scene for five to ten minutes as you become more and more relaxed.

8. While relaxed, tell yourself that you can return to this place whenever you want or need to relax.

9. Then open your eyes and rejoin the real world.

You can find guided visualization audios for absolutely free on iTunes or YouTube (I often convert YouTube videos to audio using free online converters). One of my favorites is Yoga Nidra, which not only walks you through guided imagery in a relaxing setting but can also bring you through an entire sleep cycle without you actually falling asleep!

YOGA

Since it was first developed by ancient sages in India, yoga has been accepted as an integral practice for restoring and elevating the energetic frequency of the body. The formal system of yoga teaches that all matter in the cosmos is vibrant with life. Because of this, if your intention is to send out as much positive energy as possible, one good place to start is by moving your body in a way that generates the type of energy you want to be sending. It turns out that research backs this up: when mindful, proper yoga is performed with focused breathwork in a formal meditative setting (in other words, not with goats and babies and not drenched with sweat while your heart rate screams through the roof from a hot yoga practice), there can be a significant shift into relaxed oscillating brain wave patterns and a downregulation of the sympathetic nervous system.

I spend several minutes each day, usually during my morning stretch routine or while in the sauna, going through a few easy yoga flows borrowed from hatha yoga (one of the better forms of yoga for dropping into a meditative state). I visit a yoga class or follow along with a yoga DVD a few times a month, and once or twice a year, I attend more intensive yoga retreats for a deeper dive into this potent energy healing tool.

Finally, for a more intense form of yoga that incorporates movement, dynamic breathing techniques, meditation, and chanting, give Kundalini yoga a try. It is one of the more difficult but more energy-vibrating forms of yoga I've learned!

Spirituality and Healing

In his book *Unfinished: Believing Is Only the Beginning,* Rich Stearns presents the concept that there are three choices you can make about the story of your life.

The first choice is to believe that there is no story—that "everything we see and experience is totally random and without meaning. There is no truth. We are just a meaningless species on a meaningless planet in a meaningless universe. There is, therefore, no God and no real defining purpose to our lives." This idea prompts us to "pursue happiness instead. Find peace in your insignificance, and just let your anxiety go. Learn to savor the likely truth that the sum total of human achievement won't even register in the grand scheme, so you might as well just enjoy whatever talents you have. Use them to make yourself and others happy, and set aside any desire to be great or outstanding."

But, Rich points out, this has consequences for how we perceive right and wrong and how we treat each other: "What happens when your actions and decisions come into conflict with mine? Since we are both just 'tiny flecks of talking meat' spinning in the 'same hodgepodge of primordial goo,' there is really no such thing as right or wrong, so the only mechanism to resolve our disputes is force or power; survival of the fittest. If you really believe that human beings are no more than flecks of meat, then taking a human life has no more significance than picking a mushroom or squashing an ant."

I don't know about you, but choice #1 seems pretty depressing to me, and it's not what I want to teach my kids or the story by which I live my own life.

The second choice is to make up your own story and develop your own set of beliefs and values, without expecting others to abide by them. People who make this choice, Rich says, don't believe in absolute truth. And they can be "both monsters and saints. They could be drug dealers or human traffickers as easily as they could be homemakers or schoolteachers. ... Usually they share the fairly universal human goal—happiness. It's just that some pursue it through violence and crime and others through hard work and education. Some even find it in helping their fellow man and being generous."

But in the end, Rich says, these people are simply marking time: "For seventy or eighty years they move from one event to the next, like balls in a pinball machine, bouncing off bumpers with lights flashing and bells ringing all the way. They are busy racking up points and bonuses until the ball finally goes down the drain, the noises stop, and the lights go out. Game Over!"

Because a world of everyone making up their own story creates great potential for chaos and entropy, I'm not a fan of choice #2 either.

And then there's the third option: to become part of a greater story. When you are part of a greater story, you have a purpose, a role to play—without you, the story would not be the same. Rich writes, "Doesn't it make sense that our story has an author ... ? Doesn't it also follow that this same Author/Creator gave life to each and every character in his story—to you and to me— and that he created each one of us with unique gifts, talents, and personalities; and that he placed us within his story in both space and time?" Yes, Rich acknowledges, choosing to believe that you're part of a larger story and were created by its author requires a leap of faith. But he also says it's just common sense. "Doesn't it make more sense to believe that our story has an Author than to believe that everything we see and experience is meaningless and without purpose?"

And that third option, the choice to believe that we are living out an amazing, exciting, enchanting adventure and a magical story written for our lives—to me, that's a pretty dang good way to vibrate at a higher energy level.

So what does all this have to do with creating an unstoppable immune system? I like to think about this in the same way that the excellent book *The Healing Code* explains in great detail: Each of our sicknesses and diseases ultimately arise from stress. To control stress, you must steer your overall energy towards a state of positivity and hope, and to do this, you must engage in the crucial spiritual disciplines that maintain your focus on caring for the most important element of your being, the element that can repair your body from the inside out: your soul.

These spiritual disciplines are intimately linked to a belief in a higher power and include fasting, meditation (including periods of silence and solitude), prayer, worship (including being with others, singing, and having positive relationships), expressing gratitude, and finding purpose in life.

PRAYER

There's a reason that prayer and meditation go hand in hand with a belief in a higher power: they're often used to connect and communicate with that higher power. Along with morning spiritual reading, deep breathing, and gratitude journaling, I always start my day with the following prayer:

> *Father in heaven,*
> *I surrender all to You.*
> *Please turn me into the father and husband You would have me be,*
> *Into a man who will fulfill Your great commission,*
> *And remove from me all judgments of others.*
> *Grant me Your heavenly wisdom,*
> *Remove from me my worldly temptations,*
> *Teach me how to listen to Your still, small voice in the silence,*
> *And fill me with Your peace, love, and joy.*
> *In the name of Jesus,*
> *Amen.*

My family and I also pray with gratefulness over our meals, pray each day for each other and for those whom God has placed on our hearts, and finish each day with prayer for a restful night's sleep. This means that we live the entire day while conversing with a higher power. It's a settling and peaceful way to live your life, knowing that—pardon the slight cheesiness of this statement—the Big Guy is on your side.

GRATITUDE JOURNALING

When you introduce conscious, mindful gratitude into your day, positivity will begin to pour into your life—along with all the other scientifically proven physical, mental, and spiritual benefits of gratitude, as well as a greater amount of empathy and charity, two personal attributes that allow you to achieve a higher state of consciousness.

Daily gratitude has been proven by science to make you healthier and happier. Grateful people experience fewer aches and pains and report feeling healthier than other people. Grateful people are more likely to take care of their health. They exercise more often and are more likely to live longer. Gratitude reduces a multitude of toxic emotions, ranging from envy and resentment to frustration and regret. Research confirms that gratitude increases happiness and reduces depression, and writing in a gratitude journal has been shown to both strengthen the immune system and help you sleep better and longer.

So I start off each day by opening my gratitude journal and answering three questions (although there's nothing wrong with simply thinking of something you're thankful for instead). These questions are designed to enhance my spiritual life, relationships, physical health, and mind.

1. What am I grateful for today?

It's quite simple, really. Wake up, take a deep breath, close your eyes, and dwell on positive experiences from the past twenty-four hours, and then ask yourself, "What am I grateful for?" You'll often find it is the simplest of things: the birds you hear outside, the sunlight streaming through the window, the pitter-patter of a child's feet going up or down stairs, the soft skin of your lover in bed next to you, or simply the refreshed feeling of having experienced a solid night's rest. Then simply write down what first comes to your mind.

Sometimes this can be a bit difficult: you don't have a great night of sleep, you wake up with the sniffles, your phone is blowing up with texts, or it's a dark, stormy day outside. This is when the magic of gratefulness takes over: as you consider what you're grateful for, you're suddenly able to find the silver lining in any situation, like how wonderful your toes feel when you wiggle them! For example, two nights ago, I woke up groggy, having gotten just four hours of sleep. The day was cloudy, my wife was out of town with the kids, and I felt less than stellar. But as I took a deep breath and closed my eyes, I felt a surge of gratitude for the simple ability to take in air through my nose and my mouth. And what did I write down? "I am grateful for the wonderful complexity of my lungs and how efficiently they delivered oxygen to my body with that single breath." It's that easy!

2. What truth did I discover in today's reading?

This question assumes that you read the Bible or another spiritual text every morning before your gratitude journaling. By writing down the answer, you will often discover important truths that you might otherwise have missed. In addition, when you read with the intent to find truth, meaning, or inspiration, you discover far more and pay much closer attention to what you're reading.

Here's an example: Recently, I felt frustrated that I did not have enough time to work on my novel. My reading for the day was Psalm 25, which states in verse 3, "Let no one who waits on you be ashamed." After reading that, I realized that sometimes waiting is a good thing. Sometimes we have no choice about the things we must wait for, but we certainly do have a choice about how we wait. I realized that rather than waiting in fear, apathy, or shame, we can wait in patience and gratitude while seeking God's wisdom, strength, and direction. So I wrote in my journal, "Sometimes waiting is a good thing." That's it. Short and sweet.

If I hadn't been seeking some kind of truth while reading, I would have been far more likely to read quickly through that section without realizing the truth I discovered.

A few other quick tips for this second question:

- Don't pursue too many truths. Homing in on a single truth that speaks to you makes it far more likely that you'll dwell on that one truth the rest of the day.

- Make the truth succinct. Resist the urge to write an entire essay and stick to a single, simple sentence.

- Don't bite off more than you can chew. I read a few verses of the Bible, a single passage of the tiny devotional *Our Daily Bread*, or a few pages of an inspirational book. If I tried to read more, I simply wouldn't have the time for a morning reading habit. And if you read for too long, you won't have much time left over for journaling, identifying someone you can help or serve, or narrowing down your truth for the day.

3. Who can I pray for, help, or serve today?

Instead of focusing on myself—asking "What can I achieve?" or affirming, as Stuart Smalley famously quipped on *Saturday Night Live,* "I'm good enough, I'm smart enough, and doggone it, people like me"—this question is entirely focused on others.

I find that thinking of others is one of the most valuable, meaningful, and rewarding ways to start my day. When you begin this practice, you will find yourself meeting more neighbors, inviting friends over for dinner, volunteering in your local community, engaging in deeper relationships with your loved ones, and approaching your entire day with a refreshing, unselfish attitude.

And this too can be simple. Yesterday, I rolled over and looked at my wife, Jessa, lying there next to me. I was overwhelmed with a feeling of gratitude about how much she does for me, our household, and our family, and I was overcome with the desire to really be there for her that day. So I jotted down her name in my journal, and for the rest of the day I went out of my way to pray for and serve her—in this case, by recruiting the boys to help me make her dinner so that she could relax. Another time, when I realized that our annual church program to feed children at a local poverty-stricken elementary school was kicking off, I wrote down the name of the school principal and said a prayer for him. Later that day I called him to see if there was anything I could help with to get the program moving along—all steps I probably would have neglected to take if I had not started my day with a spirit of service!

That's it: simply write down one thing you are grateful for, do your day's reading, jot a note about the truth that you've discovered, and think of one person you can pray for, help, or serve that day. (In full disclosure, I have created a Christian Gratitude Journal that walks you through this entire process with zero guesswork, in a beautiful little hardcover journal that I have to admit I'm pretty dang proud of. Check it out at christiangratitude.com.)

PURPOSE

I'm going to end this chapter with my final, most potent tip for increasing your energy vibration and the vibrations of all people around you, and it is this: identify your purpose in life and enable yourself to achieve that unique purpose the very best of your abilities. Allow me to share with you my purpose in life, which I've memorized and clearly defined: *To empower people to live an adventurous, joyful, and fulfilling life.*

See, when it comes to being happy and living a long time, what matters is not your forty-eighth ayahuasca trip, six-pack abs, a better WOD time, the perfect diet, or any other recent infatuation of the health, wellness, and longevity movement. All flesh and blood eventually dies. The fastest track athlete will eventually be defeated by muscle loss, neural degradation, and arthritis. The most beautiful supermodel in the world will not be on the cover of the *Sports Illustrated* swimsuit issue when she's ninety-seven years old. Even wealthy, powerful CEOs will eventually be betrayed by their bodies and die.

What is actually contributing most to your energy vibrations at any given moment isn't your beauty or your fitness or your accomplishments—it's your soul. Your spirit. Your ability to be truly boundless. I even have a tattoo on my shoulder, emblazoned onto my skin when I was just twenty years old, expressing this: it's the Japanese symbol for ki, also known as chi, soul, spirit, chakra, prana, and the invisible, boundless life force that flows through all of us. Caring for this all-encompassing energy of my body is how I live my life.

True and lasting happiness is not achieved by external circumstances, your thoughts, your intentions, not even your feelings, but by your inner soul. In his book *Soul Keeping*, John Ortberg defines the soul as the aspect of your whole being that coordinates, integrates, and enlivens everything else. He writes that we all have two worlds: an outer world, which is visible and public and obvious, and an inner world that may be chaotic and dark or gloriously beautiful. In the end, the outer world fades, and all you are left with is your inner world.

Ironically, the more obsessed we are with ourselves, our fitness, our cognitive performance, our finances, and our food, the more we tend to neglect our souls. When your soul is not centered and right, you tend to define yourself by your accomplishments, your physical appearance, your title, or your social circles and friends. But then, when you lose these, you tend to lose your identity. I've experienced this myself when I've gotten injured or sick or had a poor race, and subsequently I felt like I was losing my happiness and transitioning to a lower level of energy vibration because I was losing my identity as an athlete. Perhaps this is why one of my favorite Bible verses says, "What does it profit a man to gain the whole world and forfeit his soul?"

So how do you connect with and care for your soul? Start by asking yourself: What is the core part of you that you want folks to talk about at your funeral? In other words, what is your purpose? If you're not clear on this, ask some people who know you well to describe why they think God put you on earth and what skills and talents seem to flow naturally from you. Ask them what should be written on your gravestone. Ask them what they think your purpose is. I'll hazard a guess that it's not that you were the best exerciser, or that you followed an amazing, flawless diet, or that you had gorgeous skin or made oodles of money.

But it's not enough to simply identify your purpose. To truly connect with and care for your soul, you must then connect with your inner self. Ask yourself this one question: "What aspect of my life can I change today that will allow me to care for my soul so that I can achieve that purpose?"

Maybe it's starting a meditation practice. Maybe it's stepping into a church. Maybe it's mending a torn relationship. Maybe it's stopping to breathe. Maybe it's dropping a relentless pursuit of a better body and brain and realizing that to truly achieve deep, meaningful satisfaction in life, you must care for the most important part of you, the part that will exist for eternity, and live your life based on your core purpose. No matter what it is that must change, you'll find that you must often change your environment and your habits. This might mean staying in bed an extra ten minutes to write in a gratitude journal, ditching Netflix to hang out with your family, or spending a Saturday volunteering at the homeless shelter rather than going on a two-hour bike ride or doing back-to-back workouts.

So let me ask you this: What is your purpose? And how alive is your soul so that you can fuel that purpose? Now, take a deep breath in through your nose and out through your mouth. Feel your spirit. Feel your soul. Feel it? It's there—it may be shriveled up and dry and neglected, but it's there, ready for you to grow and nurture it. Take one more deep breath in through your nose, then smile and breathe out. You are an amazing soul. You are here for a purpose. If you still need help identifying or developing your purpose and your personal why, I recommend you read the books *Discover Your True North* by Bill George and *Claim Your Power* by Mastin Kipp, as well as visit TheWhyStack.com, StartWithWhy.com, and WhyInstitute.com. You can also look into a Strengths Finder or DISC Assessment test (visit BoundlessBook.com/15 for links). Finally, though it may seem like a depressing exercise, writing your own obituary in a few paragraphs can help you identify how you want to be remembered and what your core purpose is.

THE LAST WORD

The fact is, the modern-day immunity marketplace is flooded with supplements and herbal formulas claiming to cure the common cold or to make the human body heavily guarded against illness, but it can be difficult to sift through the bold marketing and fake supplements to find what's truly useful. But you're now equipped with everything you need to know to defy the odds of getting sick and create an unstoppable immune system via research-proven but little-known supplement, food, and lifestyle strategies, along with the spiritual disciplines that can make your immune system stronger and more robust.

Should your head be spinning with the wide variety of ways you can support your immune system, here's a simple example of how to weave many of the strategies in this chapter into a cold and flu season protocol:

- Eat a wide variety of fermented foods. (I particularly recommend making the wonderful yogurt from Dr. William Davis on page 364.)

- Place several drops of thieves oil in an essential oil diffuser in your office, home, or bedroom and run the diffuser all day long.

- Each morning, take a handful of colostrum capsules, a teaspoon of mushrooms, a dropperful of oregano oil in a glass of water, or all three. Take a shot of RESTORE prior to each meal.

- Have a piping-hot cup of organic bone broth with lunch or dinner. Add even more immune support by stirring in a teaspoon of medicinal mushrooms.

- If you're exposed to sickness, continue using the strategies above, but also sip on elderberry juice or use elderberry tincture three times a day and take zinc lozenges, vitamin C, and echinacea.

- Whether you're sick or not, don't stop moving. Try to engage in low-level physical activity, even if it's just an easy walk in the sunshine or a bit of bouncing up and down on a trampoline. If you're too sick to move, consider resting with infrared blankets, an infrared sauna, or a Biomat to keep lymph fluid circulating.

- Consider a quarterly IV infusion of high-dose vitamin C from a local functional medicine practitioner.

- Regularly practice the spiritual disciplines, including meditation, silence, solitude, study, prayer, worship, and belief in a higher power. Don't underestimate the power of the mind and belief patterns to heal the body.

Finally, no discussion of the immune system would be complete without addressing a question I'm asked nearly every day: What would I do if I found that I had cancer? While I am not a physician and this should not be taken as medical advice, I can tell you that without a doubt that if I were diagnosed with cancer, I would incorporate recommendations that I have learned from Dr. Thomas Cowan, along with Dr. Thomas Seyfried, Dr. Nasha Winters, and many others—most notably these:

- Follow a ketogenic diet that is low in protein and rich in organic plant foods (primarily juiced using a Norwalk juicer), with a limited amount of carbohydrates (20 to 30 g per day) and sixteen to eighteen hours of fasting per twenty-four-hour cycle.

- Frequently consume hydrogen-rich water, deuterium-depleted water, and Quinton hypertonic water solution.

- Drink 2 to 6 cups of organic bone broth each day, along with medicinal plants and mushrooms, most notably chaga, ashitaba, turmeric, burdock, mistletoe, and melatonin and the glycoside extracts of the digitalis and strophanthus plants.
- Use NR, NAD, NADH or NMN daily (see chapter 19 for more details).
- Get frequent infusions of high-dose vitamin C and ozone blood replacement IV therapies.
- Frequently use Rife therapy, PEMF therapy, and hyperthermia using technologies such as the Royal Rife machine, Pulse Centers PEMF massage table, and the Biomat.
- Frequently use a hyberbaric oxygen therapy chamber.
- Spend twenty to forty-five minutes in an infrared sauna every day.
- Completely eliminate non-native electromagnetic fields, such as WiFi and Bluetooth, and any significant smartphone use.
- Perform a complete environmental detoxification audit of personal care products, household cleaning chemicals, lighting, air, and water (see chapter 20 for more details).
- Consider high-dose T cell therapy.
- Perform a complete emotional detoxification focused on gratitude, prayer, meditation, relationships, and de-stressing.

While this list is by no means exhaustive, it would be my non-negotiable list for myself and the advice I'd give to any loved one who was interested in cancer prevention or cancer management. I'd also visit CareOncology.com for a list of practitioners who can offer alternative forms of immunotherapy based on Dr. Thomas Seyfried's work and research into the concept of press-pulse cycling for cancer.

ONE THING YOU CAN DO THIS WEEK

Your lymph system responds quite well to the g-forces generated during exercise and, more notably, when bouncing on a trampoline. But another technique for enhancing the movement of lymph fluid is even easier: plant both feet on the ground and let yourself bounce up and down while wiggling your hands and fingers. Do this for five minutes tomorrow morning when you wake up and notice how your entire body feels more energized and awake. This whole-body shaking technique is actually an ancient qigong practice!

For bonus points, begin gratitude journaling in the mornings, or at least write down or think of one thing for which you're immensely grateful.

For citations for all the research studies mentioned in this chapter and a deeper dive into the topics of this chapter—including links to podcasts, blog posts, recommended tools and supplements, and much more—visit BoundlessBook.com/15.

QUANTIFIED SELF

HOW TO TEST, TRACK, AND INTERPRET BLOOD, SALIVA, URINE, AND POOP

I shifted awkwardly on the toilet seat, using one porcelain-planted hand to steady myself while I held a small paper collection device shaped like a hot dog tray (complete with red-and-white checkered squares) in the other. It had been ten minutes, and not a single particle of fecal matter had materialized from my backside. I squirmed, grimaced, then finally managed to squeeze out a marble-sized speck of poo onto the tray.

A handful of brochures and poop-collecting instructions were splayed out on the bathroom floor in front of me, along with a small plastic storage container for my tiny turd. Based on the photograph on the tube, my deposit was large enough. I could now finish my duty in an actual, civilized toilet bowl, thank-you-very-much. With a sigh of relief, I dropped my sample into the tube and settled back on the toilet seat, slightly apprehensive about repeating this procedure on days two and three, and wondering what my wife would think of the prepaid FedEx shipping bag full of my poop tubes laid neatly next to her homemade kimchi in the refrigerator.

From sniffing peanut butter in an attempt to drip massive amounts of saliva into a tube for DNA analysis, to spraying urine into a giant orange bucket I carried around for twenty-four hours for a University of Connecticut lab experiment on athletes, to giving a dizziness-inducing nineteen full tubes of blood for a plasma longevity panel, in my quest to discover the best ways to self-quantify everything happening inside the human body, I've done just about anything to test and tracked just about everything.

Not a single day goes by that I'm not asked about the most important parameters to track if you want to fully analyze and optimize the performance of your body and brain. In our modern era of "the internet of things," Web 2.0, and a dizzying number of self-quantification devices, it can be confusing and frustrating to figure out what to measure when it comes to blood, biomarkers, metrics, and beyond—and even more confusing and frustrating to figure out what to do with all the data.

After testing, tracking, and interpreting biometrics from self-quantification devices, along with blood, saliva, urine, hair, and poop, I've found the tests and tracking tools that give you the most bang for your buck without producing oodles and oodles of unnecessary data. This chapter will explain the 20 percent of self-quantification efforts that give you 80 percent of the valuable data and results, and the best way to figure out exactly what is going on inside your body on a daily basis.

While there are literally hundreds of blood, urine, and saliva measurements you could use to track your health, and scientific advances are constantly making more and more test markers available, I'm going to share with you the best, most reliable indicators of health and the best tests for determining whether you are venturing into the land of nutrient depletion, gut issues, the wrong diet for you, and overtraining, or whether there are hidden missing components that you can optimize through diet, lifestyle, or supplements.

THE 11 BEST BLOOD BIOMARKERS TO TEST

When it comes to testing your blood, I'm a fan of paying the closest attention to the biomarkers that are associated with aging. After all, if you can control for these blood values, you can be relatively confident that you're going to maintain not just a reduced rate of biological aging but also superior overall health.

If you care at all about how well you're doing in the longevity game, you're curious how fast you're aging, or you want to quantify the efficacy of your healthy-eating and healthy-living efforts, it's worth paying attention to each of the following parameters. This list is by no means comprehensive, but it includes the biomarkers that I consider the most important to track. Please keep in mind that lab reference ranges are flawed and do not take into account your physical activity levels and exercise goals, your current diet, your health history, and many other factors—so be sure to pay attention to the next section, on "When Normal Ain't Normal," because "normal" lab values are often not what they seem, and you don't want to take unnecessary steps to correct an issue that really isn't an issue.

When Normal Ain't Normal

When a doctor orders a test like a blood or saliva panel to look for health-related biomarkers, he or she compares your results to the results of the average population, which are known as a reference range or reference interval. This allows a physician to see how your test results compare to what's considered normal. About 80 percent of doctors' recommendations, diagnoses, and prescriptions are based on lab tests and their reference ranges. But reference ranges may not be as normal as they are supposed to be. In this context, "normal" doesn't necessarily mean "ordinary" or even "optimal." "Normal" refers to how the values from an average population create a range or distribution of numbers on a graph.

NORMAL CURVE

About 5 percent of people fall outside the reference range of any test, yet they may be perfectly healthy.

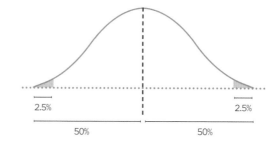

When values are placed on a graph, the average value lies in the middle, and half lie on the left side of the average (the lower half of the range) while the other half lie on the right side (the higher half of the range). These values account for 95 percent of the population. Once 95 percent of the population is accounted for in a reference range, any remaining values are considered to be the tails of the curve on a graph, resulting in about 2.5 percent of the measured population falling outside of the reference range on either side.

Here's the first reason why reference ranges can be problematic: there's no universally applicable range for most lab test results. Different labs can use different ranges, so if you go to one lab for, say, a blood test, you might get results that suggest you're perfectly healthy, but if you get the same test at a different lab, your result might be "abnormal." Most labs don't even carry out their own research to establish reference ranges but instead use those provided by test manufacturers. Labs are supposed to perform twenty sample tests to verify that the manufacturers' ranges are accurate, but most labs don't even perform this step!

Granted, reference ranges can be useful because they give fixed values for biomarkers from relatively healthy populations, which gives health-care providers a basis for analyzing your personal results, diagnosing conditions, and prescribing treatments. Ranges also give you, the patient, a chance to see how your biomarkers measure against those of tested populations. But ranges don't account for large population research, which often suggests completely different ranges for diagnosing disease and mortality risks. Reference ranges also don't account for genetic individuality and differences in environment but instead act as a blanket, one-size-fits-all approach to diagnosing. The ranges are based on "healthy" populations, but these can be hard to define or find because the tested population may include people with undiagnosed diseases or conditions that affect their results. And, again, just because a certain range of values is considered normal doesn't mean that those values are optimal—it just means those are the average values of the population that was tested.

The second reason why laboratory reference ranges need to be viewed with a wary eye is that they don't necessarily reflect levels that would help you go from good to great; they simply reflect the absence of disease. For example, thyroid-stimulating hormone (TSH) is often not flagged as high until it reaches levels above 4.0, but many people—although they may not have full-blown hypothyroidism—can feel sluggish or show signs of low metabolism or low thyroid activity with levels as low as 2.0. The same can be said for testosterone. The reference ranges on a lab test often don't flag a result as low unless it's so low that it's a sign of hypogonadism; the reference ranges don't necessarily allow for high libido, fast exercise recovery, or increased physical performance, which all require higher levels of testosterone, so an "average" testosterone result would be too low. In these two scenarios, you may look at your test and think your thyroid and testosterone are just fine when, in fact, they should actually be addressed if your goal is peak performance.

Another reason why reference ranges frequently don't represent optimal ranges is that they are often applied to both men and women when, instead, men and women should ideally have separate ranges. For example, aspartate aminotransferase (AST) and alanine aminotransferase (ALT) are liver enzymes that are used to measure liver function, liver damage, and nonalcoholic fatty liver disease. One reference range allows for AST to vary from 10 to 40 U/L (units per liter) and ALT to vary from 7 to 56 U/L for both men and women. But research indicates that while this may be a "normal" range, it's far from ideal for either men or women. Several research reports on liver enzymes suggest that for men, ALT shouldn't exceed 30 U/L, and for women, it shouldn't exceed 19 U/L. One study performed to determine upper cut-off values for AST and ALT states that in men, ALT shouldn't exceed 22.15 U/L and AST shouldn't exceed 25.35 U/L, while in women, ALT shouldn't exceed 22.40 and AST shouldn't exceed 24.25. Dr. Bryan Walsh, a board-certified naturopathic physician and the man behind the Walsh Detox protocol described in chapter 13, claims that ALT and AST shouldn't be much higher than 20 and that their reference ranges in men and women should be different.

While the reason why ideal ranges for AST and ALT are different for men and women is a matter of speculation, one study suggests that hemoglobin may be responsible. High hemoglobin levels are strongly associated with elevated ALT levels in men, and hemoglobin is typically lost through bleeding. Since men don't have a monthly menstrual cycle by which they lose regular amounts of blood, they typically have higher hemoglobin levels than women, possibly resulting in higher levels of liver enzymes.

So if you order a blood test and your results fall outside of the "normal" range, that doesn't necessarily mean you're sick or have a higher risk of getting sick. After all, reference ranges come with built-in bumpers on either side to allow for 5 percent of the population to have out-of-range biomarker values, and 5 percent can be an enormous number of people, and may include you.

With all that in mind and a healthy skepticism in place, let's look at the most important biomarkers and what they mean.

1. RBC Magnesium

Accurately measuring magnesium levels can be difficult. Magnesium is found primarily within your cells (intracellular), but most blood tests for magnesium measure what is outside the cells (extracellular), so they may not detect a significant deficiency. Despite this fact, most physicians measure magnesium with a simple blood test, and many people are then informed that their levels are normal. But to get an accurate reading, you need to measure intracellular magnesium levels, which can be done by testing red blood cells.

A red blood cell (RBC) magnesium test can provide an earlier indication of magnesium deficiency than a standard magnesium blood test. This is because when levels are low, the body pulls magnesium from red blood cells. So a standard magnesium blood test may show normal levels while an RBC magnesium test gives a far more accurate picture of low magnesium. The ideal range for RBC magnesium levels is 6.0 to 6.5 mg/dL; the normal reference range is 4.2 to 6.8 mg/dL. RBC magnesium measurements can help predict important longevity markers such as insulin sensitivity and likelihood of hospitalization. High levels of RBC magnesium can predict physical performance and potential for sarcopenia (muscle deterioration) as you age.

While you can request an RBC magnesium test during a visit to your doctor or health-care provider, you can also order one yourself through an independent lab, such as LabCorp or Direct-Labs, or get the test as part of the comprehensive blood panels I designed for men and women, which are available through WellnessFX and include RBC magnesium measurements (visit BoundlessBook.com/16 for links to these tests).

Finally, as an alternative to RBC magnesium testing, some physicians will test magnesium by scraping some cells from the tongue and smearing them onto a slide, which is sent to a lab to be tested for magnesium. A lab called Intracellular Diagnostics offers this test, and it is just as accurate as an RBC magnesium test.

2. Estradiol

Some of the most important hormones to test for in both men and women are estrogens, particularly estradiol. (I'll address full hormone panels later in this chapter.) Estrogens aid in regulating bone mass and strength by stimulating bone-forming osteoblasts and inhibiting bone-absorbing osteoclasts. This type of bone support is crucial for reducing age-related fractures and maintaining healthy production of new blood cells as you age. Interestingly, when women are treated with exogenous estrogens, reductions in bone mass and increases in bone turnover can be reversed, suggesting that estrogens have a potent bone-protective effect.

Estrogens also protect against oxidative stress and participate in the antioxidant system by decreasing the expression of NADPH oxidase, an important source of cell-damaging superoxide radicals, and increasing the availability of nitric oxide, an antioxidant naturally produced in the body. In addition, estradiol stimulates the activity of antioxidant enzymes, such as glutathione peroxidase, in mitochondria. Since mitochondrial respiration produces reactive oxygen species, which cause oxidative damage, this activity of estradiol results in less oxidative stress from normal metabolic processes; this may be part of the reason that women's life expectancy is generally longer than men's. Estrogens can also stimulate muscle repair and regenerative processes, likely by acting as antioxidants and mitigating oxidative damage, leading to greater muscle strength and preventing fall-related fractures.

Ideal estradiol levels vary for men and women, ranging in men from about 10 to 82 pg/mL (one picogram, pg, is one one-trillionth of a gram). Levels in women vary depending on the point of their menstrual cycle they are in when tested:

- Less than 50 pg/mL during menstruation
- Up to 200 pg/mL during follicular development
- Up to 400 pg/mL just before ovulation

In women, estradiol levels dip just before the release of the ovum and peak again during the luteal phase and then reach their lowest point at the end of the luteal phase.

There are a few options for testing levels of estradiol, but they're not all created equal. Blood testing is the least effective method because it provides only a snapshot of your hormones levels at the exact moment you had your blood drawn. Since your hormone levels change throughout the day based on your normal circadian rhythm, this doesn't give you a full picture. A salivary panel, known as an adrenal stress index, comprises four or five salivary measurements performed throughout the day and gives you a more accurate idea of how your hormones are fluctuating during a twenty-four-hour period. However, the gold standard for hormone testing is a urine test known as the DUTCH test, which tells you not only what your hormones are doing over a twenty-four-hour cycle but also the upstream and downstream metabolites of those hormones. This tells you if you are deficient in certain hormones, if your hormones aren't being metabolized properly, or if they're being metabolized too rapidly. You can order a DUTCH test online at dutchtest.com and an adrenal stress index online from DirectLabs or other online lab test websites.

3. High-Sensitivity C-Reactive Protein

Over two dozen research studies have proven that baseline levels of the inflammatory marker high-sensitivity C-reactive protein (hs-CRP) in healthy men and women are highly predictive of future risk of cardiovascular ailments, including heart attack, diabetes, stroke, sudden cardiac death, and peripheral arterial disease. Research also suggests that hs-CRP levels predict repeat coronary events in people with heart disease and that the outcome of patients following a heart attack is closely correlated with hs-CRP levels. Ultimately, individuals with high levels of hs-CRP have a risk of cardiovascular problems about two to three times higher than the risk of those with low, optimal levels.

In my opinion, an hs-CRP test for inflammation, combined with a basic lipid panel, is the best way to evaluate your risk for heart disease. By eating a diet high in anti-inflammatory herbs, spices, and nutrients (especially turmeric and fish oil) and avoiding overtraining, excessive stress, and toxin exposure, I personally try to keep my hs-CRP below 0.5 mg/L, and I prefer to have it below 0.2 mg/L. You can order an hs-CRP test through your doctor or health-care provider, through Amazon, or through an independent lab, such as DirectLabs.

4. Triglyceride-to-HDL Ratio

Otherwise known as the atherogenic index of plasma (yep, that's a mouthful), a high triglyceride-to-HDL ratio (meaning a high number of triglycerides relative to your HDL cholesterol) is one of the best indicators of your risk for heart disease. This test has the added benefit of predicting lipoprotein particle size and insulin resistance, two other important markers for longevity. In one study in elderly women, the triglyceride-to-HDL ratio predicted all-cause mortality, meaning it predicted the risk of not only cardiovascular mortality but also the overall risk of dying from anything.

There are, of course, a host of additional studies on this ratio, including a study that shows that triglyceride-to-HDL ratio is one of the best predictors of the risk of death from coronary heart disease or cardiovascular disease. A ratio of 2 or under is good, but like most of my healthiest clients, I aim for 1 or under. Anything above 4 is typically a very unfavorable scenario.

In my clients and myself, I consider the following three variables to be the biggest issues to pay attention to for an overall picture of your lipid and cholesterol health:

- **Trends:** Triglycerides should ideally go down over time, while HDL should trend upward.

- **Total cholesterol-to-HDL-C ratio:** Lower is better and usually indicates fewer atherosclerotic LDL cholesterol particles. HDL-C specifically refers to the cholesterol carried within HDL particles.

How to Change Your Triglycerides

If your triglycerides are elevated, generally about 150 mg/dL, implement the following strategies:

- Consume high amounts of monounsaturated and omega-3 fats and little sugar and starch (e.g., low-carb Mediterranean-style diet).

- Supplement with vitamin C.

- Supplement with fish or krill oil.

- Eat more olive oil.

- Add fenugreek seeds to your meals.

- Supplement with ashwagandha.

- Get more prebiotics and probiotics from fermented foods and supplements (see chapter 13).

- Eat fruit in moderation, preferably small, dark-colored berries.

- Exercise before meals (brisk walking is particularly effective).

If your HDL is low, generally below 60 mg/dL, implement the following strategies:

- Eat more olive oil.

- Eat more eggs.

- Follow a low-carb or ketogenic diet.

- Eat more anthocyanin-rich foods, such as blueberries, blackberries, pomegranates, eggplants, red cabbages, and other dark-colored fruits and vegetables.

- Stick to a low-to-moderate alcohol consumption.

- Cook with coconut oil and/or add it to meals.

- Eat more fatty fish.

- Get more aerobic exercise.

- **Triglyceride-to-HDL-C ratio:** Lower is better and usually indicates fewer and larger LDL particles (which are less damaging). Ideally, this ratio should be 1 or lower. HDL and triglyceride levels can be measured by your doctor, but you can also order panels yourself through LabCorp or DirectLabs and then compare the results of the HDL panel to the triglycerides panel to determine your ratio. HDL and triglycerides are also typically measured on a lipid panel, which I'll talk about below.

5. Blood Lipids (Cholesterol and Triglycerides)

An advanced cardiovascular and lipid panel goes beyond the typical cholesterol test to help uncover early risk factors for heart disease. Many people don't realize it, but a cholesterol test is important long before you feel old or sick. A basic lipid panel measures fats and fatty substances in the blood, such as LDL, HDL, total cholesterol, and triglycerides, while a full lipid panel goes far beyond the basics and includes LDL particle sizes.

LDL particle size is crucial because research has shown that small, lower-density LDL cholesterol is more inflammatory and toxic to blood vessels than larger, fluffier LDL, and that a high level of lipoprotein(a)—a type of small LDL particle that inflames your blood and makes it "sticky" and more prone to clotting—indicates the presence of the most dangerous blood lipids. A comprehensive lipid panel can reveal the amounts of the different types of cholesterol particles in your blood and give you a far more accurate profile of your cardiovascular risk than standard cholesterol tests.

In most cases, a doctor or medical textbook will give you the usual one-size-fits-all "normal" cholesterol and lipid ranges, such as the following:

Total cholesterol	Less than 170 mg/dL for those under twenty years old, and less than 200 mg/dL for those aged twenty or older
HDL cholesterol	Greater than 45 mg/dL for those under twenty, and greater than 40 mg/dL for those twenty or older. In women aged twenty or older, normal values are greater than 50 mg/dL.
LDL cholesterol	Less than 110 mg/dL for those under twenty, and less than 100 mg/dL for those twenty or older
Total-cholesterol-to-HDL ratio	Less than 5.0 mg/dL
Non-HDL cholesterol	Less than 120 mg/dL for those under twenty, and less than 130 mg/dL for those twenty or older
Triglycerides	Less than 75 mg/dL for those aged nine or younger, less than 90 mg/dL for those aged ten to nineteen, and less than 150 mg/dL for those twenty or older

While these numbers are approximations that can give very general guidance for improving health or avoiding cardiovascular disease, the fact is that cholesterol values tend to fluctuate depending on diet, exercise, genetics, and lifestyle. Dave Feldman of CholesterolCode.com has developed a new paradigm for understanding cholesterol that looks at the effects of fatty foods. Dave initiated very large changes to his lipid markers through a series of self-experiments in which he changed only his dietary fat intake and kept every other lifestyle- and exercise-related factor constant. His Feldman Protocol has now been used by over two hundred people who follow his work. The protocol involves eating a high-fat, low-carb diet with large quantities of fatty food for a few days, and the results from most people show, paradoxically, a corresponding drop in total and LDL cholesterol numbers.

Dave refers to this as an inversion pattern, and his lipid energy model suggests that high intake of dietary fat, especially when that fat is being used for energy by a very active person, can cause the liver's production of LDL (low-density lipoprotein) to go down because fewer lipoproteins are needed to transport fatty acids through the body and because triglycerides and fatty acids are being used so rapidly as a fuel. In other words, lean, active people eating a high-fat diet may see their LDL drop.

But this may not matter anyway because LDL can actually be a poor measurement of cardiovascular risk when compared to two other important lipid markers: HDL cholesterol and triglycerides. In studies that stratify all three, HDL and triglycerides appear as the clear risk indicators, while LDL becomes nearly irrelevant. When HDL is high and triglycerides are low, risk for cardiovascular disease is very low, regardless of LDL levels.

Ultimately, cholesterol can be confusing. If you want to become a cholesterol expert and understand everything you need to know about lipids, I highly recommend my friend Dr. Peter Attia's "The Straight Dope on Cholesterol" series of articles and his five-part interview series with Dr. Thomas Dayspring, both available at PeterAttiaMD.com. As explained in detail in that series, LDL particle count and size are particularly important compared to simply LDL cholesterol, and your lipid panel should ideally be an NMR panel—a blood test that directly measures the amount of LDL circulating in the body and counts the number of LDL particles using nuclear magnetic resonance technology. Ideally, total LDL particles should be less than 1,000 nmol/L, total small LDL particles less than 600 nmol/L, LDL size greater than 21 nm, HDL size greater than 9 nm, and VLDL (another kind of lipoprotein) less than 0.1 nmol/L.

6. Omega-3 Fatty Acids

The fatty acids present in your blood are worth examining because a higher proportion of omega-6 linoleic acid can predict earlier death and physical and cognitive decline. This is because linoleic acid can make red blood cells more susceptible to oxidative damage, which ages the cells and impairs their ability to deliver oxygen. At the same time, older individuals with low levels of omega-3 fatty acids decline physically more quickly than older adults with higher levels. A low omega-3 fatty acid count also predicts smaller brain volume and cognitive decline, even in older adults who don't possess any other symptoms of dementia. And finally, the more omega-3 fatty acid in the red blood cells, the lower your risk for colon cancer—and the higher the omega-6, the higher the risk for colon cancer.

The ideal dietary ratio of omega-6 to omega-3 is 4:1, although many antiaging and functional medicine practitioners suggest a 1:1 ratio or higher in favor of omega-3. (The average American eats a ratio ranging from 12:1 to 25:1!)

There is also an important caveat. The omega-6 fatty acid in plants and vegetable oils is linoleic acid, but the omega-6 fatty acid that you ultimately use in your body and that you get from animal foods is arachidonic acid. The omega-3 fatty acid that is found in plants and vegetable oils is alpha-linolenic acid, but the omega-3 fatty acids that you ultimately use in your body and that you get from animal foods are EPA and DHA. Now here's one thing that a lot of folks don't realize: despite all the talk about the ideal omega-6-to-omega-3 ratio, most of the data on this ratio is based on animal experiments in which the animals were fed only fats found in plants and vegetable oils, specifically linoleic acid and alpha-linolenic acid.

The enzymes that convert linoleic acid into arachidonic acid are the same enzymes that convert alpha-linolenic acid into EPA and DHA, so too much intake of one fat may use up more of the enzymes and hurt the conversion of the other, resulting in an even greater omega-6-to-omega-3 imbalance. But it's important to understand that unless you're a vegan who is only getting fats from plants, this doesn't matter, because the arachidonic acid, EPA, and DHA found in animal foods, particularly foods such as eggs, liver, and fish (and, even if you are a vegan, algae) don't need to compete for the enzymes—they're already usable and don't need to be converted. So, ultimately, you need to pay more careful attention to omega-6-to-omega-3 ratios only if you are eating a vegan diet. Excessively limiting omega-6s could actually be harmful to the mitochondrial membrane—meaning, don't completely swear off seeds, nuts, and other important sources of omega-6s!

An omega index test is offered by labs such as OmegaQuant, Great Plains, Quest, and WellnessFX. This test examines the EPA and DHA in red blood cell membranes, then calculates an index. For example, if you have sixty-four fatty acids in a cell membrane and three are EPA or DHA, then you would have an omega-3 index of 4.6 percent. An index of 8 percent or higher is ideal. Most people have an index around 6 percent or below, and in the US, most people are at 4 percent or below—the highest risk zone. This translates to a 90 percent higher risk of sudden cardiac death!

Finally, your ratio of stearic acid to oleic acid, also known as your saturation index, is another important marker to check. Stearic acid is a saturated fat, and oleic acid is a monounsaturated fat. A lower saturation index (less stearic acid and more oleic acid) is linked to reduced risk of several aging-related diseases, including nonalcoholic fatty liver disease, prostate cancer, colon cancer, and gallbladder cancer. The normal index for both adults and children is 0.97 to 1.02.

Lipid panels can be ordered through your doctor or health-care provider or through independent labs like DirectLabs and LabCorp.

7. Testosterone and Free Testosterone

Several studies have proven that low testosterone (low T) is associated with increased mortality. One study showed that low T levels are associated with increased mortality in male veterans. Another study showed that low T is associated with increased mortality over a twenty-year time span, independent of metabolic syndrome, diabetes, and prevalent cardiovascular disease (but this can be attenuated by adjustment for inflammatory markers IL-6 and C-reactive protein, making yet another case for keeping your inflammation low, especially if you have lower T).

One report concluded that low T may be even more dangerous than previously thought and lead to a greater risk of death. That study tracked nearly eight hundred men, fifty to ninety-one years old, living in California. Their T levels were measured at the beginning of the study, and their health was then tracked over the next twenty years. The men with low T had a 33 percent greater death risk over the period of the study than the men with higher T.

In addition, low T can drastically affect the quality of your life as you age. Symptoms reported by the low-T men in the twenty-year study included decreased libido, erectile dysfunction, fatigue, loss of strength, decrease in bone density, and decreased muscle mass. These men tended to be overweight or obese and had higher risk of cardiovascular disease and diabetes. Indeed, men with the lowest T, below 241 total serum level, were 40 percent more likely to die!

Once T is produced by the testes (in men) or the ovaries or adrenal gland (in women), it enters the bloodstream as free T, which is the bioavailable form of T that your body can use. Normally, about 98 percent of this free T is bound to either albumin or sex hormone binding globulin (SHBG). While about 55 percent of albumin-bound T can be used, SHBG-bound T is not readily bioavailable.

When it comes to T deficiencies, it is important to understand that having high total T levels does not mean that you will also have high levels of bioavailable free T. Some men have total T levels ranging from 300 to 800 ng/dL, but their free T levels are often as low as 2, 3, or 4 ng/dL (often less than 1 percent of total T!). This can occur because some of the 2 percent of total T that remains in a free form can be converted into hormones like estradiol and DHT.

While you do need some amounts of estradiol and DHT (DHT is especially important in the brain because it promotes neurogenesis), when too much of your free T is converted into these hormones, you can suffer from low levels of bioavailable T, which are associated with the health issues outlined above and an increased risk of death. This excess conversion is often linked to deficiencies in minerals like lithium, magnesium, and manganese, so you should ensure that you're eating plenty of dietary sources of these minerals, such as nuts, dairy, red meat, and leafy greens for lithium; legumes, avocados, and dairy for magnesium; and whole grains, nuts, and leafy greens for manganese. Environmental chemicals can also be a major contributor to excess T conversion; I'll explore that more in chapter 20.

So what ratio of free T to total T should you aim for? Ideally, you want at least 2 percent of your T to be free, and this usually means that as a ratio, your T levels should be at least 1:49 free T to bound T. In other words, if your total T is, say, 500 ng/dL, then your free T levels should be about 10.2 ng/dL. The upper accepted levels for free T peak at 27 ng/dL, but it is important to note that this upper limit is simply the result of available measurements and does not reflect the maximum amount of testosterone that a healthy human can maintain. This is why it is important to also pay attention to qualitative variables like libido, recovery, and erectile function.

For men, ideal levels of free T typically range from 4.6 to 22.4 ng/dL, and ideal levels of bioavailable T (which includes albumin-bound T and free T) range from 110 to 575 ng/dL. For women, ideal levels of free T range from 0.02 to 0.5 ng/dL, and ideal levels of bioavailable T range from 0.5 to 8.5 ng/dL. (You can delve into even more resources on the link between T and overall health and longevity in a very fascinating article by Dr. Jeffrey Dach that's linked to on BoundlessBook.com/16.)

If you are testing your testosterone levels, testing DHEA as well can add insights. The largest amount of hormone produced by the adrenal glands is actually in the form of DHEA, which is a precursor to estrogen, progesterone, and testosterone. Symptoms of DHEA deficiency usually include fatigue, cognitive impairment, depression, decreased libido, and recurrent infections. Fortunately, DHEA is relatively easy to measure. But when DHEA is measured, the results should be correlated to age to be meaningful. For example, men around the age of twenty should have high levels of DHEA (around 1,200 mcg/dL). But by age ninety, the level is usually closer to 180 mcg/dL. A thirty-year-old man with a DHEA level of 250 mcg/dL would technically fall "within the normal range" of 180 to 1,200, but as you can imagine, this is a problem, since it's nowhere near optimal and can actually indicate adrenal insufficiency and significant hormone imbalances. Women's ranges vary considerably with age as well. For example, in twentysomething women, ideal DHEA levels are from 145 to 395 mcg/dL, before declining to 45 to 270 mcg/dL in the thirties, with levels further dropping to 32 to 240 mcg/dL in the forties.

Finally, even though I've emphasized that free T is important, new research indicates that total T may not be as bound and inactive. While traditional medical orthodoxy has promoted the idea that sex steroids bound to SHBG are biologically inactive, it turns out that testosterone, even when bound to SHBG, can still have effects on tissue. A protein called megalin can actually allow SHBG-bound testosterone to interact with cells for repair, recovery, and other anabolic effects of testosterone, but this occurs only in the presence of adequate amounts of vitamin D_3 and cholesterol, which is likely why sunlight and a high intake of healthy fats can be so beneficial for libido and energy!

Similarly to estradiol and estrogen testing, the best way to test hormone levels such as testosterone and DHEA is not via a blood test or salivary test (although salivary tests are more accurate than blood tests if performed four or five times throughout the day), but via a comprehensive DUTCH test—see page 402 for more.

8. IGF-1

I first discussed the "sweet spot" for insulin-like growth factor 1 (IGF-1) in chapter 9. As I explained there, IGF-1 promotes the growth and repair of skeletal muscle, the growth of new neurons, and better cognitive function. However, lower levels of IGF-1 result in increased longevity. In animal studies, genetically engineering the animals to be IGF-1 deficient results in 50 percent longer life spans. So the key is to find the sweet spot for IGF-1.

Recommended levels of IGF can vary widely, but in an eye-opening hormone replacement therapy podcast interview I conducted with antiaging physician Dr. Richard Gaines, he advised that the sweet spot for IGF-1 is between approximately 80 and 150 ng/mL. You can order an IGF-1 blood test online through LabCorp or Lab Tests Online.

9. Insulin

Low fasting insulin can be a crucial marker for longevity and indicates an important variable called glycemic variability, which is how often and how much your blood sugar levels fluctuate throughout the day. In chapter 8, I talked about the extreme importance of glucose regulation and glycemic variability when it comes to longevity, and insulin is intimately tied to these variables.

For example, cancer patients who eat the highest amount of insulin-producing foods experience worsened cancer and increased overall mortality. Furthermore, high insulin levels can predict cancer mortality, even when controlling for variables such as diabetes, obesity, and metabolic syndrome. In older adults with type 2 diabetes, the level of insulin use also predicts mortality.

The trick is not to eliminate insulin altogether but to keep insulin levels within certain limits. My friend Dr. Joseph Mercola recommends "a normal fasting blood insulin level … below 5 [uIU/mL], but ideally … below 3." You can order a blood insulin test through your doctor or health-care provider or online through LabCorp or DirectLabs.

10. Complete Blood Count with Differential

A complete blood count with differential, also known as a CBC, is often used as a broad screening test to determine an individual's general health status. It can be used to screen for a wide range of conditions and diseases and to help diagnose various conditions, such as anemia, infection, inflammation, a bleeding disorder, or leukemia. The CBC evaluates the three major factors that circulate in the blood:

- White blood cells (WBC), which defend against infections and cancer and also play a role in allergies and inflammation. WBC count is a count of the total number of white blood cells in a person's blood sample, as well as the number of the various types of white blood cells: neutrophils, lymphocytes, monocytes, eosinophils, and basophils.
- Red blood cells (RBC), which transport oxygen throughout the body. RBC count tells the number of red blood cells in a person's blood sample. Other factors in this part of the panel include hemoglobin, hematocrit, MCV, MCH, MCHC, RDW, MPV, and PDW.

Hemoglobin measures the total amount of the oxygen-carrying protein in the blood, which generally reflects the number of red blood cells in the blood. Hematocrit measures the percentage of a person's total blood volume that consists of red blood cells. Mean corpuscular volume (MCV) is a measurement of the average size of a single red blood cell. Mean corpuscular hemoglobin (MCH) is a calculation of the average amount of hemoglobin inside a single red blood cell. Mean corpuscular hemoglobin concentration (MCHC) is a calculation of the average concentration of hemoglobin inside a single red blood cell. Red cell distribution width (RDW) is a calculation of the variation in the size of RBCs.

- Platelets, which form blood clots at a site of damage to stop bleeding. Platelets are measured as part of the RBC test. The mean platelet volume (MPV) is a calculation of the average size of platelets. Platelet distribution width (PDW) reflects how uniform platelets are in size.

In an article in the *Journal of Hospital Medicine*, it was reported that the most impressive predictors of mortality to be derived from a CBC are burr cells (a type of red blood cell with spike-like surface projections), nucleated red blood cells (NRBCs, red blood cells with nuclei), and absolute lymphocytosis (an increase in the number of lymphocytes in the blood). In the analysis, burr cells and NRBCs were associated with mortality rates eight to ten times higher than that of the average hospital patient. There are anecdotal reports in the literature of burr cells being associated with "ominous prognosis" and more robust statistical analyses showing NRBCs to be associated with increased mortality. Lymphocytosis has also been reported as a mortality risk in patients, especially those with trauma and emergency medical conditions. The analysis shows that all three of these findings are strong, independent predictors of mortality.

In addition, one study reports that men and women with above-normal WBC counts could face an increased risk of death at an earlier age, particularly from cardiovascular disease. Even people with normal WBC counts may not be out of danger; counts at the high end of the normal range are also associated with increased risk of illness and death. Basically, the risk of cardiovascular mortality increases as WBC counts increase, and the increased risk of mortality associated with high WBC counts is maintained over forty years of follow-up!

For total WBC counts, a healthy range is between 5 and 8 cells per liter. Higher counts often indicate infection, and lower often indicate a depressed or suppressed immune system. And again, consistently high WBC counts translate to an increased risk of death at an earlier age, particularly from cardiovascular disease.

Here's a more detailed breakdown of what to look for in a WBC panel:

	EXPECTED	HIGHER VALUES INDICATE	LOWER VALUES INDICATE
Neutrophils	40–80%	Viruses, autoimmunity, or detoxification challenges	Drug reaction, autoimmunity, aplastic anemia, bone marrow cancers
Lymphocytes	20–40%		Autoimmunity, hepatitis, flu, or other viral or bacterial infection
Monocytes	0–7%	Liver dysfunction, prostate problems, or recovery from an infection (or Epstein-Barr virus)	Hairy cell leukemia or bone marrow damage (but only if there's a low value on multiple tests)
Eosinophils	0–3%	Food sensitivities, environmental allergies, or parasites	Stress, steroid use
Basophils	0–1%	Histamine intolerance	Stress, allergic reaction, steroid use, hyperthyroidism

You can order a CBC through your doctor or medical provider or order it online through LabCorp or DirectLabs.

11. Iron

Iron is an important nutrient for almost all life. It forms hemoglobin, making it necessary for the transportation of oxygen in blood. It comprises proteins throughout the body and regulates cell growth and differentiation. It even helps maintain brain function, metabolism, endocrine function, and immune function and plays a role in the production of ATP, your body's primary energy source. But while iron seems to be the darling of many in the health and medical industries and iron deficiencies are frequently tested for, iron toxicity is rarely addressed.

Because many people are convinced that iron is a panacea, it can be found in everything from multivitamins to fortified, whole-grain breakfast cereals. Problem is, if you consume too much iron, you can develop iron overload. Hemochromatosis is a disease characterized by an accumulation of dangerously harmful levels of iron. This can be an especially concerning issue for men (in women, menstruation helps rid the body of excess iron) and for sedentary individuals, who don't turn over as many red blood cells and as much iron as active individuals, particularly endurance athletes.

Basically, as your cells produce energy through normal metabolism, they create low, manageable levels of a toxic by-product of oxygen called superoxide. Enzymes convert superoxide into hydrogen peroxide, which is then converted into water and oxygen. But when iron interacts with superoxide or hydrogen peroxide, it leads to a chemical reaction that produces a free radical known as a hydroxyl radical. Hydroxyl radicals can be extremely harmful to your cells, and if you are consuming excess iron or have excess iron in your bloodstream, you can produce high levels of these radicals, leading to age-related chronic conditions such as cancer, heart disease, and diabetes, and neurodegenerative conditions like Alzheimer's and Parkinson's. Think of this as "rusting" your body.

There are two biomarkers that will reveal if you have excess iron. The first is a protein called ferritin. When your iron levels are sufficient, the protein hepcidin is secreted by the liver and signals the cells in your gastrointestinal tract to block the absorption of iron. It also signals your body's other cells to bind their iron to ferritin, which acts as an iron storage mechanism. If your ferritin levels are high, then you may have too much iron in your body. People with hereditary hemochromatosis have a genetic inability (based on their HFE gene) to effectively use hepcidin to regulate iron levels, so they are highly susceptible to iron overload. A typical reference range used by most laboratories for ferritin ranges from 200 to 300 ng/mL for both women and men, but the actual ideal levels for adult men and nonmenstruating women are between 30 and 60 ng/mL, and you don't want to be below 20 ng/mL or above 80 ng/mL.

If you're a woman and are still menstruating, you are more likely to suffer from iron deficiency than iron overload, so if you experience fatigue, paleness, shortness of breath, headaches, dizziness, heart palpitations, dry or damaged hair and skin, restless legs, or mouth swelling during your period, you likely need to consume more iron. If you have no symptoms and your biomarker levels are within the ideal range, then your iron levels are probably being sufficiently regulated by your menstrual cycle. If you're a man, you'll likely only experience issues with low ferritin or low iron if you're a heavily training athlete or you're not eating any red meat.

Another biomarker to track for iron is gamma-glutamyltransferase (GGT). GGT is a liver enzyme involved in the metabolism of the antioxidant glutathione, as well as the transport of amino acids and peptides. Originally tracked to determine the extent of alcoholism and liver damage, GGT is also highly interactive with iron and can be used to track levels of excess free iron (unbound iron in your blood). In fact, GGT has been shown to be the single most predictive measure of early death by any cause. If you have both high ferritin and high GGT, you have a significantly increased risk of chronic disease because it means that you have both excess free iron (indicated by GGT) and excess stored iron (indicated by ferritin) that keeps those free levels elevated. As with ferritin, the reference ranges for GGT that are considered "normal" in men and women are not the ideal levels. In men, "normal" GGT levels are allowed to range all the way up to 70 U/L (units per liter), but ideal levels are less than 16 U/L. For women, normal levels range up to 45 U/L, while ideal levels are less than 9 U/L.

You can request ferritin and GGT tests through your doctor or order them online through LabCorp or DirectLabs. Conveniently, to reduce excess iron levels, all you need to do is give blood two or three times per year, reduce your intake of red meat, or take up some form of frequent cardiovascular exercise, or all three. Men and postmenopausal women are particularly at risk for developing iron overload because they don't lose a significant amount of blood once a month, so if you fall into one of those two categories, then consider giving blood a few times per year. If you can't give the liter of blood that's normally drawn, then you can have 2 to 6 ounces of blood drawn once every few weeks.

The Bottom Line

So there you have it. Sure, you should certainly pay attention to variables such as love, stress, relationships, diet, fasting, grip strength, and more. But you should also track the important biomarkers listed here, which can give you early warnings about accelerated aging and increased risk of mortality. The only blood test not included above that I still highly recommend if your goal is to track your biological aging process is a telomere analysis. You can learn more about that test, and telomeres in general, in chapter 19.

HOW TO TEST YOUR HORMONES

Because hormone levels fluctuate throughout the day, the gold-standard method for testing your hormones is the DUTCH urine steroid hormone profile, which is performed via multiple collections throughout the day—all made in the comfort of your home. It is the most cutting-edge way to truly see what's going on with your hormones because it doesn't just measure hormones but also hormone metabolites, the molecules that remain during metabolism of hormones.

Measuring both hormones and their metabolites can give you or your health-care practitioner a much better overall picture of hormone production. For example, someone whose salivary test shows low cortisol could discover through a DUTCH urine steroid hormone profile that they have normal cortisol production but high levels of metabolites—in other words, they produce enough cortisol, but it's getting broken down very quickly. There are also some metabolites that are important markers for cancer risk and can only be measured in urine.

With serum (blood) and saliva hormone spot-testing, it's possible to track variations in hormone release throughout the day—and this is a great way to measure how your hormones change during a twenty-four-hour period. In contrast, a standard twenty-four-hour urine collection many physicians use reflects your total hormone output in a twenty-four-hour period. But by using the DUTCH urine steroid test, you get the best of all worlds: blood, saliva, and urinary results with just a urine collection. The DUTCH test measures the following:

- Free cortisone (a corticosteroid related to cortisol)
- Creatinine (a by-product of creatine breakdown)

- Free cortisol. Most circulating cortisol is bound to albumin and corticosteroid-binding globulin; less than 5 percent is unbound. Only free cortisol can reach the enzyme transporters in the kidneys, liver, and other organs involved in excretory and metabolic clearance.
- Tetrahydrocortisone, a-tetrahydrocortisol, and b-tetrahydrocortisol (all metabolites of cortisol breakdown)
- DHEA (precursor for estrogens and testosterone; see page 398)
- The progesterone metabolites a-pregnanediol and b-pregnanediol
- The androgen metabolites etiocholanolone, androsterone, testosterone, 5a-DHT, 5a-androstanediol, 5b-androstanediol, and epi-testosterone
- The estrogen metabolites estrone, estradiol, estriol, 2-OH-estrone, 4-OH-estrone, 16-OH-estrone, 2-methoxyestrone, and 2-OH-estradiol
- 6-OH-melatonin-sulfate (the major, active metabolite of melatonin)

Testing with DUTCH is easy. When you order it, you are sent a collection kit straight to your front door, and the kit includes five easy-to-use filter paper devices on which you urinate. You then use the enclosed prepaid label to send them back to the lab. Your DUTCH results will have helpful, actionable tips for adjusting some of the lesser known metabolites.

HOW TO TEST FOR FOOD SENSITIVITIES

I prefer to use Cyrex Labs for food-sensitivity testing because their tests are highly accurate, consistent, and based on the latest research and development in food-sensitivity analysis. Unlike outdated tests that test only one form of a given food, Cyrex tests for multiple forms of foods (raw, cooked, and processed) and food cross-reactions, and identifies only foods that challenge your immune system so you can reduce the load on your immune system by minimizing exposure to those foods.

I particularly like Cyrex because it produces fewer false positives than other food sensitivity tests. It's quite popular these days for health enthusiasts to order tests advertised as ALCAT tests (you can even buy them on Amazon!). Many of these tests use an enzyme-linked immunosorbent assay (ELISA), which tests allergies and sensitivities to a variety of common allergens, or an antibody assessment panel that tests for IgG and IgA. I had this panel done on myself and discovered that I can't tolerate dairy from cows (but not from goats) and chicken eggs (but not eggs from other fowl, such as ducks).

Considering the amount of omelets, raw-dairy yogurt, raw-dairy cheese, Greek yogurt, and protein bars containing whey from grass-fed cows that I was consuming at the time, it was impossible to ascertain which came first, the food sensitivities or the high levels of antibodies circulating in my bloodstream because I was eating those foods. And herein lies the problem with blood-based food-intolerance testing: the presence of antibodies to certain foods does not necessarily mean that those foods are causing a harmful immune reaction. It more likely means that those are the foods you eat the most often or have eaten the most recently.

In fact, people who were allergic to milk or eggs as kids but eventually outgrew those allergies (which is fairly common) tend to have more antibodies to those foods. In other words, the presence of antibodies is linked to an *increased tolerance* for those foods, not a decreased tolerance. Yet when you test yourself, you may receive a long and foreboding list of foods to avoid (often hundreds of them!) when they may not be your problem.

This is why, for the best accuracy, I recommend the Array 3, Array 4, and Array 10 tests from Cyrex Labs, which will give you plenty of information without producing false positives or giving you a frustrating, extremely long list of foods that you can't eat. This is due to many reasons, including these:

- Food that's been heated above 118 degrees Fahrenheit experiences changes in its protein structure and, thus, its antigenicity. Cyrex screens for raw and cooked forms of common foods on their Array 10.

- Some antigens are cross-reactive, meaning that antibodies developed for one food also respond to another food. Cyrex tests for reactivity to these cross-reactive antigens, as well as for reactivity to pan-antigens like parvalbumin and latex hevein.

- Instead of testing only for reactivity to individual proteins, Cyrex also tests for reactivity to food combinations.

- Many food products, especially gluten-free foods, substitute gums for gluten to hold the food together. Cyrex tests for sensitivity to these gums.

- Binding isolates like lectins and agglutinins tend to affect specific tissues. Cyrex tests for sensitivity to these isolates.

- Cyrex measures your reactivity to artificial food colorings.

- Oils that were once thought to be uncontaminated by proteins actually contain hidden proteins called oleosins. Cyrex tests for reactivity to oleosins.

- Meat glue is used to hold meat together (it's crazy what food manufacturers do these days, huh?). So in addition to testing for reactivity to meat, Cyrex also tests for reactivity to meat glue.

- Some people produce more IgA or more IgG. Cyrex combines the two into one panel to reduce the chance of missing reactivity.

On your results, Cyrex gives three ranges of results: "normal," "equivocal," and "out of range." "Normal" indicates an immune response within the accepted range, "equivocal" is one standard deviation away from a normal result, and "out of range" is two points of deviation from normal.

You should consider any "out of range" result to mean that the food is provoking a serious immune response. An "equivocal result" is also significant and may mean you are just beginning to exhibit an immune reaction to a food, and temporary elimination of that food—as well as addressing issues such as a leaky gut or implementing other strategies from chapter 13—is a very good idea. If you test positive for immune sensitivity to many foods, remove only the ones you react to the most (the "out of range" scores) and begin a protocol to restore tolerance. After several weeks, you can test again, and if fewer foods come back positive, it's a sign you are on the right track.

The Cyrex Array 10, also called the Multiple Food Immune Reactivity Screen, measures reactivity to 180 food antigens, including reactions to foods in cooked, raw, and/or modified forms. This can then help you customize which foods to eat and avoid. Of all the Cyrex panels, I consider it to give you the best bang for your buck when it comes to food-sensitivity testing. Other useful Cyrex panels include Array 4 (gluten-associated cross-reactivity), Array 11 (chemical immune reactivity), and the Cyrex Array 10C, which combines all of their best food-allergy tests into one highly informative panel that evaluates over 180 different food antigens and cross-reactivities.

You can't order these Cyrex tests yourself, but a physician can order them for you. (BoundlessBook.com/16 includes a short list of doctors who have the test available for purchase on their website; you usually still need to call their office.)

A new way to test for food allergies is via a microbiome panel, which can give clues about food allergy or intolerance risks based on gut flora. Research has shown that people with food allergies experience differences in their gut flora, which, in turn, suggests that changes in your gut microbiome impact the development of allergies and intolerances. A normal human microbiome includes a wide range of bacteria, including enterobacteriaceae, bacteroides, lactobacilli, and bifidobacteria, and reduced numbers of these microbes has been shown to impair the immune system, leading to allergies or intolerances.

For example, reduced levels of lactobacilli and increased levels of *Staphylococcus aureus* are correlated with milk and egg allergies. Reduced numbers of *L. casei*, *L. paracasei*, *L. rhamnosus*, and *Bifidobacterium adolescentis* have been associated with egg white allergies and allergies to cow's milk. Lower levels of actinobacteria, proteobacteria, and bacteroides have also been correlated with general allergies and intolerances. Research has also suggested that if you have poor gut flora diversity, you may be predisposed to intolerance of gluten, FODMAPs, and histamines. When it comes to gluten in particular, certain bacterial strains can aid your digestive system in breaking down gluten proteins, which means that if you lack these strains, you're more likely to have a gluten intolerance. SIBO (small intestine bacterial overgrowth) is known to result in FODMAP intolerances and is caused by a lack of beneficial gut bacteria. Similarly, an overgrowth of histamine- or enzyme-producing bacteria that interferes with histamine metabolism can result in histamine intolerances. (Later in this chapter, I'll talk more about how to test the bacterial diversity in your microbiome.)

Finally, many symptoms of food allergies or intolerances are actually brought on by mold and mycotoxin exposure. Using laboratories such as Quest Diagnostics and LabCorp, a functional medical practitioner can measure levels of c4a, TGF-beta-1, MSH, VIP, VEGF, MMP-9, and leptins, and these give a snapshot of how the immune system may have been impacted by mold toxicity. Markedly elevated levels of c4a, TGF-beta-1, MMP-9, and leptins and low levels of MSH, VIP, and VEGF all point in that direction. You can find a physician well versed in this type of testing on the website SurvivingMold.com, and chapters 4 and 20 address how to manage mold and mycotoxin exposure.

HOW TO TEST FOR MICRONUTRIENT DEFICIENCIES

Sometimes you need to take a deep dive into the smaller variables that a basic blood test doesn't look into, such as amino acids, fatty acids, antioxidants, minerals, metabolites, enzymes, inflammatory markers, and more. For this, you can use a special panel called an ION profile, also known as a micronutrient blood test.

This test is a combination of advanced nutritional analyses that measure levels of organic acids, fatty acids, amino acids, vitamins, minerals, and antioxidants. Over time, deficiencies in these compounds can cause a variety of chronic health conditions, and if you struggle with things like poor sleep, less-than-stellar workouts, brain fog, appetite cravings, sore joints, or other "mysterious" issues, this profile can help to elucidate deficiencies in micronutrients and other small components that other basic blood tests simply can't discover.

The Micronutrient Blood Test ION Profile (also known as the Nutreval) from Genova, which is actually a combination of blood and urine testing, includes functional deficiency marker testing for vitamins B_1, B_2, B_3, B_5, B_6, B_{12}, and folic acid, vitamins A and E, beta-carotene, coenzyme Q10 essential elements, amino acids, fatty acids, organic acids, lipid peroxides, and homocysteine. It also tests for a variety of nutrient, detoxification, and cell regulation markers, as well as bacterial and yeast/fungal compounds.

Several of the more common deficiencies, particularly in those who do not eat a widely varied diet consisting of whole foods, include vitamin D, vitamin B_{12}, vitamin A, iron, iodine, magnesium, and calcium. But, as you learned in chapter 13, this can vary widely from person to person based on biochemical individuality.

HOW TO TEST YOUR GUT

There are approximately 40 trillion microorganisms living in your gut, where they make up your gut microbiome. They help you digest your food, produce beneficial and harmful chemicals, control infections from pathogens, regulate your immune system, and even control your emotions (ever have a "gut feeling"?). Some of these microorganisms have been implicated in maintaining optimal health, while others can contribute to many chronic conditions, including diabetes, obesity, Alzheimer's, Parkinson's, coronary artery disease, psoriasis, lupus, and autism. By taking care of your 40 trillion microbe friends, you can maximize your wellness and potentially prevent disease.

One way to figure out what's going on with your gut bacteria is via a full sequencing of your gut microbiome using a service called Viome, which I talked about in chapter 13. But while identifying the microorganisms in your gut is important, you can gain the most insight into your gut when you also understand the function of those microorganisms (this is called "gut microbiome gene expression"). This is because the microbes in your gut produce thousands of chemicals, called metabolites, that affect your overall wellness. Viome identifies the metabolites produced by the microbes in your gut and provides personalized diet and lifestyle recommendations to fine-tune the function of your gut microbiome to minimize the production of harmful metabolites and maximize the production of beneficial ones.

As explained in chapter 13, every person is biochemically unique. As a result, you process macronutrients (fats, protein, and carbohydrates) differently than others do. Because of this, as part of the "poop test kits" that they send you in the mail, Viome also sends you a special "nutritional challenge" shake and asks you to take a series of measurements after drinking it, which they use to determine how quickly you regain your gut flora balance and how you metabolize different macronutrients. When they combine the results of this nutritional challenge test with your poop test results, Viome can tell you your ideal macronutrient ratio and make dietary recommendations that are unique to you. They'll also give you a full list of the microbes in your gut—bacteria, viruses, yeast, fungi, bacteriophages, and all other living microorganisms.

In addition to a Viome test for your complete gut microbiome analysis, I'm also a fan of the Genova GI Effects Comprehensive Profile, which I also discussed in chapter 13. Because it goes beyond the bacteria that Viome analyzes and also tests for yeast, fungi, parasites and other microorganisms, I consider this to be the gold standard for gut testing if your goal is not necessarily to analyze the biome but to instead identify markers that could be causing acute or chronic gut issues.

Finally, at the time of this writing, a new company called Onegevity Health has released an at-home stool test for the microbiome that uses a different form of gut biome testing than the Viome panel—a form called "shotgun sequencing." Although the company is new, their initial research indicates that they are getting very impressive data on the bacteria in the gut, and since the company is owned by Thorne, which makes supplements, they are able to make targeted supplement recommendations, along with food and lifestyle recommendations, based on your results. Onegevity also plans to add food delivery services based on your specific results, along with additional at-home tests for blood and saliva.

HOW TO TEST YOUR GENES

You're no doubt familiar with 23andMe, the genetic testing service that can analyze your saliva and then give you detailed information on your ancestry and certain genetic variables that affect your health. Problem is, even though I'm a big fan of getting a 23andMe test, the good folks at 23andMe only test for a limited number of genetic factors, and legally, they can only release a limited amount of health information, which means that you must download your raw data from 23andMe (it is very easy to do this) and then upload that data to other websites that can give you much more actionable information than 23andMe can.

Ben Lynch's online genetic analysis service, StrateGene, analyzes your raw genetic data from 23andMe for a host of different so-called dirty genes—just one example of the useful information you can glean once you upload your raw genetic data to a third-party analysis website.

DNAFit is another good service to upload your genetic data to, especially if you're active and want to know more about how to exercise and how to eat. DNAFit can determine your response to a selection of key genetic markers associated with health, fitness, nutrition, and athletic performance, and it provides an in-depth analysis of up to forty-five key genetic variants, allowing you to tailor your training and nutrition choices to play to your genetic advantage. The DNAFit Nutrigenetic report uses DNA data to provide information about your response to carbohydrate and fats; detoxification (phase 1 and phase 2) ability; antioxidant capacity; omega-3 and vitamins B and D needs; salt, alcohol, and caffeine sensitivity; lactose intolerance; and celiac disease predisposition. The DNAFit Fitness report uses DNA information to provide information regarding your response to power training versus endurance genetics, aerobic (VO_2 max) response, recovery profile, and injury risk.

While StrateGene and DNAFit are two of my favorite third-party services to which you can upload your 23andMe data, there are a host of other useful services for analyzing your genetic data, including Genetic Genie, MyHeritage, LiveWello, Gene Food, and many others. If you are looking for genetic or epigenetic information on chronic health conditions, Tree of Life (ToLHealth.com) is a fantastic option because they do their own genetic testing. This is because 23andMe recently quit testing for nine thousand genes that correlate with chronic health conditions. So Tree of Life looks at everything from breaks in your heme pathway to potential iron dysregulation.

At the time of this writing, I've recently finished a more advanced genomics test from Youtrients in Canada, which tested me for far more genetic variables than I was able to access in my 23andMe test. During the follow-up evaluation, which you can listen to as a podcast at BoundlessBook.com/16, you learn how whole genome sequencing (WGS) has become more affordable but is still the most expensive option at around $1,000. But if you want a more comprehensive look at your genes, then WGS is the way to go because every single base from all of your chromosomes is analyzed.

Should You Train Based on Your Genetics?

You've seen it before: there's that guy or girl at the gym who has been training only half as long and half as hard as you and seems to be making twice the gains and getting twice the results. They must be on steroids, right? Not necessarily. It's possible that they're simply performing the exact number of sets and reps and using the precise weights that are appropriate for their genetics, while you're possibly training with a strategy that flies completely in the face of your own genetics.

While sports scientists have long suspected that elite athletes are born and not necessarily formed in the gym, a growing body of research studies are now revealing literally dozens of genetic variants that are linked to highly individualized training responses and sport-related traits. Elite sports coaches from countries such as Russia and China are now taking this to the next level by selecting the right candidates for the right sports and then personalizing each athlete's training based on their unique genetic profiles.

One recent study from Europe impressively demonstrated that matching your genotype with the appropriate training modality can lead to a far to more effective resistance training protocol. The researchers set out to develop an algorithm that would allow athletes to achieve greater results in response to high- or low-intensity resistance training programs by predicting each athlete's potential based on the power and endurance qualities of their genetics using fifteen performance-associated gene polymorphisms.

In the study, athletes completed an eight-week high- or low-intensity resistance training program that was either matched or mismatched with their individual genotype (based on information such as whether they appeared to be genetically equipped with slow-twitch or fast-twitch muscle, levels of mitochondrial density, repair and recovery mechanisms, and antioxidant production). They were given pre- and post-training performance tests for both explosive power and endurance capacity. The study was double-blind, and both researchers and athletes were unaware of the "genetic potential status" of each individual athlete, which was determined by an algorithm developed by DNAFit.

The results were astounding. Training according to your genes produced impressive results. Those with the power genotype who trained with high-intensity, low-rep training and those with the endurance genotype who trained with low-intensity, high-rep training had performance gains up to 610 percent greater than the participants who trained with the opposite training protocol from what their genetics dictated! Nearly 82 percent of the low or non-responders in the study were from the genetically mismatched groups who were training using the wrong training program for their genetics.

The researchers summarized that "matching the individual's genotype with the appropriate training modality leads to more effective resistance training" and that "the developed algorithm may be used to guide individualized resistance-training interventions." The big takeaway is this: if you do indeed get a DNAFit test that tells you how you should be training based on your endurance or power responder profile, you'd most likely benefit big-time from paying attention to those recommendations! For example, I am nearly 90 percent on the power responder scale, and my body fares far better for both performance and recovery when I train with heavy weights in an explosive manner as opposed to light weight with high reps, whereas my friend and endurance responder Kelly Starrett noticed huge performance breakthroughs when he adopted the opposite approach.

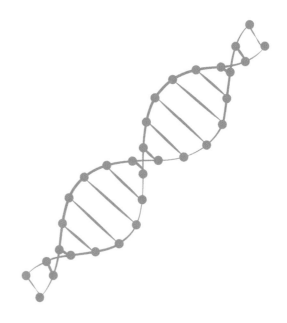

Then there is whole exome sequencing (WES), offered by companies such as Helix, which sequences only the regions of DNA that code for proteins, which still accounts for approximately 2 percent of the whole genome. In contrast, genotyping, which is what services such as 23andMe and Ancestry.com do, gives you access to only about 0.03 percent of your genome.

In the case of my testing with Youtrients, I discovered a host of useful and actionable information, including the fact that neither I nor my twin boys (who were also tested) are able to adequately produce vitamin D in response to sunshine, meaning that we should all supplement with vitamin D and eat vitamin D–rich foods. We also produce lower-than-normal levels of BDNF (indicating a need for brain-boosters such as lion's mane extract consumption, infrared sauna, intermittent fasting, and aerobic exercise), carry the gene for APOE ε3/4 (indicating that we should be careful to avoid excess consumption of saturated fat and should instead favor a Mediterranean-style diet with more monounsaturated and polyunsaturated fats) and, finally, do not produce much endogenous glutathione (indicating a need for glutathione supplementation). Armed with this data, we can lower our genetic risk factors with smart lifestyle decisions.

Of course, it is important to understand that this fix was specific to me, and none of the strategies that I used should be considered a blanket treatment or cure-all for everyone. What works for one person may not work for another, which is why testing is so important.

HOW TO TEST BLOOD GLUCOSE AND KETONES

Knowing how your body is responding to its fuel can be key to understanding why you're having trouble losing weight, why you're crashing during a workout, or whether your diet is correctly keyed in to your individual needs. That's where blood glucose monitors and ketone meters come in.

Testing Your Blood Glucose

While a single blood test using an inexpensive blood glucose monitor from any drugstore or health website can give you a static snapshot of your blood glucose levels, nothing beats a continuous blood glucose monitor for truly determining how your diet is affecting one of the most important parameters of your health and fitness: glycemic variability.

A continuous glucose monitoring system (CGM) is just what it sounds like: a system that monitors your blood sugar continuously, twenty-four hours a day. A sensor is inserted right beneath your skin and attaches to a transmitter that sends the data to the receiver. You are then able to see your blood sugar level at any point with the receiver or a phone app.

The sensor is inserted under the skin of your abdomen or on the back or your arm and is typically worn for seven to fourteen days straight. (In my opinion, if you are eating your normal diet and you eat the same things regularly, you'll know everything you need to know about your blood glucose after two weeks and can stop testing at that point, unless you're wearing the CGM for medical reasons.) If your diet widely varies or you're simply a supremely curious self-quantifier, you can of course wear a CGM continuously (I wore the Dexcom G6 for an entire year!). This sensor reads glucose levels in the interstitial fluid below your skin's surface, and the transmitter it's linked to sends this information wirelessly to a receiver or smartphone app (or an insulin pump, if you're diabetic and using one). This means that at any given time during the day or night, you can look at your phone or receiver and see how your blood glucose level is trending, and you can even receive instant notifications if it gets too high or too low.

In CGM studies of healthy people, a normal fasting blood sugar is approximately 83 mg/dL or less, and in very metabolically healthy, active individuals, it's in the mid to high 70s. Unfortunately, most doctors accept anything under 100 mg/dL as normal, but studies have shown that people with fasting blood sugar levels above 95 have more than three times the risk of developing diabetes than people with levels below 90.

Even more important than fasting blood glucose is the amount of time your blood sugar is elevated over the level known to increase disease risk, which is about 140 mg/dL. Ideally, after a meal—even a high-carb one— blood sugar should rise to around 120–130 mg/dL for about forty-five minutes and then drop, reaching less than 100 mg/dL by the two-hour mark.

One caveat is that if you are eating a very-low-carb or ketogenic diet, you may see elevated fasting blood glucose levels. This is because low-carb diets cause a natural drop in insulin levels and some amount of insulin resistance. When carbohydrates are restricted, fatty acids are freed up for use as a fuel, which means that in the long term, muscles have less need for sugar and thus become less sensitive to insulin. So if you eat a low-carb or ketogenic diet and have a somewhat high fasting blood sugar (e.g., above 90–100), this is not important, and you should instead pay closer attention to your postprandial blood sugar levels.

The two most popular CGMs—both of which I've experimented with and found to work well, especially when covered in kinesio tape or some kind of elastic bandage for high-intensity workouts, races, swimming, or sauna exposure—are the Dexcom and the FreeStyle Libre. Admittedly, I was nervous about using a continuous blood glucose monitor because I worried that with my active lifestyle, it would constantly become detached from my body, that it would become water-damaged, or that the extremely small sensor needle would become bent. But as long as I am careful to tape the CGM prior to intense physical activity, it seems to stay attached well and continues to take good readings (this is especially true for the more expensive but far more accurate Dexcom G6 model). The Simpatch adhesive patch for Dexcom works particularly well.

Testing Your Ketones

In addition to blood glucose, ketone levels can offer good insight into your body. Ketones, you'll recall from chapter 4, are produced during fatty acid breakdown, and your ketone levels reflect how efficiently you are burning fat, or how efficiently you are producing energy, even in the absence of high blood glucose levels. Assuming you do not possess genes that would make you respond deleteriously to a high-fat, low-carb diet (as explained in chapter 13), ketosis can be a powerful nutritional approach to switching your metabolism to prioritizing fat as a fuel while also increasing cognitive and physical performance. (Incidentally, even if you're not achieving ketosis via a high-fat, low-carb diet, you can still amp up ketone production with intermittent fasting or another form of calorie or carbohydrate restriction.) Many people assume that if they are eating low-carb or fasting, they are in ketosis, but actually measuring ketones can be useful, especially if you're just getting used to a new diet or supplement and are trying to determine whether it increases ketone production. Ideal blood levels of ketones to indicate if you are in a state of ketosis range from at least 0.5 millimolar up 3.0 millimolar.

There are actually three testing methods for ketosis because there are three forms of ketones in your body: acetoacetate, which can be tested in your urine; acetate, which can be tested in your breath; and beta-hydroxybutyrate, which can be tested in your blood.

Let's begin with acetoacetate. The way ketones get into your urine is if they are "spilling over" in excessive amounts. This means that if there is an excess of ketones or if you are not utilizing ketones efficiently, they can be dumped into your kidneys to be excreted in your urine as acetoacetate. The way to measure these excess amounts of ketones is through a urine strip, which changes colors relative to the number of ketones in your urine (usually the darker the purple color on the strip, the more ketones you have).

Unfortunately, this is not always a reliable test. Once your body is in a keto-adapted state and you're efficiently using ketones for fuel, you will see progressively lower levels of ketones that are reading on the strip. This is misleading: you may actually be in a deep state of ketosis and using almost all the ketones your body is producing, but the strip says you have low ketones because there are fewer ketones spilling over into your urine. So urine strips can be a cheap and effective testing method if you are just starting to get into ketosis, but they aren't viable for long-term or consistent testing once you've been consistently in ketosis.

Acetone (also called acetate) is the second ketone body and is produced by gas exchange in your lungs. Acetone has been found in research to correlate very closely to levels of beta-hydroxybutyrate in the blood and can be measured directly with a breath ketone meter. One of the key advantages of a breath meter for testing ketones is that it is reusable and usually involves a one-time purchase of a device such as a Ketonix, Keyto, or LEVL.

Finally, the primary ketone body that you use for energy (or can take as an exogenous ketone supplement) is beta-hydroxybutyrate, or BHB. Here's how BHB is used for energy: upon entering a cell, it is converted to acetoacetone, which is ultimately converted to acetyl-CoA. Acetyl-CoA is then used in the Krebs cycle for the production of ATP.

A blood test for BHB can be done easily at home the same way people with diabetes check their blood glucose. You simply prick your finger and squeeze a drop of blood onto a strip, and a small handheld reader tells you the level of BHB in your blood. This is the most direct and accurate way to measure your level of ketones. The downside to using a blood ketone meter is that some people may have a strong aversion to needles and blood, and the testing strips are expensive, usually $5 to $10 per strip (although a newer device called Keto Mojo has dropped the price of strips down to $0.99 each). The blood level of BHB is measured in millimolars, or mmol. Studies have shown that the optimal ranges of BHB levels for ketosis are between 0.5 and 3.0 mmol, although this varies based on activity levels, time in ketosis, fat-burning efficiency, and other factors.

So how do I personally test my ketones? Although I wear a CGM (the Dexcom G6) to monitor my blood glucose, I'm not a fan of the hassle or expense of constantly measuring blood ketones. Instead, I use a device in my office called a LEVL to monitor my breath ketones.

Clinical research has demonstrated a correlation between the amount of acetone detected in the breath, blood ketone values, and body fat burned, making breath ketone testing a reliable indicator of ketosis fat loss. A breath ketone–measuring device such as the LEVL detects trace amounts of acetone in your breath when your body is burning fat. You simply breathe into it, and your breath is captured and then analyzed by LEVL's nanosensor, providing you with an instant measurement of your body's acetone concentration.

When you first shift into a lower carbohydrate intake, your body increases the amount of fat it burns relative to the amount of carbohydrates, and your breath acetone concentration ramps up. This happens over the course of three to seven days, until you reach an elevated level of breath acetone. If your diet becomes higher in calories or carbohydrates, your body will become less dependent on fat for energy, resulting in a drop in acetone concentration over one to two days.

I prefer this method of measuring ketones because it's quick and easy. It does not measure blood mmol concentrations, but I still find it far easier and more convenient than blood testing for ketones.

HOW TO TRACK YOUR READINESS FOR STRESS

No one can perform at their best 24/7/365, because both mental and physical readiness varies from day to day. This means some days are perfect for challenging your body and mind, and other days should be focused on easy, restorative, relaxing activities. Ideally, this is something that should be quantified and tracked. In chapter 12, I explained the idea of a "readiness score," which indicates how recovered I am and how well my body is responding to the demands of daily life. It's a very sleek and efficient way to test the body's recovery status and overall wellness without the need for imprecise subjective evaluation, time-consuming questionnaires, or extensive testing, and it requires just one simple piece of hardware, the Oura ring. I'm now using the readiness score as one of the few key daily metrics I glance at (the other is sleep, and when I'm trying a new diet, food, or supplement, I keep an eye on my blood glucose and ketones). The readiness score allows me to answer important questions such as these:

- Is my nervous system ready to take on the day?
- Should I take it easy today in my workouts or go all-out?
- How much stress can I handle today?
- Should I get extra sleep tonight, or take a nap today?
- Have recent lifestyle or environmental changes significantly affected me?

All of these questions can be quickly answered by glancing at my readiness score first thing in the morning. If my daily stress load and recovery are in balance, then usually my readiness score is high. I use the same method with the clients and athletes I coach to give me intelligent data that I use to structure their training for the week—even occasionally pushing the athletes in training through low periods of readiness followed by big bouts of recovery so that they can super-compensate and bounce back even stronger (a training method called "periodization").

It's true that the state of your body and mind can give you subtle hints about your readiness. For example, are you relaxed or tense? Is your mind crystal clear or covered in fog? Do you feel healthy or a bit under the weather? But these are mainly subjective evaluations of your readiness. An objective evaluation is also important, which is why getting a personal readiness score is something I do each morning by quickly glancing at the smartphone app that connects to the Oura ring.

As you'll recall from chapter 12, the readiness score ranges from 0 to 100 percent and is based on specific metrics tracked by the Oura ring. A general rule of thumb is that if your readiness score is above 85 percent, you're ready to meet the day's more stressful physical and mental challenges, and if it's below 70 percent, you might want to consider concentrating more on recovery.

HOW TO TRACK YOUR SLEEP

What is the right amount of sleep for me? How fast did I fall asleep? Did I go through a normal series of sleep stages during the night? Am I sleeping well? Until this new era of self-quantification came upon us, outside of sleep laboratories, it was very difficult to answer these questions objectively.

The problem with sleep monitoring is that traditionally, most people didn't have tools with which to track sleep accurately outside sleep clinics. Without a measuring device, you cannot really know whether you have had enough deep or REM sleep. In addition, it can be tough to remember how well you slept, say, a couple weeks ago, or to generate a realistic view of how your sleep trends with your diet, supplements, and exercise. This is important because your "sleep history" can have a significant effect on your readiness score. In addition, it's easy to misinterpret sleep quality: having a feeling that you slept like a log doesn't necessarily mean that your sleep was actually restorative, and training through a low readiness score or a low sleep score can cause an impending injury or illness to rear its ugly head, even if you subjectively felt as though you were ready for stress. I've seen this happen over and over again in both myself and in clients and athletes I train who decided to just listen to their body instead of listening to their body *and* using better self-quantification through science.

If you don't know what your sleep quality is, you cannot act proactively. In the worst case, this can lead to a situation where you start to learn more about your sleep only after you've developed some sort of a sleeping disorder, such as severe sleep apnea or insomnia, and need to consult a sleep clinic or find yourself addicted to sleep supplements or medications. Even if you do go to a professional sleep clinic or sleep lab, you're usually only there for a night or two of sleep analysis, and the sleep-tracking devices there can be quite uncomfortable to wear, thus giving you inaccurate data (go ahead, just try to get a normal night of sleep in a lab with a bunch of electrodes attached to your head).

It probably comes as no surprise to you that I swear by the Oura ring as my favorite accurate yet unobtrusive sleep-tracking device: it doesn't disturb sleep, but its highly accurate sensors quietly measure body signals such as resting heart rate, heart rate variability, respiration rate, body temperature, and movement during sleep, along with tracking all your sleep cycles. You can grab your sleep metrics in an easy-to-read format and visualizations from the smartphone app, along with guidance on what the different metrics mean and how you can improve your sleep quality with time. Oura uses the following parameters to calculate your sleep score:

- **Total sleep:** This shows you the total amount of sleep you achieved the previous night, including light, REM, and deep sleep. It's important to realize that the total time you spent in bed does not necessarily equate with the amount of total sleep.

- **Efficiency:** Put simply, efficiency means the percentage of time you spent sleeping while in bed. The longer you slept, the more efficient your sleep was. In general, a sleep efficiency score of 85 percent or above shows that you fell asleep quickly enough (in less than twenty minutes) and didn't wake up too often during the night.

- **Disturbances:** Disturbances are the other side of the efficiency coin and show the total time you spent awake during the night. Disturbances such as wake-ups, get-ups, and restless time during your sleep can have a big influence on your sleep quality, resulting in less-restorative sleep. This can be one of the primary reasons behind daytime sleepiness. Obviously, many things can cause your sleep to be interrupted, but variables such as stress, noise, sleep companions, light, room temperature, infections, drinking too much (alcohol or even water) so that you get up to pee during the night, and later evening activities (exercise, screen time, heavy meals) are all on the list of potential suspects.

- **REM sleep:** As you know from chapter 7, REM is short for "rapid eye movement." This is the stage of sleep that is associated with dreaming, memory consolidation, learning, and creativity. It ideally makes up about 20 to 25 percent of your total sleep time, but that tends to decrease with age.

- **Deep sleep:** Deep sleep, or NREM sleep, is considered the most restorative and rejuvenating stage of sleep. This is the stage when muscle repair and growth takes place, your body is relaxed, your blood pressure is lower, and it's harder to wake you up. The amount of deep sleep varies between nights and individuals, but on average, adults should spend 15 to 20 percent of their total sleep time in deep sleep. This percentage also tends to decrease with age. Simple practices such as daily physical activity and avoidance of heavy meals and alcohol before bedtime, long naps, and caffeine in the afternoon can increase your amount of deep sleep, as can following all the sleep hygiene tips in chapter 7, such as sleeping in a cool, dark room with limited sound interruptions.

- **Sleep latency:** This is the amount of time it takes for you to fall to sleep. Sleep latency is highly variable, but a rule of thumb is that it shouldn't take you more than fifteen to twenty minutes to fall asleep. There are many reasons that your sleep latency might decrease, including exposure to too much blue light at night, a late dinner, and consumption of alcohol too close to bedtime. Bear in mind, too, that dozing off in less than five minutes can often indicate that you are sleep deprived or that you didn't sleep enough the previous night.

- **Sleep timing:** As you learned in chapter 7, every human has a biological clock aligned to day and night cycles. All of our essential biological processes, such as body temperature, hormone releases, and hunger, operate on twenty-four-hour cycles known as the circadian rhythms. As you also learned in that chapter, there are significant differences in our rhythms. Some of us are morning oriented, some are evening people, and others are somewhere in-between. But regardless of orientation, having consistency in your rhythm and your sleep timing is important (for example, I go to bed at approximately 10 p.m. most nights and am up at approximately 6 a.m. most mornings). In addition, having the midpoint of your sleep somewhere between midnight and 3 a.m. is preferable from a sleep quality point of view.

The Oura ring uses all of the parameters above calculate your daily sleep score. The score ranges from 0 to 100 percent, and as a rule of thumb, the higher it is, the better and more restorative your sleep.

How I Use My Sleep Data

Let's take a look at how to practically use the data you can glean from a sleep system like the Oura, shall we? Before writing this chapter, I opened up all my app data. Two nights ago, I was in bed from 10:31 p.m. until 7:29 a.m. Pretty impressive, eh? Makes me a good little sleeper. But upon taking a closer look at my sleep data,

I can see a few concerning issues, including these:

- I spent a good hour of that time awake.

- I spent five hours and thirteen minutes of that time in light sleep (59 percent of the total night of sleep!).

- My lowest resting heart rate of 39 bpm occurred at about 4:30 a.m., nearly two hours later than my lowest resting heart rate normally occurs, and was three beats higher than my normal lowest resting heart rate of 36 bpm.

So although one would think upon first glance that I had a complete rock-star night of sleep, that's far from the truth. As a matter of fact, this morning I received a warning that my readiness score is low and that I may not be recovered fully from the previous day's activity. Interestingly, the previous day's activity was a three-hour horseback ride, an activity my body definitely was not used to and which it needed additional recovery time for.

Pretty interesting, eh?

By adjusting my activities the next night—avoiding screen time after 9 p.m., eating a light dinner, not drinking a second glass of wine, and taking a magnesium bath to both relax me and bring my core temperature down—I achieved a sleep score of 97 percent, with my lowest heart rate during sleep being 34 bpm (nice and low for me), achieved at my ideal time of 2:30 a.m. I spent 27 percent of the night in deep sleep and only 5 percent awake, and I was even congratulated the next day by my smartphone Oura app on sleeping "like a bear in the winter." I had a high readiness score and high physical activity recommendation for the day.

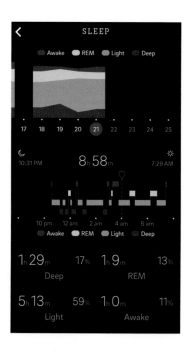

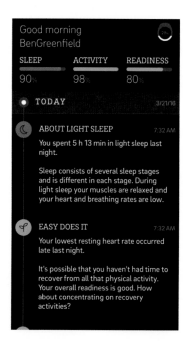

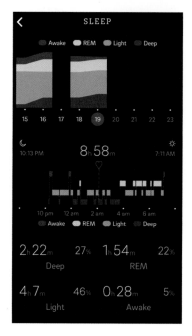

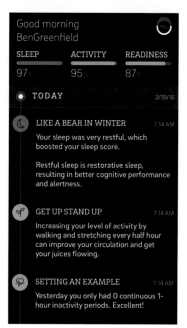

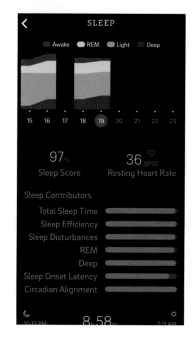

HOW TO FIND A GOOD PHYSICIAN

Finally, should you be concerned after testing and want to visit a medical practitioner who is able to intelligently interpret and help you to fix your lab values, I cannot recommend highly enough that you work with a functional or integrative medicine practitioner. These doctors act a bit like detectives by employing lab work, comprehensive medical histories, and a broad knowledge of the human body to gather information and reach a diagnosis. This is the foundation of functional and integrative medicine: having a well-trained physician identify the root cause of your symptoms and then address it, whether it's infection, nutrition, metabolism, a toxic burden, genetic factors, lifestyle, emotions, or relationships.

There are a number of kinds of medical practitioners who work in functional and integrative medicine, including the following:

- **Medical Doctor (MD):** Not all MDs specialize in functional or integrative medicine, but those who do go through a traditional medical program and then follow that with additional training.

- **Doctor of Osteopathic Medicine (DO):** Like an MD, a DO, who is trained at an osteopathic medical school, offers a host of services, including prescribing medications. They can even become surgeons. Osteopathy is a type of alternative medicine that emphasizes manual readjustments, myofascial release, and other physical manipulations of muscle tissue and bones, so DOs tend to focus on the body as a whole.

- **Doctor of Chiropractic (DC):** Usually, we think of chiropractors as those who treat orthopedic dysfunction, but they can also practice functional and integrative medicine. But they can't prescribe medications, so they'll typically work with an MD or recommend one if you need traditional treatment.

- **Doctor of Naturopathic Medicine (ND):** Most of these doctors avoid drug prescriptions and surgery. Instead, they focus on natural health-supporting agents. Often, a functional or integrative medical practitioner with an MD is also trained as an ND, and this can be a very good combination.

Here are my recommended resources for finding the perfect physician for you:

- American Academy of Anti-Aging Medicine (www.a4m.com)
- Institute for Functional Medicine (www.ifm.org)
- American Association of Naturopathic Physicians (www.naturopathic.org)
- Paleo Physicians Network (www.paleophysiciansnetwork.com)
- American College for Advancement in Medicine (www.acam.org)
- Re-Find Health (www.re-findhealth.com)
- Wild Health (www.wildhealthmd.com)

Many of the physicians in these networks, if they're not in your region, will be willing to offer telemedicine and work with you from a distance via online lab review dashboards, phone, and Skype.

THE LAST WORD

If all this testing sounds a bit overwhelming, please remember that the goal is not to spend each day hunched over a tube while spitting saliva, filling beakers full of blood in a laboratory, or pooping into a tray every time you use the bathroom. Here's what the ideal, simple self-quantification scenario would look like:

- **DNA test:** Once in a lifetime
- **Comprehensive blood test:** Once per year
- **Gut microbiome test or stool panel:** Once per year or whenever the gut seems to significantly change in function or health
- **DUTCH test:** Once per year or when feeling fatigued with no explanation, particularly if libido is low
- **Food allergy test such as Cyrex:** Once per year or whenever the gut seems to significantly change in function or health
- **Readiness and sleep tracking:** Daily
- **Ketones and glucose testing:** Optional, but ideally performed on a daily basis when adopting a new diet or when attempting to evaluate how different food groups affect glycemic variability or ketones
- **Micronutrient test:** Optional, but to be performed if concerned about energy levels or health issues, or when you want to dial in supplementation and diet protocol even more thoroughly

Two final resources that I think are quite excellent guides for educating yourself on how to interpret your own lab tests and address common deficiencies are Dr. Chris Masterjohn's "Testing Nutritional Status: The Ultimate Cheat Sheet" and Dr. Bryan Walsh's functional medicine and bloodwork interpretation courses. You'll find links to both at BoundlessBook.com/16.

ONE THING YOU CAN DO THIS WEEK

It's time to start self-quantifying. You don't have to buy a fancy, $10,000 full-spectrum blood test from a longevity institute—considering how inexpensive and accessible DNA testing is, it can be a perfect place to start. So invest in yourself. This week, order a simple, at-home DNA test. If you've already gotten one, open up your results, look at your disease risks, and see what you can do to address them proactively. For example, if you have a higher-than-normal risk of prostate cancer, you can start getting more lycopene from a fresh tomato every day. Or if you have a high risk of type 2 diabetes, you can begin saving any carbohydrates that you eat for after an exercise session, when your blood sugar levels won't be as prone to fluctuation. You get the idea. DNA testing is probably one of the less expensive and more informative tests in this chapter.

For citations for all the research studies mentioned in this chapter and a deeper dive into the topics of this chapter—including links to podcasts, blog posts, recommended tools and supplements, and much more—visit BoundlessBook.com/16.

SUPERMODEL

MAXIMIZE YOUR SYMMETRY AND BEAUTY

I was reading the book *Deep Nutrition* by Dr. Cate Shanahan when I first realized some shocking facts about beauty and symmetry—facts that we tend to ignore in our politically correct modern Western culture infatuated with fairness for all, but facts that are nonetheless incredibly relevant to anyone who is trying to reinvent their body or health.

In the book, Dr. Shanahan explains that the way we look speaks volumes about our health because of the idea that form implies function. But the entire subject of optimizing appearance is incredibly emotionally charged; physicians even pretend that disfiguring birth defects and other developmental malformations are unavoidable. However, if doctors and nutritionists were willing to explore the connection between beauty and health, every child would have a better chance to grow up healthy. From cheetahs to babies to doctors, all animals fundamentally equate symmetry and attractiveness with health and fertility.

In her book, Dr. Shanahan talks about a California surgeon named Dr. Stephen Marquardt who was interested in whether the beauty and symmetry of a human could be quantified. In his research, Marquardt kept running across mathematical formulas and rules of symmetry in painting, photography, writing, architecture, and other art forms. He eventually created a formula for evaluating the beauty-health connection based on the principles of symmetry described by ancient Greeks.

At the core of these mathematical principles of beauty is a set of numbers named the Fibonacci sequence. As you extend this mathematical sequence out to infinity, a golden ratio forms that was originally used by the Egyptians and Greeks to design perfectly balanced works of structural art, such as the Great Pyramids and the Parthenon, which mystify architects even today. If you think back to high school math, you may be more familiar with the golden ratio as symbolized by the Greek letter phi. Phi was even worshipped in ancient Egypt and Greece as a fountainhead of eternal beauty called the divine ratio.

Leonardo da Vinci was also obsessed with these geometric relationships and the structure of the human form, and his Vitruvian Man sketch of a man superimposed on a circle and a square illustrates these same mathematical sequences, which he used in his quest for discovering the ultimate human symmetry.

But back to our friend Dr. Marquardt. In his pursuit of the perfect human face, he discovered that the golden ratio is uniquely capable of generating a special kind of symmetry called dynamic symmetry, which is based on a balanced, crystalline-like structure. In John Cleese's BBC series *The Human Face*, which features Marquardt's research, a symmetrical mask based on dynamic symmetry is superimposed over photos of people society has deemed beautiful, such as Marilyn Monroe, Halle Berry, and Elizabeth Taylor. The mask fits each face perfectly, revealing that these celebrity icons and many others—including the movie stars, professional athletes, and supermodels we consider to be attractive—all fall into this same bucket of mathematical proportion. So much for beauty being in the eye of the beholder, eh?

It turns out that beautiful people don't just randomly happen but instead are products of DNA strands that are naturally driven to create dynamic, symmetric geometry during bone formation and tissue growth. Whether it is the shape of a pine cone, the segments of insect bodies, the spiraling of a seashell, the symmetry of a leaf, the bones of your fingers, or the size of your teeth, everything that relies on order and symmetry follows specific rules of math and physics encoded in living matter everywhere. A new field called biomathematics is now confirming that recurring patterns seen throughout nature are more than just coincidences, that phi and the Fibonacci sequence are capable of producing intricate patterns that can emerge spontaneously given the correct starting conditions (such as human DNA), and that the health of a biological organism is largely dependent on its symmetry.

This idea of healthy form being intimately tied to healthy function can be highlighted in the work of researchers who studied the effect of four dominant female body types on life span. They categorized women based on body shape: banana, apple, pear, and the rarest of shapes, the coveted hourglass. The women with the most attractive of the four body types, the hourglass, not only lived longest but also were the healthiest. Statistics consistently show that a longer, slimmer waist and wider hips correlate with reduced rates of infertility, osteoporosis, cancer, cognitive problems, aneurysms, diabetes, and more. Research has also shown that women with less symmetrical faces are less healthy and more susceptible to depression and other emotional instabilities.

Of course, the same holds true for men. Research has shown that women are more attracted to men with more symmetrical features. In fact, one study demonstrated that during sex, women have more orgasms with men whose bodies and faces are more symmetrical, regardless of the level of romantic attachment to the men or the men's sexual experience. Another study showed that men with asymmetrical faces are, like women, more prone to experience greater levels of anxiety, depression, headaches, and even GI problems. Other studies show that for both men and women, the less symmetrical someone's body is, the more aggressive the person tends to be when provoked in any way.

In her book, Dr. Shanahan also uses the example of a brain, which has the same organizing force that helps to calculate the sculpting of a beautiful face. She describes how, within the jelly-like matrix inside our skulls, neurons in the human brain form bifurcating tendrils called dendrites, each of which looks like tiny branches coming off a well-proportioned, graceful tree. Just as a mathematical ratio delineates the branch formation, symmetry, and growth of plants and thus helps them capture more sunlight, the same dynamic symmetry may allow our brains to pack in as many nerve connections per cubic inch as possible, making the best use of the limited real estate between our ears. This is a perfect example of how every healthy part of every living thing follows the same basic formula for growth to promote proper function.

Our desire for beauty and symmetry is not simply a matter of vanity. The way we look speaks volumes about our health because form implies function, which means that less attractive faces and bodies can be less functional. Children with suboptimal skull structure may need glasses, braces, or oral surgery, whereas children with more symmetrical cranial architecture won't. For example, narrow nasal passages irritate the nasal mucosae, increasing the chances of rhinitis and allergies. And furthermore, when the airway in the back of the throat is improperly formed, a child may suffer from sleep apnea, which starves the brain of oxygen during sleep, oxygen that is needed to develop normal intelligence.

Of course, asymmetry can occasionally work to a human's advantage. For example, a glance at any annual "Body" issue of *ESPN the Magazine* reveals the forms of some of the best athletes on the face of the planet, reflecting each athlete's success in their particular sport. The jumpers have long, gangly legs with disproportionately large butts; the swimmers have oddly short legs with enormous, winglike latissimi dorsi; and the basketball players have narrow chests and waists and freakishly long arms.

The inherent pleasure we seem to derive from looking at attractive people may offer insight into how the brain works. Just think about it: if beautiful human faces and bodies share the same dynamic symmetry as the connections in our brain, then they may trigger a greater dopamine and pleasure response than observing objects with less symmetry, such as an ugly witch from a fairy tale book or the Hunchback of Notre Dame.

If we can instinctively recognize the form-function relationship and use the presence or absence of dynamic symmetry to gauge health, then we are likely to make better judgments about who is more attractive, who is healthier, who is more fertile, who would be the fittest or safest mate, and, in modern culture, who might be best primed to receive a better job, command a higher salary, make the team, or get the bonus. Science has shown that, whether we want to or not, we really do judge a biological book by its cover, and nowhere is this truer than in our ability to perceive slight symmetrical differences and subtle nuances in our fellow humans' faces and bodies. Although it's contrary to the modern notion that it's unfair that some people might be inherently more attractive than others, the truth is that some people are more symmetrical and, thus, more beautiful than others.

Even from birth, we are naturally attracted to pattern and symmetry. Researchers studying infants have discovered that babies gaze at symmetrical faces longer and learn to recognize them faster. Later in life, during puberty, our brains begin to associate certain patterns with sexual promise, enabling us to select the fittest mates.

So it turns out that, as unfair as it may seem, symmetry and beauty can result in a more successful career, higher income, more social success, and a potentially easier life. This confession may sound like a callous platform for vanity and bullying, but it's based primarily on a physiological genetic principle that we modern humans have inherited from our ancestors. Press a publisher, a judge, a casting director, or a news reporter hard enough, and you may get them to confess that good looks matter in their fields more than they'd like to admit. As irrelevant as these facts are to the contemporary "we're all beautiful in unique ways" philosophy, they are incredibly relevant if you're trying to reinvent your body or your health, or if you want to give your child the highest chances of health and success. I'd say that's a pretty good reason to pay close attention to what you're about to discover in this chapter!

HOW TO ASSESS AND QUICKLY FIX YOUR OWN PERSONAL BODY SYMMETRY

Before delving into the host of tips, tricks, and hacks you can use to increase your own personal symmetry and take advantage of your newfound understanding of the extreme importance of symmetry, let's go over a few self-assessment symmetry tests so that you can get a sense of how well your body is currently aligned.

First, stand in front of a mirror with your arms at your side, pinkies turned in and thumbs turned out, and look at your shoulders. Is one shoulder higher? Does one rotate inside more than the other? Your shoulders should be symmetrical and square—if they aren't, it means they're imbalanced.

While in the same position, look at your hands in the mirror. Do you see the backs of your hands or your thumb and forefinger? Is it difficult to keep your pinkies in and your thumbs out? If you see the backs of your hands, or if you have the urge to rotate your hands forward (if holding the position feels difficult or unnatural), your shoulders are internally rotated.

Now, take off your shoes, stand in the same position, and close your eyes. For thirty to sixty seconds, pay close attention to how your body weight is distributed on your feet. Is there more weight on one foot than on the other? Is your weight forward on the balls of your feet or farther back toward your heels? Is it on the inside or outside of your feet?

Open your eyes and look down. You want both feet to point straight ahead, with the toes of each foot drawing even with those of the other. If your feet turn out, it likely means that your hips and lower leg muscles aren't engaging the way they should. If your feet turn in, you may have excessive internal hip rotation or supination (a turning-inward of the foot).

To see how simple adjusting your symmetry can be, even without going back in time and selecting new parents, learning proper posture early in life, or spending your childhood barefoot or in minimalist shoes, you can perform a few simple symmetrical alignment exercises before reassessing your posture.

Exercise 1: Sitting Arm Circles

This exercise rebalances your shoulder joints by moving the shoulders through internal and external rotation.

1. Place a chair in front of a mirror so that you can watch your shoulders. Start by sitting in the middle of the chair with your feet pointed straight ahead, 4 to 6 inches apart.

2. Relax your stomach and roll your pelvis forward to create a small arch in your low back. Hold this position during the entire exercise.

3. Squeeze your shoulder blades back and extend your arms straight out from your sides at shoulder level.

4. Curl your fingertips to your palms, as if you're making a fist, and point your thumbs out straight ahead. As you do this, keep your arms straight and at shoulder level.

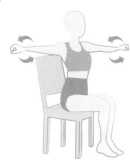

5. With palms facing down and thumbs pointing straight forward, rotate your hands up and forward in 6-inch shoulder circles for thirty reps.

6. Now reverse direction, with palms facing up and thumbs pointed backward. Rotate your hands up and backward in the same small shoulder circles for thirty reps.

7. Keep your arms at shoulders level throughout the entire exercise.

Exercise 2: Sitting Elbow Curls

This next move promotes scapular retraction and helps to pull your shoulders and upper back muscles into place for a tall, proud posture.

1. Stay in the seated position with your pelvis tilted forward, back slightly arched, and stomach relaxed. Curl your fingertips to your palms and point your thumbs out. Place your knuckles at your temple with your thumbs pointed down toward the ground.

2. Pull your elbows back and then close them together in front of your face, as though you are flapping your wings. Keep your elbows up at shoulder level the entire time. Keep your head still and erect. Continue to open and close your elbows with your knuckles at the temples for thirty reps. Be sure to bring your elbows all the way back, as if you were sitting up against a wall and trying to get your elbows to touch the wall. When you bring your elbows together to touch in front of your face, try to keep them as high as possible.

Exercise 3: Kneeling Ankle Squeezes

These squeezes promote hip stability through bilateral engagement of the external rotators of the hips and can "turn on" a weak butt.

1. Kneel with a pillow or block between your ankles and feet. Keep your pelvis tilted forward and stomach muscles relaxed throughout the exercise.

2. Focusing on using your glutes and pressing through the entire inner edges of your feet, squeeze and release the pillow or block between the entirety of the inner edge of your ankles and feet for thirty reps. Keep your upper body relaxed and look straight ahead.

Exercise 4: Supine Foot Circles and Point Flexes

This exercise targets the muscles of the lower leg and foot and can assist with ankle, knee, and hip symmetry and function.

1. Lie on your back with one leg extended and the other leg pulled up toward your chest. Clasp your hands behind the flexed knee. Keep the foot that is on the floor pointed straight up toward the ceiling, with your thigh muscles relaxed.

2. Circle the foot of the leg you're holding in one direction for thirty reps and then reverse direction for thirty more reps. Make sure the knee stays absolutely still, with all movement coming from the ankle, not the knee. Make the biggest, fullest circles you can possibly make with your foot. Imagine that you're scraping out the inside of a bowl with your foot.

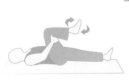

3. Do thirty reps of pointing and flexing that same foot, bringing the toes of the elevated leg back toward the shin to flex, then reversing direction to point the foot forward.

4. Switch legs and repeat.

After these four simple exercises, you can now reassess your posture. First, stand in front of the mirror and check the position of your hands and shoulders. Do you notice any difference in your shoulder alignment or hand positioning? Next, close your eyes and check in on the weight distribution between your feet. Finally, glance down at your feet. Are they closer to being straight?

These exercises are derived from a practice called Egoscue, which is a fantastic form of alignment that I'll talk about more later in this chapter. If you sprinkle these moves into your morning movement routine (see chapter 21 for more details on how to create this routine) on a consistent basis, you'll note continued improvements in alignment, symmetry, and function throughout the day.

HOW TO EAT YOUR WAY TO SYMMETRY

Before you hit the weights, stretch with bands, do yoga, and foam-roll to tackle asymmetries, it's important—for both yourself and any children in your life—that you begin with an understanding of how to eat your way to better symmetry. The Weston A. Price diet is well known for providing the average human body with most of the biochemical constituents necessary for better bones, skin, nails, teeth, hair, and overall health.

So who was this guy? Dr. Price was a well-known, well-respected dentist practicing in Cleveland, Ohio, from the 1920s to the 1940s. His works were widely published in prestigious, peer-reviewed journals, and he even experimented in his home laboratory, evaluating the nutrient content of different foods.

Price wanted to know how diet impacted human physiological growth and development. In the 1930s, he traveled all over the world to study Pacific Islanders, Australian Aborigines, the Inuit, Swiss Highlanders, South American Indians, and New Zealand Maori. Even at that point in history, many indigenous populations hadn't been exposed to the Western diet of highly processed, low-nutrient-content foods like white flour and sugar. Typically, these people, who consumed the nutrient-dense diets their ancestors had eaten for generations, were handsome and had broad faces, wide dental arches, exceptionally aligned teeth, and no tooth decay.

But when these groups began consuming white flour, sugar, and nutrient-poor Western foods, within a single generation, their faces grew narrower, their dental arches became irregular, their teeth became overcrowded, and tooth decay ran rampant. Price determined that these growth abnormalities and infections were due to poor nutrient availability and absorption. He also believed that Western dietary patterns promote the development of allergies and airway obstruction. This, in turn, leads to mouth breathing, poor tongue posture, and the resulting growth of long, narrow faces (which, as you'll learn in this chapter, can be reversed via breathwork and nutrition). But it all began with diet.

Price also found common factors in the traditional diets of the above-mentioned people groups that promoted the childhood growth of strong, straight, and symmetrical features. He found that traditional cultures even had special preconception diets, often one and even two years before birth, ensuring the mothers had adequate storage of crucial vitamins, minerals, and nutrients. These diets—and the modern Weston A. Price diet, which I recommend to just about every woman who is expecting or trying to conceive—usually included some combination of grass-fed meats and organ meats such as liver, eggs from pastured chickens, raw milk and butter, cod liver oil, fish eggs, fermented foods such as cheese, yogurt, and sauerkraut, soaked nuts and properly prepared grains, wild plants, and fresh fruits and vegetables. These foods supplied important nutrients essential for proper infant development, particularly vitamins A, D, E, and K_2. As a matter of fact, the last three women I've assisted with nutrition during their pregnancies, following the Weston A. Price guidelines, have all given birth to beautiful, perfectly healthy, and symmetrical babies weighing more than 10 pounds.

Back when Price was still practicing, experts frequently blamed poor facial and physical symmetry on racial mixing. Even modern orthodontists blame poor symmetry and development on everything from genetics to thumb-sucking to consuming soft foods. All of these variables may indeed affect symmetry, but Price discovered that the largest variable responsible for asymmetry issues is the steep decline in nutrient density in modern diets. In particular, his studies led him to the conclusion that facial narrowing takes place because the fat-soluble vitamins A, D, E, and K_2 become deficient in the diet.

Current research backs up Price's theory. In rats, researchers have demonstrated that deficiencies in vitamin K_2 during pregnancy cause facial dysmorphology. During fetal development, K_2-dependent proteins concentrate in the nasal septal cartilage to assist in proper growth of facial bone structure. If the fetus doesn't receive enough K_2 during weeks six to nine of gestation, this cartilage calcifies early, causing a condition called maxillonasal dysplasia, or the underdevelopment of the maxilla (the upper jaw). This is pretty important when you consider the fact that the shape of the maxilla bone determines the shape and symmetry of the entire middle third of the face! K_2 also requires vitamins A and D to function properly, so these three nutrients are critical for the proper growth of a fetus's facial bones.

As Dr. Shanahan points out in *Deep Nutrition*, this also means that to have the most symmetrical children, adequate time is needed between babies to allow a mother to replenish these vitamin stores before growing the next child. She also reveals a surprising body of research that backs up what Price discovered: children in multiple countries who aren't exposed to high levels of fat-soluble vitamins (vitamins A, D, E, and K_2) when they're young or in the womb tend to have weak bone structures and significant facial asymmetry.

In addition to vitamin K_2, let's take a look at the importance of vitamin A for symmetry. Vitamin A is certainly necessary for vision and is often marketed as a supplement for eye health, but the truth is that less than 1 percent of the vitamin A you eat is used in this way. Much of the vitamin A you consume is instead used to maintain the morphological health and function of epithelial tissues in your body, including your skin and the lining of your gut. Not only that, but vitamin A is also directly involved in maintaining normal phenotypic expression, which is the observable characteristics expressed by your genetic code. By depriving yourself or your kids of sufficient vitamin A, you might be causing not only less-than-beautiful skin or an unhealthy gut but also improper genetic expression, which has obvious implications for physical symmetry, function, and beauty.

Vitamin D is another perfect example. A study done on the effects of deficiency in this fat-soluble vitamin, in the absence of exposure to direct sunlight or artificial substitutes for sunlight, concluded that vitamin D plays a key role in the deposition of calcium in bones, which means that a deficiency of these nutrients can result in rickets, osteomalacia (softening of the bones), and abnormal or asymmetrical bone structure. Vitamin D plays a particularly important role in the strengthening of bones, as well as the absorption and mobilization of calcium throughout the body. Once the prohormone vitamin D_3 has been produced by the body or consumed in the form of vitamin D–rich foods, it's processed first by the liver and then by the kidneys, where it reaches its hormonal form. This form of the vitamin acts through a nuclear receptor to perform calcium absorption, phosphate absorption in the intestine, calcium mobilization in the bones, and calcium reabsorption in the kidney.

Finally, there's the fat-soluble vitamin E, which is necessary for circulation and tissue repair and healing, and which may slow the aging process because of its potent ability to quell free radicals. Anyone who has eaten an appreciable amount of modern, processed vegetable oils likely requires high amounts of vitamin E to combat the damage these polyunsaturated fats can cause. Vitamin E is found in animal foods such as butter and organ meats, and in plant foods such as nuts and seeds, legumes, and dark-green leafy vegetables.

By focusing on foods on the Weston A. Price diet, you'll build better bones, better teeth, better hair, skin, nails, and beyond. That's right: if you currently have poor bone density, facial asymmetries, tooth decay, dry hair, or brittle nails, you can change all of these, even if you are already out of childhood. In addition, if you introduce these same foods into your children's diet, they'll grow to be taller, more attractive, more symmetrical people. This is exactly why we're raising our twin boys on grass-fed butter, sardines, liver, raw dairy, fermented foods, and a host of other beauty-producing foods. There has never existed in our home a version of a kids' meal, such as macaroni and cheese, peanut butter and jelly sandwiches, or pizza. These foods were never an option, and if you didn't want liver pâté with your salmon and hollandaise sauce, you could simply go to bed hungry. Because their palates developed for real, nutrient-dense food, when we eat out, our boys turn down the children's menu of chicken wings, mini burgers, and french fries and instead choose the complex, natural, organic, fat-soluble-vitamin-rich foods from the adult menu. As a result, their jaws are symmetrical, their teeth straight, their bones solid, and their brains well-functioning, and they carry themselves as more reliable, capable, and strong humans. Does this mean that they may get better jobs, their salaries may go up, and their coworkers and friends may look up to them more, due to their height and symmetry? While I won't deny there are a host of other factors that also affect societal success, I do believe that food choices play a significant role.

You'll find a link to a more thorough explanation of Price's diet on BoundlessBook.com/17, but here are some of the basics:

- Unprocessed whole foods
- Pasture-fed meats and animal foods like beef, game animals, lamb, poultry, and eggs
- Wild, non-farm-raised fish, fish eggs, and shellfish
- Full-fat dairy products from pasture-raised cows. Ideally, these should be raw and/or fermented products like raw milk, yogurt, kefir, cultured butter, raw cheeses, and fresh and sour cream.
- Liberal use of animal or animal-derived fats, including lard, tallow, egg yolks, butter, and cream
- Traditional oils like extra-virgin olive oil and expeller-pressed sesame oil, and limited amounts of expeller-pressed flaxseed oil, as well as coconut oil, palm oil, and palm kernel oil
- Cod liver oil, enough to provide 10,000 IU of vitamin A and 1,000 IU of vitamin D. It's less well-known and less popular, but emu oil can also accomplish this.
- Organic fresh fruits and vegetables
- Soaked, sprouted, or sour-leavened whole grains, legumes, and nuts. These processes eliminate antinutrients like phytic acid and enzyme inhibitors.
- Frequent consumption of lacto-fermented fruits, vegetables, drinks, and condiments

- Homemade beef, chicken, and lamb stocks made with the bones of non-GMO animals, as well as stock made with wild fish
- Filtered water for both drinking and cooking
- Unrefined salts and a wide range of herbs and spices
- Homemade salad dressings made with extra-virgin olive oil, raw vinegar, and limited amounts of expeller-pressed flaxseed oil
- Moderate use of traditional, natural sweeteners such as raw honey, maple sugar, maple syrup, dehydrated cane sugar juice (sold as rapadura sugar), stevia powder, and date sugar
- Strictly moderate consumption of unpasteurized beer and wine
- Cooking these foods in cast-iron, stainless-steel, glass, or high-quality enamel pots and pans

But symmetry doesn't stop with food. Even with a perfect diet and our best attempts at adequate nutrition, certain habits can result in distortion of the dental arches and facial asymmetries, as can movement patterns and lifestyle habits. Let's begin with one that we explored in chapter 3: breathing.

HOW TO BREATHE YOURSELF TO BETTER SYMMETRY

You've already discovered a host of valuable breathing tips in chapter 3—but what I didn't emphasize in that chapter is how darn important the practice of Buteyko breathing and the type of breathwork I first learned from *Oxygen Advantage* author Patrick McKeown are to your overall symmetry, your physical performance, and, surprisingly, your sleep quality.

When you look at the facial and jaw formation of the vast majority of top-class athletes and Olympic champions, such as Roger Federer, Rafael Nadal, Steve Hooker, Sanya Richards-Ross, and Usain Bolt, what's immediately noticeable is the forward growth of the face and wide, symmetrical jaws.

One likely reason for this prevalence is that high-level athletic ability and success depends on having an open, well-formed airway, which, in turn, depends on symmetrical facial structure. Interestingly, the most decorated Olympian of all time, Michael Phelps, is one of the few athletes of his caliber who does not possess a strong, forward jaw and a wide facial structure—but he's also participating in a sport heavily dependent on mouth breathing.

In chapter 3, I explained that—as detailed by the late Dr. Konstantin Buteyko and author Patrick McKeown—the best, most natural way to breathe is through the nose, although many children, especially those with autoimmune issues such as asthma, heavy mucus, or nasal congestion, tend to breathe through the mouth. Unfortunately, young children who develop a mouth-breathing habit typically develop asymmetrical faces and poor jaw and tooth alignment. This is because mouth breathing impacts facial growth in a couple of ways. It can cause the face to grow lengthwise and become long and narrow, and it inhibits the full development of the jaws, which shift slightly back from their ideal positions, reducing the openness of the airway.

You can try a little experiment to see how this works: close your mouth, stick your chin out, and breathe deeply in and out through your nose. Pay attention to how the air freely and naturally flows down and back out behind your jaws. After that, retract your jaw and pull your chin in toward your neck and throat as far as you can, and try taking another breath. Most likely, you'll feel like your throat is too narrow and restricted for you to breathe properly. This is the same effect that poorly developed facial and jaw structures have on the airway.

In contrast, nasal breathing enhances smell, improves oxygen absorption in your lungs by increasing nitric oxide production in the sinuses, warms and humidifies the air you breathe before it reaches the lower airway, and helps filter impurities from the air via the hairs and cavities within the sinuses. But the benefits don't stop there, because nasal breathing is also responsible for proper craniofacial development, temporomandibular joint function, head posture, and overall facial symmetry. As you can imagine, when nasal breathing does not occur because we are stressed, sick, or have developed mouth-breathing and shallow chest-breathing habits, the body is forced into a series of reactions that prioritize getting oxygen into our blood, including sleep-disordered breathing, which is becoming pandemic in children and directly affects their growth, development, academic performance, behavior, and much more. Think of the classic hyperactive, bratty kid with an annoying personality, a runny nose, and a constantly wide-open gaping jaw. This isn't actually a stereotype—it's a reality.

One reason nasal breathing significantly affects facial symmetry is that the forces exerted by the lips and tongue can actually influence facial development. As you breathe in, the lips and cheeks exert a slight inward, sucking pressure as the tongue exerts an opposite force. But when you breathe through your nose, the tongue should lay naturally against the roof of the mouth, pressing against the roof of the mouth and causing it to grow wide and U-shaped, just like the tongue. This creates room for all your teeth.

Patrick himself has pointed out to me studies that were performed on young monkeys in which the researchers forced the monkeys to mouth-breathe. As might be expected, the monkeys developed facial abnormalities and crooked teeth, which also happens in human kids. This is why so many people need to have their overcrowded wisdom teeth removed later in life.

Now, try mouth breathing. You'll find it quite difficult to rest your tongue in the roof of your mouth. Instead, the tongue of a mouth breather tends to rest near or on the floor of the mouth. The top jaw therefore isn't shaped by the tongue resting against it, leading to the research-proven development of a V-shaped mandible, narrow facial structure, and crooked teeth. On the other hand, a nose-breather's jaw is typically square, wide, and jutting forward to the point that the chin sticks almost as far forward as the tip of the nose. The classic comic-book illustration of a dominant male, such as Superman, Wolverine, or Mr. Incredible, often conveys strength by displaying a rugged and exaggerated jaw, while many comic-book villains have narrow faces and recessed jawlines! Just watch any cartoon or read a comic book to see what I mean. For the same form-implies-function reasons I addressed earlier, a strong jawline is considered healthier and more attractive.

When the jaws are set back and the airway is smaller, there is poor definition of the cheekbones as the face sinks downward, the nose becomes asymmetrical, and upper back and neck postural changes occur that result in decreased muscle strength, less chest expansion, impaired breathing, disrupted sleep, and even subpar athletic performance. When kids develop a mouth-breathing habit instead of breathing through their noses, the tongue isn't in the correct position to act as a natural form of braces and cause the teeth to grow straight. But the bigger concern isn't actually how crooked the teeth are: it's that crooked teeth are a sign that you have a restricted airway. This leads to poor oxygenation throughout your entire body, causing far more serious problems than an ugly mouth.

Dr. Mark Burhenne, author of *The 8-Hour Sleep Paradox* and an authority on dental health, points out in his blog, AskTheDentist, that humans are developing smaller jaws and smaller airways than our ancestors had, and this prevents us from reaching and sustaining deep, restorative sleep. He also believes that—in addition to mouth breathing, prolonged bottle-feeding, sippy cups, and the consumption of soft, processed foods—autoimmune-induced food allergies cause nasal congestion that further impedes proper jaw and facial development.

Burhenne has noted that when the jaw and face are not properly symmetrical, the airway is compromised. Normally, as you approach the deepest stages of sleep and your body goes limp, your jaw falls back and your tongue relaxes. But the tongue normally doesn't block your airway because of the ample room created by a fully developed jaw, wide arch, nasal breathing, and proper swallow reflex.

However, in a modern era of mouth breathing, poor intake of fat-soluble vitamins, allergies, and poor oxygenation, we struggle to get good sleep because of sleep apnea. When you are in deep stages of sleep, the muscles that keep your airway open go limp. The tongue muscle softens and becomes a wide, floppy lump at the back of the throat, and in those with sleep apnea, it falls back into and partially blocks the airway. At the same time, the airway narrows and can potentially become too flaccid to support normal breathing. In extreme cases, the airway becomes so narrow that breathing can stop completely.

Each time the brain has to deal with these breathing interruptions, it halts its entry into deep sleep, and your body is never able to complete stages of deep and restorative sleep. You toss and turn, talk in your sleep, kick your legs, grind your teeth, or snore, which are all signs your body is attempting to reopen your airway for more efficient breathing. These interruptions keep you from achieving the ideal stages of deep, restorative sleep. It is now known that sleep disturbances and sleep apnea, a growing issue in younger and younger populations, are a contributing factor to chronic diseases such as Alzheimer's, cancer, heart disease, diabetes, ADHD, mood disorders such as depression, and cognitive learning disorders.

There are two primary methods to see if you have sleep apnea:

- Use a continuous pulse oximeter to monitor your oxygenation levels during a night of sleep. If they drop dramatically at several points throughout the night, you are likely experiencing sleep apnea.

- Get a sleep study polysomnography. A physician usually prescribes this test. If yours won't, there are decently accurate alternatives to conventional sleep studies, such as Knit Health, which provides you with a twenty-one-day sleep assessment for $99.

To remedy sleep apnea and acquire the airway our ancestors had while obtaining optimum airway efficiency, there are several steps you can take:

- Go listen to all my podcasts with Dr. Joseph Zelk on obstructive sleep apnea, including his tips and offer for a customized sleeping mouthpiece. We also discuss the use of continuous positive airway pressure (CPAP) therapy, which uses a hose and mask to deliver constant and steady air pressure. (You'll find links to these podcasts on BoundlessBook.com/17.)

- Consider mouth taping during a night of sleep, using tape specifically designed for sleeping made by Somnifix. (See chapter 3 for more on mouth taping.)

- Regularly perform all the posture- and symmetry-fixing strategies spread throughout this chapter, including a monthly postural assessment.

- Get regular jaw realignment therapy or some form of massage work on your jaw, face, and neck muscles.

- Pay attention to the information on sleeping position in this chapter, and consider converting to a side sleeping position, which can result in fewer sleep apnea issues.

- If you must sleep on your back, shop for a specially designed back-sleeping sleep apnea pillow that you can use to position your neck so your airway is more likely to stay open. A zero-gravity mattress and bed frame can also work well.

- When your tongue and other tissues in your throat fall back and block your airway, a small device called a hypoglossal nerve stimulator can help.

In addition, here are a few more tips for you and the kids in your life:

- If your kids spend a lot of time sucking their thumbs or letting their mouths hang open, it's a guarantee that their faces will grow differently than how nature intended. Avoid thumb-sucking, extended bottle-feeding, sippy cups, and mouth breathing as much as possible.

- Look into and learn more about orthotropics, an orthodontic alternative and treatment focused on proper and harmonious facial development.

- While looking into orthotropics, avoid orthodontics, since getting braces and especially headgear to straighten teeth can significantly compromise your airway.

- For any dental work, use a holistic dentist. Holistic dentistry, also known as biological dentistry, is the equivalent of complementary and alternative medicine for dentistry.

- Consume foods rich in vitamin K_2, such as egg yolks, liver, butter, and natto, or consider a K_2 supplement. (For more on the importance of K_2, read *Vitamin K_2 and the Calcium Paradox* by Dr. Kate Rheaume-Bleue.)

- Chew each bite of food twenty-five to forty times (yep, you read that right) and, rather than giving your young children high amounts of pureed foods such as applesauce, cottage cheese, milk, and yogurt, feed your them whole, unprocessed foods that they can chew. When you chew, consider the impact of your posture on the motion of chewing. Studies have shown that keeping your head upright, as opposed to reclining or slouching forward (e.g., being hunched over your phone as you chew), activates more mastication muscles. A forward, slumped head posture pulls the food away from the back of mouth, which disrupts the natural rotary motion of chewing. (To see what I mean, try to tuck your chin against your neck and swallow.)

- Complete one of my favorite Ayurvedic cleansing practices, which I consider to be both a detoxification technique for the mouth and exercise for the jaw: oil pulling (see page 448).

For correct development of the jaws, face, and airway, and to ensure proper oxygenation through the upper airway, it is imperative that a child habitually breathes through the nose and that you make every attempt possible to also engage primarily in nasal breathing, even during difficult exercise sessions. This is the entire thesis of my friend John Douillard's book *Body, Mind, and Sport*, and I highly recommend you give it a read to learn a host of drills that teach you the same techniques John used to breathe through his nose during difficult workouts and even during entire Ironman triathlons. Of course, all of Patrick McKeown's books and his ButeykoClinic.com and ButeykoForKids.org websites are also excellent resources for learning more.

Patrick McKeown was part of a recent study on the Buteyko method at the University of Limerick to determine the method's efficacy as a therapeutic treatment for rhinitis, or inflammation and irritation of the nose, in asthma patients. The results? Patients experienced a whopping 70 percent reduction in symptoms like snoring, difficulty during nasal breathing, nasal stiffness, poor sense of smell, difficulty sleeping, and forced mouth breathing. In the box on the following page is one of the primary exercises Patrick taught to participants in the study. It is the same exercise I often perform during my breath-hold walks, as detailed in chapter 3.

1. Take a small, silent breath in and a small, silent breath out through your nose.

2. Inhale as much air as you can without excessive straining, then pinch your nose with your fingers to hold your breath.

3. Walk as many paces as possible with your breath held.

4. When you resume breathing, do so only through your nose. Try to calm your breathing immediately.

5. After resuming your breathing, your first breath will probably be bigger than normal. Make sure that you calm your breathing as soon as possible by suppressing your second and third breaths.

6. You should be able to recover normal breathing within two to three breaths. If your breathing is erratic or heavier than usual, you have held your breath for too long.

7. Wait for a minute or two before repeating the breath-hold.

8. Repeat this exercise five or six times until your nose is decongested.

Generally, this exercise will unblock your nose even if you have a head cold. But as soon as the effects of the breath-hold wear off, your nose will likely feel blocked again. By gradually increasing the number of steps you can take with your breath held, you will find the results continue to improve. When you are able to walk a total of eighty paces with your breath held, your nose will be free permanently. Eighty paces is an achievable goal, and you can expect to progress by ten paces per week.

Each week, Patrick teaches this exercise to groups of five-to-ten-year-old children, many of whom have serious breathing difficulties. Within two to three weeks, most children are able to walk sixty paces with their breath held, and some children quickly achieve up to eighty paces. Try it yourself and see how you do!

THE MOST IMPORTANT BODY PART FOR BETTER SYMMETRY

I have a confession to make. I am very, very uncomfortable when I am standing around at a party or social gathering wearing shoes. I don't like shoes. As a matter of fact, I avoid shoes anytime I can, and as a result, I have large, flat, tough, calloused, highly functional feet that get me no compliments on aesthetics but that I know can tackle just about any surface on the face of the planet. See, when it comes to overall body alignment, there's no body part more important than your feet.

Two of the smartest folks I know in the realm of adjusting your beauty from the ground up are the brilliant biomechanist Katy Bowman, author of *Whole Body Barefoot*, and podiatrist Dr. Emily Splichal, author of *Barefoot Strong*. I've learned from both these women, whose books I highly recommend, the extremely crucial role the feet play in posture and symmetry. So why are the feet so darn important?

First, it's important to understand that 25 percent of your body's bones are located in your feet, and that these delicate entities that support your whole body have thousands of nerves on their soles that can affect nearly every organ and part of your body. So if you aren't standing correctly on your feet, it can have a negative impact not just on your overall posture but also on your organs and health. For instance, foot researcher and nutritionist Norman Walker posits that if women consistently wear heels that are over 2 inches high, their digestive system can be thrown out of alignment; it can contribute to constipation and poor digestive function. Thousands of years of Chinese medicine are based on foot reflexology, which involves the stimulation of different areas of the foot to eliminate toxins, improve circulation, target specific organs, and soothe nerves. One large research review summarized 168 research studies and abstracts from journals and meetings from around the world and found that reflexology can increase blood flow to kidneys and the intestines, decrease blood pressure and anxiety, reduce pain in AIDS patients, control peripheral neuropathy due to diabetes mellitus, kidney stones, and osteoarthritis, and even produce a positive effect on type 2 diabetes by stabilizing blood sugar. There is also a growing body of biomechanics research linking shoes with a heel significantly higher than the toe to a host of joint issues, including knee, hip, and lower back pain.

Then there's your lymphatic system. Pete Egoscue, who developed the Egoscue training program mentioned earlier in this chapter, teaches that the feet are crucial to the normal function of the lymphatic system. Just like the circulatory system, the lymph system has to pump against gravity. It drains upward, just like the veins, and muscular contractions in the feet act like tiny elevators that return waste back up your legs. The muscle contraction that takes place when your bare foot touches the ground helps the lymph nodes drain to their interlinking vessels. Egoscue also teaches that proper foot strength is crucial to balance, digestion, absorption, elimination, and bowel movements.

Problem is, any issues that you may have with your feet most likely began early in your life when Mom and Dad decided to slap a pair of big, clunky, built-up shoes on you before you headed off to your first day of school. But back in 1991, long before tales of Tarahumara runners and the growing body of barefoot and minimalist shoe research by folks like Harvard professor of human evolutionary biology Daniel Lieberman (the grandfather of the barefoot running movement, who once took me on a seven-mile barefoot run through Boston), Dr. Lynn T. Stahel pointed out in his paper "Shoes for Children: A Review" that optimum foot development can only occur with a barefoot, uncoddled foot environment early in age. Staheli, who also wrote several books on pediatric orthopedics, explained that stiff and compressive footwear can cause deformity, weakness, and loss of mobility, and that shoe selection for children should be based on a barefoot model.

In other words, aside from times when the foot is injured or foot and sole protection are absolutely necessary—such as when strolling through big-city streets strewn with broken glass or syringes, or when at church or a wedding, cocktail party, or other social event where modern manners are a must—both children and adults should set their feet free. And in situations where shoes are required, zero-drop or minimalist footwear should be your selection of choice.

My kids rarely wear shoes. Like some kind of ancient tribesmen—or their own dad—they have ugly, calloused, tough feet. They play outside, hike, run, stand, and move primarily barefoot and wear minimalist shoes to school.

The reason it's so important to set your and your children's feet free is that the shape and density of your bones is a direct result of the loads and geometry placed on the body. So this means that the way a foot is loaded in childhood will affect the lifelong shape of the pelvis, hips, knees, back, and even the space in the chest that the lungs are in!

This is why kids with poor posture and coddled feet often grow up to be adults with poor posture. Kids who haven't had their bones exposed to a variety of loads, such as running or lifting and moving objects, have been shown to have lower bone density later in life and to suffer from flat feet. Furthermore, pediatric research is now showing that overprotective, built-up, stabilizing modern footwear can interfere with the development of proper foot strength, ankle stability, and movement patterns because the foot muscles atrophy and foot bones degrade. Another problematic effect of wearing shoes too often, especially tight-fitting athletic shoes or dress shoes with a tapered end and a small toe box, is a condition known as toe crowding, in which little space is available between the toes, resulting in the loss of balance and proper muscle function within the entire foot.

Fortunately, this is all reversible. Of course, you can't reverse it in two weeks by buying Vibram FiveFingers, getting a stress fracture, and then filing a lawsuit against the minimalist shoe company for false advertising. Just like losing weight after twenty years of poor eating, movement, and lifestyle habits, reinventing your feet takes patience. For most of my clients who wore cushioned, overprotected shoes much of their lives, it took years to transition to going fully minimalist or barefoot and to develop strong and natural feet. Fortunately, with kids, things happen faster. Because they have a greater ability to remodel bone and build muscle, children can reshape and redevelop foot structure and bones within just three months.

- Walk barefoot as much as possible, without even socks. Removing your socks allows for the development of more proprioceptive nerve endings on the bottoms of your feet.

- Be sure that when you walk, your feet point straight ahead. To test this, you can find straight lines on the floor or sidewalk and see how closely your feet align to the line. Most people walk with their toes slightly turned out, which can interfere with the proper use of muscles and ligaments in the feet, knees, and hips.

- Choose shoes that are super flexible or minimalist. Good brands include but are not limited to Xero, Vibram, Vivo Barefoot, Happy Little Soles, Bobux, Merrell, and Nike Free.

- Play foot games yourself or with your kids to encourage motor skills and healthy foot development. For example, you can pick up marbles with your toes and then drop them into a cup, or scrunch up a towel with your toes before using your hands to return the towel back to its original position. Both are fantastic exercises for plantar fasciitis as well.

- If you get a massage, be sure that your therapist spends plenty of time on your feet. A traditional Chinese medicine practitioner well versed in foot reflexology can work on your feet as well. Look for one certified by the National Certification Commission for Acupuncture and Oriental Medicine.

- Every day, at your desk, while talking on the phone, or even while seated and eating, you can roll up and down and side to side on your feet a golf ball, lacrosse ball, or tiny foam-roller-like devices made specifically for foot massages. TheraFlow is a good brand, readily available online, and I'll include a few other key choices on BoundlessBook.com/17.

- Throughout the day, try lifting and spreading your toes and holding the position for thirty to sixty seconds. The exercise will help you develop stronger toe flexors, which are the muscles that help you lift your toes toward your shins. Studies show that the strength of these muscles is a surprisingly good indicator of your overall health. In addition, you can use Happy Feet Socks, which spread the toes and strengthen the feet. Happy Feet makes options for both children and adults.

- If you live near sand or have beach access, run and walk barefoot in the sand, which is one of the best ways to both strengthen and stretch the feet.

HOW TO HACK YOUR WORKPLACE FOR OPTIMIZED SYMMETRY

Whenever I post photos of my elaborate home office setup to Instagram, Facebook, Twitter, or other social media outlets on which trolls come pouring out of the woodwork to ridicule every last shred of my existence, I'm often torn to pieces about "how complex it all seems" and "why can't I just sit in a chair at a desk like normal people?"

Fact is, I am neither embarrassed by or shy about my unique workplace environment. Why? Frankly, because after years of finishing up a day at the computer feeling as though my eyeballs were burning out of their sockets, my back was a chunk of immovable concrete, and my elbows and wrists were throbbing with overuse pain, I now feel like a million bucks after a day of typing, calls, writing, podcasting, research, and more. In my opinion, unless you're baling hay in the hail or sucking down coal dust in a mine, you should feel healthy and full of energy after a day of productive work, not beat up, locked up, and ready to stay couch-bound for the remainder of the evening.

Although I have plenty of strategies for optimizing air, light, water, and electricity in my office—most of which you'll discover in chapter 20—in this section, I'm going to focus on workplace ergonomics: specifically, how to align a desk with a human body to lessen muscle fatigue, increase productivity, and reduce the number and severity of work-related musculoskeletal disorders, such as low back pain, carpal tunnel syndrome, and elbow tendinitis, all of which can produce biomechanical disorders and asymmetries.

Stand-Up Desk

I don't sit all day. I also don't stand all day. Instead, I switch positions as frequently as possible (about every fifteen to thirty minutes), from seated to standing to lunging to kneeling to walking to right leg up on a stool to left leg up on a stool… You get the idea. This is because standing for long periods of time has been shown to be just as bad for you as sitting for long periods of time, as anyone who has stood all day and experienced blood pooling, stiff knees and hips, locked-up back, and eventual varicose veins can attest. Enter the stand-up desk, which I talked about in chapter 12. I use a simple nonmotorized model that comes equipped with a hand crank that I can easily adjust, with the added bonus of a quick biceps workout. For a list of some of the better stand-up desk models, visit BoundlessBook.com/17.

Saddle Chair

The Salli saddle chair that holds a hallowed place in my office was designed by my friend and former competitive bareback-riding champion Veli-Jussi Jalkanen, a sixty-five-year-old Finnish inventor who plays tennis right-handed and left-handed, swims buck naked every morning in an ice-cold river, spends hours each evening planning new inventions in his giant sauna, and is obsessed with both prostate and low-back health. This guy goes by the nickname "Vessi" and is one of the most physically talented older men I've ever met. He competes in several sports on a national and competitive level, including shooting, diving, and sprinting. He still rides horses, skis, skin dives, walks extremely long distances with heavy packs, and swing dances. The guy can crank out twenty-five pull-ups, speaks multiple languages, owns several multinational corporations, and looks like he's about forty years old. Most relevant to what you're now reading, he also designed what I consider to be the Cadillac of ergonomic back- and butt-friendly chairs to keep your posture upright, your pelvis in a neutral position, and, most important for you guys out there, your balls and prostate happy and free.

Stool

When I'm not standing upright at my desk, I'm typically leaning back against a special stand-up, height-adjustable stool called a Mogo (basically, imagine a stool designed for you to lean against at an angle). It is a simple, no-frills standing desk accessory equipped with a nonslip rubber foot that works on indoor surfaces, along with a reinforced-fiberglass turf tip that keeps you stabilized on grass, dirt, and turf, making it perfect to toss in the car for the kids' soccer games. The seat collapses down and folds to take on the go, easily fitting in a backpack or suitcase, and only weighs about 2 pounds. The seat pan is designed to cradle your bum in a pelvis-friendly position, similar to the Salli saddle chair.

Manual Treadmill

I'll admit that it can be tough to type or engage in deep work while walking on a treadmill, but for phone calls, consults with my clients, Skype meetings, Kion team huddles, and other tasks conducive to talking rather than typing, you'll usually find me churning out miles on my treadmill. I tend to walk at a slow pace for two to three miles during any given workday. I opted for a manual treadmill with a curved belt for two reasons: (1) electrical treadmills are notorious for churning out massive amounts of dirty electricity, along with WiFi and Bluetooth, and (2) I wanted a treadmill that would double as a workout tool I could perform high-intensity sprints on. An added bonus is that this style of treadmill also trains your body to both walk and run with flawless biomechanics. The best models currently available are the Assault AirRunner and the SpeedFit.

Balance Board

You've no doubt seen or toyed around with balance-challenging devices and boards like a BOSU ball or a Wobble board. Problem is, these tools are so difficult to balance on that they make it hard to focus while working. I've settled on a happy medium: a beautiful, wood-finished, slightly but not overly challenging balance device called the FluidStance, which I happen to be balancing on while I type this very sentence.

Mat

There are a variety of topographical or cushioned mats that you can stand on while working to stretch and entertain your feet and tone your tiny foot muscles, and they provide you with a more comfortable surface and greater variety of standing positions than a hard floor or carpet. I have two such mats in my office: a TerraMat antifatigue mat equipped with terrain features that encourage frequent movement and a special design to engage the blood-pumping mechanism of your calves, and a kybun kyBounder mat, which was designed by former podcast guest and Swiss inventor Karl Müller after he was inspired by walking in rice paddy fields in South Korea.

Golf Ball

While there are about eight billion varieties of fancy body-massage balls and tools that you can use to massage and strengthen your feet while standing or seated, I'm partial to the perfectly sized, ideally textured, inexpensive, easy-to-find golf ball. I simply roll one around on each foot for about fifteen minutes at any given point during the workday. If I lose one, there are always plenty more to be found.

Doorframe Pull-Up Bar

In my opinion, everyone needs an easy-to-install pull-up bar in at least one doorframe of their house, their office, their garage, or all three. Even if you can't crank out a few pull-ups every time you walk under it (my rule is five pull-ups, allowing me to do thirty to fifty pull-ups on any given day), it's perfect to simply hang from with one or both arms to stretch the shoulders, decompress the spine, and traction the wrists. You'll find a multitude of options online, and I'll link to a few of my favorites on BoundlessBook.com/17.

Ergonomic Keyboard

For a long time, I was resistant to the idea of venturing beyond my simple MacBook Pro and into the realm of giant external monitors and cushy ergonomic keyboards. But after making the switch to both (see below for my monitor choice), I'll never go back. Sure, I can't easily take my ergonomic keyboard with me when traveling or use it while working on an airplane, but for cranking out several hours of writing with pain-free wrists and elbows, I'll never go back being hunched over my tiny laptop keyboard with my giant hands and fingers in a cramped-up clawed position, hunting for keys. I currently use the Ergo Pro keyboard connected to my MacBook Pro (I prefer the non-Bluetooth version to reduce dirty electricity, a concept I'll talk more about in chapter 20).

Antiglare Monitor

Do you ever get headaches after working on a computer for a long time? Eye strain? Mild irritation? Brain fog? It's not all in your head. See, just like most televisions, computer monitors flicker. Monitors have been flickering for many years, but most people don't realize this because the flicker is invisible. But the flicker is still hard on your eyes and is just one of the computer monitor issues responsible for the growing epidemic of nearsightedness and myopia—also known as computer vision syndrome.

Even fancy LCD monitors are not flicker-free, though many people think they are. These LCD monitors originally started out using something called CCFL, or cold cathode fluorescent lamps, as a backlight source for the monitor, but in recent years manufacturers have shifted to using LEDs, or light-emitting diodes. If you have one of those thin monitors, then you probably have an LCD screen with LED, and if you are unsure, you can check the model number on the back of the monitor and google it. The use of LED has numerous benefits, including lower power consumption, far fewer toxic substances because of the absence of the cathode, and some fantastic picture-quality advantages, but along with all these benefits come potential eyestrain issues that can damage and destroy your eyes over the long term.

See, when your monitor is set to maximum brightness, the LEDs are glowing at full strength. If you reduce the brightness setting, the LEDs need to emit less light, and this is accomplished with small breaks or pauses (flickers!)—the LEDs turn off for a short, nearly imperceptible time. When you reduce the brightness setting of your monitor even more, the breaks become longer. This creates a frustrating catch-22: a bright screen can strain your eyes, but the flicker created by a dimmer screen can also strain your eyes. Compared to old-school CCFL monitors, the newer LED-based monitors carry the greatest risk of giving you eyestrain, tired eyes, or nasty headaches.

My friend and software designer Daniel Georgiev, a brilliant young computer programmer from Bulgaria, has fixed this entire issue by inventing a special software called Iris that controls the brightness of the monitor with the help of your computer's video card, allowing you to have adequate brightness without the flicker. It even automatically adjusts your computer monitor's settings based on the sun's position wherever you happen to be in the world. When paired with my eye-friendly, low-flicker Eizo monitor and a decent set of blue-light-blocking glasses, I can type for hours with zero headaches or vision issues. You can learn more about this entire setup in my podcast with Daniel, linked to at BoundlessBook.com/17.

Dictation Software

Finally, I've been kicking myself for not discovering Dragon Dictation software earlier. The concept is quite simple: you talk and the computer types. Sure, after vocalizing an entire chapter of a book, an article, or an email, I still have to swoop in and do a few quick edits (even after two years of dictation, my assistant Marge's name still autocorrects to "March"), but when it's paired with a Jabra 930 headset, Dragon Dictation's accuracy far exceeds that of any other dictation software I've experimented with. It allowed me to be a hyperproductive author even when battling a bout of tennis elbow, which is what inspired me to look into voice-to-text solutions in the first place two years ago. I now dictate about 30 percent of my writing.

The Bottom Line

Are there other tactics I could use besides those I've mentioned above? Sure. I could go out and buy the fancy under-desk cycling machine I saw a few weeks ago in the back of the airline magazine, I could slap some gravity boots on the ole pull-up bar for some Batman-style decompression, and I could probably even hire a Zen master bodyworker to gently massage my tight traps while I'm hunched over the keyboard.

But what I've just shared with you are the tried-and-true tools that have worked best for me—without littering my office with every biohack known to man. For even more, listen to my podcast "The Healthy Writer: How to Keep Your Keyboard, Mouse, Laptop and Writing Habits from Destroying Your Health" and read the book *Deskbound* by Kelly Starrett—you'll find links to both on BoundlessBook.com/17.

Finally, even in the absence of a formal standing workstation or other fancy devices in your office, you can adopt a wide variety of sitting postures when working on a laptop or reading magazines, papers, or books at a coffee shop, in a living room, at a restaurant, or elsewhere. Amazingly, new research reveals that adopting a wide variety of sitting postures can help to control blood sugar and development of tendinopathies. These postures can include the following positions:

- A full squat, with heels down (stretches the back, glutes, quads, and calves)
- A high kneel (stretches the quads, Achilles tendon, and foot fasciae)
- A low kneel (stretches the feet and quads)
- A long sit (stretches the hamstrings and wrist flexors)
- A side sit (stretches the external and internal rotators of the hip)
- A cross-legged sit (stretches the hip adductors and rotators)

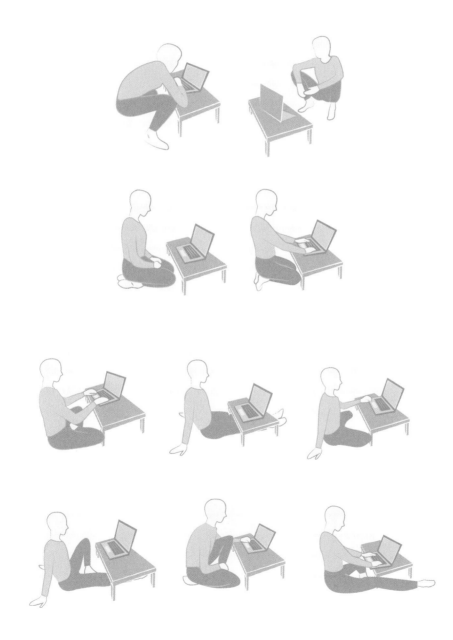

Office Stretches

Standing or sitting in one position all day while you're working can cause your joints to become stiff and subject your neck and back to long-term, chronic compression, which can lead to back pain, poor posture, and physical performance degradation. Ideally, you should switch your working positions throughout the day, take short exercise and walking breaks, or use a treadmill workstation to avoid these problems, but if you find yourself forced to be seated for an extended period of time, you can perform the following exercises to decompress your joints, improve blood and lymphatic flow, eliminate aches, and keep your energy levels higher throughout the day. When I'm at conferences or in meetings, I'll often use these stretches and poses, which take full advantage of what causes many of the problems in the first place: a chair. You don't need to perform all these stretches at once but can weave them in throughout the day.

1. Standing Overhead Reach

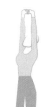

Stand with your feet hip-width apart and your toes pointing forward. Grasp your fingers together and turn your hands so that your palms face up. Reach overhead with your clasped hands and press your palms up while engaging your shoulders and core. Hold the position and take five deep breaths. Release the position, then repeat twice more.

2. Butterfly Elbows

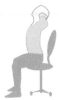

While seated, sit tall and place your fingertips behind your ears (without interlocking them). Make sure you're not applying any pressure to your neck or the back of your head. Lift up your chest and ribs and pull your elbows back until you feel a stretch across your chest. Inhale deeply, and, as you exhale, round your back, drop your chin and bring your elbows together in front of you while pressing your elbows forward to stretch out your upper back and shoulder blades. As you inhale again, return to the starting position. Repeat the movement for a total of four full reps.

3. Chair Chest Opener

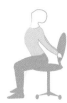

While sitting on the very edge of your chair, reach your hands back and grab the sides of the back of the chair with your thumbs pointing down. Roll your shoulders back and down, lift your chest, and elongate your neck (imagine you're pressing into the ceiling with the top of your head). To stretch out your chest, lean deeper into the movement. Take five deep breaths, release, then repeat once more.

4. Standing Chair Lat Stretch

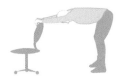

Stand about three feet away facing your chair. While keeping your knees slightly bent, bend at the hips and reach out to grab the top of the back of the chair, keeping your arms straight. Flatten your lower back and lengthen your shoulders to form a straight line from your hands to your hips. Line up your head between your arms and take five deep breaths. Release the position, then repeat once more.

5. Standing Chair Lat Twist

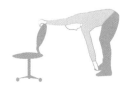

In the position held at the end of the Standing Chair Lat Stretch, with your knees slightly bent and your lower back flat, reach down with your right hand and touch your left foot. Hold this position and take two breaths, then return to the original position with both hands on the back of the chair. Twist in the opposite direction and touch your right foot with your left hand, holding for two breaths. Repeat the movement twice more on each side.

6. Mirrored Chair Pose

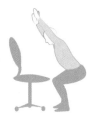

Face your chair and put your feet together. Squat and try to match the height of the chair with the tops of your thighs. While maintaining a straight spine, reach overhead with your palms facing each other. Hold the position and take five breaths. Release and repeat twice more.

7. Seated Figure 4 Hip Stretch

Sit with both feet flat on the ground. Place your right ankle across your left knee and flex your right foot. Sit tall with your back straight and lean forward while pressing down on your right knee until you feel a stretch in your hips. Hold the position and take three breaths. Release and repeat with your left ankle, then repeat twice more on each side.

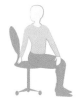

8. Seated Spinal Twist

Start by sitting with both feet flat on the ground. Put your right arm over the back of the chair, and put your left hand on your right knee. Press with both hands as you look over your right shoulder and twist your torso. To give yourself more space to twist, lean slightly forward. Hold the position and take two deep breaths. Release and repeat on the other side. Repeat the movement twice more on each side.

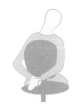

9. Bound Neck Stretch

Sit tall in your chair and reach down with your right arm (you can grasp the seat of the chair as long as you're still able to keep your arm straight). Reach behind your back with your left hand, clasp your right wrist and tilt your neck to the right. You can enhance the stretch by gently pressing your arm away from your torso. Hold the position and take two deep breaths. Release and repeat with the opposite arm. Repeat the movement twice more on each side.

10. Alternating Fingers Wrist Stretch

Sit tall in your chair and stretch your right arm straight in front of you with your fingers pointing down. With your left hand, gently pull on the back of your right hand to stretch out the top of your right wrist. Hold the position and take two breaths, then flip your right hand so that your palm faces out and your fingers point up. Pull gently on the front of your right hand with your left to stretch out the bottom of your right wrist. Hold the position and take two breaths. Stretch the top and bottom of your right wrist twice more, then repeat the movements for three reps with the opposite hand.

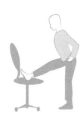

11. Hamstring Stretch

Stand about two feet away facing your chair. Place the heel of your right foot in the middle of the chair while flexing your right foot (try to point your toes upward). While keeping both knees slightly bent, put your hands on your hips and bend forward until you feel a stretch in your right hamstring. Hold the position and take three deep breaths. Release and switch to the left leg. Repeat once more with each leg.

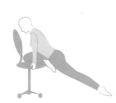

12. Chair Pigeon Pose

Stand facing your chair, bend your right knee, and place your right calf across the front of your chair while flexing your right foot (your knee should be on the chair while your foot should be off the edge). Grab both sides of the seat and step back with your left leg until your left knee and hip are straight. You can make the stretch deeper or shallower by bending or straightening your elbows. Hold the position and take three deep breaths. Release and switch to your left leg. Repeat once more on each side.

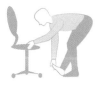

13. Single Leg Toe Pull

Stand up and face your chair. Bend forward from the hips and place both hands on the front of the seat. Reach down and grab your right toes with your right hand while keeping your left hand on the seat and slightly bending your left leg. Gently pull up on your right toes until your calf and hamstring feel stretched (try to keep your hips square and your lower back flat). Hold the position and take two breaths. Release and switch to the left arm and leg. Repeat twice more on each side.

DAILY MOVEMENT
TIPS FOR SYMMETRY

When it comes to daily movement, the three most potent movement habits I utilize for mobility and symmetry are as follows: (1) daily morning mobility snacks, (2) Foundation Training, and (3) ELDOA exercises.

Mobility Snacks

Let's begin with the first habit: mobility snacks. See, it's relatively rare that I can find the time to spend a solid ninety minutes getting a full-body massage therapy session, or even hunt down an hour for a self-inflicted deep tissue session with a foam roller, a deep tissue massage ball, a vibration tool, or any other strange tissue-mobilization devices from what my wife refers to as my medieval torture box of body tools. But while the water for my French press coffee is heating and the coffee is steeping, I can indeed find just ten to fifteen minutes to hunt down and mobilize any tight, sore, or adhered areas from the previous day's activities. With this approach, I spend 70 to 105 minutes each week fixing my body and symmetry. For example, just this morning I performed these activities:

- Rumble Roller on my shoulders (the Rumble Roller is a foam roller equipped with teeth-gritting ridges)
- Lacrosse ball on the back of each knee to mobilize the hamstring attachment in popliteal space
- Myobuddy massage tool on both wrists and inner elbows
- Elastic band traction on my right shoulder
- Rumble Roller on my left and right hips
- Peanut (two lacrosse balls taped together) up and down my spine
- Light stretching after all of the above

Each morning, the routine slightly changes, but the goal is always the same: spend just ten to fifteen minutes in a desperate act of self-love, keeping the many pieces of my body together.

Foundation Training

My second habit is Foundation Training, which, along with the third habit of ELDOA stretches, I weave in throughout my day during work breaks, when I'm in the sauna, as a workout warm-up or cooldown, or even if I have a few minutes left after my morning mobility snacks.

To understand how Foundation Training works, you must understand how gravity affects your body. Just think about all the different things that happen when gravity hits your body—specifically, gravity's ability to adversely affect the following physiological systems:

- **Respiratory system:** A compressed rib cage limits the lungs' ability to expand and diminishes your breathing capacity.
- **Digestive system:** Squashed organs don't function nearly as well as they should, and that burdens the body's ability to gain nourishment from food.

- **Circulatory system:** Squeezed blood vessels are not as efficient or as effective as they ought to be in transporting nutrients, oxygen, carbon dioxide, hormones, and blood cells to where they need to be.

- **Nervous system:** A compressed spinal cord and constricted neural pathways slow the progress of all those neurotransmitters trying to communicate from the periphery to the central nervous system—and back again—and can undermine the brain's ability to coordinate and influence all the activities of your body.

Hunching all day at a keyboard, tilting our heads forward over our phones, commuting long hours, and slouching on the couch simply magnify and aggravate these problems, resulting in poor posture that throws our bodies out of balance, causing unnecessary stress and strain that compromises our joints, restricts organ function, and weakens our force output.

So the reasoning goes something like this: If you can wake up in the morning and do something that fights all the effects of gravity and restores your body to a decompressed state that theoretically allows you to feel better and stands taller all day long, with better digestion, no low back pain, and enhanced circulation...

...why not try it?

Dr. Eric Goodman, as you may recall from chapter 3, developed Foundation Training to heal and correct back pain by training your posterior chain muscles—your shoulders, back, butt, and legs—to properly support your body. Now, many professional and Olympic athletes use his system every day to enhance performance and force output while maintaining the health of the entire spine. Fans of Foundational Training include Chad Reed, a motocross and supercross world champion; Lakey Peterson, a women's surfing champion; Tour de France cyclists; and many more.

Foundation Training is all about your core, and, as Dr. Goodman explains in *True to Form*, a book that systematizes his entire approach, your core is anything that connects to your pelvis, whether above or below it, including your hamstrings, glutes, and adductor muscles. Your functional movement capacity, your athletic ability, flexibility, balance, and strength all depend on a powerful core, and Foundation Training teaches all those core muscles to work together through specific full-body movements and breathing patterns. Foundational Training includes moves that target the following muscles:

- **Glutes:** Properly activated glutes, otherwise known as a "turned-on butt," are crucial for correct movement patterns and posture.

- **Adductors:** Your inner thigh muscles are your built-in traction system. When this muscle group remains strong, you have increased hip stability, stronger arches in the feet, and a pelvic brace that protects your back with a couple of the strongest muscles in your body.

- **Deep lower-back muscles:** These facilitate the proper integration of the posterior chain muscles and the "talk" between your glutes and pelvis.

- **Abdomen and hip flexors:** It can seem like a bit of a disconnect, but think of these front lower muscles of your body as directly affecting the mobility and function of the back lower muscles. If the front is too tight, the back will not work properly.

- **Transverse abdominis:** These deep ab muscles are your built-in bracing system, and when the transverse abdominis is tightened against the other muscles in this core group, the entire system becomes stronger.

Here's one Foundation Training exercise: the Founder.

1. Stand with your feet hip-distance apart and your weight on your heels.
2. Let your knees unlock and pull your hips back as you push your chest forward.
3. Without moving your feet, pull your heels together to activate your adductor muscles.
4. You should feel tension in your low back, adductors, glutes, and hamstrings; these muscles let you know your posterior chain is active.

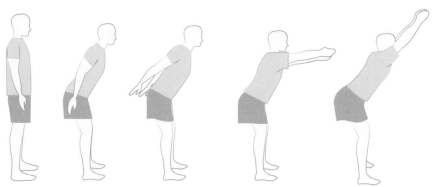

5. Chest is high with arms back and your thumbs out to the side, shoulders pulling back and down. Hold for 15 seconds.

6. Bring your arms out in front as you pull your hips away from your ankles. Hold for 15 seconds.

7. Bring your arms all the way up as you lift your chest slightly higher. Hold for 15 seconds.

Source: FoundationTraining.com. Used by permission.

Every exercise in Foundation Training is designed to include as many muscles in a given movement as possible, disperse more force throughout your body, and take friction away from your joints by placing that tension into the proper core muscles instead. Every exercise lengthens the front of your body, where the overtightened, overshortened muscles in your body are, and strengthens and lengthens the back of your body, allowing you to stand tall and to move powerfully, gracefully, and with a lot of flexibility. So what exactly is happening to your body when you implement moves like this?

1. **You turn your butt on.** The contract-and-hold nature of Foundation Training is technically a form of eccentric force dispersion, especially among the posterior chain muscles such as your glutes and hamstrings. Improved muscle tone, muscle chain integration, and more efficient muscular contractions are all consequences of this type of eccentric training. When you stimulate a muscle's ability to absorb force before you ask that muscle to generate force, it learns efficiency and proper posture. In short, you turn your butt on so that you use your glute muscles well throughout workouts, standing postures, and sitting postures during the rest of the day.

2. **You breathe more deeply.** When it comes to oxygenation, mitochondrial health, and overall nervous system strength, there is nothing you can do that is more important than breathing well. Your serratus muscles are of key significance to rib cage expansion during inspiration, and during the decompression breathing that accompanies every Foundation movement, you train your serratus musculature, particularly during the exhalation of each breath. (Important note: Your lungs are in your rib cage, not your abdomen.) Considering you breathe twelve thousand to twenty-two thousand times per day, it's pretty dang important that you execute this repetitive pattern properly.

3. **You increase innervation and blood flow to your skull.** You have important neurological and vascular tissue traveling through the area on which the base of your skull rests. To open blood flow to these areas, you must actively lengthen and increase space along the back of the neck as well as the front of the chest. The cranial nerves deserve more respect, attention, and space than they can receive in the postures associated with anterior head carriage, such as sitting at a desk or driving in a car. Foundation Training lengthens the spaces around these nerves and pulls your head and neck into a more appropriate position.

There are also a host of other benefits to Foundation Training, from improved digestion to increased force output from the powerful glute muscles, but you now know everything you need to know to explain to your loved one or neighbors why you're sticking your butt out and breathing with your hands clamped across your rib cage every morning, right?

I'm a big fan of the minimum effective dose of any body-enhancing program like this, so I personally keep the chart at right, from Dr. Goodman's book, on my phone and try to perform the list of exercises for each respective day, weaving them throughout the day. Each day's exercises take about ten minutes to incorporate.

Monday, Wednesday, Friday *3 repetitions of each*	Tuesday, Thursday, Saturday *3 repetitions of each*
1. Standing Decompression	1. Supine Decompression
2. Lunge Decompression	2. Prone Decompression
3. Woodpecker	3. Founder
4. Internal Leg Tracing	4. Woodpecker
5. Anchored Bridge	5. Woodpecker Rotation
6. Anchored Back Extension	6. Integrated Hinges
7. Kneeling Decompression	

ELDOA Exercises

And finally, there are the ELDOA exercises. Two years ago, a guy knocked on my front door. He'd flown all the way from Alabama to my house to train me in a new method of movement and deep fascial stretching that I had never before encountered, something he called the ELDOA Method. Now don't get me wrong: as you've probably already suspected, I've done my fair share of mobility training. But this guy, Jacob Schoen, spent the weekend at my house and trained me for eight solid hours, introducing me to a completely new form of extremely intensive stretching, which I now take breaks from work to do each day. It is one of the best ways to eliminate lower back pain, heal the spine, and get a full-body myofascial stretch.

"ELDOA" is a French acronym that stands for *étirements longitudinaux avec décoaptition ostéo-articulaire*, which translates to "longitudinal stretching with osteoarticular decoaptation." Yep, that's a mouthful. The method consists of postural exercises that target specific joints to decompress, relieve pain, and restore function and balance. With the primary goal of applying high amounts of internal tension to reduce pressure on the spinal discs, increase blood flow, and reduce back pain, ELDOA is based on the concept of using self-induced myofascial stretching and traction to put tension around a joint.

The method itself consists of multiple positions that maximize fascial tension around a joint, typically over the course of a series of transitions that progressively increase fascial tension and cause decoaptation at the desired spinal level (*decoaptation* is the term used to describe a reduction in compression forces at a joint). Each rep of an ELDOA stretch is held for ten to thirty seconds and performed with deep, diaphragmatic breaths. When performed correctly, these stretches literally make you feel as though you're being quartered by a horse, medieval-style, but the rush of blood to the joint, the extreme stretch, and the mobility of the body parts you stretch with ELDOA is unparalleled.

On BoundlessBook.com/17, you'll find several helpful videos of what ELDOA looks like, along with my podcast with Jacob. But I focus on three primary ELDOA stretches that give me the most bang for my buck: T6–T7 (this stands for thoracic vertebrae 6 and 7), T8–T9, and L5–S1 (lumbar and sacral vertebrae, respectively).

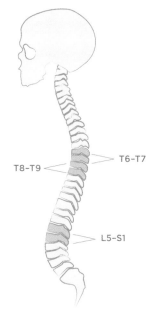

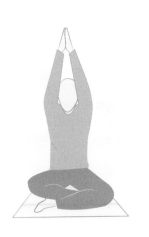

ELDOA T6–T7 stretch

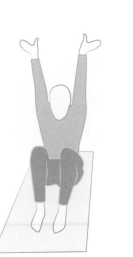

ELDOA T8–T9 stretch

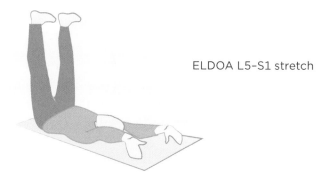

ELDOA L5–S1 stretch

Egoscue

At the time of this writing, I've begun to use a form of symmetrical training called Egoscue. Founded by Pete Egoscue in the 1970s, the Egoscue Method is a form of postural therapy designed to fix misalignment in the body. It's a series of simple exercises and stretches that restores musculoskeletal balance and symmetry, returning the body to its proper posture and bringing you back to an active, pain-free lifestyle. The Egoscue Method reeducates your muscles on how to function to maintain proper alignment. Recently, I watched with fascination as one of the Egoscue master trainers, Brian

Bradley, showed me a video of a ripped thirteen-year-old soccer player decimating his entire soccer squad by over ten seconds on a 400-meter track run. The difference between this young man and the others? He did no weight training—only bodyweight training and Egoscue.

To get a better idea of how Egoscue works, look at the five-minute video of Egoscue Train Anywhere exercises on YouTube—you'll find a link on BoundlessBook.com/17—and visit egoscue.com.

SLEEP YOUR WAY TO SYMMETRY

When I settle down for a night of sleep, my head is resting against a 650 down pillow for the ideal combination of comfort and neck and head support, and a special side-sleeping pillow is tucked between my knees for added biomechanical support. My entire body is supported on a special gel matrix called an Intellibed, which provides memory-foam-like softness combined with firm support for my long, lanky frame.

The fact is, I'm a bit of a diva when it comes to my sleep surface and sleep posture—which I'm not ashamed of when you consider the fact that I spend about one-third of my life in a bed, as most humans should. Even if you sleep just 7 hours a night, this means you lie down for over 2,400 hours each year!

An improper sleeping position is a notorious cause of bad posture and poor symmetry, resulting in a spine that isn't able to distribute forces as optimally as it was intended to, poor posture during the day after a night of bad sleep, and a body that's wracked with aches and pains. The good news is that there are sleeping positions and sleeping surfaces that promote the greatest amount of symmetry, equally distribute stress throughout the body, provide the optimal position for back health, and minimize uncomfortable compression of joints and muscles.

Your chosen sleeping posture should encourage symmetry and alignment of your entire body. Because each body type and body symmetry is highly variable, there is no single, perfect sleeping posture—but there are definite pros, cons, and best practices for each posture.

Back Sleeping

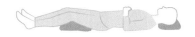

Let's begin with sleeping on your back. This position promotes symmetry the most, equally distributes stress throughout the body, and compresses joints the least. The cons? It can contribute to sleep apnea and snoring, can place more stress on the lower back, and can be uncomfortable for people with preexisting poor posture. If you decide to sleep on your back, I recommend you place a pillow underneath your knees. This will cause a slight bend in your hips and knees and allow your lower back to flatten against your mattress. This position can also alleviate any tension throughout the lower back. Try setting pillows under your knees at different heights until you find the most supportive position.

At your head, place the pillow so that it supports the small of your neck. There should be complete contact of your neck on the pillow and no contact on the backs of your shoulders. Make sure that the back of your head is in contact with the pillow, and not the top of your head. One pillow that works particularly well for back sleeping is the Neck Nest, which was designed by my friend Peter Martone. (On BoundlessBook.com/17, you'll find a discount code for the Neck Nest, along with a link to my interview with Peter on this and many of his other sleep posture tricks.)

If you're sleeping on your back, you can also place a pillow by your side to help offload the weight of your arms, and if you want to truly upgrade a back-sleeping position, shop for a zero-gravity bed or listen to my podcast on zero-gravity sleeping. Finally, if you are going to sleep on your back, when you first get into bed, try my friend Esther Gokhale's method of stretch lying:

1. Lie down on your back.
2. Bend both knees and plant your feet on the bed hip-width apart.
3. Prop your upper body up on your elbows.
4. Slowly lower yourself onto the bed one vertebra at a time.
5. Place your hands behind your head and slowly elongate the back of your neck.

6. Pull your shoulder blades away from your ears and down toward your feet.

7. Straighten out your body and allow your legs to relax to the sides.

You'll find a helpful video for this technique at BoundlessBook.com/17.

Side Sleeping

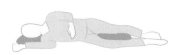

Although I nap on my back, for a full night of sleep I'm a side sleeper, and I've found that the hip-misalignment issues that can be brought on by side sleeping can be alleviated by ensuring that the spine is in a straight and neutral position while sleeping. Side sleeping reduces snoring and sleep apnea issues, and if you, like me, lie awake at night staring at the ceiling when you attempt to sleep on your back, side sleeping is a perfect alternative sleeping position. But it does increase stress on one side of the body and can have a high risk of misalignment, especially if you have wide shoulders or hips.

Proper side-sleeping alignment is also highly dependent on proper mattress support, which I'll talk about later in this chapter. For a proper side-sleeping position, first place a pillow between your legs (a quick online search for "side sleeping pillow" will give you a host of good options, and a few of my favorites are listed on BoundlessBook.com/17). This will prevent your upper legs from rotating the rest of your body. You can also support your upper arm with a pillow to offload any stress on your shoulder. For your head support, place the pillow in the small of your neck. There should be complete contact of your neck and no pillow contact on the back of your shoulders.

While a slight bend of the knees is fine, avoid the curled-up-in-a-ball fetal position, which can compress your entire body and cause bad posture and hunched shoulders. Instead, remain lengthened and elongated through the spine. It helps to imagine someone is pulling your head up to make you taller. You may not be able to stay in the same side-sleeping position throughout the night, and many people rotate from the left side to the right side, which is completely normal, although you will likely spend the greatest percentage of time on one side or the other.

Finally, the added benefit to side sleeping? Glymphatic drainage of toxins from your head (see the box on the facing page).

Stomach Sleeping

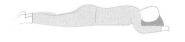

So, as you've just learned, the back and the side sleeping positions are both acceptable. But what about sleeping on your stomach? Unless you want a neck injury, a sore jaw, or a hyperextended low back, I do not recommend stomach sleeping. The only time this position is biomechanically appropriate is if your bed has a face hole in it, like a massage table, allowing you to sleep with your neck straight. While I have a couple of friends who do indeed sleep on their stomachs on a massage table, even they primarily use it for naps, not for a full night of sleep. There are simply too many head, neck, sinus, and shoulder issues that arise from attempting to spend eight hours laid out on your stomach.

Choosing the Right Mattress

Of course, no discussion about sleep would be complete without a consideration of the actual sleeping surface, a.k.a. your mattress. Until last year, I slept on a relatively spendy 100 percent organic nontoxic mattress equipped with memory foam, organic latex, and a host of other frills, including organic essential oils, hevea milk, and rare plant extracts. I was getting the ultimate in

How to Drain Your Brain During Sleep

A term that emerged in science only when research revealed its existence in 2016, *brain drain* refers to the glymphatic system, which, you'll recall from chapter 7, is a functional waste-clearance system for the central nervous system, similar to the lymphatic system for the rest of your body.

The glymphatic system facilitates the exchange of cerebrospinal fluid for interstitial fluid to clear interstitial waste from the brain parenchyma, the functional tissue of the brain (both white and gray matter). This waste is moved into venous pathways and ultimately cleared via lymphatic vessels in your cervical spine. Activation of the glymphatic pathway is controlled by the brain's arousal level. During sleep, when the brain is relatively quiet, the volume of its interstitial space expands. This increased interstitial space, when paired with a solid night of sleep, results in efficient waste removal.

Perhaps the most notable waste cleared by the glymphatic system is the soluble amyloid that can otherwise build up and accumulate as amyloid plaques in the brain. Research has shown that patients suffering from chronic impairment of the glymphatic pathway function due to traumatic brain injury are more vulnerable to neurodegeneration and have an increased chance of developing dementia and Alzheimer's. So it turns out that draining the brain is important!

Interestingly, research has also confirmed that glymphatic transport and clearance is significantly superior when you sleep on your side or your stomach. Sleeping on your stomach is not great for back health, posture, or symmetry, but sleeping on your side with a small pillow between your legs is actually an ideal sleeping position, especially if it doesn't bother your head, neck, and hips.

One other fascinating fact I noted while reviewing the scientific literature on glymphatic drainage is that any sleep medication that mimics anesthesia, including, most notably, popular sleep pharmaceuticals such as Ambien and Valium, limits glymphatic drainage—meaning that although you may be lying in bed for eight hours, you're definitely not going through normal sleep cycles, nor are you engaging in efficient waste removal.

super-soft hippie sleep, and I was also limiting my exposure to polybrominated diphenyl ethers (which can poison your thyroid gland), formaldehyde (a known carcinogen), chemical flame retardants, polyurethane foam (which releases volatile organic compounds around your body while you sleep), and bioavailable antimony, a heavy metal notoriously found in mattresses.

Problem is, although I was limiting my exposure to chemicals and toxins, I was waking up each morning with low back pain, locked-up hips, and a sore neck. In a nutshell, the mattress simply wasn't supporting my beat-up athlete's body in an ideal fashion. Upon asking my friends who are equally obsessed with a good night's sleep what mattress they recommended, I learned from my friend Katie, the famed health blogger of WellnessMama.com, of a special gel-matrix sleep surface called Intellibed.

While it's still toxin-free, the Intellibed also has a gel matrix that's designed to reduce joint pressure during sleep—by up to 80 percent compared to popular memory foam or adjustable air mattresses. It was even found to reduce bedsores and pressure wounds in hospitals. The mattress fabric stays cool during a night of sleep, which is integral to quality sleep, and provides all the comfort of memory foam with all the support of a firmer mattress. Some EMF-mitigating enthusiasts claim that the springs used in the Intellibed may be transmitting dirty electricity, but even this is only an issue if there are a significant number of electricity-producing devices scattered about the bedroom, such as WiFi routers, Bluetooth smart home apps, televisions, and other items I consider to be unnecessary in a hallowed sleep space.

In summary, whether you sleep on your back or on your side, be sure to support your body accordingly and select a mattress you're comfortable spending a third of your life on—guilt-free.

SELF-CARE ROUTINES

No discussion of beauty would be complete without a discussion of daily cleansing and care routines for your teeth and skin. You should already know the basics—wash your face every day, brush and floss your teeth regularly, don't use harsh cleansers, and so on. But here are the routines and compounds that I've personally found to be the most effective for maintaining my own healthy teeth and skin.

Oil Pulling

Oil pulling is a proven and time-honored method, particularly in Ayurvedic medicine, to remove bacteria and promote healthy teeth and gums. It can be more effective than flossing and is one of the best ways to naturally whiten your teeth, even without toothpaste or charcoal powder.

The procedure is simple: you simply swish about a tablespoon of oil, typically coconut oil, olive oil, sesame oil, or a blend of cleansing oils, in your mouth for five to twenty minutes.

This works by removing fat-soluble toxins and bacteria from your mouth when you spit out the oil and creating a clean oral environment that contributes to the prevention of gingivitis, bad breath, cavities, tooth decay, and gum infection. The *Journal of Ayurveda and Integrative Medicine* recently published a study that reviewed holistic approaches to oral health. The analysis revealed not only that oil pulling is one of the most effective natural solutions for preventing tooth decay and premature tooth loss but also that the effects of oil pulling reach far beyond oral health. For example, it may also help prevent heart disease (just google "heart disease oral health" to see what I mean), systemic inflammation, acne, and throat dryness, and it can also whiten teeth, strengthen the jaw, and, of course, help with TMJ symptoms.

Here are the exact details for correct oil pulling:

1. Do it first thing in the morning, before you brush your teeth or drink anything. I wake up, walk to the sink, put a tablespoon of oil in my mouth, and then swish for about ten minutes while preparing coffee, stretching, and performing other routine morning activities. The oil I currently use is a brand called The Dirt, which is a blend of coconut oil, sesame oil, and essential oils of peppermint, cardamom, clove, tea tree, turmeric, and rose, along with a hexane-free stevia extract, natural menthol, and rosemary extract.

2. Gently swish 1–2 tablespoons of the oil in your mouth and between your teeth for five to twenty minutes, but be sure that you don't swallow any of the oil, since it does contain toxins and bacteria from your mouth.

3. Spit out the oil in a trash can. Do not spit into the sink or toilet; it can clog the pipes. Then immediately rinse your mouth with water, swishing and spitting several times.

If you don't want an oil as complex as the one I use, you can still get plenty of benefits from coconut oil, but I recommend you add a few drops of essential oil to it for extra flavor and breath freshening, and also for the additional antibacterial benefits the oils can provide. I prefer peppermint, oregano, and/or lemon. Within one week of oil pulling each morning, you'll likely notice that you have a cleaner mouth and better morning breath.

Supermodeling Your Skin

Let's talk about what you slather—or don't slather—on your skin. The host of chemicals and harsh irritants present in most personal care products, as well as completely safe and natural solutions, will be covered in detail in chapter 20, but in this section, I'll share with you a few of the more potent skin-care compounds I've discovered and personally use on a daily basis.

To enhance the radiance of my skin, I used to smear my face every morning with extra-virgin olive oil. Olive oil? Yep, and here's why: Olive oil contains three major antioxidants—vitamin E, polyphenols, and phytosterols. These antioxidants can protect your skin from premature skin aging. Vitamin E partly accounts for the antiaging benefits of olive oil because it helps restore skin smoothness and protects against ultraviolet light. Hydroxytyrosol, a rather rare compound found in olive oil, also prevents free-radical damage to the skin, particularly sunlight damage.

Olive oil doesn't clog pores and doesn't give skin the annoying sheen that coconut oil (another natural moisturizer and skin protectant) does, and the color in a good extra-virgin olive oil can add tone and glow to the skin.

But although I often still use olive oil as a moisturizing and glow agent, particularly when I'm traveling and I've forgotten any other skin products (you'd be surprised at how simple it is to hunt down canola oil–free extra-virgin olive oil at any hotel or airport restaurant), I've recently upgraded my skin-care protocol. Why? First, I've been studying the skin microbiome quite a bit lately; as a matter of fact, just a couple of months ago I sent skin microbiome samples off to the Human Microbiome Project to get analyzed.

The long and short of it is this: Your skin is the largest organ in your body and is colonized by a diverse array of microorganisms. This is driven by the ecology of the skin surface, which is highly variable and depends on, among other things, geographic location, the health of the host (you!), and exogenous environmental factors, like whichever skin product you happen to be using.

These skin microbiota play a role in educating your immune system by passing information from the environment into your body, allowing you to better thrive in whichever geographical location you happen to be in and helping you to build a healthy and robust immune system. Yep— your skin microbiome actually changes as you travel. Fascinating, eh? In research, the human body plus all its microbes, including viruses, bacteria, fungi, and mites, has even been referred to as a superorganism.

Of course, none of the positive, immune-boosting, complexion-enhancing effects of a healthy skin microbiome will happen if you are (1) constantly bathing yourself in antibacterial soaps and cosmetic toxins; or, perhaps less well-known, (2) not feeding your skin compounds that allow your good skin bacteria to flourish.

Unfortunately, olive oil—while rich in skin antioxidants—doesn't really feed the skin microbiota. There's also little evidence that olive oil alone can help produce youthful collagen and elastin, remove wrinkles, shrink cellulite, nourish connective tissue, fade scars, kill bad bacteria, or rejuvenate damaged skin. One of the reasons you age and get wrinkles is because your body's cellular defense systems deteriorate over time, and the free radicals that are produced as part of your normal metabolic processes can overwhelm your skin's natural antioxidant defenses. Olive oil can help a little bit with this, but it isn't really a complete panacea.

So, especially as I age, I've been searching for a better solution. I've been looking for other natural oils and ingredients that not only provide antioxidants and skin radiance but also produce an antiaging, wrinkle-reducing, cellulite-shrinking, scar-removing, and, of course, microbiome-feeding effect. Two years ago, my wife Jessa, who has extremely sensitive skin that can only handle the most hypoallergenic substances; my aunt Cynthia Greenfield, a former attorney and the formulator of the Wild Mediterranean oil of oregano I use; and I, the former olive oil–obsessed giant walking pizza, set out on an expedition to source from the four corners of the planet the best organic and hypoallergenic ingredients that have been proven to reduce wrinkles, smooth cellulite, nourish connective tissue, fade scars, kill bad bacteria, rejuvenate damaged skin, give you a smooth, glowing complexion, feed your skin microbiome, and much, much more.

We received strange bottles of oils, tonics, and tinctures in the mail from all over the planet, and over the course of a yearlong quest, we narrowed down our choices to twelve natural skin-care compounds. In no particular order, here are the ingredients we've identified as the top tonics to smooth on our skin each day. Keep in mind that these should always be organic.

1. Aloe vera
2. Jojoba oil
3. Amla
4. Triphala
5. Lavender
6. Wild oregano oil
7. Geranium
8. Palmarosa
9. Turmeric
10. Juniper berry
11. Lemon
12. Patchouli

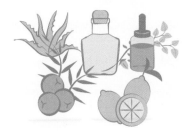

Figure out a way to combine all these in proper ratios, package them, and get them all on your skin in one fell swoop, and you've got yourself one potent antiaging skin serum.

If you don't want to source each of these on your own, I've packaged them all into one healthy, antiaging skin serum called Kion Skin Serum, which is all-organic—you'll find a link to it on BoundlessBook.com/17. I personally put one big dollop on my face and my hair each morning, paying a bit of extra attention to rub it in well over any scars and wrinkles. There are absolutely no toxic preservatives, endocrine disruptors, or chemicals in the formulation, and we've followed closely my personal rule that I won't put anything on my body or skin that I couldn't eat. It even feeds your skin microbiome and nourishes damaged hair.

Once-a-Week Mask

Aside from moisturizing with olive oil and using the skin serum above, about the only other step in my skin-care protocol is putting on a clay mask once a week. For this, I use a blend of eight nutrient-dense ingredients from a company called Alitura. The mask removes dead skin, tightens pores, promotes blood flow, and encourages the growth of new skin cells. Its ingredients include:

- **Freshwater pearl powder,** which is a natural exfoliant that has the remarkable ability to even skin tone, smooth wrinkles, eradicate sun spots, reduce redness, and mitigate irritation. It is a well-known ingredient in traditional Chinese medicine and is used in tonics to treat skin disorders and beautify the skin because of its high antioxidant, protein, and mineral content. Indeed, research suggests that pearl powder substantially increases total antioxidant capacity, particularly the activity and levels of the antioxidants glutathione and superoxide dismutase. Research also suggests that pearl powder considerably suppresses lipid peroxidation, the oxidative degradation of fats in the body. This means that not only is pearl powder a potent skin treatment, but it can also treat age-related degenerative disorders.

- **Grass-fed colostrum,** which is a potent source of a variety of nutrients, such as vitamins, minerals, amino acids, and enzymes. Colostrum is particularly high in insulin-like growth factor (IGF-1). IGF-1 is widely distributed in the skin and is concentrated in injuries, where it promotes the regeneration of the skin. Research suggests that topically applied IGF-1 stimulates collagen synthesis in skin fibroblasts, the growth of fibroblasts and keratinocytes, and angiogenesis (the growth of new blood vessels), all of which promote healthy skin elasticity and blood flow.

- **American ginseng,** which is known to eliminate impurities in the blood and facilitate skin cell oxygenation. American ginseng also contains numerous phytonutrients and has a high antioxidant content.

- **10 percent L-ascorbic acid,** the form of vitamin C that is absorbed most rapidly through the skin. With consistent use, L-ascorbic acid can fade sun spots, acne scars, and skin discoloration, and reduce the appearance of wrinkles. Topical L-ascorbic acid is also necessary for collagen production and healthy skin tone and acts as an antioxidant to eliminate free radicals in the skin.

- **Rhassoul clay,** which is rich in minerals that purify pores, balance oily skin, and exfoliate dead skin cells, making it a potent detoxifying agent. Research has shown that rhassoul clay can also improve skin elasticity.

- **Calcium bentonite clay,** or green desert clay, which contains minerals that help remove toxins and clear up the skin. It also shrinks pores and controls the overproduction of sebum, an oil produced in the sebaceous glands in the skin. Calcium bentonite clay develops a mild electrical charge when saturated with liquid, which makes it particularly helpful in extracting acne-producing toxins and metals and shrinking and tightening inflamed pores.

- **Kaolin clay,** or illite clay, which acts as an antibacterial agent. Research has shown that ion-exchanged kaolin clay can significantly reduce bacterial load, skin inflammation, and wound morphology. Kaolin clay is effective for treating irritated, sensitive skin because of its ability to purify pores, treat acne, and reduce oil production.

- **Organic kelp powder,** which is a rich source of vitamin B_{12}, vitamin E, and other nutrients that soothe and heal the skin. The sodium alginate in kelp is a topical cleanser and antioxidant that can promote a healthier complexion by penetrating pores and drawing out impurities.

All these ingredients come blended by Alitura in a powdered form, and once a week I simply mix them with a few ounces of apple cider vinegar, smear the mixture on my face and hair, and let it dry for about thirty minutes before rinsing it off with warm water, closing my pores with cold water, and finishing with a quick smear of skin serum.

Since adopting my 1-2-3 combo of this weekly mask, the daily serum, and a moisturizer like olive oil, I've been approached by complete strangers who ask me what I do to keep my face glowing and young, and by family members and close friends who have commented on the reverse-aging of my face. In other words, this stuff works, and it's far simpler than you'd think once you make it a habit!

THE LAST WORD

Phew! This chapter may have seemed overwhelming in terms of the host of methods you can use to improve your symmetry and give yourself a step up in your career, your beauty, your physical performance, your sleep, and more.

So for you and your family, let's review just a few of the biggest tips from this chapter:

- Work with a holistic dentist. Look for one who practices orthotropics, which is a specific type of facial growth guidance.

- Eat foods rich in vitamin D, like fatty fish, egg yolks, and butter, and in vitamin K_2, like natto and grass-fed butter, or consider using a D/K_2 supplement. For more on the importance of these fat-soluble vitamins, I highly recommend the book *Vitamin K_2 and the Calcium Paradox* by Dr. Kate Rheaume-Bleue.

- Chew each bite of food twenty-five to forty times, and for additional masseter hypertrophy (increasing the jaw muscle and width), consider switching to a special form of jaw-strengthening gum called mastic gum, although falim gum is also quite good. Feed your children whole, unprocessed foods that they can chew (although I recommend waiting to introduce solids until a baby is at least six months old).

- Train yourself to breathe through your nose, don't habitually mouth-breath, and practice proper tongue posture by keeping the tongue resting lightly against the top of the palate. On BoundlessBook.com/17 there is a link to an article and research by Dr. Mike Mew that focuses on how tongue forces can remodel your face and bring your maxilla bone forward, which affects your entire face and mouth structure.

- Limit stress. Cortisol shows on your face because it leads to shallow chest breathing and the tightening of the jaw and neck muscles.

- Do exercises for your posture each day. Your ears should align with your shoulders, hips, and feet, and your back should be straight. The type of forward head posture associated with mouth breathing affects your back and hips as well as your facial symmetry.

- Oil pull for five to ten minutes each morning. Be sure to spit (not swallow) after finishing, and use extra-virgin coconut oil or The Dirt brand oil-pulling oil.

- Use natural ingredients and compounds to enhance the beauty and symmetry of your skin—they make a much bigger difference than you'd think.

- Set up your sleeping environment and sleeping position to enhance symmetry during the approximate third of your life that you spend in bed.

For citations for all the research studies mentioned in this chapter and a deeper dive into the topics of this chapter—including links to podcasts, blog posts, recommended tools and supplements, and much more—visit BoundlessBook.com/17.

ONE THING YOU CAN DO THIS WEEK

Mouth breathing is a big cause of facial asymmetries. So for the next twenty-four hours, see if you can breathe only through your nose, even during exercise, unless you're doing something for which nasal breathing proves extremely difficult, such as singing, swimming laps, or getting deep into the throes of a high-intensity interval training session. In addition, review the practical tips above and identify at least three that you can implement this week.

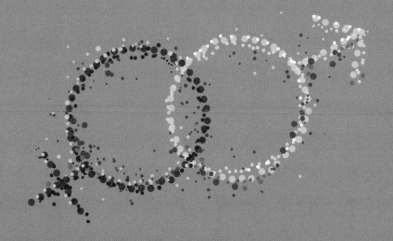

18

SEX

TANTRA, ORGASMS, LIBIDO, SEXUAL SATISFACTION, HORMONES AND BEYOND

Lying facedown and buck-naked, I grimaced and squirmed on the medical examination table. Behind me, a physician assistant clad in blue scrubs repeatedly jammed a foot-long needle in and out of my spine and butt. Each time the entire needle was fully embedded, she yanked it back out, causing a loud sucking sound to emanate from my fat tissue. "You should've eaten more doughnuts this week—there's not a whole lot of marrow back here for the stem cells."

I gritted my teeth, hoping the bruising and bleeding would subside before my foray into the OCR World Championships, just two weeks away, and pondering whether I'd made a mistake to attempt a fringe stem cell–harvesting procedure so close to my big race. But the pain from the fat-marrow-harvesting syringe was actually slightly less than I'd anticipated, possibly thanks to the pain-killing lidocaine injection seeping through my spine, or perhaps thanks to the flood of endorphins still circulating through my veins from a procedure the day before: an injection of platelet-rich plasma into my crotch, accompanied by acoustic sound wave blasting on my gonads and the use of a high-pressure digital pump to build new blood vessels in my nether regions.

Welcome to a typical weekend in my life. The harvesting of my own precious fat was meant to collect and concentrate therapeutic stem cells, which can theoretically be used to rapidly heal my body should I get hit by a bus or suffer a horrible disease. But the process can also be used—in this case along with the sexual organ injections, sound waves, and pump—as fodder for a seasonal *Men's Health* magazine article entitled (brace yourself) "New Year, New Dick."

So who the heck am I? Some kind of masochistic playboy? A man obsessed by my own crotch? An orthorexic, hypochondriac hacker preoccupied with fringe medical procedures that would keep me a teenage boy forever?

Hardly. Within a few hours of rolling off the examination table and waving goodbye to the physician assistant, I stepped onto a plane to travel home to my wife and twin boys, my serene farm in the forest, my organic vegetable garden, my goats and chickens, my hunting bow, and my quiet, peaceful daily routine. Admittedly, my home also contains tens of thousands of dollars' worth of cutting-edge, life-extending, performance-enhancing, cognition-boosting biohacks—from sound-healing machines to hypoxic training units to high-speed vibration platforms to micro-doses of plant medicines to infrared saunas to hyper-chilled endless pools and beyond. I live a life immersed in an odd yet highly thrilling marriage of ancestral wisdom and modern science, tapping each day into what it means to be fully human and reaching into every nook and cranny of full mind, body, and spirit optimization.

But among my forays into relentless self-experimentation, I really have experienced many twists on sexual health hacking. High-intensity acoustic sound wave therapy blasting my crotch? Been there, done that—multiple times, in fact. Digital penis pump? Own it. Tantric sex? Yes, even the whole reverse-orgasm concept. Gas station dick pills? Embarrassingly, yes. Red light therapy on the balls? A daily must at the office. Platelet-rich plasma injections? Sure. And, to top it all off, I underwent full sedation in 2018 for a full-body stem cell makeover, complete with cosmetic and sexual enhancement, including exosome-upgraded bone marrow stem cells from my own hips injected everywhere in my body—and I do mean *everywhere* (see chapter 12 for details).

Love on its own is a positive and powerful emotion crucial to psychological and physical health, but once love is paired with a healthy sex life and sexual health, you get a potent one-two combo for body, mind, and spirit optimization. In this chapter, you will discover not only the host of health benefits of good sex but also how much sex is too much, the ideal frequency of lovemaking and orgasms for both men and women, the best sex-supporting foods and supplements, the best sexual exercises, the best sex biohacks, and the best sex resources for further learning.

Sex is (or at least should be) an intense spiritual experience that's intertwined with happiness and longevity. Ultimately, after reading this chapter, you'll possess an intimate understanding of how to optimize hormones (a crucial component of libido and sexual performance), spruce up your sex life, and experience sexual health and satisfaction that most people never tap into.

HOW MUCH SEX IS TOO MUCH?

Of course, as great as sex is for you, that doesn't mean you need to spend every waking hour as a sex-obsessed maniac in the bedroom, the fancy hotel, and the giant heart-shaped hot tub. It turns out there are philosophies and scientific fields that address how health, longevity, and sexual performance can be influenced by frequency of ejaculation or orgasm. Admittedly, while teachings and research on the frequency of orgasm in women are scant, there is plenty of theory and research in men.

The Taoist Theory of Ejaculation

In the Eastern philosophy of Tao, there is a foundational sex guideline formulated over centuries that is repeatedly emphasized in Taoist literature: that a man must preserve and retain his semen in order to enhance his strength, health, and longevity. This Taoist philosophy maintains that men who keep their ejaculation to a minimum and retain their semen can grow stronger and have clearer minds. Men who practice this type of ejaculation control supposedly also maintain higher levels of testosterone, sperm, and semen and have a more voracious sexual appetite.

Taoist theory also teaches that semen retention via reduced ejaculation frequency strengthens the brain, claiming that the essential nutrients in semen are absorbed by the prostate when they don't seep out elsewhere, and that they can then enter the bloodstream and circulate throughout the body to nourish other tissues and organs, including the brain. Since semen and cerebrospinal fluids contain the same basic ingredients, preserving semen could theoretically nourish the brain by making more essential nutrients available to it.

These Taoist principles are built on the premise that the human body is endowed with a limited supply of primordial energy and that your life span (including your sexual life span) is determined both by the rate at which this energy is used up and by your lifestyle, which either does or does not replenish and strengthen that energy. Since a man's life force—which is commonly referred to as his *jing*—is theoretically used up with each ejaculation, ejaculation frequency should be regulated, the theory goes, to allow the body to rebuild before the jing is used up again through ejaculation.

What the Evidence Says

So what does more modern medical evidence suggest? Studies do indeed show that men experience a significant loss of zinc with each ejaculation, which is probably why eating foods high in zinc, such as pumpkin seeds, shellfish, or (my favorite) black ant powder before or after sex is recommended. Long-term excessive ejaculation may cause chronic zinc deficiency, which can lead to chronic fatigue, mental confusion, and significant loss of sexual drive. Research published by the National Institutes of Health has found that after seven days of not ejaculating, men's testosterone levels reached 145.7 percent of the baseline. There is also some evidence that when ejaculation frequency exceeds the capacity of the body to fully replenish semen, men can experience chronic fatigue, low resistance to stress, loss of sexual drive, loss of focus, and irritability.

On the flip side, a 2004 study in the *Journal of American Medical Association* concluded that ejaculation frequency does not increase the risk of prostate cancer, and there are other studies that suggest that frequent ejaculations may actually decrease the risk of developing prostate cancer. According to researchers at the Boston University School of Public Health, ejaculating at least twenty-one times a month may reduce a man's prostate cancer risk. Of course, the question remains whether in the study, men who were healthier in the first place were the ones with more ejaculations, so their health could have had absolutely no relation to ejaculation frequency.

Then there's the testosterone component. There haven't been any extremely compelling studies on sex frequency and testosterone correlation in *young men*. But one big observational study on 1,226 men aged seventy or above found that regular sex helped to diminish the decline in testosterone that occurs naturally with age. The study authors reported: "We found a consistent association among older men followed over two years between the decline in sexual activity and desire, but not in erectile function, with a decrease in serum [testosterone]. Although these observational findings cannot determine causality, the small magnitude of the decrease in serum T raises the hypothesis that reduced sexual function may reduce serum T rather than the reverse."

One small study also found out that men having sex in a sex club had, on average, 72 percent more salivary testosterone after sex (I am not endorsing sex club visits as a staple in your sexual-health routine, but just sayin'). Interestingly, men at the sex club who were only masturbating while watching sexual acts raised T only by 11 percent. The logistical questions I have about how this study was conducted are obviously numerous.

Another study showed that abstaining from sex for three weeks can slightly increase testosterone, and a follow-up study verified that—for testosterone-increasing purposes—the optimal ejaculation frequency for men is about once every seven days. The study noted that on the seventh day of abstinence, there was a 146 percent increase in testosterone production. But too long a period of abstinence—over three months—can actually suppress testosterone production. Granted, there are other elements involved with frequency of sex, such as happiness, connection, longevity, and prostate cancer risk, but it does appear that for testosterone-production purposes, having sex once a week (not masturbation, but sex with a human being) is a good frequency.

Pardon the expression, but I suspect your mind will be absolutely blown by the seriously legit biological and spiritual benefits that regularly getting busy with a partner can produce. These effects go far beyond orgasms or propagation of the human race and include the following.

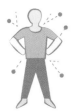

1. **A stronger immune system:** Researchers have discovered a direct correlation between sexual activity a few times a week and higher salivary levels of immunoglobulin A (IgA), an antibody that helps fight infections and the common cold. In contrast, IgA levels were lowest in people who had no sex or lots of sex (more on excessive sex later in this chapter).

2. **Less depression and stress:** Contact with semen during intercourse has an antidepressant effect on women. Regular intercourse also makes blood pressure more resilient to stress, reduces overall psychological stress, and reduces plasma and salivary cortisol while producing beneficial mental health effects.

3. **Better brainpower:** A study on rodents found that sexual activity increases neurons in the hippocampus, the section of the brain that stores memories. In addition, sex may also increase analytical thinking capabilities.

4. **Improved overall physical fitness:** Depending on how you do the act, a half hour of sex can burn through close to 150 calories (that counts for at least a couple of those chocolate-covered strawberries). By the way, the reverse is also true: frequent exercise has been shown to enhance sexual performance.

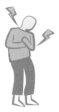

5. **Reduced pain:** Oxytocin is the trust hormone that makes you want to snuggle up to your partner after sex, and it also reduces stress and promotes feelings of calm and well-being. In addition, sex causes a release of serotonin, endorphins, and phenylethylamine, which are all hormones that generate intense feelings of pleasure while at the same time eliminating pain. This is likely why studies have shown that intercourse can stop migraines and lower the discomfort of arthritis.

6. **Improved sleep:** Following an orgasm, and even during sex, the brain releases norepinephrine, serotonin, oxytocin, and vasopressin, all of which can help you fall asleep faster and increase the amount of time you spend in deep sleep. Men are especially likely to succumb to the sleep-inducing effects of sex because the prefrontal cortex, the part of the brain responsible for interpreting and responding to new information, slows significantly in men after orgasm.

7. **Enhanced sense of smell:** After sex, the body produces the hormone prolactin. Prolactin can generate new neurons in the olfactory bulb, which is the part of the brain that controls how you understand and react to smells.

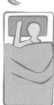

8. **Antiaging effects:** Studies have shown that couples who had intercourse three or more times a week appeared on average ten years younger than their chronological age. Orgasms also trigger the release of estrogen in both men and women, which can improve hair and skin quality, making people look more attractive.

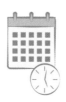

9. **Better heart health:** Research suggests that sex reduces the risk of stroke and coronary heart disease in men. Men who have sex once a month or less are 45 percent more likely to contract cardiovascular disease than those who have sex more frequently. Research also suggests that men with better overall health have higher libidos and therefore more sex overall, which creates a positive feedback loop that further builds a healthy cardiovascular system. Interestingly, results from most studies suggest that high sex frequency is positively related to later risk of cardiovascular events for men but not for women,

whereas good sex quality (a high perceived rating of sexual satisfaction) seems to protect women but not men from cardiovascular risk in later life.

10. **Regular menstrual periods:** The odorless pheromones in male perspiration can have a significant effect on a woman's mind and body. Scientists have found that women exposed to male sweat are calmer and more relaxed. These women also experience smaller changes in their levels of luteinizing hormone, which controls the menstrual cycle. The stress-reducing effect of sex is another contributing factor in maintaining regular periods.

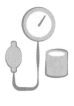

11. **Lower blood pressure:** High blood pressure can cause erectile dysfunction in men and reduced arousal and ability to orgasm in women. But multiple studies show a link between low testosterone and high blood pressure, and the spikes in testosterone associated with sexual activity may help lower blood pressure in both men and women.

12. **Possible lower risk of prostate cancer:** There is a link between regular ejaculation and prostate health. Some studies suggest sex flushes out any carcinogens in the prostate gland. On the other hand, a recent study showed that frequent sexual activity in young men (in their twenties and early thirties) could actually increase the risk of developing prostate cancer. But frequent ejaculation in middle-aged or older men (age fifty and above) decreased disease risk. In other words, the verdict is still out on this one—and later in this chapter, I'll cut through the confusion and address what frequency of sex means for your health.

13. **Lowered risk of pregnancy complications:** Frequent sexual intercourse and exposure to semen can reduce women's risk of developing a serious pregnancy complication called preeclampsia, which can cause swollen extremities, headaches, nausea, and seizures. This is because a protein found in semen called HLG-A can regulate women's immune systems.

14. **Enhanced sperm:** Studies show that men who ejaculate daily for seven days have higher-quality sperm at the end of the week, and the sperm's rate of DNA fragmentation drops from 34 percent to 26 percent, meaning it is more likely to fertilize an egg. This is likely because frequent ejaculation means that sperm spends less time in the testicular ducts and is therefore less likely to be damaged.

I find it interesting that when expressing and receiving the emotion of love and experiencing the physical act of sex are combined, it builds just about every health base you need to cover, which makes frequently loving and making love one of the most powerful things you can do to become boundless.

Then there's the whole debate about having sex before a game. When it comes to sports and competition, many Western and Eastern athletic coaches advise their athletes to not ejaculate the day of an athletic competition because it is scientifically documented that testosterone levels might drop immediately after ejaculation and theoretically diminish athletic performance. One sexual performance anecdote, mainly derived from athletes, is that sex the previous day or even many days before competition somehow hinders performance.

But this idea has actually been researched and may not really make sense. For example, one study comparing the maximal effort on a cycle ergometer test found out that having sex two hours before performance slightly diminishes recovery capacity, while having sex ten hours before the event had absolutely no effect on performance or recovery. Another study found that having sexual intercourse twelve hours prior to maximal treadmill effort didn't produce any negative effects on performance.

How It Works in Practice

So let's say you do decide to experiment with ejaculation frequency. How can you, in practical terms, pull this off (excuse the pun)? The most common system is to simply limit ejaculation to every few days. One popular theory among Tao practitioners is to base ejaculation frequency on intercourse frequency, with ejaculation occurring only two or three times out of every ten sexual encounters. One Tao theorist, Sun Simiao, recommends ejaculation no more than once every twenty days for men over fifty and no more than once every one hundred days for men over sixty. Another Tao theorist suggests that ejaculation frequency should be regulated according to the seasons; he recommends ejaculating no more than every three days during spring, twice a month in summer and fall, and not at all during the cold of winter! Many men I know, including Pedram Shojal, author of *The Art of Stopping Time*, practice reduced ejaculation frequency as a lifestyle. Pedram recommends the following frequency:

Twenties: All you want
Thirties: Three to four times per week
Forties: Two to three times per week
Fifties: One to two times per week
Sixty and above: Once a week or less, depending on health

From a practical standpoint, you injaculate rather than ejaculate by squeezing the same muscles you'd squeeze if you were trying to stop the flow of urine while breathing the energy up your spine. And if you get too close? Jam your fingers and apply pressure into your perineum, the soft tissue between your scrotum and your anus. I learned this tactic in the book *The Multi-Orgasmic Man*, which is an excellent read if you'd like to learn more.

But it's much harder than you can possibly imagine to finish a good romp in the bedroom without blowing your load. Call me a weakling, but I lasted about a month attempting sex without ejaculation. It's difficult enough for a busy father of twins to find a quiet lovemaking moment with his wife. When those times arise, I don't want to hold anything back. Cookie Monster's balls were never so blue, but patience can be a virtue. The beauty of this tactic for you male readers is that it's free, aside from the tranquilizers you might need to keep from transforming into a pent-up, angry, moody, aggressive, blue-balled man on those days you decide to have sex but not ejaculate. After having sex frequently without ejaculating, I felt like someone had handed me a double espresso, especially when it was a morning romp. I had a lot more energy during my midday workout. At night, though? I missed that cuddly, post-sex, oxytocin-induced coma. I felt like I needed to take a sedative to get to sleep postintercourse on those nonejaculation days.

So ultimately, the decision of how frequently you're going to ejaculate is up to you, but I personally find that in an era of loneliness, internet addiction, and reduced personal interactions, most human beings need to be having more sex, not less. This means that if you're going to experiment with reduced ejaculation frequency, it's important to understand that it does not mean less physical interaction or even less sex. It simply means that you may want to think twice before you blow your load every time.

A Note for Women

Interestingly, things are a bit different for women. Although women do indeed ejaculate, there isn't much research on the frequency of ejaculation in women. But there is research on the frequency of vaginal intercourse. Specifically, women who have more sex (once per week or more) have better mental health and higher levels of emotional satisfaction, higher heart rate variability, lower resting heart rate, lower levels of the inflammatory markers homocysteine and hs-CRP, and lower risk of mortality.

Unlike for men, for women, neither being sexually active nor frequency of sex is significantly related to cardiovascular risks, but the majority of data suggests that the more sex a woman has (within reason), the better—and, as you learned earlier, the perceived quality of a woman's sex life is correlated to decreased cardiovascular risk.

THE BEST FOODS AND SUPPLEMENTS FOR SEX

Whether you're doing the deed once a day, once a week, or once a month, there are proven herbs, supplements, brews, and blends that can enhance libido, orgasm, blood flow, and other determinants of sexual performance and sexual satisfaction—all without your needing to swallow a handful of the infamous gas station dick pills.

Maca

Multiple studies show that maca, a root vegetable, enhances libido in both men and women. Maca can treat sexual dysfunction caused by selective serotonin reuptake inhibitors (SSRIs), a kind of antidepressant. It can also mildly benefit men with erectile dysfunction from other causes. Moreover, preliminary animal evidence suggests that red maca might improve prostate health and reduce anxiety. My favorite way to use maca is to toss a teaspoon to a tablespoon into my morning smoothie or afternoon tea, as it bestows a nice, pleasant, nutty flavor to just about any smoothie or beverage.

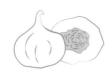

Cocoa

Low nitric oxide (NO) levels can cause blood vessels to narrow, leading to poor circulation, which can result in erections that are softer and more difficult to maintain. Just like the flavonoids in grape seeds and pine bark, epicatechin and other flavonoids in cocoa can help support NO levels, thus improving blood flow and alleviating this type of erectile

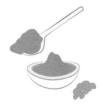

dysfunction. Chocolate and red wine used to be my backstage bodybuilding go-to for enhancing blood flow and vascularity, and a chunk of dark chocolate along with a glass of wine (which contains the procyanidins and nitric oxide precursors you'll discover shortly) after dinner is perfect if sex is in the plans.

Yohimbine

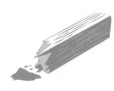

Yohimbine is an alkaloid found in the bark of the African yohimbe tree. It is a stimulant often used to increase rates of fat oxidation but has also been shown in research to increase virility and erectile rigidity. Viagra and Cialis make for better erections, but they have no direct effect on libido; yohimbine, however, can have a direct, positive effect on libido. Problem is, yohimbine can also make you extremely anxious and jittery—not a state you want to be in for a night of romance (although, interestingly, those with higher-than-normal aerobic fitness levels seem to be partially protected from this effect).

Eurycoma Longifolia and Cistanche

Eurycoma longifolia is a potent extract that's also known by several other names, such as tongkat ali, Malaysian ginseng, and longjack. Evidence supports its traditional use as a libido enhancer for both men and women, and in addition to its aphrodisiac effects, eurycoma can also increase sperm production and may directly act as a pro-erectile agent. Ultimately, based on the existing research to date, eurycoma appears to be an effective boner pill if that's what you're looking for.

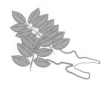

A similar compound that I've personally found much more success with is cistanche, known in Chinese herbal medicine as "the stalk enlarger" (chuckle). Legend is that Genghis Khan consumed cistanche daily. Considering the guy's stamina and that 8 percent of Asia's population are said to be his descendants (that is one in two hundred people worldwide!) and that I personally mix some up in coffee or tea before date night, it's one that I can recommend even higher than eurycoma.

Fenugreek

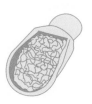

In Ayurvedic medicine, fenugreek is called "methi" (its Hindi name) and is used to increase virility. In healthy men, high doses of fenugreek appear to significantly increase libido and sexual satisfaction. Considering that fenugreek is also a fantastic digestif and a seed you can add to stir-fries, sauté with, or sprinkle on salads, it makes sense to have some in your pantry anyway.

Osthole

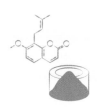

Research shows that osthole, also known as osthol and cnidium monnieri, acts on the same physiological mechanisms as sildenafil, the active ingredient in Viagra. It can enhance erectile function, specifically by stimulating the release of nitric oxide, which relaxes blood vessels and appears to increase both male and female sexual performance and arousal. It has also been shown in rodent models to raise testosterone. Interestingly, osthole may also help to control blood sugar by increasing the expression of GLUT4 sugar transporters in skeletal muscle, can improve cognitive performance by increasing the brain's plasticity and BDNF, can inhibit histone deacetylase, which can increase gene expression in areas of the brain related to memory and learning performance, and is currently being researched as an ingredient in anticancer drugs!

Procyanidins

Like the flavonoids in cocoa, procyanidins and other flavonoids in pine bark and grape seeds can help support nitric oxide levels, which helps prevent the narrowing of blood vessels and thus ameliorate certain types of erectile dysfunction. Pycnogenol, a patented pine bark extract standardized to 65 to 75 percent procyanidin, is the best-studied source of procyanidins. Grape seed extract is cheaper, but its effect on blood flow is less reliable and could take longer to develop (up to one month). To approximate the effects of procyanidins, you can just knock back a glass of a good, tannin-rich red wine. Just be careful with the alcohol, which is a great social lubricant but a known libido and sexual performance suppressor.

Nitric Oxide–Producing Foods

From arugula to watermelon to dark chocolate to red wine to pumpkin seeds, extra-virgin olive oil, beets, avocados, celery, and beyond, a host of foods can increase blood flow or enhance sexual health. While there is certainly lore out there that the best way to bump up hormones is to eat a big fatty cut of steak drenched in butter, you'll likely find that all this accomplishes is a food baby in your tummy and a slightly comatose feeling. Instead, I'd recommend this powerful sex salad recipe that includes a ton of nitric oxide precursors: to a bed of arugula and spinach, add cubed or sliced cooked beets and carrots, a handful of chopped walnuts, sautéed red onions, a few chunks of red apple, and a sprinkling of fenugreek seeds. Dress with extra-virgin olive oil and balsamic vinaigrette. Serve with a glass of red wine and a chunk of dark chocolate, then let the good times roll.

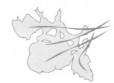

Other Supplements

Finally, if you're deficient in certain vitamins and minerals, supplementing with them can drastically affect fertility and sexual performance. These nutrients include creatine, vitamin D, vitamin K, magnesium, zinc, and cholesterol-based compounds such as DHEA. To cover your hormonal and sexual bases, I recommend supplementing daily with 5 g creatine, 2,000 IU vitamin D, 150 mcg vitamin K_2, 400 mg magnesium, 50 mg zinc, and 25 mg DHEA.

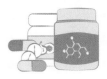

BIOHACKING THE BEDROOM

Okay, okay. Perhaps the whole dark-chocolate-and-red-wine thing is old news for you. Perhaps you've covered your vitamin and nutrient bases. Perhaps you've even gotten your hands on some avant-garde Chinese herbs. But now you want the fringe stuff: the best sexual exercises, sex workouts, and biohacks for a better sex life, with a particular focus on techniques, experiences, and stories about what I've personally experimented with. I'm about to spill the beans on everything I've tried and found success with (and there's plenty) to boost testosterone, libido, and overall bedroom performance. And ladies, don't fret: there's plenty in this section for you too. Let's begin.

1. Try Weight Lifting for Your Genitals

My friend Jordan Gray, a relationship expert and sex coach, first alerted me to the towel technique for enhancing your sexual muscles. It is literally just like it sounds: you hang a slightly wet towel over your erection and practice repeatedly contracting to lift the towel, eventually progressing to larger and wetter towels. My former podcast guest Kim Anami, who lifts everything from kettlebells to coconuts with her vagina, teaches a similar technique to women with a jade egg. My own personal version of the towel technique involves the use of the Private Gym, a magnetic resistance device designed especially for a man's junk. On BoundlessBook.com/18, you'll find a link to the nitty-gritty details of my thirty-day training block with the Private Gym. It's an entertaining read, trust me (spoiler alert: it works, but it gets exhausting after a while).

2. Sleep, but Not Too Much

Yawn. I know, I kicked this horse to death in chapter 7. But the majority of the daily testosterone release in men occurs during sleep. Fragmented sleep and obstructive sleep apnea are associated with reduced testosterone levels in both men and women. A study published in the *Journal of the American Medical Association* found out that one week of sleep restriction (five hours of sleep per night) decreased testosterone production by 10 to 15 percent! But don't sleep too much: studies have also shown that sleep's effect on testosterone has an inverted U-shaped curve. Testosterone production increases with increasing sleep duration up to ten hours, after which it decreases.

3. Get Lean, but Not Too Lean

It is generally noted in research that the higher your body fat percentage, the lower your testosterone. The correlation works especially in the direction of getting leaner, which seems to instantly raise testosterone levels. Longitudinal analyses showing that baseline hormone levels don't change anthropometric measures imply that body composition affects hormone levels, not the reverse. Yep, you read that right: being lean gives you high testosterone more than high testosterone

Women Need Testosterone Too

While testosterone is often advertised and heralded as the ultimate male hormone, women need adequate amounts of testosterone too, and it is produced by the adrenal glands and ovaries. Although their blood testosterone levels are significantly lower than men's, women start to produce more amounts of the hormone during puberty, and levels peak for most women in their early twenties (provided they're not using hormonal contraceptives, which unfortunately suppress nearly all normal sex hormone production). By the time a woman has reached menopause, she may have only half of the level of testosterone she once had.

Because testosterone not only helps maintain muscle and bone mass in women but also contributes to sex drive, monitoring and maintaining adequate testosterone levels is important for women, especially as they age. Several older women I know who use bioidentical hormone replacement therapy swear by the libido-, mood-, and sex-enhancing effects of just a touch of testosterone cream applied vaginally (it also assists with vaginal dryness).

One study in the *New England Journal of Medicine* evaluated sexuality and quality of life in women with low blood levels of testosterone. After the researchers raised the female participants' blood levels of testosterone via a medicated skin patch, their overall health and sexuality dramatically improved.

makes you lean. More body fat also usually increases aromatase enzyme activity, which converts more testosterone into estrogen. But you also don't need to be an emaciated marathoner—too little body fat can actually be detrimental to testosterone production. It has been roughly estimated that a male body fat percentage between 8 and 14 percent is optimal for testosterone production.

4. Train for Testosterone

While strength training and muscle gains often reduce body fat percentage (which leads to higher testosterone levels), they also have an independent effect on elevating testosterone. Having more muscle mass is positively correlated with higher testosterone. Lifting medium-heavy weights explosively can stimulate short-term and long-term testosterone production. Training progressively by adding more weight nearly every time you train causes your body to adapt to higher and higher testosterone levels via neuromuscular adaptations.

Follow these basic principles when strength training for optimal testosterone production:

- Lift explosively.
- Lift heavy enough, but not too heavy (to have an optimum force-velocity curve, because moving weight fast can have a good effect on testosterone).
- Use compound lifts to activate large amounts of muscle mass.
- Focus on body parts that have a high density of androgen receptor sites (particularly the chest, shoulders, and legs).
- Do sprint intervals to maximize force production in minimal time and to activate fast-twitch muscle fibers.
- Do as much work on as much muscle tissue as you can as quickly as possible.

If your gym time is limited, the dead lift and squat are, in my opinion, the king and queen of testosterone-boosting exercises. Of course, as you can probably guess, too much endurance training or chronic cardio can lower testosterone levels significantly.

Testosterone has powerful antiaging effects for women too. It is responsible for enhancing lipolysis of fat tissue, building muscle, keeping skin supple, increasing bone mineral density, and, as noted above, creating a positive mood and an improved ability to handle stress. Testosterone levels in women have also been linked to enhanced cognitive functioning.

At the same time, in both men and women, low testosterone levels have been associated with heart attack, Alzheimer's disease, osteoporosis, and depression. If you're a woman and you're cold all the time but your thyroid levels are adequate, you are likely low on testosterone. Other symptoms of low testosterone in women include sluggishness, muscle weakness, fatigue, sleep disturbances, weight gain, fertility issues, and irregular menstrual cycles.

Ultimately, for women, a little bit of testosterone—achieved in youth by following the same tips dished out to the guys in this chapter and achieved in age with a touch of bioidentical hormone replacement therapy—can go a long way toward improving looks, figure, energy level, outlook on life, sex appeal, and sexual fulfillment. According to the University of Rochester Medical Center, a woman should have a total of 15–70 ng/dL of testosterone in her blood, although there are no conclusive guidelines for what should be considered a low testosterone level in women.

5. Control Stress

Chronic stress leads eventually to chronically elevated cortisol levels in the blood. Cortisol is necessary for life, but when levels are too high for too long, it can cause diminished testosterone secretion, as cortisol and testosterone compete for similar hormonal precursors and raw materials (especially pregnenolone). In military studies, prolonged stress has been shown to significantly lower testosterone secretion. Meditation, time in nature, breathwork, evening carbohydrate refeeds on physically active days, adaptogenic herbs (ashwagandha in particular), vitamin C, and phosphatidylserine are all strategies I've personally used to kick high cortisol to the curb.

6. Eat Enough

Your body needs enough calories to produce adequate amounts of testosterone. With constant and prolonged caloric restriction, the body enters survival mode, which means that your reproductive system is not of great importance anymore—your body simply wants to survive rather than reproduce. After all, why make babies in times of stress and starvation? The body instead conserves energy for vital processes and internal organs. For optimal testosterone production and fertility, you should eat at energy maintenance or a slight calorie surplus. But, if you are overweight, research suggests that a minor calorie deficit and losing weight can elevate testosterone production.

So get lean first and then cycle in higher-calorie days for optimal testosterone production and maintenance. Losing weight slowly also appears to be a good idea because a 15 percent daily calorie deficit during weight loss doesn't seem to affect testosterone negatively (but if you're on a daily caloric deficit, it is still advisable to incorporate regular calorie refeeds, such as eating to caloric balance or slight excess on one day of the weekend).

Finally, please remember that it's just fine to tap into all the physiological benefits of fasting, particularly via daily twelve- to sixteen-hour intermittent fasts, as long as you don't think of fasting as synonymous with caloric restriction. I'll tackle fasting more in chapter 19, but if your goal is to maximize testosterone and libido, then simply go long periods of time between meals, and when you do finally eat, eat a significant number of calories—at least as many as you need to sustain your metabolic rate.

7. Nail Your Macros

Protein is especially important in the sex and hormone departments. Chronic protein malnutrition can cause low testosterone levels. The caveat is that you don't actually need as much protein as you may have been told. For most folks, the recommended daily allowance of 0.45 to 0.64 g per pound of body weight is enough for optimal testosterone production. I personally eat 0.5 to 0.7 g of protein per pound of body weight on easy exercise or recovery days and 0.7 to 0.8 g per pound on hard exercise days. Exceeding 0.8 g per pound doesn't seem to give any additional benefit, even for hard-charging athletes. In addition, the protein source is also a major factor in testosterone production. For example, a study published in the *British Journal of Nutrition* found that when healthy men replaced meat protein with soybean protein, their testosterone-to-estradiol ratio decreased significantly. Yes, you read that right: steak beats edamame, hands down.

Here's another reason not to go too far overboard on the protein: for optimal testosterone production, it seems crucial that you don't eat too much protein and that you eat enough carbohydrates and fat. One study that compared protein and carbohydrate changes and their hormonal effects discovered that when the male subjects followed a high-protein, low-carb diet for ten days, their total testosterone levels were 21 percent lower than in men who ate a high-carbohydrate, low-protein diet. Part of this is likely due to the fact that excessively low carbohydrates, particularly when paired with high levels of physical activity, can inhibit thyroid activity, raise cortisol, increase levels of sex hormone binding globulin, and generally lower endocrine function—although many of these issues can be solved by including plenty of fats in the low-carbohydrate diet, which this study did not do (as a matter of fact, adequate fats paired with either a low-carbohydrate or high-carbohydrate diet seem to do a very good job maintaining hormonal status). The high-protein diet also caused significantly higher cortisol levels (the diets were equal in total calories and fat), which is yet another reason I'm personally not a fan of exceeding 0.8 g per pound of body weight, even for building muscle or muscle maintenance: you certainly need adequate amino acids, but it doesn't take as much protein as you'd think.

Another study in strength-training men compared ratios of protein to carbohydrates to different fats and found that diets higher in carbohydrates that were paired with saturated and monounsaturated fats were associated with higher testosterone production than high-protein diets. Previous studies have also noted that men who consume a diet containing 20 percent fat have significantly lower concentrations of testosterone in the blood than men who consume a diet of 40 percent fat. Many other studies have also shown that eating enough fat is crucial for testosterone production, which makes perfect sense because cholesterol from fats is a raw, potent material for steroid hormone production.

Another study compared the testosterone-to-cortisol ratios in two groups of carb-consuming men. The study found out that the men who got 60 percent of their calories from carbohydrates had significantly higher free-testosterone-to-cortisol ratios than those who got 30 percent of their calories from carbs. This doesn't mean I endorse a 60 percent carb-based diet per se, but I stand by my recommendation for active individuals attempting to optimize hormone production to at least engage in some kind of daily or weekly carbohydrate refeed of 100 to 200 g of carbs.

Ultimately, when it comes to macros, the bottom line is this: for optimal testosterone production, you shouldn't dip too low in calories or too high, you shouldn't consume too much protein (more than 0.8 g per pound of body weight) or eat too little carbs (below 30 percent of calories) for long periods of time (especially in active people), and—whether you're eating a high-carbohydrate or low-carbohydrate diet—you shouldn't avoid saturated or monounsaturated fats.

8. Hydrate

Even mild dehydration (1 to 2 percent body weight loss) can raise cortisol levels and deleteriously affect testosterone production. In addition, the more dehydrated you are, the more cortisol and adrenaline rise and the more testosterone drops. If you are significantly sweating or in a stage of heavy exercise, drinking water becomes even more important for testosterone maintenance. (My article "10 Things Your Pee Can Tell You About Your Body" includes a few handy tips for using urine strips to quantify your level of hydration—you'll find a link on BoundlessBook.com/19.) Just be sure to steer clear of estrogen-boosting and endocrine-disrupting plastic water bottles (and anything else that contains the all-too-common additives BPA, phthalates, parabens, triclosan, and benzophenones).

9. Increase Androgen Receptor Density

Present in both men and women, androgens are hormones such as testosterone and androstenedione that are important for normal sexual organ development before birth and also sexual development during puberty. In adults, androgens play a crucial role in libido, physical performance, and sexual function, and also act as precursors to important hormones such as estrogen. Androgen receptors are what allow the body to respond appropriately to androgens. As a general rule, the more receptors you have, the better your body is equipped to respond to your hormones. Here are some of the better-researched methods to increase androgen receptor density:

- Fasting (not calorie restriction per se, but significant time between meals and a twelve- to sixteen-hour daily fast)
- Coffee or caffeine—caffeine, at a dosage of about 2 mg per pound of body weight before exercise or 240 mg per pound of body weight after exercise, can raise testosterone level significantly.
- Explosive resistance training (short, fast sessions two to three times per week)
- L-carnitine (this is a lipid transporter molecule, and supplementing with about 2 g per day can increase androgen receptor activity in cells by providing fuel for the receptors)
- The supplements mucuna (5 g or more), forskolin (250 mg of a supplement containing 10 percent forskolin taken twice per day), and creatine (5 to 10 g per day)

10. Try Electrical Muscle Stimulation (EMS)

A study on rats discovered that electrical stimulation caused a significant increase in androgen receptors and even led to an increase in muscle mass by enhancing muscles' sensitivity to androgens. In addition, a study on humans showed that electrical stimulation of meridian points increased concentrations of total testosterone and DHEA. Check out chapter 12 for details on EMS.

11. Get Red Light Therapy

I'm not really a nudist kind of guy. The last nudist beach I visited primarily featured lots of curly hair, unattractive gonads, and a disturbing volleyball game spectacle, so ever since, I've tended to stay away from nudist beaches and bars. But on one particularly sunny spring day, while on a camping trip, I decided to sunbathe nude in the forest. I lay out in my hammock with my drawers tossed to the forest floor, my crotch proudly displayed to the bright, blue sky, basking in the glorious feeling of warmth on my balls. I pondered whether this was some kind of little-known biohack I was tapping into. After all, enough people expose their crotch to the warm rays of the sun that there must be some benefit to it, right? I had to find out.

As a man on a constant quest to optimize my brain and body, including my own balls, I decided to look into the health effects of UV light on the genitals. To my surprise, some studies have actually demonstrated that exposing the torso or the testes to light can potentially increase testosterone. In fact, studies on the effects of light on the testes go way back to 1939, when researchers exposed various parts of men's bodies to UV light. They found that men's testosterone levels went up by 120 percent when the participants' chests were exposed to UV light, and they went up by 200 percent with UV exposure to the genital area (this was the same study former professional baseball player Gabe Kapler cited back in 2015, when he advocated for tanning your testicles in a blog post that later went viral).

To be fair, the results of the 1939 study are eighty years old, so it's possible that the effects of sunlight on your nuts have been overstated. But assuming it is good for you, there's one major problem with it: most dudes don't have the time, desire, or year-round exposure to sunlight to step out into the backyard buck-naked (not to mention that most guys have something called neighbors, many of whom have access to phones and can call the police). Ultimately, moseying through the neighborhood on a sunny day with your pants jacked down isn't a practical way of getting your daily dose of testosterone.

So I delved back into the research and messaged the one guy I consider to be an expert in all things testosterone and sperm-count related: my Finnish friend and physician Dr. Olli Sovijärvi, who studied at the University of Helsinki. I originally met Dr. Sovijärvi when speaking at a biohacking conference he hosts in Finland. Turns out that since those initial sunshine studies, many more studies have investigated the effects of direct sunlight on the torso, which increases a human male's testosterone levels by anywhere from 25 percent to 160 percent, depending on the individual.

Sunlight directly on the testes reportedly has an even more profound effect, boosting production in Leydig cells (the cells that produce testosterone) by an average of 200 percent. Olli went on to inform me that some animal studies have linked light, particularly a special form of light called red light, to increased testicular function. (It's important to note that this is not exactly proven science: one red light study conducted on rams, for instance, was inconclusive.)

The theory is this: While sunlight has many beneficial effects, such as vitamin D production and improved mood, it is not without its downsides. Too much exposure to sunlight, particularly to sensitive areas like the skin around your precious ball sac, can create sunburn, excess radiation, inflammation, and damage. And let's face it: you don't want a shrunken, shriveled, dehydrated dick, no matter how impressive the tan.

Although it's part of the light spectrum you receive from sunlight exposure, isolated red light is different from sunlight. Visible red light is comprised of light wavelengths in the range of 600 to 750 nm, while infrared ranges between 700 nm and 1mm. According to red light therapy proponents, these forms of red light work to stimulate ATP production, increase the energy available to the cell, and, in particular, increase the activity of the Leydig cells in your testes.

It's important to note that there are currently no light therapy devices on the market cleared by FDA for the enhanced production of testosterone (although a few treatments, like LED red light beds, have been approved by the FDA for narrow uses, like wrinkle reduction). That said, the treatment is generally considered low-risk, so the products like the one I tried do not require FDA clearance. It also should be noted that most (but not all) of the existing clinical research related to testosterone production and sperm mobility stems from animal studies, not studies involving humans.

There is also another caveat to this, and this is the part where Olli just about scared my pants off (or, more appropriately, back on). Many types of lamps and bulbs sold for red light therapy (such as incandescents, heat lamps, and infrared lamps that generate red light at greater than 1000 nm) give off a significant amount of heat and can actually fry your testicles. So you have to be careful when you use red light therapy—unless self-castration with a red heating lamp from Home Depot is on your wish list.

The good Dr. Olli then went on to inform me that each night, he lies down on his couch, pulls down his pants, and hugs a big long panel of red infrared light from an LED source at 600 to 950 nm. It sounded just like hugging a giant, warm teddy bear (a hard and uncomfortable teddy bear that's plugged into a wall outlet and is generating enough red light to turn the entire room into a video arcade).

I was convinced. The morning after my conversation with Olli, I ordered something called a Joovv (pronounced "Joove") light (which you may remember from chapter 12). This was the red light he personally recommended and used himself, and I didn't want to play around with frying my balls to a crisp with a cheap knockoff, so I spent the big bucks (a grand total of $995) for what the website described as a full-body LED red light therapy device.

When my Joovv arrived the next week, I hoisted it downstairs to my office, leaned it against my stand-up desk, pulled down my pants, and flipped it on.

I jumped back as best I could with my underwear wrapped around my ankles. Holy hell. Not only was the red light panel itself as wide as my torso and nearly five feet high, but the light coming out of this thing was freaking blinding. I fumbled for the little sunglasses that were included with the light panel and slapped them on. There, much better (although I later learned that sunglasses aren't necessary and that this form of light can actually be therapeutic for the eyes).

No longer feeling like I was staring into the depths of a semitruck's red brake lights, I simply stood there, naked. I replied to a few emails, then checked my watch. Five minutes. That should be good. After all, according to good ole Dr. Olli, five to twenty minutes is the sweet spot for red light exposure to your gonads, and I didn't want to overtrain or excessively fry my little fellas on their first foray into the wonderful world of red light.

The rest of the morning, my crotch felt warm. Alive. So I did it again. Glancing out my office window to make sure the lawnmower guy wasn't tooling around in the grass, I pulled down my drawers and bathed myself in the heavenly, warm, tingly glow, this time for eight minutes.

That night, my wife and I made love. Admittedly, I felt—well—a heavenly, warm, tingly glow in my crotch. Nice.

Two days later, I waited until the evening, then wandered downstairs. I rubbed my hands together, took a deep breath, and flipped on my Joovv. I called my mom to see how her day was going (she had no clue what was going on below the phone). Ten minutes. I read a blog post. Fifteen minutes. My crotch grew warmer and warmer, but in a pleasant, day-at-the-beach sort of way. I finished an email. Twenty minutes. Mission complete.

That night was date night, and I was a rock star.

I sat at dinner, horny, my penis pulsing, staring across the table at my wife and feeling like I'd popped a couple of Viagra. Later, I blew the biggest load I could recall in recent memory.

And from that point on, for nearly the past seven months, I've stuck with twenty minutes of red light exposure on my crotch each day. Actually, I'm afraid to do more. I suspect there must be a law of diminishing returns, and I don't want to wind up with my dick looking like a leather handbag. But in the meantime, it is now a daily habit to pull down my pants at my desk, flip on my Joovv, and get my red light on.

12. Seek Out Cold

One study conducted in 1988 in Finland investigated serum levels of hormones, including testosterone, in men after they spent two hours in a cold room (50 degrees Fahrenheit). Although testosterone didn't go up, cortisol decreased, which could free up more raw material for testosterone production. In addition, heat exposure on the testicles has been shown to reduce testosterone levels (one study on over six thousand men showed that sperm quality and volume are higher in the winter).

Then there are anecdotes from Chinese and Russian powerlifters who ice their balls after training and before competitions, bodybuilders who swear by dipping their junk in cold water to increase testosterone (google it and prepare to take a deep dive into the ball-icing forums), and even a device called the JetPack, which claims, "Your Balls which Produce nearly All of Your Testosterone Don't Get Enough Cold!"

But before you rush out to buy a cold pack for your balls, you can simply do the following:

- Take cold baths and showers.
- Wear loose boxers or go commando (this is also good for blood flow to your nether regions).
- Sleep naked or wear loose pajamas (no undies).
- Avoid sitting for long periods of time.

13. Take Targeted Mineral Supplementation

Research has shown that supplementation of the mineral boron at approximately 10 mg per day can increase free testosterone and decrease estrogen levels (it can also lower levels of pro-inflammatory cytokines). Since boron accumulates in the gonads, long-term use may produce the best benefits.

Iodine is another essential mineral (which means it must be acquired via diet). The thyroid gland absorbs iodine from the blood to make thyroid hormones, so about 15 to 20 mg of iodine is concentrated in thyroid tissue and hormones. In addition, 70 percent of the body's iodine is distributed in other tissues, such as mammary glands, eyes, salivary glands, and testicles. Lack of iodine in the body can cause hypothyroidism, and hypothyroidism can lead to low free-testosterone concentrations.

One proposed explanation for the high occurrence of hypothyroidism and hypogonadism in men today compared to decades ago is the increase in environmental toxic halogens, such as fluoride, chlorine, and bromine. When concentrated in the body's tissue in high amounts, these can replace iodine's locations inside the cells—most notably in thyroid cells and the Leydig cells in the testes.

So it is critical to have enough iodine in your system to optimize testosterone production. Some male biohackers I know even paint their testicles with the highly concentrated Lugol's iodine to get better testicular absorption! One iodine protocol—it's not proven by science, but many fitness forums claim it doubles testosterone—is a blend of selenium, magnesium, vitamin C, oral iodine, a B vitamin complex (which provides cofactors for ATP), and salt. The hypothesis for this therapy seems legit (replace minerals, vitamins, and iodine), but I've seen neither clinical nor animal studies.

14. Try Pulsed Electromagnetic Fields (PEMF)

Dirty electricity emitted from mobile phones, microwave ovens, WiFi routers, and other devices has been reported to affect biological systems, causing, for example, inflammation, radiation damage, and hyperthermia (heated tissue). What's especially concerning is that many folks keep their microwave-emitting smartphones in their front or back pockets, often quite close to testicles or ovaries. A number of studies have demonstrated clear relationships between smartphone use and reduced sperm count and sperm quality. These signals can also disrupt the Leydig cell population and testosterone concentration, along with hormonal balance in women.

PEMF may assist with rebalancing the neuroendocrine system, including hormone production. One study on rats showed that after microwave radiation—which caused oxidative stress and lowered testosterone production—PEMF therapy for sixty days helped the poor rats to bounce back so successfully that testosterone levels ended up even higher than before.

So if you know that you are being exposed to dirty electricity, especially near your nether regions, the use of a small PEMF device near your crotch (such as the FlexPulse, discussed in chapter 6) or a larger device for whole-body PEMF treatment (such as the Pulse XL Pro table from Pulse Centers, which I discussed in chapters 6 and 16) may be a good idea indeed.

15. Do Sex-Specific Exercises

Sex can be simultaneously the most pleasurable and the most stressful experience that you share with another human being. You've probably snickered before at that guy or gal at the gym who's thrusting their hips repeatedly towards the ceiling, but they're actually onto something. From grinding to thrusting to grunting to lifting to planking, there are some essential exercises that can help improve your sex life and sexual performance.

I'd recommend you begin by improving both the strength and endurance of your hip flexors, abdominals, and spinal erectors, all of which are muscles engaged in thrusting, circular hip motions and which stabilize your body in a number of different sex positions. Some of the best moves include barbell squats, Zercher squats (there's a video on BoundlessBook.com/18), glute bridges, hip thrusters, reverse hyperextensions, front planks, narrow-grip push-ups, reverse-grip chin-ups, and of course, the ab wheel rollout (trust me, it's incredibly effective and one of my go-to exercises for recovery in between, say, a set of squats and a set of overhead presses). One of the best authorities on glute exercises is Bret Contreras, who recently wrote a book called *The Glute Lab*, which I highly recommend.

There's something to be said for Kegel exercises too, in which you squeeze and contract the same muscles you'd squeeze if you were trying to stop the flow of urine, tightening and relaxing these muscles for intervals of two to five seconds for ten to fifteen reps at a time, several times a day. As I've learned from podiatrist Dr. Emily Splichal and biomechanist Katy Bowman, it's important to train these muscles not in isolation but rather in conjunction with their supporting musculature, most notably the transversus abdominis. This is best achieved by imagining that the area just a few inches below your navel is the center of a clock, with 9 in front of you and 3 behind you, and you are attempting to draw in 9 toward 3 and noon toward 6 while at the same time squeezing your Kegel muscles. It sounds complex, but it works, and when done right you feel your entire lower abdominal musculature contract in unison, rather than only your Kegels.

With just a few hours a week devoted to exercise, you can indeed improve your sex life significantly. Should you want to add in a bit more Eastern, Taoist-like breathwork to take things to the next level, orgasmically speaking, then see the sidebar on tantric sex on page 475.

Finally, to develop even better breathwork, more flexibility, and more cardiovascular endurance, along with a better ability to move energy throughout your body (which especially enhances intercourse), give Kundalini yoga a try. When it comes to sex, I've found that to be the most helpful form of yoga.

16. Inject Your Penis with Stem Cells

In 2017, the European Association of Urology published trial results showing that stem cells can restore sufficient erectile function to allow previously impotent men to have spontaneous intercourse. It worked for eight of twenty-one patients, and it's the first time that such therapy has enabled men suffering from ED to have sex without needing other medicines, injections, or implants. The Danish researchers utilized the same fat-sucking, stem-cell-harvesting procedure that cost me a cool $8,000 at the US Stem Cell Clinic, which covered about thirty vials.

Before committing to a penile injection as yet another form of self-immersive journalism to see if a guy can go from good to great in the sex department via just a little bit of better living through science, I reviewed the risks. If it was done incorrectly, I could suffer serious infection, nerve damage, and complete loss of sexual function, going from ramrod straight to wet-noodle saggy. Then again, I am relentless self-experimenter who makes a living pushing the boundaries of sound judgment (I once installed blue-face-hypoxia-producing devices in my office to train for the Spartan Agoge, a 38-below-zero adventure race in Vermont). Call me reckless—a few of my editors sure did—but I'm not one to let reasonable fear get in the way of a fun story.

First, some of my adipose tissue was removed in a process called autologous adipose-derived adult stem cell transplantation. Afterward, it was spun in a centrifuge to remove waste and create a bloody stew rich in mesenchymal stem cells—the type that can transform into other types of cells, such as bone cells, cartilage cells, or muscle cells. The stem cells were then isolated using a filtration process, and, just before injection, would be added to my own platelet-rich plasma (PRP) and activated with a low-light laser. A roughly decade-old technique used to concentrate growth factors from blood platelets, PRP has been shown to accelerate healing of tendinopathy and arthritis in joints, as well as wounds and surgical sites.

Straight-up PRP injections can be used to treat the penis, but in this newer technique, PRP is blended with stem cells for their regenerative benefits. The injection can occur on the same day as the harvest. But in my case, according to the physician assistant, I was way too skinny (ahem, I prefer "shredded") to get enough fat tissue. My stem cells needed time to multiply.

After returning home, I looked up stem cell and antiaging clinics in eastern Washington and northern Idaho. Most of the phone calls started like this: "Hi, have any of your physicians ever injected stem cells into a penis?" I didn't want a rookie with trembling hands dropping a syringe of my expensive stem cells, nor did I want someone's first time to be with my penis.

"Well," the receptionists typically said, "we do joints and skin procedures, but—"

"Thank you! Have a great day!" Click.

Finally, on my fifth call, the office manager at Lenoue Integrative Medicine in Spokane told me, "Yes, Dr. Pasma has performed this several times. Do you have access to your stem cells?"

Eight weeks after being harvested, my baby Frankensteins were ready to be shipped. The US Stem Cell Clinic sent me an order form, conducted a virtual swipe of my credit card for $300, and voilà: there was a knock at my front door at 7 a.m. on the morning of my injection. Bleary-eyed, I opened it and found a smiling, freckle-faced FedEx driver holding a potential holy grail of sexual vigor. Two hours later, clutching my precious stem cells with both hands, I shouldered open the glass doors at Lenoue Integrative Medicine. An unshaven twentysomething with messy hair and wearing blue scrubs and orange tennis shoes looked up from behind the counter.

"Hi, can I help you?"

I cleared my throat and glanced around nervously, hoping to find a gray-haired professional in a lab coat or a studious nurse in a clean white frock—anyone other than this apparent frat boy.

"I'm Ben Greenfield. I'm here for...you know...the injection."

He smiled broadly and extended his hand.

"Mr. Greenfield! We've been expecting you. I'm Dr. Pasma!"

Gulp. I reached over the counter and shook his hand, hoping it had been thoroughly washed and looking for even the slightest sign of a tremor. But I could find no excuse to back out now. After unveiling my stem cells—two small, unimpressive syringes sat on ice at the bottom of a large Styrofoam box—I completed a few pages of paperwork and soon found myself in the exam room.

First, Dr. Pasma gathered a vial of blood from my arm, to be spun in a centrifuge and blended with my stem cells. Fifteen minutes later, he returned with a handful of syringes and an iPad. "So, what kind of music do you want to listen to?"

I shrugged at the unexpected question but thought to myself, *The kind of that induces deep focus and concentration, doc.* When I opened my mouth, I said, "Deep house, I guess?" With techno beats thumping in the background, I fell backward on the table and jacked down my pants. Remember this the next time your doctor needs to check anything below the belt: it's like jumping off a cliff into the ocean—the longer you wait, the more awkward and difficult it becomes. In my year of "dicksperiments," I had mastered the drill: wear loose pants, preferably no underwear, and expose yourself as if it is the most natural thing in the world.

The next few minutes went by quickly. Dr. Pasma injected a nerve block into the right and left sides of my penis. A few seconds later, he took the two syringes of stem cells, mixed them with plasma, and injected one into each side of my corpus cavernosa. I sighed with relief—this guy was no slack, just a fast-working professional. The entire procedure took less than five minutes.

As I pulled up my pants, he held out another syringe. "You want this?" he asked, smiling.

I furrowed my eyebrows. "You didn't inject all the stem cells?"

"Nah, this is just leftover plasma. But it makes a great facial moisturizer."

So is this alternative-medicine junk science, or junk science?

"For men without any symptoms of erectile dysfunction, stem cell injections in the penis are unlikely to cause any benefit but are more likely to cause harm," says Dr. Alex Shteynshlyuger, the director at New York Urology Specialists. "We know that the injection of medications into the penis predisposes men to a small risk of scar formation called Peyronie's disease, which can lead to erectile dysfunction, bent penis, and shortening and narrowing of the penis. While the risk from a few injections is small, it is not a pleasant risk for men who have no problems to start with."

Dr. Shteynshlyuger also said that penile stem cell injections currently being marketed to men should really be called "god-knows-what injections," because there is no quality control to determine what kind of cells are being used and no scientifically valid method of injecting a specified dose. While the hope is that these presumed stem cells lead to penile regeneration, there is no assurance that they won't become abnormal cells, such as scar tissue cells or precancerous cells.

I didn't know this until several months after the procedure, but I had already started questioning things the day after my stem cells were harvested in Florida. That's when the FDA issued the US Stem Cell Clinic a warning letter for violating safety protocols and, in the words of FDA commissioner Scott Gottlieb, MD, misleading "vulnerable patients into believing they are being given safe, effective treatments that are in full compliance with the law." (The clinic says that procedures "in which a patient's own cells are reinjected back into the patient is based on sound science and is conducted by a licensed healthcare professional in a safe environment. However, FDA claims that the clinic's procedure constitutes drug manufacturing, and thus must be approved by FDA. We do not agree.")

But what about my positive findings?

Three hours after the stem cell/PRP injection in Spokane, my dick was black and blue. The next morning, before I left town for business, I had a quickie with my wife. I felt firmer, bigger even, and the orgasm was mind-blowing. Afterward, upon seeing the bruising on my penis, my wife said, "That must've hurt." It did. A little.

Four days later, back home from my trip, we went at it again. By now the bruising had vanished, and the sex was even better. We have lived together going on fifteen years, and although she has rarely uttered a word about the size of my penis, she remarked, as I emerged from the shower one morning, "Is that swelling from the surgery, or is it just growing? It's bigger."

According to New York–based urologist Dr. David Shusterman, these sound like the benefits of PRP—also known as a Priapus shot or P-shot—which should always be administered by a urologist to minimize bruising.

"PRP is effective for ED and will increase penis size and firmness during an erection," he says. "The difference between stem cells and PRP is that PRP is better studied and is, in my opinion, safer for now. The introduction of stem cells can attract a number of types of cells that are not needed or beneficial. PRP attracts the cell types needed for regeneration of the tissues. Stem cells may offer another treatment option over time, but stem cell therapy is currently more experimental."

Should my genitalia turn gray, fall off, or explode, I will cry, curse myself, and be sure to let everyone know. For now, I just have to figure out how I'm going to tell my children that Dad spent a hefty portion of their college fund on his dick.

17. Be a Man

As described in the book *The Way of the Superior Man* by David Deida, not only is expression of masculine essence key to being a true and complete man, but suppression of masculine activities—such as competition, fighting, hunting, lifting weights, leading your family, caring for your woman, building a legacy, and spending time with other men—can actually suppress biological functions, including testosterone production.

I've made it a point over the past several years to deeply explore what is often referred to as the "manosphere," an informal network of podcasts, blogs, forums, and websites about optimizing masculinity. While I'm opposed to the popular manospheric idea that men "don't need women" and can operate independently without a feminine essence or a feminine presence in their lives (often referred to as "MGTOW," short for "Men Going Their Own Way"), and I'm also not a fan of the infatuation with pickup artistry that's so prevalent in the manosphere community, I've certainly found many of the resources within the manosphere to be incredibly motivating and educational, inspiring me to be a stronger man and better father and husband. Some of the better resources and books I've discovered include the following:

- The Rational Male book series by Rollo Tomassi
- *The Way of the Superior Man,* by David Deida (his book *Dear Lover: A Woman's Guide to Men, Sex, and Love's Deepest Bliss* is an excellent companion book for women)
- *Wild at Heart,* by John Eldredge (his book *Captivating* is a good companion book for women)
- *Be a Man*! by Larry Richards
- The 21 Convention YouTube channel, 21 Studios

Although not a manosphere resource per se, one of the most life-changing processes I've ever embarked on for enhancing my sense of legacy is the Lifebook process, which I completed with my wife. The Lifebook is a remarkable life-envisioning system that empowers you to achieve not just one or two of your life's biggest goals but all of them—and rapidly. During the process, you create an entire book that outlines in great detail your vision, strategy, beliefs, and premises for twelve different categories: health and fitness, intellectual life, emotional life, character, spiritual life, relationships, parenting, social, financial, career, quality of life, and life vision.

If I, God forbid, were to get hit by a bus tomorrow, someone would be able to hand my children my Lifebook and say, "Here. Here is your dad, in a book. This is everything he stands for, believes in, and values, and everything he would have wanted to teach you about life." You can learn more about the Lifebook at BenGreenfieldFitness.com/Lifebook.

18. Consider Testosterone Optimization Therapy.

No discussion of hormone optimization would be complete without addressing the confusing and controversial world of hormone replacement therapy for testosterone. One of my friends and one of the most knowledgeable guys I know, Jay Campbell, is my go-to resource on this topic, and his book *The Testosterone Optimization Bible* and my podcast with Jay (which you can find at BenGreenfieldFitness.com/Jay) are my sources for everything testosterone-related.

Testosterone is the lifeblood and the foundation of all things related to male health. In fact, suboptimal testosterone levels may be responsible for a seemingly endless list of diseases, including these:

- Depression
- Inflammation
- Infertility
- Obesity
- Heart disease
- Prostate diseases
- Diabetes
- Metabolic syndrome
- Insulin resistance

Using testosterone optimization therapy (TOT) is no different than using a health-promoting substance like aspirin, caffeine, or antibiotics. Exogenous testosterone has been successfully used to treat hypogonadism since its recognition as an essential biological molecule for male health in the 1930s, which won researchers the Nobel Prize for Chemistry.

The rewards of optimizing your testosterone levels via TOT are often dramatic and completely transformative. The men who go down the route of therapeutic administration ultimately classify their lives in two different phases: life before TOT and life after TOT. Here's just a sample of the ways in which testosterone can improve your mindset and physical health

- It's clinically proven to boost confidence levels, especially among potential sexual partners who are evaluating your potential as a mate.
- It improves mental outlook and resiliency, allowing you to remain more composed and tactical in stressful situations.
- It increases assertiveness, leading to greater certainty and faster decision-making.
- It reduces body fat.
- It increases muscle mass.
- It improves heart health.

- It helps treat depression.
- It improves memory and helps protect against Alzheimer's.
- It fights chronic inflammation.

As a man, your health (and your testosterone levels) are in your hands! Don't be like the millions of men worldwide who are doomed to low testosterone levels and suboptimal living. You can learn much more in *The Testosterone Optimization Bible* by Jay Campbell and on BoundlessBook.com/18.

THE LAST WORD

Let's finish with just a few of the best sex resources for more learning, including the most cutting-edge, proven, helpful books and programs I've found on sex. Here's what both my wife and I have found to be excellent resources:

- *The Multi-Orgasmic Man*, by Mantak Chia and Douglas Abrams
- *Men Are from Mars, Women Are from Venus*, by John Gray, PhD
- *How to Be a Great Lover* and *The Great Lover Playbook*, by Lou Paget
- *The Way of the Superior Man, Dear Lover*, and *Finding God Through Sex*, by David Deida
- *The 7 Principles for Making a Marriage Work*, by John Gottman
- Kim Anami's Sexual Salon, KimAnami.com
- Jordan Gray's sex and relationship counseling, JordanGrayConsulting.com
- Jon and Missy Butcher's Category 13 videos, JonAndMissy.com

Tantric Sex

Tantric sex, or tantra, is a slow, intimate form of sex that leads to a better connection between you and your partner. While there is no one singular way to do tantric sex, the simplest way is to slow down, control your breathing, and be cognizant of your body in every moment. When it comes to becoming multiorgasmic, especially as a man, cultivating this skill is simpler than you might think.

Set aside some time to masturbate yourself to arousal, and then consciously raise and lower your arousal level, alternating between nine and five on a scale of ten. Consciously use your breathing to circulate the sexual energy throughout your body. Do this for thirty to sixty minutes a couple of times per week, and you will become intimately aware of your ejaculatory point of no return. Once you're familiar with this arousal zone, you'll be able to ride the edge of this orgasmic precipice and experience multiple orgasms in no time. But let's be clear: don't think of each orgasm as a ten after a ten after a ten, but rather as riding the edge of a nine-point-five for seconds and eventually minutes at a time without having to pause for a break.

If you want to become proficient in the art of being multiorgasmic, it generally takes anywhere from one to three months of consistent practice. I learned this tactic from the book *The Multi-Orgasmic Male,* and when I first began trying it, I noted an increased connection and intimacy with my wife, more orgasms, greater sexual stamina, and more powerful orgasms. On the other hand, while the long game between the sheets sounds enticing, sometimes I don't like the feeling of holding back and being less animalistic. When I do it right, though, my body and mind seemed to blend, and the sensation is pure bliss.

The unfortunate truth is that in today's hookup culture, it's too easy to focus on the carnal aspect of sex and miss out on the deeper connection that lies just beneath the surface. But there's a reason physical intimacy is so alluring. There's an implicit promise of an emotional and spiritual relationship, which affects both your mental state and your physical satisfaction as much as doing it does.

Improving your physical sexual performance with the supplements, foods, and hacks listed in this chapter is a great way to start spicing up the bedroom, but you can really amp up your sexual experience by allowing for and nurturing powerful spiritual satisfaction through one of the most intimate physical experiences that humans can engage in. You'll discover an astounding amount of boundless energy pouring into your life.

ONE THING YOU CAN DO THIS WEEK

The next time you plan on having sex, forsake any big, rich, heavy, fat-filled, supposedly testosterone-producing meal such as steak, and instead eat a simple meal of blood-boosting foods like an arugula salad with beets, cubed watermelon, pumpkin seeds, extra-virgin olive oil, and a bit of dark chocolate or red wine.

Already eating the right foods? Then move on to connection and breath. During lovemaking, look into your partner's eyes, take deep breaths, and imagine the energy from each breath moving up your spine and washing over your head, then traveling down the front of your body and to your sex organs. You'll notice a powerful surge of boundless sexual energy!

> For citations for all the research studies mentioned in this chapter and a deeper dive into the topics of this chapter—including links to podcasts, blog posts, recommended tools and supplements, and much more—visit BoundlessBook.com/18.

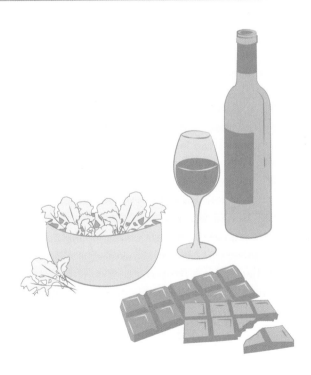

19

LONGEVITY DECODED

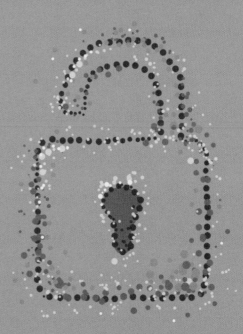

ANCESTRAL WISDOM AND MODERN SCIENCE TO MAXIMIZE HEALTH AND LIFE SPAN

Demographers, epidemiologists, gerontologists, and other researchers on aging have long puzzled over the theoretical question of the maximum human life span, along with the host of proposed practices that could help us achieve that potential. In the past decade alone, we have seen a veritable laundry list of tactics we can use to make ourselves more age-resistant, from nutrients, vitamins, and pills—including vitamin D, aspirin, metformin, magnesium, pterostilbene, resveratrol, blueberry extract, nicotinamide riboside, and rhodiola—to lifestyle practices such as shivering our asses off; self-imposed starvation; fecal transplants; strict veganism; injections of growth hormones, testosterone, stem cells, exosomes, and the blood of younger healthy humans; and, speaking of younger humans, simply having more children.

The fact is, compared to the biblical Methuselah, who purportedly lived to the ripe old age of 969, we do not seem to be moving the antiaging dial much. Researchers estimate that in the US today, the average adult life expectancy is still only about seventy-seven—and, disturbingly, that's now plummeting due to high rates of chronic diseases (many of which are preventable with simple lifestyle changes you'll learn about in this chapter). Despite the Chinese lore of the recently perished, allegedly 256-year-old Li Ching-Yuen, the longest-lived person on record is Jeanne Calment of France, who died in 1997 at 122 years and 164 days old.

Then there's a Jamaican woman named Violet Brown, who died in 2017 at 117. (She claimed her secrets to longevity included church, no pork, no chicken, and no rum!) At the time of this writing, the oldest person alive is Kane Tanaka of Japan, aged 115 years and 336 days.

But when we observe nature, some amount of immortality, or at least a significantly longer life span, appears to be achievable. Take the naked mole rat, for example. The naked mole rat's cells themselves seem to make proteins—the molecular machines that make bodies work—more accurately than human cells do, preventing it from developing age-related illnesses like cancer

The 256-Year-Old Man

Imperial Chinese government documents from 1827 congratulate Li Ching-Yuen on his 150th birthday, and documents from 1877 congratulate him on his 200th birthday. This Chinese herbalist and martial artist died in 1933 and claimed to have been born in 1736, although other records suggest he was actually born in 1677.

Is this possible? The longest confirmed life span on record is that of Jeanne Calment, who lived to be 122, and Li Ching-Yuen is reported to have lived to be 256, more than twice as long as Madame Calment! It strains credulity, but let's take a look at his life, shall we?

Li Ching-Yuen began his career as an herbalist at ten years old. He spent the majority of his life in the mountains of China eating a diet of herbs and rice wine and gathering plants and herbs, including wild ginseng, goji berries, lingzhi mushrooms, gotu kola, and he shou wu. These herbs are known to have potent longevity benefits, but are they enough to lend someone 256 years of life?

Surprisingly, Li Ching-Yuen did not ascribe his incredibly long life to his diet or even to his practice of qigong. While on his deathbed, Li said, "I have done all that I have to do in this world." In the West, aging is seen as an enemy to be conquered and overcome with technology and supplements. In fact, there's an entire philosophy, transhumanism, that holds that the human race can, through science and technology, evolve beyond its current physical and mental limitations. Li's last words suggest a very different outlook on life. He recognized that he had certain tasks to complete in this life, and when he had performed them, he willingly lay down to rest, knowing that he fulfilled the entirety of his life's purpose.

Li also gave longevity advice that flies in the face of the modern, hard-charging, go-hard-or-go-home outlook that many people subscribe to. When asked by the warlord Wu Pei-fu what the secret to long life is, Li is said to have replied, "Keep a quiet heart, sit like a tortoise, walk sprightly like a pigeon, and sleep like a dog." Li believed that the calmness and peace of mind with which he approached daily life contributed the most to his longevity.

Perhaps there is something to be learned from such a calm, long-lived man. Setting aside whether he was really 256 years old at his death, it seems pretty obvious that he did live a very long time and proved that there is much more to longevity than injecting yourself with all sorts of bizarre concoctions and engaging in the latest biohacks.

and Alzheimer's. And unlike in humans, the way these ugly little creatures handle glucose doesn't seem to change with age, reducing their susceptibility to diseases like diabetes. The naked mole rat also possesses genes that allow it to process oxygen more effectively than other rodent species, which may contribute to its impressive twenty-to-thirty-year life span.

The naked mole rat is not the only animal scientists are now probing to pick the lock of long life. With a rampant metabolism and a heart rate of one thousand beats per minute, the hummingbird should, on paper, be riddled with rogue, DNA-destroying free radicals, but the tiny birds seem relatively bulletproof against heart disease. Then there are lobsters, which seem to have evolved a protein that repairs the telomere tips of their chromosomes, allowing for a decreased rate of telomere shortening that most animals are incapable of achieving. (Recall from chapter 9 that telomeres become shorter each time the cell divides; once they're short enough, the cell can no longer repair and undergoes accelerated aging or, worse, becomes cancerous).

Consider Adwaita, the giant tortoise from India who died of liver disease in 2006. At the time he died, he looked just as young as a spry teenage tortoise—but carbon dating of his shell showed that he was over 250 years old. Some clams and oysters also don't seem to experience an increased risk of mortality as they age. For example, measuring the growth rings of one ocean quahog revealed that it had lived 507 years, and annual growth rings of other bivalves reveal an average life span of over 400 years. Even certain trees enjoy extreme longevity: a bristlecone pine named Methuselah in California is 4,851 years old!

Finally, as if rats, hummingbirds, lobsters, tortoises, clams, and trees were not enough to make us longevity-seeking humans a bit jealous, we mustn't forget one animal on earth that may hold the master key to immortality: *Turritopsis dohrnii,* also known as the immortal jellyfish. Most jellyfish, when they reach the end of their lives, die and melt into the sea, but not the immortal jellyfish. Instead, it sinks to the bottom of the ocean floor and its body folds in on itself—assuming the jellyfish equivalent of the fetal position—and regenerates back into a baby jellyfish in a rare biological process called transdifferentiation, in which its old cells somehow transform into young cells. The stem cells that allow for this continuous self-renewal express high levels of FOXO genes, which also play a key part in human longevity.

So is there a human equivalent to the immortality powers these animals seem to have tapped into? Many in popular antiaging and longevity circles have suggested that, in the next several decades, we could indeed unlock the secrets to living to approximately 120 to 140 years old. Indeed, many biohackers and antiaging enthusiasts such as Peter Diamandis, Elon Musk, Dave Asprey, Tony Robbins, and even li'l ol' me are striving to live longer than 160 years.

This chapter will not only teach you many of the advanced longevity secrets of the fringe biohackers but also reveal everything you need to know about why the world's more traditional longevity all-stars not only live longer but also tend to live better. They have strong connections with their family and friends. They are active. They wake up in the morning knowing that they have a purpose, and the world, in turn, reacts to them in a way that propels them along. An overwhelming majority of them enjoy life even in old age. They share common behavioral and lifestyle characteristics—such as close family relationships, avoidance of smoking, a plant-based diet, moderate and daily physical activity, social engagement, and participation in a community that includes people of all ages—even though they are all from different areas of the world and of different races, nationalities, and religions.

After spending nearly two decades immersed deeply in the health, fitness, nutrition, and longevity industries, I have come to the realization that embracing both modern science and ancestral wisdom can allow one to live a long and healthy life whose span rivals and even exceeds that of our ancestors. That is why my children and I forage for wild plants (a longevity tactic you'll learn more about in this chapter) but do so using a plant identification smartphone app that allows us to identify everything from mushrooms to plants with incredible accuracy—we can tap into a bit of better living through science so that we don't get poisoned or make fatal mistakes that our ancestors might have made while foraging. It's also why I own a quaint and simple, off-the-grid, barn-style home in the forest where we grow most of our own food, yet I fill that barn with tens of thousands of dollars' worth of modern antiaging biohacking equipment. And it's why, the last time I disappeared into a seven-day high-country elk bow-hunt in the mountains of Colorado, I had a neurofeedback brain-training device neatly tucked away in my camouflage backpack.

In this chapter, you will discover exactly how to live a happy, long, and fulfilled life with one foot planted in the realm of ancestral living and the other foot planted in the realm of modern science and biohacking. Granted, there are entire books and fantastic websites—most of which I have read word for word—that could fill thousands of pages of antiaging advice. My favorites are linked to on BoundlessBook.com/19. But for the purposes of this book, I have decided to give you the best of the best: the techniques I have personally tried, the tactics that are steeped in research, and the strategies that have thousands of years of practice behind them. So you can think of this chapter as a cookbook for longevity that gives you all the low-hanging fruit and teaches you all the basics of living a long and happy life while also exposing you to the more advanced practices that have emerged in the past several years.

But first, before I get into life-extending strategies, it is important to understand exactly how we age in the first place.

HOW WE AGE

There does not appear to be one single cause of aging. When I interviewed antiaging pioneer and impressively bearded Aubrey de Grey on my podcast, he outlined seven separate aging mechanisms his SENS Research Foundation (the acronym stands for "Strategies for Engineered Negligible Senescence") has identified and researched: mutations in chromosomes, mutations in mitochondria, junk inside cells, junk outside cells, cell death, protein cross-linking, and cell senescence (a phenomenon in which a cell can no longer divide but does not die, which would let other cells divide). Many longevity scientists would argue that plenty more than seven aging mechanisms exist, including my friend Dr. Harry Adelson, who theorizes that aging is due to a loss of available stem cells, and Dr. Michael Rose, who argues that aging is related to our loss of reproductive usefulness as we age.

These mechanisms are important to understand because, in order to truly enhance longevity, we should ideally address each and every element that might be causing us to grow old too soon. As you'll see, most are related to a simple accumulation of damage: breakages in the molecular machinery of cells, an accumulation of metabolic waste products that your body cannot break down, and the failure of biological systems that are increasingly unable to cope with the damage. Over time, this damage can affect every cell in every organ, structure, and tissue. Let's take a closer look at how this damage process affects the biological systems in your body.

Bones and Skeletal System

In men, bone density starts to diminish at age thirty-five. In women, this process occurs even earlier, with peak bone density occurring at around age thirty, and postmenopausal women experience an accelerated rate of bone loss. The foot arches become less pronounced, contributing to reduced height. The discs that separate your vertebrae lose fluid, which aggravates this effect even more. The long bones of the arms and legs become brittle due to mineral loss. Joints become stiffer and less flexible and can lose some of their fluid, causing the cartilage to rub together and wear out. Calcification, the depositing of minerals in and around some joints, also occurs.

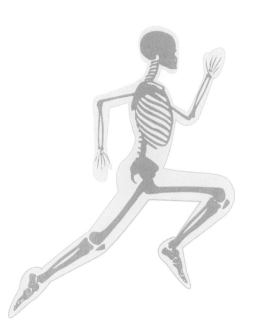

After thirty, skeletal muscle mass declines more than 20 percent in both men and women in the absence of triggers such as regular exercise, muscle loading, adequate protein, and, based on recent research, heat stress. With this gradual muscle loss, known as sarcopenia, strength and flexibility decreases, along with coordination, balance, and height. The deterioration of the central nervous system can also lead to a reduced ability to recruit muscle fibers. Posture deteriorates, and the overall risk of bone breakage increases. The gradual breakdown of the joints can lead to inflammation, pain, stiffness, and even physical deformities such as a hunched back or bowlegs.

Physical activity—particularly stressing the muscles and long bones of the skeletal systems—can help to slow many of these aging mechanisms, as can regular sauna exposure, healthy protein intake, and pulsed electromagnetic field therapy (discussed in chapters 6 and 12).

Digestive System

As digestive activity gradually slows with aging, you are more likely to get constipated frequently, which can often be exacerbated by medications, such as proton pump inhibitors and antibiotics, and by medical conditions, such as diabetes and irritable bowel syndrome. The muscle contractions that push food along your digestive tract can slow down with aging, causing waste to move more slowly through the colon, and the longer it takes to move through the colon, the more water it loses, which exacerbates constipation. Lower physical activity levels in older people can also contribute to the effects of constipation.

A condition known as diverticulosis can develop, which occurs when small pouches in the lining of the colon bulge through weak spots in the intestinal wall. This can lead to gas, bloating, cramps, and even more constipation. A more severe form of this condition, diverticulitis, occurs when the pouches become inflamed, leading to abdominal pain, cramping, fever, chills, nausea, and vomiting. Cancerous or noncancerous polyps can also form in the colon. Gastroesophageal reflux disease (GERD) is the most common age-related gastrointestinal disorder and occurs when stomach acid rises into the esophagus, causing heartburn and other symptoms.

Natural digestive enzyme production decreases with age, leading to a loss of protein absorption, which can further aggravate sarcopenia. Enzyme depletion even outside the digestive system can also be an issue, since enzymes are responsible for constructing, integrating, transporting, providing, and eliminating a host of nutrients and toxins. Research has shown that people who have a chronic disease or poor energy levels tend to have fewer enzymes in their blood, urine, and tissues.

Chewing food more thoroughly, eating adequate fiber and fermented foods, supplementing with digestive enzymes, and consuming amino acids—along with implementing the strategies in the gut and immune-system chapters of this book (chapters 13 and 15)—can all help to slow the aging of the digestive system and depletion of enzymes.

Respiratory System

Maximum lung capacity and maximum oxygen utilization (VO_2 max) decrease gradually after about age twenty-five, especially if you're not frequently exercising. You also experience decreases in measures of lung function such as vital capacity (the maximum amount of air that can be breathed out following a maximum inhalation), a weakening of the respiratory muscles, and a decline in the effectiveness of lung defense mechanisms, including reduced numbers of white blood cells on the surface of the lung alveoli.

As the muscles and tissues around your lungs, particularly the diaphragm, weaken, you experience a decreased ability to breathe enough air in and out, as well as a decreased ability to keep airways sufficiently open. The alveoli can lose their shape and become looser and more dysfunctional. Even the skeletal changes in the spine and ribs can impact the effectiveness of your respiratory system, and the part of the brain that controls breathing may also lose some of its function as you age.

All of these changes in the lung tissue can cause air to become trapped in the lungs, making it harder to breathe. Decreased lung capacity negatively impacts overall health in several ways. For example, one study that followed 5,200 individuals for three decades demonstrated that lung volume was the greatest predictor of health and longevity!

Regular cardiovascular exercise and the adoption of the type of breathwork practices and protocols described in chapter 3 can help to support the aging respiratory system.

Urinary System

After about age thirty to forty, two-thirds of us undergo a gradual decline in the rate at which our kidneys filter blood. The kidneys begin to lose tissue, and the number of filtering units known as nephrons decreases. The blood vessels that supply the kidneys can harden, further impairing the kidneys' filtration rate.

The bladder wall loses its elasticity, meaning it cannot hold as much urine as before, and the muscles controlling the bladder begin to weaken. The urethra can become blocked by an enlarged prostate gland in men or by a prolapsed (fallen) bladder or vagina in women. A loss of bladder control is quite common for women, especially around menopause, and medical conditions such as diabetes or a history of voluminous endurance sports can also contribute to this incontinence.

Simple strategies to control these issues include deep pelvic core training, adequate hydration and mineral intake, limited consumption of dehydrating foods such as alcohol and caffeine, and avoidance of excess protein.

Reproductive System

For women, menstrual cycles stop at around age fifty-one and the ovaries halt production of estrogen and progesterone. The ovaries also stop producing eggs, and after menopause, you can no longer become pregnant. Vaginal walls become thinner, drier, less elastic, and possibly irritated, which can often cause sex to become painful. The risk of vaginal yeast infections increases, and the external genital tissue and breast tissue thins. The pubic muscles can lose tone, resulting in a prolapsed vagina, uterus, or bladder.

Men do not experience a major change in fertility with age, but testicular tissue mass decreases and testosterone gradually declines, along with blood flow to the reproductive organs. Sperm production falls, though it doesn't stop. The volume of ejaculated fluid often remains constant, but there are fewer living sperm in it. The prostate gland enlarges as some of the prostate tissue is replaced with scar-like tissue. Men can also experience problems getting an erection. Based on the theory that reproductive uselessness can accelerate aging because we are no longer able to propagate the population, it is important to maintain regular sexual activity with age and even utilize many of the sexual enhancement biohacks from chapter 18, such as acoustic sound wave therapy, infrared therapy, or stem cell injections.

Endocrine System

The hypothalamus, located in the brain, produces hormones that control the other structures in the endocrine system. Although the levels of these regulating hormones stay the same as you age, the responses of the other endocrine organs to those hormones can diminish.

At thirty years old, human growth hormone begins its regression in both men and women and declines at a rate of around 14 percent per decade. When women transition into menopause, progesterone, testosterone, and estrogen levels begin to fall. At fifty, thyroid activity begins to decrease, and hyper- or hypothyroidism may develop.

Also at fifty, men may begin to experience andropause (the male version of menopause, most notably accompanied by a decrease in testosterone). In both men and women, a decline in DHEA (a potent hormonal precursor) can cause increased vulnerability to a variety of cancers. At sixty, as insulin production decreases and insulin cell receptor sensitivity lowers, the ability to metabolize sugar declines, and insulin resistance or diabetes becomes more prevalent. At seventy, hormones that protect against the loss of calcium in bones decline, making osteoporosis more prevalent.

One reason that the natural hormone replacement industry is now booming is that it can be effective for mitigating many of the endocrine issues that occur with age. However, more ancestral practices, such as organ meat consumption, regular sex, care for the gut, and the avoidance of modern plastics and endocrine-disrupting chemicals, can be equally effective strategies.

Circulatory System

At around forty years old, your heart muscles thicken and blood vessels stiffen, which can cause the heart to fill with blood more slowly (this can often occur earlier if you're a hard-charging athlete). This forces the heart to work harder to pump blood through the vessels and can lead to high blood pressure and other cardiovascular problems, such as cardiac arrhythmias. The receptors that monitor blood pressure when you change positions can also deteriorate, which can cause dizziness when you stand up from sitting or lying down. This process can be further exacerbated by calcification, or excess calcium deposits, in the body, which manifests as the stiffening of joints, plaque buildup on the teeth, a hardening of the arteries, impaired brain function, and general aches and pains. Many individuals over sixty have enlarged deposits of calcium mineral in their major arteries, often caused by a lack of minerals in the diet, dehydration, limescale in tap water, and even synthetic calcium supplements.

Abnormal heart rhythms can develop, leading to arrhythmias like atrial fibrillation. The heart's natural pacemaker, which controls the rate of the heartbeat, can develop fibrous tissue and fat deposits in some of its pathways and lose some of its cells, resulting in a slower heart rate. The walls of blood vessels, especially the smaller capillaries, can thicken, resulting in a slower rate of exchange of nutrients and waste products. The blood itself can change: the total water content of blood falls, and your ability to produce new red blood cells and certain white blood cells deteriorates.

The circulatory system also includes the lymphatic fluid that circulates through the body, and if the lymphatic circulation stagnates, toxins can accumulate and immune cells are not delivered to the areas of the body where they are needed most, resulting in the deterioration of immunity and a weakened ability to fight infection and disease.

Regular cardiovascular exercise, hydration, regular exposure to heat and cold, and the lymph-fluid-circulating strategies from chapter 15 can all help to stave off these issues.

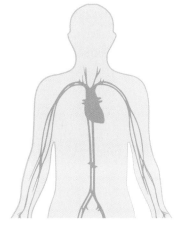

Nervous System

The nervous system doesn't decline with age as dramatically as some of the other systems, but during normal aging, some nerve cell structure and function is indeed lost, which causes messages to be sent more slowly. Waste products can collect in brain tissue, causing plaques and tangles. The most severe decline in mental function is a result of diseases such as Alzheimer's and other forms of dementia, which some doctors attribute to these plaques and tangles. (Plaques are actually a part of the immune system and release antimicrobial agents to deal with bacterial, viral, or fungal infections in the brain, but over the course of a lifetime they can accumulate in neural tissue, which causes cognitive decline.) Even diabetes can affect thinking and behavior in older individuals.

By age forty, the lenses in the eyes begin to stiffen, resulting in vision impairment, particularly when focusing on near objects. Hearing loss might develop, which occurs sooner in men than in women, and memory also tends to worsen.

By paying close attention to and implementing the strategies found in chapters 1 through 7, you can significantly support your nervous system and keep these issues at bay.

Skin

Stem cell production and stem cell availability both decline with age, and one result of this is that the skin's epidermal cells slow in their reproduction. Melanocytes, which produce pigmentation, decrease in number while the remaining cells increase in size. This can cause thinner, more translucent skin, as well as large pigmented spots like liver spots. Skin injuries, tearing, and infections become more frequent as skin integrity deteriorates.

Loss of fat and collagen in the underlying tissues can cause skin to sag and wrinkle, and the connective tissue loses its strength and elasticity, a process known as elastosis. The blood vessels in the skin become more fragile, and bruising, bleeding under the skin, cherry angiomas, and other conditions become more common. The skin becomes dry and itchy as the glands that produce oil reduce their production levels. The fat layer beneath the cutaneous layer of skin thins, leading to an increased risk of skin injury and a reduced ability to maintain consistent body temperature. Sweat glands produce less sweat, making it harder to cool off and increasing the risk of overheating or developing heat stroke.

Stem cell–supporting strategies, along with the beauty tactics from chapter 17, can help to keep all this from occurring or minimize these effects.

Underlying Causes

So what are the underlying causes of this type of full-body, systemic damage that occurs with age? There are a variety of factors that can aggravate or accelerate age-related deterioration, but the following processes are the major culprits.

CHRONIC INFLAMMATION

Inflammation can often go on for years without your noticing until accelerated aging and disease suddenly set in. As a matter of fact, of the ten leading causes of mortality in the US, chronic inflammation contributes to at least seven:

- Alzheimer's disease
- Stroke
- Chronic lower respiratory disease (asthma)
- Cancer
- Diabetes
- Heart disease
- Influenza and pneumonia

GLYCATION

Glycation occurs when sugars in the bloodstream attach to proteins to form harmful molecules called advanced glycation end products (AGEs). The more sugar in your diet or the more chronically elevated your blood sugar levels, the more likely it is that AGEs will develop, which can cause inflammation and cell membrane damage that can result in the development of degenerative diseases such as diabetes, atherosclerosis, chronic kidney disease, and Alzheimer's disease.

METHYLATION DEFICITS

Methylation—the process of transferring a methyl group from one molecule to another—is a crucial biological process that's involved in removing toxins, growing and repairing cells, and metabolic functioning. Methylation deficits are linked to a number of health conditions, including diabetes and cancer, and are caused by a variety of factors, including stress, nutrient deficiencies, and genetics.

DEGRADING MITOCHONDRIA

A growing number of cell biologists have proposed that the number and functionality of mitochondria can determine your potential for longevity, and one major theory of aging—the free-radical theory—posits that the oxidation of cells by reactive oxygen species (ROS) plays a leading role in the weakening of vital functions in aging organisms. The mitochondrial interior has been researched and found to be particularly susceptible to this oxidation. In addition, since mitochondria exhibit less damage in women than in men, scientists have speculated that the health of mitochondrial DNA might be a factor in why women live longer than men.

Poor lifestyle factors, such as bad air, unclean water, artificial light, electrical pollution, inflammation, a nutrient-poor diet low in antioxidants, lack of exercise, and many, many others, can contribute to poor mitochondrial status.

The Most Important Data to Track

Because of the dangers of chronic inflammation and glycation, I am convinced that the two most important markers you can track for overall health and longevity are your levels of inflammation and your glycemic variability. For inflammation, hs-CRP is a simple value to track (see chapter 16 for more details), but an advanced inflammatory panel from a company such as Quest Diagnostics can also test markers such as myeloperoxidase, Lp-PLA2, dimethylarginine, oxidized LDL, prostaglandins, and fibrinogen. For glycemic variability, blood glucose and hbA1c are the best markers, although a continuous glucose monitor, such as the Dexcom G6, can give even better data. Chapter 16 has more details on tracking your biomarkers, including sections on hs-CRP and continuous glucose monitors.

Overmethylation and Undermethylation

For the carnivores out there those who just have to have their meat, the meat eaters who say, "I like my steak. I like my steak with eggs," there is a problem. Most meat, particularly muscle tissue, contains high amounts of methionine, which is a potent methyl donor. Over the next few paragraphs, you will learn what exactly a methyl group is, why it may be bad for you to overconsume strong methyl donors, and how to eliminate the side effects of overmethylation or undermethylation.

A methyl group is a carbon atom attached to three hydrogen atoms. It is an abundant organic compound that is derived from methane. Normally, methyl groups are attached to larger molecules, but on their own, they can be a methyl anion, methyl cation, or methyl radical. Methylation occurs when a methyl group is taken from one compound or molecule and is transferred to another—for example, a methyl group can be added to your DNA from a methyl donor like methionine. The process is largely responsible for switching genes on and off and silencing viruses. When your body experiences normal methylation, less desirable genes, such as those that code for cancers and autoimmune diseases, are switched off while helpful genes are switched on. Methylation is also required for cell division, neurotransmitter synthesis and metabolism, detoxification, cellular energy metabolism, the formation of protective myelin sheaths around neurons, and early central nervous system development.

The critical functions of methylation mean that when the process malfunctions, your body can go haywire quickly. Undermethylation is a state of low methylation, either because your body is unable to adequately transfer methyl groups or because you're not consuming enough methyl-donating compounds or foods. Overmethylation is a state of high methylation. Neither of these states is necessarily bad (undermethylation, for example, is often associated with attention to detail, slight perfectionism, and high levels of personal accomplishments), but they both have the capacity to cause different kinds of mental and physical stress.

Because it can keep serotonin levels low, undermethylation can cause you to be a dopamine-seeking, hard-charging high achiever. It can lead you to pursue perfection and achievement and has been associated with obsessive-compulsive tendencies, a low tolerance for pain, and ritualistic behaviors. A state of undermethylation can also make people more susceptible to depression.

Overmethylation is associated with creativity and sensitivity. If you are prone to overmethylation, you probably exhibit high levels of empathy for others but also experience sleep issues, food and chemical sensitivities, hyperactivity, panic attacks, and a tendency to gain unwanted weight. Overmethylation has also been highly correlated with schizophrenia.

If you are prone to undermethylation, you will do well with a high intake of muscular meats. Because you do not have enough methyl groups being transferred to places that need them—like your DNA—you might need to consume a higher amount of meat to compensate, especially if you consume high quantities of plant matter and folate, as these do not supply sufficient amounts of methyl groups necessary for good health in undermethylators. In addition, folate acts as a serotonin reuptake promoter. Drugs like antidepressants and selective serotonin reuptake inhibitors are received very well by undermethylators, so any compound like folate that exerts the opposite effect could be devastating to undermethylators.

If you are prone to overmethylation, the last thing you need is a higher intake of methyl donors like muscle meat (such as daily servings of steak and chicken). This would be an instance where vegetarianism or a largely plant-based diet could be beneficial. If you are an overmethylator, you need to consume adequate amounts of protein, but don't become an extreme carnivore and load up most of your plate with cuts of animals and the rest of the plate with one-tenth of an inch of vegetables (that ratio should actually be reversed!).

As a word of caution, the only way to know for sure whether you are prone to undermethylation or overmethylation is to undergo DNA testing via a testing service such as 23andMe or, for even more targeted data, a company like StrateGene, Youtrients, or TreeOfLife.

FATTY ACID IMBALANCES

Fat is a vital nutrient, and the human body needs an optimal ratio of omega-6 to omega-3 fatty acids to support normal cell membrane function in aging cells. As you have already learned, a diet high in omega-6 (often because of a high intake of vegetable oils) and low in omega-3, DHA, and monounsaturated fats can create deficits or imbalances in fatty acids.

IMMUNE DYSFUNCTION

Autoimmune diseases develop when your immune system turns on itself, resulting in inflammation and organ and cell damage. Autoimmune diseases—which include rheumatoid arthritis, lupus, multiple sclerosis, thyroid disease, and inflammatory bowel disease—are becoming increasingly common, especially in an era of chemical exposure, antibiotic overuse, and unhealthy guts.

TELOMERE SHORTENING

Telomeres are the segments of DNA at the end of our chromosomes, often compared to the plastic tips of shoelaces that keep the laces from fraying. Telomeres prevent chromosomes from becoming damaged or tangling with one another. When chromosomes do become damaged, this can cause the destruction of genetic information, leading to cellular malfunction, which increases your risk of disease and overall mortality.

Telomerase is an enzyme that lengthens telomeres and keeps them from wearing out too fast or too early and can be deleteriously affected by lack of exercise, chronic stress, low plant consumption, and a lack of mindfulness practices such as meditation and yoga.

DNA EXPRESSION

Geneticists and oncologists have long recognized that overexposure to environmental assailants such as chemicals and radiation can cause DNA damage and affect the way genes are expressed. Nutrient depletion and other environmental factors, such as electrical pollution and poor air, light, and water, can also alter gene expression. Researchers have also demonstrated that our genes can respond to our conscious thoughts and emotions and even our unconscious beliefs.

If you feel that you are constantly fighting an uphill battle against the aging processes of damage and degradation, you are right. Fortunately, basic and natural habits to enhance longevity have long been studied, and many directly affect the exact biological mechanisms involved in aging. Consider this chapter to be your guidebook to managing and mitigating the issues you have just read about, beginning with the longevity basics, then progressing to the more advanced tactics and biohacks.

12 ESSENTIAL HABITS TO ENHANCE LONGEVITY

Dan Buettner wrote the book *The Blue Zones* with the goals of discovering which populations in the world had the highest number of centenarians (people who live to be over one hundred) and teaching the world how to use the lessons from these populations. The five Blue Zones where Buettner and his team of researchers discovered the longest-living people on earth were Okinawa, Japan; Sardinia, Italy; Nicoya, Costa Rica; Ikaria, Greece; and the Seventh-Day Adventists in Loma Linda, California. Buettner discovered several characteristics that the people in these zones shared, such as these:

- A lack of smoking
- A high intake of wild plants
- A regular intake of legumes, usually prepared using ancestral methods such as soaking, sprouting, or fermentation
- Constant moderate physical activity, not as isolated exercise sessions or gym workouts but as a natural part of life (e.g., gardening, yard work, walking, and bicycling)
- Healthy family relationships and social engagement (despite less use of social media, people are extremely socially active and integrated into their communities)

Other key characteristics Buettner identified were low-to-moderate alcohol intake (especially wine and other fermented beverages), caloric moderation and fasting, a strong life purpose, low amounts of stress, and engagement in a spiritual discipline, religion, or belief in a higher power.

So how can you practically implement these habits into your own life? Here are a few potent and highly effective strategies, and some of the more common roadblocks I have seen people run into during my own consulting and coaching.

1. Don't Smoke

Your telomere length is measured in base pairs, which are the building block units that make up the ladderlike rungs of DNA. In childhood, telomeres are about fifteen thousand base pairs long, but by the time we reach old age, they have shortened to about three thousand base pairs, which equates to a loss of about two dozen base pairs per year. The oxidative damage inflicted by smoking a pack of cigarettes every day destroys an additional five pairs each year. So if you smoke for forty years, it can rob you of more than seven years of life (obesity has a similar effect: the telomeres of obese women can be as much as 240 base pairs shorter later in life than those of lean women, which is roughly equivalent to about a loss of about nine years of life).

Granted, there are some cases in which smoking can be beneficial. Think back to chapter 5's discussion of smoking or vaping loose leaf tea, organic tobacco, essential oils, and marijuana. In moderation, the stress-reducing and energy-enhancing benefits of this practice likely outweigh any cons derived from exposure to heated, potentially carcinogenic compounds, especially when vaping. In addition, as you learned in chapter 5, it really isn't the nicotine in cigarettes or cigars that is harmful.

But unless you have been living under a rock, you are no doubt aware of the dangers of chronic smoking. Cigarette smoking causes almost *half a million deaths each year*, nearly one in five of all deaths in the United States. Secondhand smoke isn't much better, causing frequent and severe asthma attacks, respiratory infections, ear infections, sudden death in children and infants, cancers like coronary cancer in adults, and, highly relevant to what you'll discover about longevity later in this chapter, extreme hampering of effective stem cell mobilization (the movement of stem cells to other areas of the body from their storage in bone marrow). In other words, don't smoke—period. As much as possible, limit your exposure to secondhand smoke. Not only that, but because air pollution has been directly linked to a decrease in telomere length, act proactively: if you live in an apartment complex, work in an office, or frequent areas that expose you to airborne pollutants, then use HEPA air filtration, houseplants that filter the air, and other air cleanup tactics you will find in chapter 20. In addition, increase your intake of whole-food, plant-based antioxidants or full-spectrum antioxidants from supplements.

Undoing the Damage of Smoking

The negative effects of smoking are well known, and it is therefore not surprising that one feature of Blue Zones is a lack of smoking. Downsides to smoking include:

- Habit formation from the effects of nicotine on the central nervous system

- Withdrawal symptoms like anxiety, irritability, depression, headaches, and sleep problems when you try to quit

- Emphysema, the irreversible destruction of the air sacs in your lungs

- Chronic bronchitis, the permanent inflammation in the lining of the breathing tubes of the lungs

- Lung cancer

- The constriction and damage of blood vessels, which can lead to peripheral artery disease

- Hypertension, a condition of chronically elevated blood pressure

- Increased risk of stroke

If you have been smoking, the good news is that much of the damage can be reversed. The first thing to do is to stock up on supportive nutrients and supplements for the moment you quit. When you quit smoking, your adrenal glands, which secrete antistress hormones, must adapt to the lack of nicotine and other addictive chemicals. You can support your adrenals with adaptogenic herbs or supplements such as St. John's wort or ginseng. Research has shown you can minimize the damage to your arteries by taking a taurine supplement once a day for two months. Since smoking also damages skin collagen and elastin, eat a diet rich in proanthocyanidins, a phytochemical found in red wine, grapes, apples, blueberries, black currants, hazelnuts, pecans, and pistachios. The polyphenols found in kale and sprouts can also repair your lungs' alveoli and bronchioles, so a former smoker's diet should contain high amounts of these foods too.

When it comes to risk of smoking-related diseases such as esophageal and lung cancer or cardiovascular disease, Dr. William Li's excellent book *Eat to Beat Disease* points out specific antioxidant-rich compounds that can lower the risk of these diseases, such as black raspberries, extra-virgin olive oil, and fermented forms of soy such as miso, natto, and tempeh. In addition, one study examined the effects of drinking four cups of green tea per day on the stem cells and blood vessels of smokers, and noted a 43 percent increase in endothelial stem cells over two weeks, along with a 29 percent increase in vascular function.

Once you give up smoking, your body will begin to respond immediately. Six hours after quitting, circulating levels of the poisonous gas carbon monoxide will decline, and your heart won't have to work so hard to pump oxygen. Within twelve weeks, your lung function will significantly improve and coughing, sinus congestion, shortness of breath, and fatigue levels will all decline. During this time frame, your lungs' hairlike cleaning structures called cilia will regrow, similar to the way that the intestinal cilia can become restored and renewed after you stop eating an inflammatory diet. After three months, your sexual performance will improve as testosterone levels normalize. After nine months, your risk of heart and cardiovascular complications will fall. After one year, it will be like you never smoked, especially if you use the strategies above.

Other dietary strategies that can help to reverse the effects of smoking include these:

- Foods high in vitamin E, like eggs, nuts, and dark leafy greens

- Foods high in CoQ10, like salmon, beef, broccoli, and avocado

- Vitamin-C-rich foods that contain high amounts of bioflavonoids, like grapefruit, spinach, and citrus fruits (especially kiwi)

- Foods rich in vitamin B complex, like dark leafy greens, eggs, fish, and liver

- A full-spectrum multivitamin rich in antioxidants

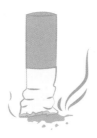

2. Eat Plants

Aside from the Seventh-Day Adventist population of Loma Linda, California, most centenarians are not vegans or vegetarians. But most do follow a predominantly plant-based diet, usually because they depend on their own homegrown or locally grown foods. Long-lived Sardinians, Nicoyans, and Okinawans tend to consume nutrient-dense produce they grow in their own gardens and supplement them with smaller amounts of animal protein, along with traditional staples like legumes, ancient grains (such as quinoa, amaranth, and millet), sweet potatoes, and corn tortillas.

Plants deliver plenty of fiber, including insoluble fiber, a natural anticancer agent, antioxidants, oxidized cholesterol reducers, blood-clotting factors, and essential minerals. Perhaps most notably, plants—especially wild plants, as I'll explain later in this chapter—possess natural built-in defense mechanisms that subject the body and gut to mild amounts of stress, causing a hormetic response that can allow the body to better mount its own antioxidant defenses. Thus, trace amounts of saponins in quinoa; lectins in soy and potatoes; gluten in wheat, rye, and barley; anthocyanins in berries; resveratrol in grape skins and red wine; EGCG in green tea; sulforaphane in broccoli and other cruciferous vegetables; catechins in cacao; and other controversial compounds are actually good for you. Even plants' phytochemicals, which contribute so many of the benefits of a plant-heavy diet, induce a mild, hormetic cellular stress that precondition your body to respond better to other, more severe stressors. One excellent book that explores this topic is *Eating on the Wild Side* by Jo Robinson, which even advises cutting up or tearing apart plants such as kale several hours before eating them. This action causes the plant to believe it is being attacked by a wild animal and to amp up its natural defense mechanisms, which then mildly stress your body upon consumption.

In many of the Blue Zones, red meat is typically eaten only a few times a month—notably during holidays and festivals—although sheep's or goat's milk, eggs, and fish are eaten often, usually two or three times per week. The animal products that are consumed tend to be raised locally, grass-fed, pasture-raised (or wild-caught, in the case of fish), and free from many of the harmful substances commonly used in conventionally raised meat and dairy, like antibiotics and growth hormones. Author Michael Pollan's recommendation to "eat food, not too much, mostly plants" is sage advice, especially for those genetically predisposed to thrive on a higher vegetable intake and lower meat intake.

When you do consume meat, rather than simply consuming the muscle, which inevitably contains high levels of methionine and low levels of glycine, which can be a mortality risk factor, consume the glycine-rich offal, such as the organ meats, marrow, and bone broth. If, for gut health or immune reasons, you plan to follow a plant-restricted diet such as the carnivore diet, consider tapping into the cellular resilience benefits that plant intake can bestow by engaging in other forms of mild stress, such as frequent sauna visits, cold thermogenesis, fasting, smart amounts of exercise, and exposure to sunlight radiation, and eat plants low in natural defense mechanisms or plants treated to deactivate their defense mechanisms (read Dr. Steven Gundry's book *The Plant Paradox* to learn more about this strategy).

Finally, if you have existing gut issues such as IBD, diverticulosis, or diverticulitis, you may want to be careful with excessive fiber intake from plant matter and should instead choose herbs and spices over "big-ass salads" and giant kale smoothies.

3. Avoid Processed and Packaged Foods

Refined carbohydrates, artificial flavors, processed vegetable oils, and natural sweeteners are very rare in longevity hot spots. It's not that those living in the Blue Zones never let themselves enjoy guilty pleasures; it's just that their guilty pleasures are typically antioxidant-rich treats such as local red wine (one to two glasses per day), sake, coffee, herbal tea, or simple desserts such as nuts, cheese, and berries or grapes. Soda, sports drinks, candy bars, and packaged baked goods—including giant bags of sweet potato chips or bottles of sugary so-called superfood kombuchas—simply are not prevalent in these diets. You also won't find these populations consuming high amounts of popular so-called health foods that you find in the healthy-foods section of many supermarkets, convenience stores, and airport newsstands, such as packaged dried fruits, trail mix, energy bars, and other items that notoriously include blood-sugar-spiking or inflammation-producing compounds such as vegetable oils and simple carbohydrates, often deceptively labeled as "organic sunflower oil," "cane sugar," or "agave syrup."

What Did Your Ancestors Eat?

Ancestral dieting seems to have become quite sexy of late. As we learn more about genetics and how diet is controlled by and impacts genetic expression, it seems to make sense that you should eat what your ancestors ate. After all, you have inherited a set of genes that developed and adapted to specific environments and diets, so it seems worth maximizing that genetic potential.

For example, in my case, as someone from predominantly Northern European ancestry, I eat plenty of fermented foods, meats, fish, eggs, berries, and raw dairy, without a large intake of citrus fruits or other foods my ancestors would not have encountered in their local habitat. If you are of Scandinavian origins, your ancestors had good access to fish rich in omega-3s and vitamin D, so you likely need a diet higher in fish and vitamin D for optimal longevity.

Certain genes can also influence these decisions. For example, MTHFR mutations that create a poor ability to methylate tend to cluster in regions and populations where a group's traditional diet was rich in folate. In a study of people in sixteen different regions of the world, Mexicans, Hispanics, Italians, and Chinese were more likely than others to carry MTHFR mutations that increased the need for dietary folate. So if you have Chinese heritage, or your grandparents migrated from Italy, or your dad was Hispanic, you should probably eat more folate-rich foods, such as leafy greens, organ meats, and pastured egg yolks.

Or take the AMY1 gene, which codes for salivary amylase production. Salivary amylase digests starch and carbohydrates, and the more AMY1 copies you have, the more salivary amylase you produce when you eat carbohydrates—and the more likely it is that your ancestors ate relatively high amounts of starch, and the more likely it is that you can handle a slightly higher carbohydrate intake. Populations that are traditionally more agricultural, such as Japanese and continental Europeans, or populations that are high-starch foragers, such as the Hadza tribe in Tanzania, have all been shown to possess more AMY1 copies than populations that consume less starch, such as those in areas of Turkey and the Congo. If your ancestors came from a region that ate more carbohydrates, you can likely thrive on natural starches such as sweet potato, yam, plantain, other roots and tubers, fruit, and rice.

One final example is the lactase persistence gene. Lactase is an enzyme that enables an adult to digest lactose without getting gut distress, diarrhea, and all the other mayhem that can happen with lactose intolerance. As you can imagine, cultures that have not traditionally raised dairy livestock, including those in Asia, Africa, and most of India, rarely carry the lactase persistence gene. In contrast, if you are of European descent, you are probably lactose tolerant.

Eating according to your ancestry is fascinating, isn't it? For an even deeper dive, I recommend reading *Returning to an Ancestral Diet* by Dr. Michael Smith and *The Jungle Effect* by Dr. Daphne Miller.

Instead, nutritional evaluations of diets in the Blue Zones have revealed a high consumption of whole, real foods that your great-grandparents would have recognized and a nutritional profile very similar to the Mediterranean diet. The diets include plenty of herbs such as thyme and rosemary, foods low on the glycemic index and free from added sugar, healthier starches such as purple potatoes, yams, taro, or lentils, and foods high in natural fats such as extra-virgin olive oil and fish.

The way I like to think about this is to look into what your ancestors would have eaten, including investigating your genetic history using a service such as 23andMe to see where your ancestors lived, and then to eat a genetically appropriate diet based on what your ancestors would have consumed.

4. Eat Legumes

A legume is a dry fruit contained within the shell or pod of a plant; the most well-known are beans, peas, peanuts, and alfalfa. Beans, in particular, seem to reign supreme in many Blue Zones. In Nicoya, black beans are eaten in large quantities. In the Mediterranean, lentils, garbanzo beans, and white beans are popular. In Okinawa, soybeans are eaten frequently. This raises an eyebrow among many nutritionally savvy folks, especially in an era of the popular Paleo diet, which frowns upon beans and legumes because they contain high amounts of gastric irritants and natural plant defense mechanisms such as phytates and lectins. But the fact is, legumes are rich in plant protein, vitamins, minerals, appetite-satiating and gut-supporting fiber, and, just as significantly, slow-burning carbohydrates that do not cause a large amount of glycemic variability.

It is unclear whether the longevity gained from legume consumption is conferred by the inclusion of slow-release carbohydrates with the exclusion of blood-sugar-spiking refined carbohydrates such as white flour, or whether the nutrient density of legumes is what makes them so special. I suspect it is both. If you want to include a daily dose of legumes in your diet, I recommend you use the same ancestral preparation techniques used in longevity hot spots, including sprouting, fermenting, and soaking. You'll find instructions for preparing a wide range of legumes on Boundlessbook.com/19.

5. Incorporate Low-Level Physical Activity Throughout the Day

You won't find many longevity hot spots engaged in soul-crushing CrossFit workouts or long, teeth-gritting forays on an elliptical trainer or stairmill. Centenarians in the Blue Zones tend to lead very active lives, yet they rarely set foot in a gym or complete a formal exercise program. Instead, being active is simply built into their life: they walk on average five to six miles a day, farm, garden, spend time in nature, do many chores with their hands instead of machines, and tend to engage in spurts of high-intensity movement or structured movement through enjoyable exercise that rarely involves pounding away on a treadmill or inching under a barbell for a squat. These spurts involve activities such as yoga, tai chi or qigong, hiking, and games or social sports, such as soccer.

Take Dr. Shigeaki Hinohara, a Japanese longevity expert and physician who died at the ripe old age of 105. In a *New York Times* story on Dr. Hinohara, he described daily habits such as always taking the stairs (two steps at a time) and carrying his own packages and luggage (my own rule: I carry my bags through every airport and up hotel stairs as high as the fourth floor). Incidentally, in case you are interested in what this fellow ate, 130-pound Hinohara's diet was relatively spartan: coffee, milk, and orange juice with a tablespoon of olive oil for breakfast; milk and a few biscuits for lunch; vegetables with a small portion of fish and rice for dinner; and exactly 3.5 ounces of lean meat twice per week.

In chapters 9 and 16, you can learn plenty about how I hack my environment using everything from a standing desk to kettlebell swings to replicate the kinds of movements involved in gathering, gardening, and hunting throughout the day, despite being relegated to a traditional post-industrial office setting. In stark contrast, my wife Jessa spends her days hauling alfalfa for the goats, feeding the chickens, pushing around wheelbarrows full of compost and rocks, chopping wood, fixing fences, planting trees, raking, shoveling, pulling weeds, and gardening. Admittedly, I am a bit jealous of her routine because she spends most of the day in the sunshine and fresh air working with her hands in an ancestral way, but at the end of the day, we have both achieved a similar amount of low-level physical activity.

Think about it like this: unless you are a professional athlete or one of your primary goals in life is to train for and complete a triathlon, obstacle course race, CrossFit qualification, or some other modern-day equivalent of a battle that requires you to train like a warrior, visiting the gym at some point during the day should be an option, not a necessity. Research backs this up, showing that it doesn't matter how hard you exercise at the beginning or the end of the day if you have your butt planted in a chair for eight continuous hours during the rest of the day.

6. Prioritize Social Engagement

In most of the Blue Zones, strong relationships come naturally because social connectedness is ingrained in the culture. Compared to most hyperconnected Western societies, they tend to be much more engaged with, conscientious toward, and helpful to each other and more willing to empathize, express feelings, and wear their emotions on their sleeves.

For example, Okinawans have *moais*, which are groups of friends and families who live together their entire lives, spending time talking, cooking together, and supporting each other. Sardinians often finish their days in a local bar, where they meet their friends for a glass of red wine. Seventh-Day Adventists in California mingle with one another weekly or even daily during religious services and the observation of the Sabbath.

Family is also very important for people living in the Blue Zones. For example, during their daylong Sabbath celebration each week, the Seventh-Day Adventists focus on family, God, socializing, and spending time in nature. Nursing homes and hospice care are rare in the Blue Zones because people are expected to honor, value, and take care of the elderly, especially older family members. As a result of their pivotal role in society, elders are far more likely to have a social network, frequent visitors, and trusted caregivers, resulting in less stress, more purposeful lives, and, ultimately, a longer life span. As a matter of fact, I feel that the pros of prioritizing social relationships and family dinners, even if it means occasionally staying out past your bedtime or eating late at night, outweigh the cons of the possible disruptions to your circadian rhythm (especially because you can limit nighttime artificial light exposure by donning a pair of blue-light-blocking glasses or consuming a family dinner by candlelight).

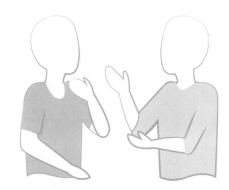

7. Drink Low-to-Moderate Amounts of Alcohol, Especially Wine

In four of the five Blue Zones, people engage in moderate and regular alcohol consumption. Take the Sardinians, for example. They are famous for their regular consumption of a regional red wine called cannonau, a dry wine that contains two to three times the flavonoid content of other wines. Not familiar with cannonau? It is known elsewhere and more popularly as grenache. Consuming wine with or before a meal can improve the absorption of the artery-scrubbing flavonoid antioxidants in the wine, and studies have shown that the consumption of wine as part of a Mediterranean diet can reduce the risk of cardiovascular disease and cancers. Regular low-level physical activity boosts these benefits even more. According to a study performed by the European Society of Cardiology, moderate wine drinking and regular physical activity is a potent combination for cardiovascular disease prevention. Indeed, Sardinian shepherds often walk up to five miles a day to tend to their flocks—and carry along a lunch of unleavened bread, fava beans, pecorino cheese, and a local cannonau wine.

You are no doubt familiar with resveratrol, a polyphenol found in the skin of grapes that may protect the body against the oxidative damage that increases the risk of cancer, heart disease, and dementia. Resveratrol can also combat the formation of the plaque found in the brains of dementia patients. This may be why the weekly consumption of alcohol is associated with better cognitive function in old age. Plenty of additional research backs up the link between wine intake, reduced stress, and longevity (and as I'll explain later in this chapter, certain compounds very similar to resveratrol can be used in a more concentrated supplement form).

This type of frequent, moderate alcohol consumption is one of my own nightly habits—most often accomplished via a digestif and bitters-rich Moscow mule, a shot of a clean-burning alcohol such as gin or vodka on the rocks with a splash of lemon and hefty dose of bitters (a drink I affectionately call a "Ben and Jitters"), or a glass of organic, biodynamic red wine. As a matter of fact, I have one drink just about every night and very rarely have two or more drinks, and since I began this practice six years ago, I have never once been drunk or experienced a hangover (aside from my very brief holiday stint investigating hangover pills for a *Men's Health* magazine article).

Don't care for alcohol or have a history that makes it something you need to be careful with? The good news is that tannin-filled, antioxidant-rich beverages such as coffee and tea may confer similar benefits. Sardinians, Ikarians, and Nicoyans all drink copious amounts of coffee, and people in every Blue Zone drink tea, including Okinawans, who nurse green tea for much of the day, and Ikarians, who thrive on the frequent consumption of a tea made with rosemary, wild sage, and dandelion. On BoundlessBook.com/19, you'll find links to some blog posts that provide more information on the benefits of coffee and tea consumption, but in a nutshell, these types of tannin-rich compounds seem to directly decrease the rate at which telomeres shorten, even after adjusting for confounding variables.

8. Restrict Calories and Fast

Caloric restriction (CR) is a reduction in caloric intake that is not associated with malnutrition or starvation. Long-term CR has been associated in multiple studies with better weight management and slowed aging, as well as a reduced risk of diseases related to metabolic health, such as type 2 diabetes, heart disease, and cancer. But for active athletes, exercise enthusiasts, or people who already have a healthy body-fat percentage, long-term CR can have some downsides, particularly making one cold and hungry because of a drop in metabolism and lean muscle mass. Who wants to live a long time if you have low libido and look like a poster child for an antistarvation campaign? Sure, if your goal is rapid weight loss or you are morbidly obese with lots of stored fat to burn, CR is a good strategy to accelerate fat loss, but even that strategy should be combined with periods of time during which you provide your body with ample calories and nutrients, such as a weekly refeed.

Intermittent fasting (IF) is probably the most popular way to get the benefits of caloric restriction without starving yourself. At its most basic, IF simply involves alternating cycles of eating and fasting, but the term encompasses many kinds of fasting, including these:

- **Time-restricted feeding:** consuming all food within a three-to-twelve-hour window each day, so you fast for at least twelve hours daily
- **Alternate-day fasting:** fasting for twenty-four hours, then eating normally for twenty-fours, then fasting for twenty-four hours again, and so on
- **Eat-stop-eat:** fasting for twenty-four hours once or twice a week
- **Fasting-mimicking diet:** consuming small amounts of food, about 40 percent of your usual calories, for three to five consecutive days
- **Feast-famine cycling:** eating according to the seasonal availability of foods
- **Warrior diet:** fasting during the day and eating a huge meal at night

I'll talk in more detail about a fasting-mimicking diet and feast-famine cycling later in this chapter.

Research suggests that in mice, IF can prevent and reverse obesity and metabolic problems, even when the mice eat an unhealthy diet. Researchers at the Salk Institute for Biological Studies performed an experiment that appeared in the journal *Cell Metabolism*. During the thirty-eight-week study, the scientists fed groups of adult male mice one of the following diets:

- High-fat
- High-fructose
- High-fat and high-fructose
- Regular mouse kibble

The caloric intake for each group was the same, but in each group, some of the mice could eat whenever they wanted while others were restricted to feeding periods of nine, twelve, or fifteen hours. On weekends, some of the time-restricted mice were allowed to cheat and eat whenever they chose. Halfway through the study, a few of the unrestricted mice were moved to the time-restricted groups.

By the end of the study, the unrestricted mice of each diet group were obese and metabolically ill. On the other hand, each diet group's mice that were restricted to nine or twelve hours of feeding per day were lean and healthy, even if they had been allowed to cheat on weekends. In addition, the unrestricted mice that were moved to the time-restricted groups had lost some of the weight they had gained! In other words, it doesn't matter whether a diet is high-fat, high-sugar, or both, or whether the diet is high-calorie. The most effective factor in maintaining a lean body is eating all of a day's meals within a short period, preferably somewhere in the range of eight to twelve hours each day.

Research also suggests that IF is effective in people, promoting fat loss and improving insulin sensitivity. Fasting also allows your gut to heal if you have been consuming gluten, gliadin, or other gut irritants, although these benefits, and the many longevity-related benefits of fasting, reach peak effectiveness after sixteen hours of fasting.

Centenarians in locations like Nicoya, Sardinia, and Okinawa are unlikely to use fasting-related terms like *time-restricted feeding*, but they do tend to eat relatively small portions of whole foods, consuming a low-to-moderate-calorie diet by being mindful of their hunger and avoiding calorie-dense, fat- and sugar-laden processed and packaged foods. Okinawans practice the traditional cultural rule of *hara hachi bu*, which means eating until they are about 80 percent full. Most meals are consumed within an eight- to twelve-hour window, referred to by researchers as a "compressed feeding window"—which perfectly matches the "new" 16-8 diet.

So why do all these different forms of fasting seem to work so well? The most recent research on fasting suggests that it all comes down to mitochondria, the tiny cellular power plants. Inside our cells, mitochondrial networks generally alternate between "fused" and "fragmented" states. Calorie-restricted diets and fasting promote homeostasis and induce a healthy fluctuation between fused and fragmented states, allowing mitochondria to live longer by cycling between a natural growth and repair process. They also increase fatty acid oxidation, which leads to fewer free radicals and less damage to your cells and the mitochondria contained within them.

In chapter 12, I detailed my own daily and weekly fasting practices—which are designed to make sure I get adequate nutrients for my active lifestyle—and explained who should be particularly careful in their approach to fasting. Later in this chapter, I'll talk about my two favorite longer-term fasting practices.

My podcast with Dr. Jason Fung (linked to on BoundlessBook.com/19) is an excellent resource that takes a deep dive into fasting, as is Dr. Fung's comprehensive book *The Complete Guide to Fasting*. Later in this chapter, I outline in detail two of my favorite forms of longer-term fasting.

9. Possess a Strong Life Purpose

An eleven-year NIH-funded study that investigated the correlation between having a sense of purpose and longevity showed that those who expressed a clear purpose for their life lived longer than those who did not, and those with purpose also stayed immersed in activities and communities involved in fulfilling that purpose. This idea of purpose is even expressed in idiomatic terms in Blue Zones: Okinawans refer to purpose as *ikigai* (translated as "reason for being"), and Nicoyans call it *plan de vida* ("reason to live").

I recommend that you know your purpose and be able to express it in one succinct sentence. My purpose in life is to empower people to live an adventurous, joyful, and fulfilling life. Need help identifying your purpose? A manual to identifying your life's purpose, such as Mastin Kipp's *Claim Your Power*, can help. If you want to begin as simply as possible, start with my friend Mark Manson's advice and simply choose to "do stuff that makes you forget to eat and poop."

10. Have Low Amounts of Stress

It is a well-known and heavily researched fact that chronic stress leads to inflammation and serves as the foundation for nearly every age-related disease. Centenarians in most of the world's longevity hot spots do not avoid all stress but do have built-in systems that allow them to manage stress on a daily basis. For Sardinians, this might mean having a glass of wine and a social dinner with family or friends at the end of the day. For Seventh-Day Adventists, it could involve a quiet nature walk on the Sabbath. For Okinawans, it is the concept of *taygay* (translated as "easygoing personality"), which is based on the idea that life simply unfolds at its own pace. In Okinawa, if an event is scheduled to begin at noon, *taygay* may mean that people on Okinawan time begin showing up thirty minutes to an hour later, which isn't necessarily something I recommend if you don't want to get fired from your job. But you get the idea: ruthlessly eliminate haste and hurry from your life. For the best stress-reducing tips, including breathwork strategies, my most potent tactic for stress, which relies on zero supplements or fancy hacks, revisit chapter 3.

One breathing concept that was not explored in chapter 3 is quite fascinating and directly tied to longevity. My friend and former podcast guest Anders Olsson has studied animals' life spans in relation to their energy expenditure, metabolism, and oxygen utilization. In his fantastic blog post "Breathe Less, Live Longer," he notes that a common denominator for long-lived species such as the naked mole rat, the bat, the short-beaked echidna, the bowhead whale and the Greenland shark is that they have slow respiration and a high tolerance for carbon dioxide (CO_2). A fast and shallow breathing pattern corresponds to low CO_2 tolerance, while deep relaxation and breathing low and slow corresponds to a high tolerance for carbon dioxide.

Anders teaches two ways to increase the levels of carbon dioxide in your body: (1) reduce your outflow of CO_2, and (2) increase your production of CO_2. When you slow down your breathing, less CO_2 is lost via exhalation, and when you perform rigorous physical activity, more CO_2 is produced. A great method to train yourself for CO_2 tolerance is to combine the two by performing low-intensity physical activity (e.g., a brisk walk or bodyweight strength training) while breathing only through your nose. Over time this CO_2 tolerance training resets the breathing center in your brain stem and allows you to tolerate higher and higher levels of CO_2, which in turn may help you to live a longer life. (To learn more about Anders's research, check out the link on BoundlessBook.com/19.)

11. Engage in a Spiritual Discipline or Religion, or Believe in a Higher Power

In chapter 15, I described how much more meaningful and hopeful life can be when we believe that our story has a great Author, rather than believing that everything we see and experience is meaningless and without purpose, or that we are simply a bunch of chunks of spiritless flesh and blood floating through space on a giant rock before eventually dying and passing away into nothingness.

While many would scoff at the belief that there are gods and demons, spirits and angels, and even one single almighty creator of the planet, research has shown a connection between longevity and faith. One study analyzed the relationship between religious practice, stress, and death in middle age, and controlled for socioeconomic factors, health insurance status, and healthy behaviors. The researchers found that churchgoers have a significantly lower risk of dying, and after adjusting for age, sex, race, and chronic medical conditions, churchgoers were 46 percent less likely to die in the follow-up period after the study compared to non-churchgoers. Non-churchgoers had significantly higher rates of blood pressure and a higher ratio of total cholesterol to HDL cholesterol, along with a significantly higher mortality rate.

It turns out that data from the Blue Zones backs this up. All but 5 of the 263 centenarians Dan Buettner interviewed for his book belonged to some faith-based community. Research also shows that attending faith-based services at least four times per month can add four to fourteen years to life expectancy. In all Blue Zones, centenarians were part of a religious community. I can't sum it up any better than Buettner, who concluded that "people who pay attention to their spiritual side have lower rates of cardiovascular disease, depression, stress, and suicide, and their immune systems seem to work better.... To a certain extent, adherence to a religion allows them to relinquish the stresses of everyday life to a higher power."

In the Bible, 1 Peter 5:7 recommends that we "cast all our cares upon Him," and in multiple other verses of the Bible, we are told not to be so stressed about the common things the rest of the world tends to fret about, like food, water, and shelter. Being able to trust in and talk to a higher power is certainly something that has given me a great deal of hope, confidence, clarity, peace, and direction in life. Frankly, I believe that a religious practice that includes spiritual disciplines such as fasting, meditation, prayer, silence, solitude, worship, and study contributes even more significantly to longevity than a salad of wild plants, a glass of red wine, or a dose of sunshine. If I had to choose just one section of the Bible that best explains to how to optimize your health and longevity through simple religious practices and commonsense morality, it would be Proverbs 3. I keep a four-minute audio recording of this chapter on my mp3 player and listen to it at least once per week.

12. Remain Reproductively Useful

This last natural strategy for optimizing longevity simply makes logical sense: don't become reproductively useless. In other words, the more consistently you can send your body and brain the message that you are still a valuable, contributing member of society, particularly when it comes to the propagation of your species, the longer nature will want to keep you around. Don't retire. Don't quit learning new things. Don't surround yourself with older, sedentary people in a nursing home or hospice setting. Instead, continue to have sex, have children, or both.

Take, for example, the tiny town of Acciaroli, Italy, where one in eight citizens is over one hundred years old. The elders in this particular Blue Zone are not your average centenarians—they are healthy, consistently happy, and, you guessed it, horny. In the findings of a recent study on why these residents live so long is the observation that sex is rampant among them. Incidentally, the study also noted that the high consumption of parsley, sage, and rosemary, all of which are aphrodisiacs, is prevalent in this region.

Let's take a closer look at what research has to say about this. In a fascinating paper on proposed models of aging, one form of aging—referred to as the Kirkwood and Holliday model—describes mortality as increasing in direct correlation to decreasing fertility (a drop in hormones, childbearing, and frequency of sex). According to this model, the more an organism invests in the maintenance of their own biology (such as feeding and physical activity) compared to propagation of their species (such as mating rituals and reproduction), then the faster aging may actually occur. Basically this model posits that the majority of an organism's expendable energy should be focused on reproduction and that when it comes to prioritizing your antiaging efforts, having sex or making babies trumps taking care of your body in other ways! A form of this model is also known as the reproductive potential hypothesis, which maintains that life-span regulation has evolved in such a way as to maximize individual reproductive success, and research has indeed shown that women who bear children later or simply bear more children experience enhanced longevity.

The benefits of regular sex and childbearing seem to be backed up by laboratory research from Dr. Michael Rose, who explained his theories on the evolution of aging to me at a cocktail party at the Ancestral Health Symposium (you'll find a link to his website on BoundlessBook.com/19). Dr. Rose proposed that aging is not a positively selected, programmed death process and has not evolved for the good of the species, as many would think. Rather, aging exists because natural selection is weak and ineffective at maintaining survival, reproduction, and cellular repair as we enter old age. In a paper published in *Philosophical Transactions of the Royal Society B*, he described how senescence (age-related deterioration) is detrimental to reproductive success. The damage that occurs during aging clearly shortens our life span, but longevity can also be shaped by selection for an increased number of what are called lifetime reproductive events, or the number of times you reproduce or attempt to reproduce.

In his book *Does Aging Stop?* Rose suggested that aging can indeed stop or plateau in the later stages of life, pointing to the demographic data in his large-scale fruit fly experiments as well as data on humans, both of which support the hypothesis that acceleration in death rates can halt in later life. While Rose had plenty of tips for enhancing this plateau, including the controversial idea that grain and agriculture consumption could accelerate age-related damage, one of his more potent suggestions was to have plenty of children and plenty of sex early in life, then continue to have children as late as possible, or at least to engage in frequent sexual intercourse to as ripe an age as possible. For multiple reasons, I am a fan of this idea, although I don't see any issues with using contraception so you don't have dozens of children running around your house, which I suspect might trigger a stress-related law of diminishing returns when it comes to longevity.

The quite possibly fabled but intriguing Li Ching-Yuen, who purportedly lived to the ripe old age of 256, was said to be a much-loved figure in his community, marrying twenty-three times and fathering over two hundred children. If it turns out that the story of Yuen is true, he may be the best example of the fact that maintaining reproductive usefulness with age could be an excellent idea indeed.

ADVANCED ANTIAGING BIOHACKS AND STRATEGIES

While the daily practices above are incredibly important for a long life, the fact is that we live in an era in which those basic antiaging tactics can now be combined with the more advanced tactics and biohacks used by the longevity and antiaging community. In this section, I will offer more advanced tactics that you can implement for longevity, including some practical recommendations.

Because many of the health, antiaging, and longevity strategies I am about to explore may seem—and often are—fringe, out of the ordinary, or even mildly excessive, allow me to clarify my take on the concept of implementing as many techniques as possible to enhance the quantity and quality of your years: *I am not a transhumanist.*

I do not believe that immortality for its own sake is a noble pursuit, nor do I believe that we as humans are capable of attaining a perfect body or brain. I do not believe that grasping at straws to hang on to every last shred of life, especially when driven by a fear of death, is a healthy way to live. I have witnessed many colleagues, friends, and antiaging-industry leaders spend too much of their precious time biohacking their bodies to live longer while simultaneously sacrificing time with their family and friends, a robust spiritual practice, and simple enjoyments, such as learning to play the harmonica or creating a beautiful watercolor painting or gardening with their children.

I am a Christian, and therefore I believe in a natural cycle of birth and death, followed by the ultimate resurrection of our bodies into a state of heavenly glory, unlike anything we would ever be able to accomplish here on earth. But importantly, I also believe that each and every person, including you, was born with a unique purpose, set of skills, and calling, and that to achieve that purpose to the very best of your ability, you must equip yourself with a sound body and mind and take steps to ensure you don't come down with cancer when you are fifty or have a heart attack when you are sixty or lose your memory when you are seventy because you made poor decisions about your health earlier in life.

In other words, the longer you are on this planet, the better able you are to fulfill your purpose in life, whether that's inspiring others to greatness, discovering the cure for cancer, making beautiful art, or writing books that delight children around the world.

Furthermore, I believe that God has surrounded us human beings with wonders and mysteries in both the natural world and the scientific domains that allow us to engage in better living via a marriage of ancestral wisdom and modern science, and that to ignore our ability to garden, forage, and create new tinctures, capsules, oils, devices, machines, and techniques that allow us to live healthier and longer is to neglect a big part of what it means to be an intelligent human being who is far different from the rest of the animal kingdom. It is to neglect our unique ability to explore, to invent, and, ultimately, to create.

So now that I'm off my soapbox, let's dive into some of those very discoveries, strategies, and inventions.

1. Longer-Term Fasting

I've talked already about time-restricted feeding and the other kinds of fasting protocols that fall in the "intermittent fasting" category and all the reasons you may want to make fasting a daily practice. But for the purposes of overall wellness and longevity, I am also a big fan of the following two longer-term fasting approaches.

FEAST-FAMINE CYCLING

My friend Dr. Dan Pompa calls the ancient healing strategy of seasonal diet variation based on food availability a feast-famine cycle. Many ancient cultures and modern Blue Zones follow this kind of pattern of fasting and feasting.

Humans have not always had grocery stores and Uber Eats services that provide food of all kinds 24-7. Instead, we have traditionally been forced to eat seasonally according to what plants are in season, what animal protein is available, and what nutrients are needed most at different times of year. For example, in the winter, many Native American tribes would give their dogs the muscle meat and subsist themselves primarily on fats, especially the organ fat from the kidneys, liver, and gut, because what they cherished most was the caloric density and nutrients from the organs. In the summer, these same tribes would eat more roots and berries, prickly pears, beans, pods, mustard seeds, cholla blossoms, acorn squash, pumpkins, and a variety of gourds—a much higher percentage of carbohydrates than in the winter, when consumption of saturated fats reigned.

In his book *Nutrition and Physical Degeneration,* Weston A. Price described this Native American practice this way:

> [Native Americans] cycled between the summer cultivation of starches and fruits and far greater reliance on fats from animals (particularly organ meats and marrow) during winter. ... The successful nutrition for nine months of the year was largely limited to wild game, chiefly moose and caribou. During the summer months the Indians were able to use growing plants. During the winter some use was made of bark and buds of trees. I found the Indians putting great emphasis upon the eating of the organs of the animals, including the wall of parts of the digestive tract. ... These Indians obtain their fat-soluble vitamins and also most of their minerals from the organs of the animals. An important part of the nutrition of the children consisted in various preparations of bone marrow, both as a substitute for milk and as a special dietary ration.

How it works: Science has shown that periods of caloric restriction and seasonal feast-famine dietary variations promoted health in indigenous cultures by forcing the body to use fat instead of glucose as a primary fuel during the winter months. This also gave the digestive system a rest and gave cells a chance to engage in the natural cell turnover known as autophagy.

How to do it: Dr. Pompa's 5-1-1 strategy, which combines seasonal eating with cyclic ketosis, is a great place to start. For five days of the week, follow a lower-carb, ketogenic diet (outlined in chapter 13) or, especially if you are attempting to lose weight, a calorie-restricted diet, primarily consisting of foods that are available locally and seasonally. One day of the week, fast for twenty-four hours (from dinnertime to dinnertime). The remaining day of the week, have a feast day, eating any of your favorite healthy food—especially carbohydrates—ad libitum, until you're full.

The 5-1-1 rule can be modified based on body fat, schedule, and physical activity levels. For some, a 4-2-1 or 2-2-3 approach works even better. Bonus points if you eat seasonally as you implement this approach, such as by eating more carbohydrates in the warmer months and more proteins and fats in the colder months: fresh fruits and berries in the spring, tubers and squash in the fall, heavier cuts of meat and fermented foods in the winter, and so on.

FASTING-MIMICKING DIET

Fasting usually involves abstaining from everything but water and perhaps black coffee and tea—no calories are consumed for the length of the fast. However, another effective approach to fasting was developed by Valter Longo and is outlined in detail in his book *The Longevity Diet:* the fasting-mimicking diet.

The fasting-mimicking diet (FMD) allows you to fast while consuming a minimal number of calories, so you can supply your body with nutrients while getting the benefits of fasting.

There are two ways you can implement an FMD:

- Alternate-day modified fasting, which is eating minimal calories every other day for a twenty-four-hour period

- An extended FMD, which is the program Longo advocates in his book and which involves consuming minimal calories for five consecutive days

As a word of caution, like other forms of IF, an FMD may be harmful for people who already have little body fat, the elderly, and children.

How it works: A typical alternate-day fast requires you to completely fast for a full twenty-four hours, then eat to satiety for the following twenty-four hours. It seems to be more effective than daily caloric restriction for maintaining long-term weight loss and allows your body to enter a powerful state of autophagy during the fasting stages. Fasting for longer periods, from three to five days, can stimulate adaptive responses such as autophagy, weight loss, and a long-term reduction of IGF-1, glucose, and markers of inflammation and aging.

An FMD produces many of the same physiological effects as these kinds of fasts but still provides your body with optimal nourishment, without activating the pro-aging pathways, including the growth hormone, insulin, and insulin-like growth factor 1 (IGF-1) pathways, which are activated by normal diets. When you follow an FMD, your body does not recognize that it is being fed and so believes that it is in a period of fasting. This can strengthen the immune system by triggering it to replace old T cells to combat particular invasive microbes; it can also improve insulin sensitivity.

How to do it: An FMD is low in calories and particularly low in protein. Longo's formula is based on meals of about 360 calories each: 9 percent from protein, 44 percent from fat, and 47 percent from carbohydrates. The diet is followed for five consecutive days; there are three meals on the first day that amount to a total of 1,090 calories, and two meals on each of the next four days, amounting to a total of 725 calories each day. However, you don't have to follow this protocol for five consecutive days—you can also alternate between normal eating days and low-calorie FMD days.

Longo owns a company called L-Nutra that premeasures and prepackages these meals as Prolon meal kits, which consist of vegan foods from natural sources. Should you choose to follow Longo's FMD diet, you can use these kits for a five-day protocol once per quarter for impressive longevity results.

However, I am not convinced that the minimalist meal kits Longo's company sells are necessary, and although they're convenient and done-for-you, they are also relatively low on the nutrient-density scale compared to fresh, whole foods. But with wild plant intake and small doses of superfoods such as spirulina, chlorella, bone broth, berries, seeds, or nuts—along with a few biohacks such as essential amino acids and ketone esters—you can easily put together your own minimal-calorie alternative to the packaged version.

One excellent example of a DIY approach can be found for free at FMDrecipes.org, which contains a full list of recipes for an FMD diet, based on Longo's research. For example, the Eggplant Pâté with Vegetables simply involves blending tahini, eggplant, oil, and lemon juice in a food processor, then adding salt, cumin, and fresh garlic to taste, and serving with a pile of vegetables. The Hearty Red Cabbage Slaw requires chopping cabbage, carrots, cilantro, and an apple in a food processor, then tossing the mixture with chopped nuts, pureed avocado, salt, pepper, lemon, lime, and garlic. While these recipes are not affiliated with Dr. Longo or his lab, they follow the macronutrient proportions laid out by his research and can help you achieve your FMD goals.

Dr. John Douillard also just released a five-day Ayurvedic cleansing approach to an FMD, which is, in my opinion and based on my own trial with his products, the best of both worlds: it combines a done-for-you diet that is shipped to your house with a real-foods approach. This protocol, called a "Kaya Kalpha" cleanse, includes daily consumption of the Ayurvedic cleansing stew Kitchari, which Dr. Douillard ships in dried packets to your home, along with a selection of ghee, herbs, and spices to maximize lymphatic drainage during your fast. I've tried both the Prolon kit and the Kaya Kalpha cleanse and have felt more clean energy and fewer appetite cravings with the latter approach to an FMD.

Finally, as a word of warning, it is usually not recommended to follow an FMD—or any form of fasting—for more than a few days at a time.

2. Hormetic Stress

While chronic exposure or overexposure to stress can result in inflammation and even life-threatening conditions, hormetic stressors are acute stressors that stimulate a favorable and beneficial adaptive response following brief exposure. These types of stressors range from the fasting protocols outlined above to exposure to cold, heat, or pathogens, to brief, intense bouts of exercise.

Many scientists believe that if you do not expose yourself to different hormetic stressors, your body may never develop an adequate adaptive response to high levels of oxidative stress (remember that the free-radical theory of aging posits that aging is the result of oxidative damage to our cells). Here's how it works: when you experience a hormetic stress, it signals your body to enter a stress-resistant mode that tells your cells that it is probably not a good time to grow old and die. For examples, rats forced to swim in freezing-cold water every day tend to live longer. Giving worms electric shocks, restricting their calories, keeping them cold, and briefly exposing them to heat makes them live longer—with these techniques, researchers have made roundworms live up to ten times longer! On the other hand, mice raised in a sterile environment free of pathogens do not live nearly as long as mice that are exposed to bacteria and viruses in a dirtier environment.

Some practical ways to experience hormetic stress each day include lifting heavy stuff (refer back to chapter 9), not stuffing yourself with antibiotics (this can even mean not using antimicrobial or antiviral essential oils every day), engaging in hot-cold contrast therapy (such as alternating between hot and cold water when taking a shower—refer back to chapter 12), eating plants with a high polyphenol content (many of the beneficial compounds found in plants are actually noxious and stimulate a hormetic response), drinking wine for its polyphenols and similar compounds, such as tannins and anthocyanins, and even consuming alcohol for its own sake (small doses of ethanol may initiate a stress response). Below are a few of my favorite forms of hormesis.

HYPERBARIC OXYGEN THERAPY (HBOT)

HBOT delivers high-pressure air that is 100 percent oxygen, typically via a full-body chamber or a face mask. These higher pressures enhance oxygen delivery to every tissue in your body. HBOT is often used to treat decompression sickness, infections, air bubbles in your blood, and wounds that are not healing as well as they should due to diabetes or radiation injuries.

How it works: Oxygen binds to the protein hemoglobin in your red blood cells. HBOT results in a ten-to-twenty-fold increase in blood plasma oxygen levels, including a significant increase in red blood cells. It also promotes tissue repair, the formation of new blood vessels (angiogenesis), wound healing, and the controlled release of reactive oxygen species in damaged and infected tissues, which can stimulate a beneficial hormetic response. HBOT may also have antifungal effects, caused by the reversal of fungal growth and the restoration of a normal immune response. Finally, the slight increase in free radicals and ROS from HBOT induces a hormetic response that can build cellular resilience, and the treatment may also induce mitochondrial biogenesis and DNA repair.

How to do it: After suffering a concussion, I spent sixty to ninety minutes a day for multiple days immersed in over two atmospheres of high pressure inside a hyperbaric chamber (you can often find one near you by googling the name of your city plus the term *hyperbaric oxygen*.) I can now simulate a full twenty-four hours in a hyperbaric oxygen chamber by doing a thirty-minute cycling workout twice per week while using a hyperoxia (or hypoxia) device called a LiveO2, which I talked about in chapter 11.

WILD PLANTS

Humankind has foraged for food, medicine, and health-enhancing compounds for thousands of years. In fact, it is entirely possible that there are plants growing right in your own backyard that can be used to enhance digestion, increase cognitive performance, and improve endurance. You just have to know how to use them.

A wild plant is any noncultivated plant or herb that, when consumed, lends some kind of benefit to your immune system, digestive system, cardiovascular system, or nervous system, or even several of these systems at once. Plants that grow wild are exposed to more environmental stressors than much of the domesticated produce you find in the aisles of the grocery store, and they can pass on their built-in stress-resilience factors to your body when you consume them. Take mint, for example. The dainty, mild taste of the small mint leaves I can buy in a small plastic container from the grocery store absolutely pales in comparison to the intense flavor and potency of the beat-up wild mint that grows in the forest behind my house—and the latter confers far more benefits.

How it works: Fruits and vegetables contain potent compounds that improve your health in a variety of ways, including phenols, polyphenols, phytochemicals, chlorophylls, and cytokines. The scientific term for this is *xenohormesis*, which simply means that environmentally stressed plants can produce compounds that can confer stress resistance and survival benefits to animals that consume them. These xenohormetic plant compounds can, when ingested, improve longevity and fitness by activating your stress response.

There are thousands of such plants that you can forage and consume. Clover, cattail, chicory, greater burdock, amaranth, field pennycress, plantain, kelp, fireweed, and even the lowly dandelion in your backyard are just a few examples.

How to do it: A local wild-plant-foraging class or meetup is a good way to get up to speed on what is growing wild in your area, and a trip to your local farmers market for ugly, dirty, bitter, sour, and misshapen produce can also leave you with a whole canvas bag or burlap sack chock-full of xenohormetic goodies. The trick is to eat as wide a variety of wild plants and herbs as you can by mixing them into teas, smoothies, stir-fries, salads, and other dishes throughout the week. If you are on the go or don't have time to forage, one of my favorite resources for organic, heirloom wild plant extracts and powders is Dr. Thomas Cowan's Vegetable Powders (you'll find a link on BoundlessBook.com/19).

As a general rule, if you cannot clearly identify a plant or herb and are not sure if it is poisonous, do not consume it. Stay away from plants that have milky or discolored sap; spines, fine hairs, or thorns; beans, bulbs, or seeds inside pods; a bitter or soapy taste; foliage that looks like dill, carrots, parsnips, or parsley if you aren't 100 percent certain of the identification; almond scents in the woody parts and leaves; grain heads with pink, purplish, or black spurs; and three-leaved growth patterns. Two apps that I've found to be particularly helpful for identifying wild plants are FlowerChecker, which gives you access to a team of live botanists, and PlantSnap, which uses artificial intelligence for plant identification.

HYDROGEN-RICH WATER

Hydrogen-rich water is essentially purified water infused with molecular hydrogen (H_2 gas dissolved in the water). In chapter 12, I explained that I use this form of hydrogen to improve my recovery and performance. I drink hydrogen-rich water from an H_2-water generator and travel with hydrogen tablets (Quicksilver Scientific and Water & Wellness are two good sources). Other good ways to get hydrogen-rich water include the H2Bev molecular hydrogen drink, although this is less travel-friendly because it's a canned beverage, and the hydrogen tablets from Drink HRW. Molecular hydrogen medicine capitalizes on the therapeutic benefits of hydrogen, which has both antioxidant and cytoprotective effects. It is nontoxic, even at high concentrations, and diffuses rapidly among your cells.

How it works: Molecular hydrogen has been shown to produce a profound improvement on stem cell availability, decrease the rate at which telomeres shorten (which are one of the major biomarkers for aging), and activate the same SIRT1 pathways targeted by sirtuin-rich foods such as blueberries and green tea, which results in improved mitochondrial function. It also increases the expression of antioxidative enzymes in the Nrf2 pathway, indicating that the mild hormetic stress caused by H2 increases resilience in cells stressed with excess oxidation from sources such as airline travel or heavy exercise. I'm personally convinced that very few modern nutritional interventions rival the anti-inflammatory and antioxidant benefits of hydrogen-rich water.

How to do it: Molecular hydrogen is usually consumed via tablets, canned hydrogen-rich water, or machines that generate hydrogen-rich water. There is no current upper limit of toxicity for hydrogen-rich water; I personally consume about 40 ounces of the water per day from the machine in my home and drink two or three 6-to-8-ounce glasses (two hydrogen tablets per glass) per day when traveling. Because molecular hydrogen also inhibits NADPH oxidase (NOX), an enzyme that can lower your levels of NAD (a molecule explained in detail later in this chapter), you can compound the beneficial effect by pairing hydrogen-rich water with other natural NOX inhibitors you'll find in this chapter, particularly foods such as pomegranates, blueberries, grapes, green tea, and berberine.

For a potent combination of NOX inhibition and hydrogen, there is even a liquid fermented beet product infused with hydrogen-rich water, available in a small, BPA-free can, that you can purchase from my friend Dr. Mercola (there's a link on BoundlessBook.com/19). Interestingly, in most cases, you'd benefit from the performance-enhancing benefits of beets by swishing them in your mouth so that your mouth bacteria enhance the conversion to nitric oxide, but hydrogen water actually does this for you, so no swishing is required. Fermented beets and hydrogen-rich water are a match made in heaven.

BHB SALTS

A BHB salt is a compound that consists of sodium (Na+), potassium (K+), and the ketone body beta-hydroxybutyrate (BHB). These salts are involved in the transcription and upregulation of the enzymes in your body's natural antioxidant pathways. They are also believed to induce ketosis and provide the same longevity benefits as caloric restriction. They can serve as a primary source of fuel for the liver, heart, diaphragm, and other tissues, and even act as an alternative fuel supply for our bodies when blood glucose levels are low.

How it works: Impaired mitochondrial function often results in excessive production of reactive oxygen species (ROS), which is involved in the development of many chronic diseases, including cardiovascular disease, diabetes, neurodegenerative disorders, and cancer. Moderate levels of mitochondrial ROS, however, have been shown to protect against chronic disease by upregulating mitochondrial capacity and endogenous antioxidant defenses. This phenomenon is called mitohormesis, and it's induced through exercise or dietary modifications such as a ketogenic diet—anything that increases reliance on mitochondrial respiration.

The consumption of BHB salts elevates BHB in a way that expands the benefits of nutritional ketosis beyond what could normally be achieved with carbohydrate restriction because it increases levels of available ketones higher than what you may be able to naturally achieve by simply restricting carbohydrates. BHB salts enhance antioxidant activity by inhibiting class I and IIA histone deacetylases, regulators that repress the transcription of the FOXO3a gene, a key gene involved in cell autophagy and inflammation. The metabolism of BHB salts also causes a negative redox potential (a greater tendency to accept electrons) of the NADP antioxidant system, which can scavenge free radicals. Adding BHB to cultures of *C. elegans* worms has been shown to extend their life span, and higher doses of ketone bodies may also extend human life spans.

How to do it: Add one to two servings of a BHB salt powder to a morning smoothie, blend it into a coffee or tea concoction, or consume it preworkout or during a workout, preferably combined with essential amino acids and electrolytes. There are a variety of companies now producing BHB salts, and you'll find links and discounts on BoundlessBook.com/19 to several, including Ancient Nutrition, Perfect Keto, KetoBlitz, and KetoForce. For a more efficient and effective way to deliver ketones into the body, you can also use ketone esters (see page 511), although they are far more expensive—$15 to $30 per serving compared to $2 to $4 per serving for ketone salts.

COLD THERMOGENESIS

Cold thermogenesis (CT) is the practice of intentionally exposing parts of the body to cold to induce an adaptive, beneficial hormetic response. CT practices include cold baths, cold showers, ice soaks, going outside on a cold day, keeping your house cold, or spending time in a cryotherapy chamber. Years of research have shown that cold exposure can cause significant increases in metabolism and calorie-burning, increase insulin sensitivity, reduce systemic inflammation, improve sleep and recovery, and potentially fight certain types of cancer. In summary, cold thermogenesis is a potent method to promote overall longevity and health.

How it works: As I talked about in chapter 8, CT is most often championed as a weight-loss strategy because it helps burn fat. Cold exposure also shuts down inflammation caused by exercise and wounds and activates the sympathetic, fight-or-flight nervous system, which regulates the mobilization and metabolism of stored fat.

But CT also enhances longevity, as does any exposure to hot or cold that mildly stresses the body. We can see this in many animal studies. For example, in 1986, a researcher at Washington University immersed lab rats in cold water for four hours each day. The rats burned so many extra calories that they ate twice as much as control rats, but they weighed less and lived 10 percent longer. Two decades later, researchers at the Buck Institute for Aging Research exposed lab worms to repeated heat shocks, and these worms lived 10 to 20 percent longer, largely by generating a surge of a protective compounds called heat shock proteins.

Many other animal studies have also shown that animals live longer when exposed to hormetic stresses such as starvation, toxins, radiation, infections, heat, and cold. It seems to be a universal adaptation—for instance, in general, when cold-blooded animals are exposed to cold, their metabolisms slow and they live longer, but when warm-blooded animals are exposed to cold, their metabolisms speed up to maintain body temperature, and they also live longer. It appears that both responses are part of an ancient genetic mechanism that senses temperature and slows aging as a survival mechanism. The theory goes that when something in the environment, such as a famine or cold snap or epidemic, is killing off part of the population, the rest of the population responds by getting tougher and living longer.

How to do it: Rather than spending the time and expense to hunt down a cryotherapy chamber, I take a cold shower or jump into a cold pool, lake, river, sea, or my home cold pool setup for at least two to five minutes twice a day. This type of cold-water immersion has repeatedly been shown to be superior to cryotherapy for tapping into the many benefits of cold. Many of my clients who are too busy to get wet wear a Cool Fat Burner vest or a Cool Gut Buster belt for thirty to sixty minutes per day while they are working.

Finally, one to two times per week, I recommend a longer ten-to-twenty-minute cold soak or ice bath that brings you to a state of shivering, or a series of two to three rounds of two-to-three-minute cold baths interspersed with two-to-three-minute sessions of Wim Hof or box breathing

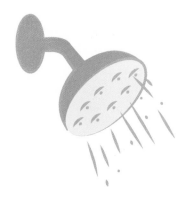

(see chapter 3). These longer, more intensive, and colder soaks can significantly enhance the conversion of white fat to brown fat (a key part of how CT helps burn fat—see chapter 8 for details) and can also be used as a quick hangover cure, cognitive boost, or what I consider to be a "cup of coffee for your entire body." But this kind of extended exposure can be overly stressful if done too often, so I recommend limiting it to one or two sessions per week. Interestingly, the genes responsible for enhancing life span in response to cold also seem to be activated by eating Japanese horseradish (wasabi). So perhaps a post-CT visit to your local sushi joint may also be in order.

HYPERTHERMIA THERAPY

As the name implies, hyperthermia therapy involves exposure to high temperatures and can include dry sauna, infrared sauna, heating mats, hot tubs, hot springs, sauna suits, or exercise on a hot day. Traditionally, hyperthermia therapy has principally been used to treat cancer, but the heart health and cellular resilience processes that it triggers make it a strategy for increased life span as well. While overheating and entering a state of extreme hyperthermia, in which your body temperature rises too high, is incredibly dangerous, controlled heat exposure is a powerful way to improve your longevity and well-being.

How it works: A recent study on hyperthermia published in *JAMA Internal Medicine* describes typical sauna use by Finnish adults—more specifically, the Finnish practice of frequent sessions in a dry, hot sauna heated to between 170 and 176 degrees Fahrenheit.

In this groundbreaking study, over 2,300 middle-aged men from Finland were divided into different groups based on how often they used a sauna: once a week, two or three times a week, or four to seven times a week. They were also sorted according to the duration of their typical sauna session: fewer than eleven minutes, eleven to nineteen minutes, or longer than nineteen minutes. After two decades, the researchers found that the higher the frequency of sauna use, the lower the risk of sudden cardiac death, fatal cardiovascular disease, and all-cause mortality. Compared with short sauna sessions (less than eleven minutes), men who spent between eleven and nineteen minutes in the sauna had a 7 percent lower risk of sudden cardiac death. For those with even longer sessions—nineteen minutes or more—the risk of sudden cardiac death was much lower (52 percent lower risk).

Why does a sauna provide such powerful medical benefits? The researchers pointed to previous studies that suggested the heart rate increase triggered by heat exposure may mimic the cardiovascular stress of exercise, and they also suggested that frequent sauna use could improve lung capacity. But there's also another factor involved.

Hyperthermic treatment of up to 120 degrees Fahrenheit for a wet sauna and between 158 and 212 degrees Fahrenheit for a dry sauna has been shown to cause a significant expression of heat shock proteins (HSP) in muscle. HSP have been implicated in longevity and aging in many species because they chaperone misfolded or newly synthesized proteins, protect cells from protein misfolding, and strengthen the immune system. The induction of HSP could potentially maintain protein homeostasis and improve longevity by refolding damaged proteins, which accumulate during aging and are toxic to cells. A decrease in HSP in aging is associated with the disruption of cellular homeostasis, which causes cancer, cell senescence, and neurodegeneration. The triggering of HSP is also correlated with 30 percent more muscle regrowth after a week of physical immobilization. That means that if you can't weight train, you have a recovery day, or you are injured, you can still maintain muscle using heat therapy. Sauna therapy can also increase oxygen consumption and red blood cell production following exercise, improve stress resistance, and aid in the detoxification of chemicals and heavy metals.

How to do it: At least twice per week (though you can do this every day), try to get into a dry sauna (at 170 to 180 degrees Fahrenheit), wet sauna (at 110 to 120 degrees Fahrenheit, and make sure the water is filtered), or infrared sauna (at about 130 to 160 degrees Fahrenheit) for fifteen to forty minutes, or until you achieve a noticeable rise in heart rate, sweat production, or both.

If you don't have access to a sauna, consider saving harder workouts for the afternoon heat of the day, perform your normal workout wearing multiple layers of clothing, or even drive home from the gym with the heater on full blast or the a/c turned off in your car. For a more relaxed and passive form of hyperthermia, I take my daily nap on a Biomat, which I increase to its maximum temperature for a combination of hyperthermia and infrared exposure, and I often lounge on the mat while reading or stretching. Performing some of your hyperthermia in a state of parasympathetic nervous system activation—instead of simply exercising while hot—may enhance the detoxification effects.

Hyperthermia can also be a very useful strategy for decreasing cold and flu duration, and one trick I use if I feel as though I may be coming down with something is lying on my back on the floor of an infrared sauna for a longer, forty-five-to-sixty-minute session, or I'll wrap my body in blankets (the silver Mylar space-age-looking blankets work quite well), lie on my Biomat, and sweat in a parasympathetic, nearly comatose state of meditation for forty-five to sixty minutes. If you opt for a wet sauna or steam room, ensure that any water piped into that room is filtered for elements such as chlorine or fluoride.

Finally, keep in mind that the sauna culture in Finland is far different from that in many other countries. For example, when I make my annual foray to Finland and visit the Finnish Sauna Society (an experience I highly recommend), they aren't tapping on their phones, chatting, watching a built-in sauna TV, or doing anything else. They're simply sitting silently, breathing and meditating, and then socializing in the cold air outside the sauna. I suspect that these regular moments of relaxation and fellowship are significant contributors to the longevity-enhancing effects of the sauna that have been demonstrated in Finnish men.

UVA AND UVB RADIATION

UVA and UVB radiation, along with UVC radiation, comprise the UV radiation that is given off by the sun. As you no doubt know, sunblock is designed to minimize exposure to these rays because they can cause cellular damage and even lead to cancer. But when you expose yourself to low, controlled levels of UVA and UVB radiation, you can actually trigger a hormetic stress response. As with cold and heat exposure, it is about finding and using the right amount of exposure.

How it works: One of the primary ways that UVB exposure enhances health is by elevating levels of 25-hydroxyvitamin D, the major circulating form of vitamin D, in people with low baseline levels. Vitamin D is essential for protein, bone, and calcium homeostasis, and a deficiency in 25-hydroxyvitamin D is associated with an increased risk of age-related chronic diseases, including Alzheimer's, Parkinson's, cognitive impairment, and cancer, so UVB exposure has a wide range of health benefits. UVA exposure, on the other hand, generates nitric oxide, which reduces blood pressure and can act as an antimicrobial.

The benefits of UV radiation don't stop with UVA and UVB. It is well known that inducing low or intermittent levels of repairable damage in cells and tissues—such as occurs with UV exposure—is a good thing because it triggers short-term bursts of more aggressive cellular maintenance, and the end result is a net gain in the quality of the cellular environment—meaning fewer damaged proteins. In one fascinating study from the 1980s, researchers assessed the effects of radiation hormesis on both young and old dogs. They reported a gain of remaining life expectancy of 15 percent in older dogs and 50 percent in younger dogs. Some of the short-lived bird species in Chernobyl have developed enhanced anticancer mechanisms by producing higher levels of antioxidants to protect their DNA, and one Taiwanese study even noted a hormetic response in humans exposed to cobalt-60 radiation! While I don't think this means you need to go pitch a tent at the base of Chernobyl, these studies, along with several others, do indicate that low-intensity ionizing radiation is a hormetic stressor.

How to do it: They're often vilified as cancer chambers, so you may be surprised to learn that tanning beds, especially those outfitted with UVB bulbs, can be a good way to get UV exposure. A lot of people sell used tanning beds online, mostly because they consider tanning to be unhealthy;

a used tanning bed, including the bulbs, will usually cost you between $1,500 and $2,000. Higher-end tanning beds are a lot more expensive but not necessarily better—most contain plenty of useless options, such as Bluetooth and aromatherapy.

Once you have a tanning bed, I recommend outfitting it with a type of lamp called a Wolff Dark Tan II Plus, which combines the highest UVB rating with the lowest UVA rating (UVA rays may be more carcinogenic than UVB rays), or another good lamp called a Collatan Maxi Twist. Some high-end tanning beds emit UVA, UVB, and red light, such as the Ergoline 1600 from Europe, but these cost well over $30,000. There are online resources for more healthy done-for-you UVB tanning bed options, and on BoundlessBook.com/19, you'll find links to these as well as to links for good lamp and bulb options.

Should you decide to forgo the tanning bed, the most natural way to get low-level doses of UVA and UVB radiation is with multiple ten-to-thirty-minute sessions of exposure to sunlight, particularly between the hours of 10:00 a.m. and 4:00 p.m. This can be as simple as saving your daily phone calls or podcasts or audiobooks for a walk in the sunshine or having lunch outside with as much skin exposed as possible. If your skin burns, it is a telltale sign you have gone far past the level of healthy hormesis.

Incidentally, there is some research on the benefits of exposing your body to red and near-infrared light before and after UV ray exposure, particularly with respect to skin protection and vitamin D production, so getting evening sunlight (which has more red and near-infrared rays) and using light-producing devices such as infrared panels in conjunction with sun exposure can be a good biohack for limiting any potential sun damage. A similar effect can be obtained by taking the supplement astaxanthin.

Finally, for heaven's sake, please moderate your use of sunscreen, which *Outside* magazine has called the "new margarine" because, although it was once considered convenient and safe, it is now associated with a growing number of issues, such as vitamin D and nitric oxide deficiencies, increased risk of blood clots, and high blood pressure. Please also pay close attention to the discussion of lighting in chapter 20, which has plenty more about how light can help or hurt your health, depending on how you use it.

3. Caloric-Restriction Mimetics

Earlier in this chapter I talked about the health benefits of limiting the number of calories you eat each day. Caloric-restriction mimetics (CRMs) are simply drugs or other natural compounds that mimic the benefits of true caloric restriction.

RAPAMYCIN

Rapamycin, also known as sirolimus, is a medication traditionally used to coat coronary stents, prevent organ transplant rejection, and treat a rare and difficult-to-pronounce lung disease called lymphangioleiomyomatosis. Rapamycin also inhibits excess activation of immune T cells and B cells by reducing their sensitivity to interleukin-2, specifically by inhibiting the mTOR signaling pathway, which is a master regulator of cell growth and metabolism—this inhibiting effect is similar to the effects of caloric restriction. Since mTOR inhibition is synonymous with longevity, rapamycin is now being studied and utilized by many longevity enthusiasts as an antiaging compound.

Rapamycin is produced by the bacterium *Streptomyces hygroscopicus* and was isolated for the first time in 1972 by Canadian researchers from samples of *S. hygroscopicus* found on Easter Island. It was given the name rapamycin after the native name of the island: Rapa Nui.

How it works: Rapamycin is known as an antibiotic and immunosuppressant. But in mammals, rapamycin also targets the mTOR signaling pathway. As DNA or cells become damaged, stimulation of growth pathways in those cells leads to aging and eventually cell death. MTOR pathways, among others, drive this type of aging. By inhibiting these pathways, rapamycin slows the aging process.

Downregulation of the mTOR pathway has been implicated in various human diseases like cancer, diabetes, obesity, neurological diseases, and genetic disorders, and because it inhibits mTOR, which also increases the cleanup process of cellular autophagy, rapamycin has been shown to help treat certain diseases.

How to do it: Rapamycin can be taken orally, either as a tablet or in a solution. Although the ideal dosage ranges from 0.5 to 2 mg, the proper dosage can vary because absorption varies from person to person, so blood levels are measured to make sure that each person has the right dose for their condition. It's best to have a medical professional keep track of blood levels following ingestion.

Rapamycin is one of the more recent and more powerful of the compounds that extend life span in rats, but because it can suppress the immune system, it also appears likely to increase the risk of infectious diseases and even diabetes. It also has side effects that limit its usefulness for longevity. Additionally, mice fed rapamycin often suffer testicular atrophy, and some of the other possible adverse effects include impaired wound healing, lung toxicity, reduced immune function, and an increased risk of cancer—so I am still on the fence about it. However, some smart practitioners, such as my friend Dr. Peter Attia, use rapamycin successfully in their practices by closely monitoring dosing schedules and selectively targeting specific anabolic and catabolic pathways with cycling dosage. So under the care of a good functional medical practitioner, you can likely use it with less risk.

But there is also a natural substance called spermidine that has been shown to induce similar cellular autophagy effects as rapamycin with no known side effects. Researchers have given animals oral supplements of spermidine and found that they lived longer and were less likely to have liver fibrosis and cancerous liver tumors, even when genetically predisposed to those conditions.

Spermidine is found in high concentrations in wheat germ, dark leafy greens, pears, whole grains, mushrooms, and smelly, fermented cheeses, and it can be purchased as a supplement. You can read plenty more about spermidine's role in autophagy in the book *Glow 15* by my friend Naomi Whittel.

METFORMIN

Metformin (Glucophage, Glumetza, Riomet, and Fortamet are some of its brand names) is a modern pharmaceutical that is often advertised as being able to extend life "for a nickel a pop." It belongs to the biguanide compound family, a chemical group that has been used to treat diabetes since the 1950s. Metformin is synthesized from the guanidine, which is found in French lilac and was used in medicine as early as the Middle Ages. The synthetic versions belong to a family of drugs known as biguanides, and the star member is metformin. It was first approved as a drug in Europe in 1957, and 37,000 tons of metformin are now produced annually, mostly in India.

Because it is an activator of the AMPk pathway and is particularly effective at improving glycemic control with a low risk of inducing hypoglycemia, metformin may seem like an ideal CRM to enhance your chances of living a long life in good health. When I first learned about metformin, I thought it might be a bit too good to be true, but it turns out that unless you overdose with metformin, or have liver or kidney issues, or you are an athlete for whom maximum oxygen utilization is important, it may be one of the safer and more effective antiaging pharmaceuticals.

How it works: Metformin improves glycemic control primarily by inhibiting hepatic gluconeo-genesis, which is the liver-based production of glucose from noncarbohydrate sources like lactate, glycerol, and certain amino acids. It also acts by opposing the action of glucagon. Glucagon is se-creted by the pancreas when blood levels of insulin and glucose fall too low and stimulates the liv-er to convert glycogen stores into glucose, which is then released into the bloodstream. By inhib-iting this process, metformin can improve insulin sensitivity and prevent hyperglycemia-induced aging brought on by the inflammation and AGE damage caused by elevated blood glucose.

Metformin can also reduce inflammation and cell death related to nonalcoholic fatty liver disease, and fibrosis, which is the thickening or scarring of tissue, particularly connective tissue, because of disease or physical stress. Finally, metformin inhibits oxygen consumption in the mitochondria, which can lower metabolism—another potentially life-extending mechanism, but one that I consider to be unfavorable for active individuals and athletes.

How to do it: Metformin is a prescription drug. Like any prescription drug, it can be ordered from online pharmacies, but this is risky, and my advice is that if you want to find out more about using it, you should speak to your doctor or health-care provider.

An effective dose of metformin for reducing the effects of hyperglycemia and acting as a caloric-restriction mimetic is 1,500 to 2,000 mg per day. Should you decide for forgo the pill, you may be interested in a slightly less concentrated version in a goat's rue supplement or French lilac tea, both of which are full of many of the same active ingredients as metformin.

KETONE ESTERS

Ketones have been studied for faster weight loss and reduced hunger, enhanced cognitive perfor-mance, blood glucose regulation, better mental focus, lower risk for disease, and lower inflamma-tion, and now there is a growing body of research on their longevity benefits too.

Ketone supplements are often referred to as "exogenous ketones." Endogenous ketones are ones your own body creates as you restrict carbohydrates or calories and burn fat, but exogenous ketones are consumed just like any other supplement—yet they have the same benefits as endog-enous ketones. The body produces three kinds of ketones—acetoacetate, beta-hydroxybutyrate (BHB), and acetone—but the ketone found in ketone esters is BHB, primarily because research has shown that it is the ketone the body can use most efficiently.

Unlike BHB salts, which I talked about earlier in this chapter, ketone esters consist of the BHB ketone itself without any salts or other compounds bound to it. This allows the body to use the ke-tones more quickly, which raises blood ketone levels more significantly than MCT oil or BHB salts.

Most of the use of ketone esters has been limited to laboratory research, but they are moving into the commercial spotlight, and the world's first two ketone ester drinks, HVMN Ketone and KetoneAid KE4, are now on the market.

How it works: You get the same life-extending properties of caloric restriction and fasting by being in a state of ketosis, so ketones—whether exogenous or endogenous—qualify as a caloric-restriction mimetic. The drop in insulin and insulin-like growth factor receptor signaling that happens when you're in ketosis increases the transcription of genes that encode antioxidant en-zymes, such as catalase, glutathione peroxidase, and superoxide dismutase, as well as hundreds of other genes—which makes ketosis an effective method for combating free-radical damage.

Earlier in this chapter, in the section on BHB salts, I explained why the ketone body BHB improves autophagy, reduces inflammation, and eliminates free radicals. It's particularly effective when delivered in the ester form. Ketone esters also have the ability to power mitochondria in aging individuals who have a more limited ability to use glucose for energy, making them a power-ful, multimodal choice as a longevity-enhancing compound.

Is There a Dark Side to Metformin?

As Tim Ferriss reported in his book *Tools of the Titans*, metformin is widely used among CEOs, Silicon Valley executives, billionaires, and world-class performers for its antiaging properties. Among metformin's fans are Robert Hariri, CEO of cellular therapy company Celularity; Craig Venter, genetic sequencing pioneer and cofounder of Human Longevity; Ray Kurzweil, futurist and inventor; and Ned David, molecular biologist and cofounder of Unity Biotechnology.

But many people are concerned about potential problems with this supposed wonder drug. In recent years, evidence has accumulated that metformin may not be all it's cracked up to be.

For example, metformin falls into a category of biguanide molecules that can increase the generation of lactate, which then enters the circulation and produces lactic acidosis. Phenformin, another member of the biguanide family, was a popular medication for diabetes but was withdrawn from clinical use in the 1970s because it caused severe lactic acidosis. Although phenformin is associated with a ten-to-twenty-fold greater incidence of lactic acidosis than metformin, metformin's effects are still significant.

Problem is, the 1940s study that linked metformin to lactic acidosis looked at patients who were already in end-stage renal failure and also were obese and diabetic. Several other studies have shown that lactic acidosis rarely happens in normal patient population groups. While metformin is contraindicated in those with renal impairment, the reported incidence of lactic acidosis in clinical practice is very low (fewer than ten cases per hundred thousand patients).

Although metformin has been the most commonly prescribed drug for the treatment of type 2 diabetes for more than five decades, its bioenergetic mechanisms remain largely unknown. This ignorance has triggered many endeavors to uncover how exactly it works—but the results are often contradictory. One study found that while metformin may play a big role in managing cardiovascular risks, it doesn't necessarily improve hyperglycemia and, on average, has little effect on insulin requirements for diabetics. And while there were two deaths in the placebo group, there were five among the patients taking metformin.

Metformin may be beneficial for cardiovascular health when used on its own. But one study found that combining metformin with sulphonylurea (another common diabetes medication) may result in an increased risk

of mitochondrial dysfunction, cardiovascular complications, and all-cause mortality. However, this study looked at morbidly obese diabetics who were using anywhere from 6 to 9 g of metformin per day—three to five times the usual dose. Other studies show it's actually the opposite: that metformin may reverse mitochondrial dysfunction.

Many people are also concerned that metformin can cause vitamin B_{12} deficiency—at least one study has found that it stimulated vitamin B_{12} malabsorption. Decreased B_{12} concentrations can cause increased homocysteine concentrations, which is (surprise!) an independent risk factor for cardiovascular disease, particularly in individuals with type 2 diabetes. During the fifty-two months of the study, B_{12} concentrations in the metformin group got progressively lower over time, and this can result in macrocytic anemia, neuropathy, and mental changes. The same can be said for metformin's effect on folate levels, especially in women. But, of course, both B_{12} and folate are incredibly simple compounds to supplement with, and they can easily be stacked with a metformin protocol to avoid deficiencies.

Another study looked at the relationship between metformin, exercise, and blood glucose levels and found that an earlier study had showed that combining metformin and exercise had the same benefits for diabetes as metformin alone and exercise alone. In fact, exercise and metformin may have contradictory effects on diabetes. First, metformin reduces blood glucose levels, but exercise tends to increase levels of glucagon, the hormone that deals with low blood sugar by mobilizing the body's stored carbohydrates. When the two are combined, glucagon concentrations rise as the body tries to compensate for the effect of metformin. Second, by increasing the heart rate, metformin has the potential to elevate rating of perceived exertion even at lower exercise intensities, which means it could lead to the prescription of lower exercise workloads than are commonly recommended. There is also a study out of Taiwan showing that in diabetics, taking metformin for long periods of time (twelve years or more) can nearly double the risk of Alzheimer's and Parkinson's—but, like the studies on lactic acidosis, this study involved the heavy use of metformin for extended periods of time.

And then there's a concern about liver toxicity. In one person with nonalcoholic fatty liver disease, metformin was pegged as the cause of jaundice, nausea, fatigue, and unintentional weight loss—the drug had caused abnormalities in liver enzymes. Another case involved a seventy-three-year-old Japanese woman who experienced fatigue, jaundice, nausea, vomiting, anorexia, and abdominal pain due to severe hepatotoxicity that resulted from metformin. But once again, like the person with nonalcoholic fatty liver disease, the patient already had a compromised liver.

Next comes metformin's potential impact on exercise performance. One study showed that metformin can decrease VO_2 max (–2.7 percent), peak heart rate (–2.0 percent), peak ventilation (–6.2 percent), peak resting energy expenditure (–3.0 percent), and actual exercise duration (–4.1 percent). While these reductions are certainly slight and potentially nonsignificant for the average exercise enthusiast, they do suggest that for a professional athlete (especially a professional endurance athlete), the use of metformin may spell the difference between a first-place finish and not even making the podium. A more recent study highlighted that metformin has also been shown to hamper endurance and limit mitochondrial proliferation in response to an exercise protocol.

Finally, there's the concern that metformin causes GI upset. But this seems to happen only in people with bacterial imbalances in the gut (as discussed in chapter 13) and may occur because metformin is working directly to alter the microbiota. Research is now showing that metformin can actually alter the gut composition in a favorable manner by increasing levels of several different short-chain fatty acid bacteria. It may also decrease inflammation in the gut in a manner that increases insulin sensitivity and lowers blood glucose.

With all of this back-and-forth on metformin, I decided to get the opinion of my friend Dallas Clouatre, a well-established author and consultant in alternative and complementary medicine, and my guest on the podcast episode "How Low-Fat Diets Make You Fat" (he also, incidentally, introduced me to a very effective alternative to metformin: bitter melon extract). Here's what he had to say:

My thoughts on metformin are that it is interesting but overhyped. Keep in mind that it works primarily on the liver (which contributes to 30 percent of glucose clearance from meals) and not on the peripheral tissues (70 percent of glucose clearance). It likely does promote a longer "health span" given that lowering insulin and IGF-1 along with mTOR, typical of caloric restriction and of those who naturally live to extreme

old age, is usually a good thing. Of course, any item that keeps insulin levels low along with keeping blood glucose in the low-normal range will lower mTOR. Downsides of metformin include reduced efficacy with advancing age, reduced efficacy with prolonged use, and GI tract issues in some individuals. Given that rehabilitation of the mitochondrial electron transport complex [which is deleteriously affected by metformin] is a normal function of a good night's sleep, for me, it is difficult to suggest the chronic intake of a drug that works by gumming up a natural process of the body.

I'll sum it up here: don't use metformin if you have liver or kidney issues, and definitely don't overdose on metformin. If you get gut discomfort while using metformin, consider waiting it out to see if your gut flora becomes balanced and your symptoms subside, which typically takes eight to twelve weeks. If you use metformin, supplement with vitamin B_{12}, and if you're a woman, monitor your folate levels and consider supplementation with a good multivitamin that contains a natural form of folate like methyltetrahydrofolate (MTHF). Finally, if you're a professional athlete or aerobic performance is very high on the totem pole for you, I'd avoid metformin.

For myself, my current habit of taking bitter melon extract is working just fine to control my blood glucose levels, but because metformin appears to have several beneficial side effects beyond blood glucose control, I may begin supplementing with it in the future. However, I encourage you to look into natural alternatives that can have similar blood-sugar-stabilizing and longevity-enhancing effects. You'll discover many such compounds in this chapter.

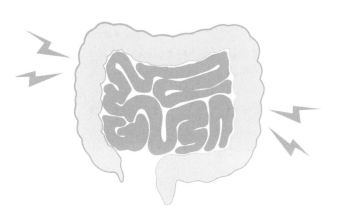

Additionally, in the presence of high glucose concentrations, ketone esters significantly increase the rate of muscle glycogen synthesis following exercise. One study pointed out that consuming ketone body esters leads to a state of pure ketosis unaccompanied by the elevation of free fatty acids, which could prove to be beneficial in treating certain neurodegenerative diseases such as Alzheimer's and Parkinson's.

Ketone esters can also inhibit NF-kB, a proinflammatory transcription factor that regulates the expression of over five hundred genes involved in cellular transformation, survival, proliferation, angiogenesis, inflammation, and more. Inhibiting the NF-kB signaling pathway has been shown to reverse several aspects of aging, most notably cardiac hypertrophy, a condition in which the heart muscle thickens due to genetics, excess exercise, or chronically elevated blood pressure. NF-kB can block the production of stem cells in older individuals, and since NF-kB increases significantly with age, particularly in the hypothalamus, it is regarded as a pro-aging compound. Downregulation of NF-kB has been shown to significantly extend life span, memory, strength, skin quality, and more.

Because they are in a D-BHB configuration that does not require them to be bound to a salt, ketone esters are known to raise blood levels of BHB more than BHB salts or MCT oils. When consumed in a drink, the ester bonds in a ketone ester are broken by gut enzymes, releasing butanediol and D-BHB into the blood. Butanediol is an alcohol that is structurally similar to BHB and is metabolized by the liver to form D-BHB. All the D-BHB resulting from this breakdown travels straight into the bloodstream because the liver is unable to use ketones.

How to do it: Once per day, preferably in a fasted state, drink a serving of ketone esters. You can also combine ketone esters with a carbohydrate source such as dextrose or ribose for a potent physical and cognitive performance aid, or with an essential amino acid source for long-term stable energy, even in a fasted state. I have used this strategy during triathlons and obstacle course races with great success, but try it during training first to ensure the esters don't result in any annoying GI distress for you.

As a word of warning, no matter what you mix them with, ketone esters taste pretty horrible, so be prepared to pop some mint gum in your mouth afterward or chase them with a very small portion of fresh juice or your favorite stevia-sweetened beverage. I have successfully experimented with and use HVMN Ketone and KetoneAid KE4 drinks.

BLOOD-SUGAR-STABILIZING HERBS AND SPICES

Chapter 8 explained the importance of controlling glycemic variability and why, especially if you want to enhance longevity, you should place a high priority on lowering blood glucose levels and inflammation. In many respects, low, stable blood glucose can act very similarly to caloric restriction, which is why I consider most insulin- and blood-glucose-stabilizing compounds—including bitter melon extract, Ceylon cinnamon, apple cider vinegar, berberine, rosemary, curcumin, fenugreek, Gymnema sylvestre, and capsaicin—to be caloric-restriction mimetics. Many of these compounds also work in on anti-inflammatory compounds, giving you a double-whammy effect when you include these regularly in your diet, as is a common practice in many of the Blue Zones.

How it works: The mechanisms vary depending on the herb or spice:

- Bitter melon contains a lectin that lowers blood glucose by acting on surrounding tissues. It also suppresses appetite.
- Ceylon cinnamon lowers blood glucose and reduces inflammation, which contributes to weight gain.
- Apple cider vinegar has been shown to reduce blood glucose levels in diabetic rats, possibly because its acetic acid restricts the digestion of starch.

- Berberine exerts a hypoglycemic effect, particularly in people with type 2 diabetes, and also regulates lipid metabolism.

- Rosemary has been shown to lower blood glucose, possibly by increasing liver glycolysis.

- Curcumin, the active ingredient of turmeric, and ginger have both been shown to reduce blood sugar levels in diabetic rats.

- Fenugreek seeds, which are common in South and Central Asia, reduce fasting blood glucose levels and improve glucose tolerance.

- *Gymnema sylvestre* helps control blood sugar levels by blocking the absorption of sugar molecules in the intestines.

- Capsaicin, the active ingredient in cayenne, reduces blood glucose by increasing insulin.

- Finally, vanadium and chromium are minerals that, taken together, appear to have a blood-sugar-lowering and insulin-stabilizing effect like metformin's.

How to do it: It's not rocket science: simply fill your pantry and cupboards with a wide variety of the herbs and spices listed above. You can also use blood-glucose-controlling and insulin-sensitizing supplements such as Kion Lean, Gymnema sylvestre, or berberine before high-carbohydrate or high-protein meals. I also recommend a shot of apple cider vinegar in a couple beverages throughout the day (a splash or two of cocktail bitters can also be highly effective), ample use of Ceylon cinnamon in smoothies or shakes, and liberal use of rosemary, fenugreek seeds, ginger, and cayenne when cooking.

4. Sirtuin-Activating Compounds (STACs)

STACs are chemical compounds that affect sirtuins, which are a group of enzymes that use NAD+ to remove acetyl groups from proteins via a process that can allow for proper genetic expression, less protein damage, and extension of life span. Some of the better-researched foods and supplements rich in STACs are blueberry extract, cacao flavonoids, green tea extract, resveratrol, curcumin, black currants, and fish oil.

How it works: Sirtuins influence a wide range of cellular processes, including circadian rhythms, mitochondrial biogenesis, aging, transcription, apoptosis (cell self-destruction), inflammation, and stress resistance, as well as energy efficiency and alertness during low-calorie situations. STACs are also considered to be caloric-restriction mimetics, and in studies, they have been shown to help prevent aging-related diseases such as Alzheimer's, type 2 diabetes, and obesity.

A new compound on the STAC scene is fisetin, a polyphenol that's found in many tannic drinks, such as tea, wine, and pomegranate juice, and fruits and vegetables, including apples, persimmons, onions, cucumbers, and, in quite high concentrations, strawberries. Fisetin is a potent senolytic, which means it plays a crucial role in reducing the development of senescent cells, restoring tissue homeostasis, reducing a variety of age-related pathologies, and extending both median and maximum life span. Reducing the development of senescent cells has been shown to lead to less inflammation, less molecular dysfunction within cells, and better stem cell function. Quercetin, an antihistamine and anti-inflammatory found in dark leafy vegetables, broccoli, red onions, peppers, apples, grapes, black tea, green tea, red wine, and fruit, can also modulate senescent cell development.

How to do it: Buy blueberry or strawberry powder or fresh, organic blueberries and strawberries and use one serving per day in smoothies, on salads, or in other dishes (look for the smaller, less sugary wild blueberries, bilberries, or wild strawberries). Alternatively, you can use black currants, although they may be harder to find. Dark cacao powder or cacao nibs, curcumin powder, turmeric root, green tea extract powder, and high-quality, organic green tea leaves are also good sources of STACs, as is a daily glass of organic red wine, a resveratrol-rich supplement such as Thorne ResveraCel, and 1 to 20 g of a high-quality fish oil per day (I take 10 to 12 g of fish oil on any days on which I'm not eating a hefty portion of actual fish—there's much more on fish oil in chapter 12).

Because most of these compounds are also antioxidant-rich foods, which, when overconsumed, may excessively blunt or halt hormesis, I recommend using them like condiments, in smaller amounts, and not as staples. Furthermore, when it comes to managing blood sugar, a handful of blueberries or strawberries is reasonable, but mowing through an entire carton is not.

5. Stem Cells and Stem Cell–Supporting Foods

There's quite a bit about stem cell therapies in chapter 12. As a quick reminder, stem cells can differentiate into more specialized cells and then produce a continuous supply of cells that can heal or build tissue in specific areas of the body. Chapter 12 explained how stem cells are categorized according to how many types of cells they can turn into and how stem cells can help with recovery, but here, I'll explore the nitty-gritty details about the different sources of stem cells, including adipose tissue, bone, placenta, and more, and how they can slow aging. You can consider this section to be your quick reference guidebook on interpreting the emerging and wonderful but oft-confusing world of stem cell therapies.

After all, there is evidence that a loss of endogenous stem cells is linked to aging and that the number of stem cells in your body may act as a biological clock for aging, with fewer stem cells ultimately resulting in overall aging. This makes sense because, as we age, a large number of the stem cells in the bone marrow get mobilized for repair and recovery. This means that everyone—and especially those whose bodies need more repair and recovery, such as professional athletes, those struggling with a chronic disease, and those who have had a large number of injuries or accidents—have fewer stem cells in their bone marrow as they age. The stem cell theory of aging postulates that the aging process is the result of the inability of various types of stem cells to replenish body tissues, so tending to your stem cells is likely one of the more effective steps you can take to enhancing longevity (especially when combined with the other strategies in this chapter). Indeed, after my first intravenous stem cell injection, my biological age based on telomere measurements dropped from thirty-seven down to twenty!

BONE STEM CELLS

The two primary kinds of stem cells found in bone marrow are hematopoietic stem cells (HSCs) and mesenchymal stem cells (MSCs). Both HSCs and MSCs are tissue-specific, meaning they differentiate only into specified, genetically designated tissues. HSCs differentiate into different types of blood cells, while MSCs differentiate into bone, cartilage, fat, and connective tissue located in bone.

How it works: Blood cell turnover, which is extremely high in adult humans, requires highly efficient homeostatic control mechanisms to maintain proper blood quality and volume, and HSCs are the primary agents of this homeostasis. HSCs were the first tissue-specific stem cells to be isolated and have been used in grafts to treat a number of blood cell diseases, such as leukemias and autoimmune disorders.

MSCs have been shown to be able to sustain the growth, viability, and multipotent status of HSCs in cell cultures. They can also heal injured and diseased tissues and organs, reduce apoptosis, and modulate immune responses, and the most recent research shows that when MSCs are given to older people in an IV infusion, they increase quality of life and decrease frailty.

Contrary to popular belief, stem cells do not necessarily travel straight to the area they're needed and instantly differentiate into some new form of tissue. It would certainly be convenient if this were the case, but in my podcast with regenerative medicine physician Dr. Matt Cook, he explained that what happens most of the time is that stem cells migrate into tissue and communicate with other cells, such as cytokines and exosomes, to modulate a normal inflammatory or repair response, or to call in other cells to help—such as fibroblast cell to assist with tendon repair. This means that stem cells—whether from fat, bone, umbilical cords, or any other source—primarily work by simply causing your body's built-in repair mechanisms to work more efficiently. If it is indeed the case that stem cells primarily modulate or stimulate an immunomodulatory effect, then the age (or the length of the telomeres) of the stem cells injected is irrelevant because it's other cells that do the healing. This means that harvesting and reinjecting your own stem cells from bone or fat when you are, say, eighty could still be a highly efficacious strategy—especially when they're combined with exosomes.

Exosomes, as you may remember from chapter 12, carry messages from cell to cell and are the "active ingredient" in stem cells, and they can be targeted to a specific cell or cells to enhance particular biological processes. Exosomes are particularly effective with stem cells from bone, which has a slightly lower MSC content than fat, because they effectively upgrade these stem cells closer to the status of fat-derived stem cells.

How to do it: A multitude of stem cell clinics in the United States can harvest stem cells from your bones with a long needle that's placed into the soft center of the bone marrow, often in the hip bones. However, very few medical institutions in the United States currently offer any type of exosome therapy. Dr. Adelson at Docere Clinics in Park City, Utah, employs a large number of exosomes in his stem cell therapy, which can be used in conjunction with any of the stem cell strategies in this section or even by themselves as a potent tissue repair and regeneration aid. Interestingly, recent research has shown that plants also produce exosomes, that, upon ingestion by a human, impart positive changes on the gut microbiome and act as tiny cell-to-cell signaling molecules all on their own. (When you step back, it's quite profound how many of the expensive or complicated methods for health or longevity can be replicated at least in part by natural means: photobiomodulation panels and sunlight, cryotherapy chambers and cold water, NAD supplements and pau d'arco tea, stem cells and fasting, and now, exosome injections and plants rich in exosomes, such as watercress, rosemary, dandelion, nettle, and mint.)

As you learned in chapter 12, Docere Clinics concentrates bone marrow stem cells into a bone marrow aspirate concentrate (BMAC). This BMAC "soup" is then combined with exosomes and reinjected into any joints that need treatment or, in the case of Docere Clinic's full-body stem-cell makeover, into every joint in the body. I underwent this procedure in 2018, and within two months, I began to notice a profound improvement in recovery and overall joint mobility and comfort. I have also had stem cells extracted from the iliac crest bone in my hip and stored with Forever Labs in Berkeley, California.

FAT STEM CELLS

MSCs appear to be very similar whether they are taken from bone marrow, adipose tissue, umbilical cord blood, or any other birth tissue, such as the placenta. The main difference between fat and bone as sources of stem cells is the number of MSCs that each contains. According to Dr. Kristin Comella of the US Stem Cell Clinic, adipose tissue contains about five hundred times more MSCs than bone marrow. Bone marrow also contains high amounts of white blood cells compared to adipose tissue, so it may be more pro-inflammatory. Adipose tissue–derived stem cells (ASCs) may also have a higher immunomodulatory capacity than their bone marrow–derived counterparts, which could enhance the potential antiaging effect of ASCs.

How it works: ASCs are considered ideal for treatments and regenerative therapies. The main benefit of using ASCs instead of bone marrow–derived stem cells is that ASCs are more readily available (partially due to a worldwide increase in obesity) and can be harvested with minimally invasive, low-risk techniques. ASCs—particularly those derived from brown fat—can be used to support the new growth of bone cells, liver cells, neurons, vascular endothelial cells, heart cells, and, of course, more fat cells.

How to do it: If you are lean, you may have difficulty getting enough stem cells from your fat without a significantly uncomfortable session with a long liposuction needle (which is exactly what happened to me). The US Stem Cell Clinic in Florida is considered one of the go-to clinics for the liposuction extraction of fat stem cells, and both my wife and I have visited the clinic for this procedure. We pay the US Stem Cell Clinic a yearly fee to store our stem cells, and for a nominal fee, they can ship them to any medical clinic for either intravenous or intra-articular (joint) injections by a medical professional.

AMNIOTIC, UMBILICAL, AND PLACENTAL STEM CELLS

Amniotic fluid is the protective fluid that surrounds an unborn baby. During cesarean section deliveries, this fluid can be saved and the stem cells it contains can be harvested, resulting in about a liter of amniotic fluid containing MSCs. As explained in chapter 12, stem cells from umbilical cord blood are not as potent as others, like bone marrow and adipose stem cells, and can develop only into a limited number of cell types. Wharton's jelly is a tissue that surrounds blood vessels in the umbilical cord and contains relatively high concentrations of precursor MSCs that have increased proliferation and differentiation capabilities, especially compared with adult sources of stem cells. Placentas also contain a significant number of MSCs.

How it works: Harvesting these types of stem cells is relatively straightforward. The current procedure for harvesting amniotic fluid adds about ninety seconds to a cesarean operation and is completely safe for both mother and child. The cells can then be used to support the healthy growth of skin, cartilage, cardiac, nervous, muscle, and bone tissues. Umbilical cord blood can easily be harvested following the delivery of a baby. The stem cells it contains have been used therapeutically to treat bone marrow–related stem cell deficits. Placental stem cells are believed to be even more potent than umbilical cord stem cells: research has indicated that they proliferate and expand more easily than umbilical stem cells and have a greater immunosuppressive capacity, resulting in reduced levels of pro-inflammatory T cells. (Indeed, there are several international clinics that offer placental stem cell therapies that contain a high number of stem cells due to expansion, although it is not currently legal in the US to modify stem cells in this manner.)

How to do it: The FDA requires that any birth tissue–based stem cell product in the US, whether amniotic, umbilical, or placental, must be acellular, which means it can't be made of any living cells. If a company in the US claims that such tissue contains living stem cells, they are breaking the law, and using stem cells from these tissues could cause graft versus host disease, a condition in which your body rejects the injected tissue. This risk of tissue rejection that accompanies injecting one person's stem cells into another person's body is why I am a bit gun-shy of using or recommending birth tissue.

I also worry about viruses from these sources. Although tissue bank products are screened for diseases and screening processes are becoming more and more strict, especially in the US, these tissues are still screened only for diseases we currently know about. But every several years, it seems, we discover a new and scary virus or prion disease, such as mad cow disease, and I don't like to take any chances with foreign tissue injections because of the chance of unknown viruses or protein diseases entering my body—so I'm more likely to recommend stem cells derived from autologous tissues like your own fat or bone. One exception to this rule is Wharton's jelly, which, as mentioned earlier, is harvested from the umbilical cord wall. Because these stem cells must communicate with both the mother's and the baby's tissue, they do not result in an antibody or other immune system response when used in other subjects.

Many US clinics offer amniotic, umbilical, and placental stem cell treatments, but they're likely to be far less effective and contain a lower stem cell count than your own bone- or fat-derived stem cells, especially if they're not combined with exosomes. There are several offshore stem cell centers (Panama is one quite popular location) that use living cells from birth tissue, based on the idea that younger tissue is better. Some centers in Mexico will culture-expand your own stem cells to concentrate their efficacy, a procedure that's banned in the US by the FDA because it's considered excessive manipulation of cells.

APSCS

In the regenerative medicine field there's an increasingly popular cell line called adult pluripotent stem cells (APSCs). This umbrella category includes very small embryonic-like stem cells (VSELs), multilineage-differentiating stress-enduring cells (MUSEs), and marrow-isolated adult multilineage inducible cells (MIAMIs), among others. Since their discovery, APSCs have been widely studied because of their ability to multiply freely and become any kind of cells in the human body. But unlike embryonic stem cells, they do not have known cancer-causing properties or other potential disease risks, and in clinical application, they can be derived autologously—that is, they can be extracted from and reinjected into your own body.

How it works: APSCs are formed in bone marrow, but rather than being stored there like other bone stem cells, they are released into your bloodstream, where they circulate inactive until your body faces extreme stress, such as low oxygen, low body temperature, or significant injuries. Once active, APSCs can home in with surprising accuracy on areas of injury and degeneration to begin the repair and regeneration process. In particular, they have been found to be effective for healing bone injuries and rejuvenating organs, and they have antiaging properties. This is almost like the blood transfusions therapy discussed later in this chapter, but without the need for the blood of a young healthy donor—your own blood goes through a process that makes it young again.

How to do it: I had this procedure performed at the offices of Dr. Halland Chen in New York City (Halland actually combined this procedure with a CoQ10 and NAD IV, as well as adding exosomes to the stem cells). After a physician collects blood (Halland pulled four 60 cc tubes of it from my arm!) or bone marrow samples, ASPCs are separated from other cells via cell-processing technology. Once isolated, the APSCs are exposed to very cold temperatures to simulate hypothermia, which activates them. Finally, the physician combines the APSCs with growth factors harvested from your own platelet cells in the same blood or bone marrow sample. The active APSCs and growth factors can then be returned to your body through an intravenous injection. Once in your bloodstream, the APSCs go to work, seeking out areas of inflammation and injury.

At Dr. Chen's clinic, this process is typically done over three consecutive days. On day 1, a CoQ10 compound, which helps generate energy in the form of ATP, is infused via IV, and you receive an intramuscular injection of vitamins such as NAD to mobilize your body's stem cells into the bloodstream. On day 2, 210 mL of blood is drawn, typically from a vein in your arm, for cell processing. On day 3, your own APSCs are infused via IV, and a small portion is reserved for injection into a specific musculoskeletal region where inflammation or injury is present.

Currently, Dr. Matthew Cook at BioReset Medical in San Jose, California, and Dr. Halland Chen in New York City are the two doctors I trust to administer an APSC procedure. After I did this protocol, I noted a profound improvement in recovery, sleep, and overall energy levels.

COLOSTRUM

In chapter 15, I explained why colostrum, otherwise known as first milk or nature's first food, is excellent for repairing a leaky gut, reducing inflammation, and building muscle. It's also a powerful antiaging supplement. It serves as a concentrated source of proteins, growth factors, and antibodies that are essential for early development of newborns and beneficial for adults too. Colostrum's properties have been revered for thousands of years across many cultures. In ancient Chinese medicine, it was regarded as a potent health tonic, and for the Maasai people of Kenya and Tanzania, it has long been regarded as a crucial part of a warrior's diet. In Britain, dairy farmers refer to colostrum as "beestings," and they used any surplus colostrum to make an extra-creamy and very healthy pudding.

How it works: Colostrum is far richer in antimicrobial peptides, immune-regulating compounds, and growth factors than normal milk. It contains concentrated, low-volume forms of vital nutrients as well as lymphocytes and antibodies, and it helps to balance the gut microbiota and enhances the growth and repair of several tissue types. It also contains cytokines, which keep communication between immune cells active, and growth factors, which assist with maintenance and growth of certain body tissues, including muscle and the gastrointestinal lining. The lacto-ferrin in colostrum assists with iron absorption and is a crucial part of your immune defense system, and the growth hormone in colostrum works individually and with the other growth factors in colostrum to aid in the growth and function of gastrointestinal tissues, muscle, and more. The immunoglobulins in colostrum are small proteins that your immune system uses to seek out and destroy foreign antigens.

Finally, colostrum contains proline-rich polypeptides (PRPs—not to be confused with platelet-rich plasma, the other PRP in this chapter), important immune system regulators that encourage the growth of white blood cells and may restore balance in cellular immune functions. PRPs may defend against oxidative stress and support brain health. Studies have now shown that colostrum is a rich source of mesenchymal stem cell–like cells, and one fascinating study showed that, while colostrum alone had a considerable effect on stem cell activity, it was a combination of colostrum, yeast extract, skullcap, zizyphus (also known as jujube), seaweed, and turmeric that had the most profound activity likely to translate into therapeutic benefit.

How to do it: Because it contains few, if any, milk proteins, colostrum is well tolerated even by people who cannot tolerate lactose and dairy. That being said, colostrum from goat's milk is generally better tolerated by those who can't handle cow's milk, because human milk and goat's milk have similar nutritional and hormonal profiles.

You can use a colostrum powder in smoothies or shakes, or take colostrum capsules. Because it can be anabolic in the sense that it increases insulin-like growth factor and growth hormone levels, I don't take colostrum year-round but instead rotate it eight weeks on, four weeks off, throughout the year. In addition, if you have a bacterial overgrowth such as SIBO, colostrum can cause a die-off reaction (known as a Jarisch-Herxheimer reaction), so it's important to start with a lower dose if you have gut bacterial imbalances.

ALGAE

Algae and phytoplankton (more on phytoplankton below) are the foundations of the marine food chain, and in order to hold that position, they must be incredibly nutrient-dense. Pound for pound, algae is the most nutritionally dense food on the face of the planet—a single gram of algae contains the nutritional equivalent of 1,000 g of fruits and vegetables! Spirulina is an extremely nutrient-dense algae that forms tangled masses in warm alkaline lakes, primarily in Africa and Latin America. Chlorella is a single-celled freshwater species of microalgae that contains the highest-density chlorophyll in nature and possesses a nutrient density close to that of spirulina.

How it works: The chemical structure of chlorophyll is very similar to hemoglobin, allowing it to efficiently carry oxygen in the blood and increase your red blood cell count. There is even some recent research that indicates that a combination of chlorophyll in your bloodstream and exposure to sunlight can allow you to produce ATP without consuming any calories! By weight, dried chlorella is about 45 percent protein, 20 percent fat, 20 percent carbohydrates, 5 percent fiber, and 10 percent vitamins and minerals. Algal amino acids are unstructured, which means that your body can absorb them easily and rapidly. This type of nutrient-dense substance can easily be incorporated into a calorie-restriction or fasting protocol without compromising your overall caloric intake.

Perhaps most interesting with regard to longevity is chlorella's ability to mobilize stem cells. One study evaluated how an extract from the edible cyanobacterium *Aphanizomenon flos-aquae* (AFA), a form of chlorella, affected human stem cells in vitro and in vivo (in the lab and inside living organisms). A double-blind, randomized crossover study involving twelve healthy subjects found that chlorella helped stem cells travel to the tissues where they were most needed.

Another study demonstrated that spirulina lowered levels of a key neuroinflammatory cytokine in the hippocampus of aged rats, leading to the reversal of age-related cognitive decline and increased neurogenesis. Spirulina protected hippocampal neural progenitor cells from inflammation caused by molecules called lipopolysaccharides—which, interestingly, are often found in a high-fat, high-sugar diet. Spirulina also promoted mitochondrial respiration and the proliferation of stem cells in culture, supporting the hypothesis that a diet enriched with spirulina and similar nutraceuticals may help protect stem cells from damage.

How to do it: Not all chlorella or spirulina is created equal. Since algae is a bioremediant that can detoxify the water it is grown in and retain the toxins, you need to be careful with your sourcing. I eat about twenty to thirty tablets of chlorella and spirulina per day in the form of 100 percent organic, cracked-cell-wall algae from a company called EnergyBits, which is grown in pristine freshwater tanks.

MARINE PHYTOPLANKTON

Marine phytoplankton are photosynthesizing microalgae that grow in oceans all over the world. In addition to comprising the foundation of the entire oceanic food chain, its primary role in the ocean is to turn inorganic raw materials, such as seaweed, minerals, sunlight, and carbon dioxide, into hundreds of different nutrients, including vitamins, bioavailable minerals, all amino acids, essential fatty acids, and carotenoids. In addition, along with algae like chlorella, phytoplankton is responsible for producing up to 90 percent of all oxygen on earth. There are about forty thousand known strains of phytoplankton, and a few of these strains (particularly those mentioned below) are extremely beneficial for humans.

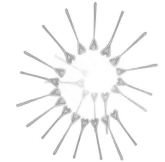

How it works: The phytoplankton strains that possess a nutritional profile compatible with human needs are dense in essential fatty acids (primarily EPA and DHA), which fuel your brain and nervous system; all amino acids, for muscle, brain, and nervous system support; enzymes and pigments that help eliminate oxidative stress and inflammation; and carotenoids, which play a role in regulating gene expression and inducing cell-to-cell communications.

A marine biologist named Luis Lubian, who was involved in an extensive study of more than forty-three thousand types of marine phytoplankton, discovered one strain of phytoplankton that is extremely nutrient-dense and well absorbed. The scientific name of this strain of marine phytoplankton is *Nannochloropsis gaditana*, or "nanno" for short. It contains the right amount and balance of amino acids, enzymes, fatty acids, minerals, and pigments, which are the building blocks our bodies use to repair DNA, produce glutathione, and generate growth hormones and stem cells. In other words, this one unique type of marine phytoplankton gives the body practically all the raw materials it needs to produce healthy new stem cells and neurochemicals.

In addition to nanno, another form of marine phytoplankton, referred to as tetra (its genus name is *Tetraselmis*), has extremely high levels of superoxide dismutase, an extremely powerful antioxidant. It is also very high in vitamin C (a strong electron donor and antioxidant) and has been shown to promote deep sleep.

How to do it: Take one or two drops of marine phytoplankton per day. I prefer Oceans Alive Raw Marine Phytoplankton, which are grown in a photobioreactor with just salt water, carbon dioxide, and sunlight, and then added to a trace mineral solution. The Oceans Alive brand contains both the nanno and tetra forms of the phytoplankton.

ALOE VERA

Aloe plants, also known as burn plant, lily of the desert, and elephant's gall, grow naturally in dry, tropical climates in Africa, Asia, Europe, and the southern and western parts of the United States. Aloe vera is a gelatinous substance derived from the fleshy leaves of the plant and has been recognized for its healing properties for at least six thousand years. A symbol of immortality, it was presented to Egyptian pharaohs as a funeral gift, and over several millennia, humans have used aloe to treat wounds, hair loss, hemorrhoids, and digestive issues.

How it works: Aloe vera contains several bioactive compounds, including vitamins, minerals, amino acids, enzymes, lignins, saponins, and salicylic acid. These, along with the other steroid-like compounds it contains—steroids, carotenoids, terpenes, and phytosterols—allow aloe vera to modulate various biological activities: it helps prevent cancer, scavenges free radicals, and exhibits antimicrobial activity by rupturing bacterial cell walls.

Aloe has been reported in several studies to improve glucose tolerance and overall glucose metabolism. For example, oral intake of aloe significantly reduced blood glucose in diabetic mice within just five days. Consumption of aloe vera juice and glibenclamide, a diabetes medication, significantly reduced fasting blood glucose within two weeks in diabetic human patients, but similar results were reported with the use of aloe vera juice alone. This is likely because the development of diabetes is accompanied by a decline in the number of circulating stem cells, and aloe has been shown to assist with mobilization of stem cells, which can migrate to the pancreas and differentiate into functional insulin-producing cells. Increasing the number of circulating stem cells has been reported to significantly improve the condition of diabetic mice and insulin-dependent human patients. Aloe vera also improves the viability of dental pulp stem cells, so it may have a significant positive effect on oral health.

How to do it: Aloe vera juice is easily consumed as a daily shot or poured into smoothies or shakes. Look for a product that is organic and at least 99 percent aloe. Often referred to on a product label as aloe vera inner leaf juice, or inner fillet, aloe vera gel is also an option, although many gels use carrageenan, which has been linked to digestive problems—a bit ironic, since aloe gel is often used to aid digestion. But when my friend Shawn Stevenson was recovering from a spinal cord injury using a host of the plant-based stem cell–support tactics in this chapter, he would eat a 3-to-5-inch chunk of aloe vera leaf multiple times per day. If you prefer to use the juice, Lily of the Desert and Nature's Way are two good brands.

COFFEEBERRY FRUIT EXTRACT

I first learned about this little-known nutrient when I interviewed Darin Olien on my podcast. Nicknamed the "Indiana Jones of Superfoods," Olien is a widely recognized exotic superfoods hunter, supplement formulator, and environmental activist who travels the planet discovering new and underutilized medicinal plants. While hiking in Africa, he came across coffeeberry fruit, which has none of the taste associated with brewed coffee beans. It's quite tart and contains three times the amount of antioxidants of powerhouse foods such as green tea and blueberries. Darin reported to me that it is one of the few plants that can increase levels of totipotent stem cells, the ones that have the potential to develop into any kind of cell in the human body (see chapter 12 for more on totipotent stem cells).

How it works: In two clinical studies, coffeeberry fruit extract has been shown to significantly stimulate brain-derived neurotrophic factor, which is responsible for the development, differentiation, and protection of neurons and is also strongly supportive of both cognitive and mental health. In addition, coffeeberry fruit extract significantly upregulates sirtuin enzymes in a manner that can offset the aging process triggered by oxidative stress and support stem cell functions, particularly when the body is under chronic or acute stress. One study observed the effects of four weeks of coffeeberry supplementation in twenty college athletes and found that postworkout antioxidant capacity was significantly higher in the group that took coffeeberry than in the placebo group. The study also found that the coffeeberry group's blood lactate levels were significantly reduced ten minutes after exercise compared to the placebo group's.

How to do it: I buy 100 percent pure Hawaiian coffeeberry extract in a powdered form, which I blend into smoothies or shakes. I typically use it as a part of my shotgun-approach morning smoothie—on BoundlessBook.com/19, you'll find a link to information about what exactly goes into this beverage, but, as you can imagine, it includes several of the supplements listed in this chapter.

MORINGA EXTRACT

Darin also introduced me to moringa, a tree native to parts of Africa and Asia. Its name is derived from *murungaii*, which is the Tamil word for "drumstick." While there are thirty different species of moringa, the most widely cultivated is *Moringa oleifera*, which is native to the foothills of the northwestern Indian Himalayas.

How it works: Moringa contains a number of antioxidants and natural antibiotics, and the phytochemicals in moringa are hepatoprotective, cardioprotective, antinociceptive (pain-reducing), DNA-protective, and antiatherosclerotic.

Different parts of the plant contain different important minerals, as well as protein, vitamins, beta-carotene, and various phenolics. In studies, extracts from the flower of the plant have been shown to cause a significant increase in the proliferation of MSCs, while the root can increase cytotoxicity to cancer cell lines, effectively killing off cancerous cells. Extracts from the leaves are known to combat high blood pressure, reduce insulin resistance, reduce inflammation, and reduce the effects of diabetes. Moringa is also one of the more powerful members of the sulforaphane family (similar to broccoli sprouts) and can increase activity of the Nrf2 pathway in a manner than significantly increases cell protection and reduces inflammation and oxidation.

How to do it: Like coffeeberry fruit extract, organic moringa leaf powder can easily be purchased online and then added to teas (I've found that it mixes quite well with green tea), smoothies, or shakes. It's one of the compounds that I add to my morning smoothie each day (the full list of ingredients can be found on BoundlessBook.com/19). If you want to get even more creative, simply take half a teaspoon of moringa powder, add a teaspoon of raw honey, squeeze in a little bit of lemon, mix them together, and add water.

The list above contains some of the top stem cell–supporting foods but is by no means comprehensive; nutrition research is constantly unveiling new compounds that enhance stem cell health and mobilization. Other notable dietary additions that may benefit stem cells include dark chocolate and other compounds rich in cacao extract, such as cacao tea; black, green, and oolong teas; foods rich in zeaxanthin, such as mustard greens, watercress, collard greens, Swiss chard, and fiddleheads; black raspberries; and even squid ink (which is used in many popular Mediterranean dishes, such as Spain's black rice and Italy's risotto al nero di seppia and pasta al nero).

6. Injections

In addition to stem cells, other injectable compounds can also have a potent antiaging effect. The following are a few of the more popular injections used commonly by longevity enthusiasts, biohackers, and antiaging medical clinics. Proceed at your own risk if you decide to inject yourself intravenously, intramuscularly, or subcutaneously. Having grown up in a family full of EMTs, I am quite comfortable whipping out needles and administering most of my own injections, especially those that are subcutaneous or intramuscular (just as a diabetic would administer insulin daily), but if you aren't comfortable with this, I recommend making good friends with a nurse practitioner or other medical professional who can assist you.

PEPTIDES

In basic terms, a peptide is simply a small protein consisting of amino acids linked in a chain. To better understand the nature of peptides, it helps to consider that proteins are made up of one or more polypeptide molecules. The proteins that we obtain through food are split by gastric enzymes into small peptides that have many different functions in the bodily systems. When administered via injection (usually subcutaneously, with the equivalent of an insulin syringe), certain peptides are particularly efficacious for joint healing, mitochondrial support, focus, energy, deep sleep, and longevity.

How it works: One of the notable properties of peptides is that they regulate the activity of certain molecules, and because of this, they influence body functions in several ways and can act like both neurotransmitters and hormones. Each organ and body function has its own unique peptide bioregulator. The characteristic of peptides that allows them to slow aging is due to the fact that they've been shown to shortcut the protein synthesis process. This means that when peptide bioregulators are active, organs can build and tissues can develop easier and faster.

In recent years, research has revealed that peptides play a significant role in the regulation of multiple mechanisms of biological aging. This branch of scientific research has led to the peptide theory of aging, which posits that changes in gene expression result in reduced protein synthesis, eventually leading to aging and the development of age-related diseases. By stimulating the body's own peptide production via peptide bioregulators, specific organs, systems or conditions in the body can be targeted by using a specific short-chain peptide to initiate greater protein synthesis.

I've personally used peptides BPC-157 and TB-500 to enhance healing and recovery. BPC-157 (body protection compound 157), which protects and heals the gut, is found in trace amounts in gastric juices. But it can also be synthesized in a lab. It can be taken in an oral supplement for a systemic effect, or injected subcutaneously or intramuscularly into or near injured or damaged tissues, where it has very powerful biological healing effects. BPC-157 is also known as a stable gastric pentadecapeptide (the name refers to the length of the peptide), primarily because it is stable in human gastric juice; can cause an anabolic healing effect in both the upper and lower GI tract; has an antiulcer effect; and produces a therapeutic effect on inflammatory bowel disease—all surprisingly free of side effects.

As demonstrated in multiple studies, BPC-157 also accelerates wound healing, and, via interaction with the nitric oxide system, protects endothelial tissue and builds blood vessels. This occurs even in severely impaired conditions, such as advanced and poorly controlled irritable bowel disease, in which it stimulates the expression of genes responsible for cytokine and growth factor generation and also collagen formation, along with intestinal anastomosis healing, reversal of short bowel syndrome, and fistula healing—all of which can be extremely frustrating issues in people who have gut pain, constipation, diarrhea, and bowel inflammation. Conveniently, BPC-157 is one of the few peptides that can be taken orally.

TB-500 (also known as thymosin beta-4) is also produced by the human body as well as by various animals. Like BPC-157, it can be synthesized in a lab and used to promote wound repair and healing, particularly because it acts on actin and myosin fibers in tendons, ligaments, and muscles (which is likely why it, along with PEMF, is a very popular healing and recovery strategy used in the horse-racing industry). It also offers many of the same effects as growth hormone, including an increase in muscle growth, improved endurance, reduced pain and inflammation (both acute and chronic), increased flexibility, and increased hair growth. Like BPC-157, TB-500 can be injected in or near any damaged muscle site and sore or injured joint with surprising healing effects, although, as I learned in my fascinating podcast with peptide researcher Jean-François Tremblay, they can act systemically, not just locally, when injected just about anywhere in the body.

Epithalon is another peptide I currently use. It is commonly referred to as the primary antiaging peptide because it is one of the very few synthesized compounds that has been shown to directly activate the telomerase enzyme in humans. Telomerase renews and elongates telomeres, the caps on the ends of chromosomes that protect DNA from damage and cancer-causing errors. A decreased rate of telomere shortening can thus be equated with decelerated aging. By activating telomerase, epithalon directly reduces the effects of time on your telomeres (there's more about herbs and plants that activate telomerase pathways later in this chapter).

Here's one way to understand epithalon's antiaging effects: After fifty to seventy divisions, cells can no longer divide and worn out, damaged, or diseased cells can't be replaced. This is called the Hayflick limit, and reaching the Hayflick limit coincides with the death of a living organism. In sufficient doses, epithalon allows cells to exceed their Hayflick limit, thus extending the life span of the organism.

One study of 266 people over age sixty demonstrated that treatment with epithalamin, the pineal gland extract epithalon is based on, produced a 1.6-to-1.8-fold reduction in mortality during the following six years, a 2.5-fold reduction in mortality when combined with thymulin (very similar to TB-500), and a 4.1-fold reduction in mortality when combined with thymulin and administered annually instead of only once, at the study's onset. Another study examined seventy-nine coronary patients over the course of twelve years and found that the group treated with epithalon enjoyed improved physical endurance, circadian rhythms, and lipid and carbohydrate metabolism compared to the control group after three years of twice-yearly treatments. The treated group also enjoyed a 50 percent lower rate of cardiovascular mortality, cardiovascular failure, and severe respiratory diseases, as well as a 28 percent lower rate of overall mortality.

In addition to epithalon, I've also injected myself subcutaneously, in my abdomen, with two particularly intriguing antiaging peptides: humanin and MOTS-c. The first, humanin, is naturally produced in small amounts by the human body. Many centenarians produce unusually high levels of this peptide, which is encoded in mitochondria and has been shown to produce strong cytoprotective actions against a variety of stressors and diseases, including oxidative stress, hypoxic damage to the brain, and oxidized LDL cholesterol. It also aids in the repair of mitochondria. The second peptide, MOTS-c, is a potent metabolic regulator that significantly decreases the risk of age-related diseases and acts a bit like "exercise in a bottle." It activates the AMPK pathway and has an exercise-mimicking effect on fat and muscle. It even induces weight loss in mice fed a high-fat diet.

How to do it: When you order peptides, they are typically in a powder form and must be reconstituted by adding sterile or bacteriostatic water, which often comes with the vial of powder. (On BoundlessBook.com/19, you'll find a link to a helpful peptide calculator that will help you do the math to know how much water to add.)

There are a number of ways you can take peptides. The most common method is to inject them subcutaneously with an insulin syringe. Injections are the fastest method and result in high bioavailability of each peptide, and although it's not as deep (and therefore uncomfortable) as an intramuscular injection, it still gets the peptide where it needs to go if you're close to the site of pain or area that needs enhanced recovery. If you're looking for a systemic antiaging effect, a subcutaneous injection near the abdomen typically suffices. Be sure to use an alcohol wipe to clean the injection site. Do not reuse the needles or mix different peptides in the same syringe.

You can also apply peptides topically to several locations on the body, including the inside of the rectum and the vagina. If you choose to apply peptides topically, you may not absorb all of the molecules, but you will still get most of the benefits. For topical application, most people mix the peptides with a cream or gel, or use a ready-made topical peptide.

Taking peptides oral typically means consuming a lozenge called a troche or spraying the inside of your mouth, although supplement companies such as Dr. Seed's are now also selling tablet versions of some peptides, including BPC-157.

Be sure that when you order peptides, you work with a high-quality source such as Peptide Sciences or a physician who is getting peptides from a high-quality source such as Tailor Made Compounding. There are plenty of helpful peptide sources on BoundlessBook.com/19, and I particularly recommend you listen to the peptide podcasts I've done with Matt Cook, Jay Campbell, Jean-François Tremblay, and Dr. William Seeds.

Finally, should you want to replicate or speak with your physician about my current peptides protocol, I've listed it below. (Note: because the world of peptides is rapidly evolving, my protocol changes nearly quarterly, but at the time of this writing, the description below is accurate.) I get most of these peptides through my physician, who orders them from Tailor Made Compounding, and I highly recommend that you visit PeptideSociety.org, the website of the International Peptide Society, to find a physician who can work with you on a peptide protocol.

- **Epithalon:** I use the Khavinson protocol, named after Professor Vladimir Khavinson, perhaps the most distinguished medical gerontology researcher in Russia. Professor Khavinson believes the limit of animal and human life span is approximately 30 to 40 percent longer than the current mean life span, and that the limit of the human life span is 110 to 120 years. The Khavinson protocol is 10 mg epithalon administered three times a week for three weeks, and that exact dosage was studied in a fifteen-year longevity study in humans that produced impressive results for controlling telomere shortening. The protocol only needs to be done once a year.

- **Delta sleep inducing peptide (DSIP):** This one needs to be used conservatively to avoid tachyphylaxis (diminishing response to successive doses of a drug, rendering it less effective). I inject 150 mcg three times a week, one hour before bed, and deep sleep levels increase by 30 to 40 percent. This can be continued for as long as it's needed, as long as it isn't used every day.

- **TB-500/BPC-157:** I take TB-500 at 1.5 mg (0.5 mL) twice weekly for full-body repair. This can be continued as long as desired. For BPC-157, I use frequent injections of 250 to 500 mcg, and during travel, I rely on the more convenient oral tablets from Dr. Seed's and take four tablets per day.

- **MOTS-c:** For mitochondrial support, I inject 10 mg once weekly. You can time this just prior to endurance exercise for added mitochondrial benefit, and repeat for up to ten weeks in a row every year.

- **FOX04-DRI:** FOX04 can sabotage the survival efforts of lingering senescent cells in old tissues, causing them to self-destruct. It has been studied in aged mice and has been shown to cause destruction of senescent cells without the unpleasant side effects of other drugs that do the same thing, while also producing a wide array of benefits that control age-related decline. I take 3 mg every other day for six days, and repeat this one to three times per year.

- **Semax:** I talked in detail about this peptide in chapter 5. It's used mostly in Russia and Ukraine for a broad range of conditions but predominantly for its studied nootropic, neuroprotective, and neurogenic/neurorestorative properties. It can be administered via nasal spray, at one spray (750 mcg) one to three times daily, or whenever cognitive enhancement is desired. I typically combine this with the transdermal cognitive peptide Dihexa.

THYMUS

The thymus is a small, irregular-shaped, fat-enshrouded gland situated at the front of the chest, between the heart and the sternum. Thymus from veal, lamb, beef, or pork is often breaded, fried, and sold in restaurants as sweetbreads. The thymus gland's primary function is to produce a type of vital white blood cell called T cells. It accomplishes this by producing cells called thymocytes, which are necessary precursors to T cells. T cells, or T lymphocytes, are critical in the maintenance of a healthy immune system.

For example, regulatory T cells maintain immune homeostasis by preventing or limiting T cell activation. Toward the end of an immune reaction, they suppress levels of other types of T cells, including effector T cells, helper T cells, and cytotoxic (killer) T cells, which are all involved in the immune system response. Memory T cells include central memory T cells, effector memory T cells, tissue-resident T cells, and virtual memory T cells. As their names imply, these memory T cells, which are found in lymph nodes and the surrounding tissues, are responsible for remembering previously encountered pathogens and developing long-term immunity and tolerance to pathogens throughout your life.

How it works: Once thymocytes are produced by the thymus, they migrate to peripheral tissues, where they act as the precursors to mature T cells. Since your body cannot properly produce T cells without sufficient precursors, supporting your thymus gland can be crucial for longevity and your ability to combat infection as you experience age-related immune system deterioration.

Indeed, research has indicated that thymus deterioration is closely associated with immuno-senescence, the degeneration of the immune system primarily due to alterations in T cell composition. The intriguing fact about the thymus gland is that its size and activity closely parallel the growth and aging processes of the body: it reaches its maximum size and activity during puberty and then slowly atrophies over time, so that after the age of sixty, it is nearly undetectable from the surrounding fatty tissues. As the thymus shrinks, your immune system deteriorates, and your body begins to lose its defenses against age-related diseases.

Interestingly, Vladimir Anisimov, a Russian gerontologist who discovered many of the anti-aging benefits of melatonin and metformin, also discovered the peptide epithalon and found that it was able to suppress cancer and extend the lives of rats and mice in a series of experiments over several decades. Even more notably, when aging humans are given epithalon, their mortality rates drop in half. Its mechanism of action seems to be via both activation of telomerase and the regeneration of the thymus. Since the thymus shrinks gradually over the latter decades of life, any compound that slows the decay of thymic tissue could induce a profound antiaging response.

How to do it: Thymus treatments are usually made from thymic extracts from cows or sheep, and they're taken orally or via intramuscular injections. Should you decide to forgo the relatively expensive intramuscular injections or "glandular" supplements that usually contain a decent dose of thymus and instead take a more ancestral route, you can make it a point to occasionally eat sweetbreads, which can be purchased online from companies such as US Wellness Meats (their beef sweetbread is quite tasty). In addition, the injectable peptide thymosin-alpha can produce similar T-cell-enhancing effects.

For information on how to purchase and use epithalon, see page 526.

PLATELET-RICH PLASMA (PRP)

Your blood consists of several components, but one of the primary components is plasma, a clear, extracellular fluid. Plasma contains a high concentration of platelets, which are small cells generated by bone marrow that play a crucial role in managing vascular integrity and regulating hemostasis (stopping a flow of blood) and can also aid in wound healing.

Platelets can be administered to a site of pain or injury to supply stem cells, protein, and other growth factors that help speed up recovery, injected into any tissue that could benefit from more blood flow (including the genitals, making PRP a popular sexual enhancement procedure), and, like stem cells, they can be used as a preventive protocol or age-reversal strategy. Platelet-rich plasma (PRP) is exactly what is sounds like, plasma that's rich in platelets, usually derived from your own blood (although corporations like the Young Blood Institute in Silicon Valley are now offering plasma from young donors).

Blood platelet levels remain fairly stable throughout middle age (twenty-five to sixty years old), but past the age of sixty, levels fall and continue to decline, and the responsiveness of the platelets themselves also deteriorates. Injections of PRP could, therefore, have antiaging effects such as supporting vascular health in older people, reducing age-related joint pain, and preventing normal age-related degradation of the skin and sexual organs.

How it works: PRP is almost always taken from your own blood. Usually, the amount of blood needed is about the same as what is normally drawn for a standard blood test—one or two small tubes. The blood is placed in a centrifuge to separate the platelets, stem cells, and growth factors from the red and white blood cells. What remains after the red and white blood cells are removed is a concentrate that gets injected into the targeted area.

I have had PRP injected into my penis to give me stronger erections and improve sexual performance (a process known as the P-shot), but the potential benefits go far beyond the bedroom.

The growth factors released after the platelets break down via a process called platelet degranulation can aid in the treatment of tendon, ligament, muscle, and cartilage injuries, as well as early osteoarthritis. Given that tissues like tendons, ligaments, cartilage, and bone heal much slower after injuries than muscle does, PRP injections can be an effective tactic for joint support, especially as the musculoskeletal system deteriorates with age. For example, I've had PRP injected into my knees (in conjunction with stem cells, exosomes, and ozone) for a very powerful joint-repairing protocol).

But PRP is best known for its role in the vampire facial (you may remember a certain Kardashian touting her vampire facial on Instagram a few years back). These PRP treatments on the face are used to treat sagging skin, fine lines, wrinkles, and scarring by promoting collagen growth underneath skin.

In addition, recently a clinic in Athens, Greece, treated 180 women by injecting PRP into the uterus or ovaries to stimulate repair of the female reproductive system. They claim to have treated twenty-seven menopausal women, of whom twelve returned to ovulation!

How to do it: Over ten years ago, my first business partner, sports medicine physician P. Z. Pearce, partnered up with me to invest in a big, fancy PRP centrifuge. Athletes would visit our facility, where we would extract their blood and then spin it in the centrifuge to concentrate the growth factors for reinjection. Just like most PRP research studies, we found that although joint comfort seemed to improve significantly after just one injection, a series of four to six injections seemed to work even better.

Since that time, Dr. Charles Runels has brought PRP to the attention of the antiaging world by developing the vampire procedures, which involve multiple injections of PRP into wrinkled, hairless, or aging areas such as the face, the top of head, or the breasts. These treatments are often combined with PRP injections into the joints. Most antiaging and beauty medical clinics now offer this procedure, and both my wife and I have had our hairlines and faces injected with a soup of BMAC stem cells, PRP, and exosomes, with a noticeable increase in complexion quality and decrease in signs of wrinkling afterward. To stave off facial wrinkling that occurs with age, my wife Jessa has done follow-up treatments of facial PRP combined with stem cells and exosomes from Dr. Amy Killen at the Docere Clinics in Park City, Utah.

As a word of caution, PRP therapy is not for everyone, and the research surrounding it is inconsistent and inconclusive. In older populations, PRP increases the risk of thrombosis and blood clots. Since platelets play a central role in the coagulation of blood, if you have a history or family history of thrombosis or blood clots, it may be better to avoid PRP therapy, unless you are looking into a plasma exchange therapy offered by the Young Blood Institute, which can actually decrease blood clotting risk and "clean out" old blood by filtering the blood and replacing the plasma with that of a healthy donor (however, this protocol is very expensive). Genetic tests will tell you whether you are at increasing risk for clotting, and you should always check with your doctor or health-care professional before getting PRP therapy.

7. Blood Transfusions

This may sound like it is taken straight from a science-fiction novel, but today, older people are injecting the donated blood of younger generations into their own bloodstreams. One company, Ambrosia, based near San Francisco, had a client base of about six hundred people near to or over the age of sixty until they were shut down by the FDA. The company was collecting screened blood from local blood banks and then selling injections to antiaging enthusiasts who were willing to pay the $8,000 fee.

The Young Blood Institute in Silicon Valley has a different approach, which they call therapeutic plasma exchange and advertise as a preventive therapy for age-associated diseases. In this procedure, a patient's plasma, which constitutes about 55 percent of total blood volume, is completely replaced by the plasma of a donor over multiple treatments. During my groundbreaking podcast interview with the founder of the Young Blood Institute, Mark Urdahl, you can hear about the fascinating clinical research currently being done on this form of plasma exchange and discover how this treatment is now being shown to reverse a staggering number of aging-related medical conditions (most notably Alzheimer's)—the podcast is linked to on BoundlessBook.com/19.

How it works: While the whole procedure may seem slightly vampiric, there are animal studies that suggest that injecting the blood of eighteen-year-olds into your own bloodstream could be beneficial. A group of researchers surgically introduced a demyelinating injury in the spinal cord of an old mouse and then exposed the cells in the area to the blood from a young mouse. The result? Some of the immune cells from the young blood helped the old mouse's own stem cells restore the damaged neurons' myelin sheaths. The study concluded that age-related impairment to the nervous system could be reversed by cells in young blood that stimulate greater regeneration signals. Another mouse study found that younger blood, when injected into older mice, introduces growth factors that are believed to have antiaging effects on heart, muscle, and brain tissue.

As for plasma exchange, a host of studies show its potential for removing circulating substances that cause disease or contribute to disease states, removing pro-inflammatory factors (like fibrinogen, IL-6, and TNF-alpha), and even increasing activity in dormant stem cells.

How to do it: Pick up the phone and call the good folks at the Young Blood Institute in Silicon Valley. Admittedly, at the time of this writing, I have not yet spent over $40,000 on young blood transfusions, nor have I committed to having all the plasma in my entire body replaced with that of some healthy college kid in Florida. Nonetheless, I am intrigued by both procedures, and I highly suspect they will become increasingly affordable and popular with time.

In the meantime, it appears that GDF11, one of the antiaging proteins activated with an infusion of young blood, is also increased by the hormone oxytocin, which is activated during childbirth, breastfeeding, and sex. It can even be purchased as a nasal spray. This promises to be an affordable alternative to a blood infusion.

In addition, several medical practitioners, including Dr. Matt Cook in San Jose, California, are now offering ozone dialysis at their practice, which is a quick and relatively inexpensive treatment that may mimic many of the blood-renewal effects of a full plasma transfusion.

8. Bioidentical Hormone Replacement Therapy

Today, many women live one-third of their lives in a state of sex-hormone deficiency. This is especially important because estrogen, which can upregulate telomerase and improve mitochondrial health, is one of the factors in the longevity advantage women have in telomere length and the cellular resilience of female aging biology. And men are not exempt from hormone deficiency: though men are subject to age-related testosterone decline and andropause, these are frequently underdiagnosed and undertreated.

Bioidentical hormone replacement therapy (BHT) is a fast track to restoring levels of hormones that naturally decline with age: the sex hormones estrone, estradiol, progesterone, testosterone, DHEA, and estriol, as well as growth hormone and insulin growth factor-1. Far different from the synthetic hormones that became vilified in the nineties for causing breast cancer in postmenopausal women, BHT involves the use of hormones that are molecularly identical to the hormones that your body naturally produces.

How it works: For women, BHT—especially when combined with peptides—appears to be far safer than synthetic hormone replacement with compounds such as progestin, which is derived from the urine of pregnant horses and has been linked to breast cancer. BHT can be combined with pharmacy compounding, which involves matching injections and pharmaceuticals to each particular patient's needs.

For men who are interested in testosterone optimization, hormone replacement therapy doesn't necessarily need to be "bioidentical" per se, since the synthetic form of testosterone is functionally identical to the natural forms produced by the body.

How to do it: Although in-depth assessments of hormone needs, ongoing hormone testing, and precise follow-up plans should be standard practice, the fact is that many antiaging clinics simply hand over injections, creams, nasal sprays, patches, and other hormone delivery mechanisms with very little systematization. For this reason, it is crucial to work with a practitioner who is willing to take the time to assess your specific needs—and you want to work with someone who uses bioidentical hormones rather than potentially dangerous synthetic chemicals such as progestin.

The best place to start is with a good functional medicine practitioner; you can find a directory at the website for the Institute of Functional Medicine (ifm.org). If your practitioner isn't well versed in hormone replacement therapy, they can direct you to someone who is. Hormones can be administered in a variety of ways, including injections, topical and vaginal creams and gels, oral pills, vaginal rings and tablets, and transdermal patches. In an ideal scenario, these are custom compounded to your specific needs, and your hormone levels are regularly tested and tracked.

One of the more effective treatments for women is the Wiley protocol, a version of compounded BHT that syncs hormones to the natural endocrine cycles of women (there's also a protocol for men). In addition, you'll find a discussion of testosterone optimization in chapter 18.

9. Mitochondrial Support

When mitochondria are stressed by inflammation or free radicals, they can kill the cell they live in via apoptosis (programmed cell death). Mitochondrial damage is a problem seen in many conditions related to aging, including cardiovascular disease, liver disease, Alzheimer's, osteoporosis, and hair loss.

Many of the strategies you have already discovered in this chapter support mitochondrial health. Here I'll explain which nutrients and supplements are known to protect against mitochondrial degradation, mitochondrial aging, and the excessive formation of reactive oxygen species (ROS), which can damage mitochondria.

NICOTINAMIDE ADENINE DINUCLEOTIDE (NAD)

Nicotinamide adenine dinucleotide (NAD) is a coenzyme that is produced by all living cells. NAD's most basic function is to receive and donate electrons during metabolic processes within your mitochondria, making it crucial for normal cellular metabolism.

How it works: NAD is involved in what are known as redox reactions, which are processes vital in all parts of cell metabolism. When glucose and fatty acids are oxidized, they release energy. NAD+, the oxidized form of NAD, picks up this energy and is then reduced to NADH during beta-oxidation, glycolysis, and the citric acid cycle. The NADH is transferred into mitochondria, where it is oxidized by the electron transport chain, which is responsible for shuttling protons across membranes and generates ATP, the energy that drives your body.

NAD+ levels markedly decline with age, creating an energy deficit that decreases the body's ability to maintain normal metabolic activity. Some of the effects of the decline in NAD+ include more chemical stress, inflammation, DNA damage, and failing mitochondria. By age fifty, most people have only half the NAD+ they did in younger years. By age eighty, NAD+ levels drop to only 1 to 10 percent of their original value. This deficiency of NAD+ predisposes the body to accelerated aging and impedes the ability to benefit from other helpful compounds, such as resveratrol and pterostilbene. NAD+ also promotes longevity by providing the same cellular benefits associated with caloric restriction and exercise, so the loss of NAD+ means the loss of these benefits.

How to do it: The gold standard for NAD supplementation is to have a large dose administered via IV in a medical or antiaging clinic (the infusion can take from one to six hours), and then to maintain NAD levels with repeat IVs, an NAD nasal spray or transdermal patch, or daily use of NR (nicotinamide riboside), NMN (nicotinamide mononucleotide), or NAD supplements (see the section below on nicotinamide riboside). The only issue with using oral supplements is lower bioavailability, particularly for neural effects, because oral supplementation does not allow any of these molecules to cross the blood-brain barrier or act on the hypothalamus to induce any positive cognitive effects.

Alternatively, NAD can be administered at home (often with the help of a nurse practitioner) via a drip IV. Masochists or the ultra-daring can even give themselves NAD through their own push IV—for a while, I did this once every two weeks from the comfort of my own home, and it took ten to fifteen minutes per session. Why do I describe this as masochistic? Frankly, mainlining this particular molecule into your bloodstream is incredibly uncomfortable, which is one reason it is usually administered over several hours—so if you opt for the quicker push IV option, prepare to feel as though your entire body is on fire while, at the same time, someone is repeatedly punching you in the gut and chest.

These days, I usually order patches from the NAD Treatment Center in San Diego, which deliver 400 to 500 mg of NAD over a five-to-six-hour period and are very easy to apply and tolerate.

NICOTINAMIDE RIBOSIDE (NR)

Nicotinamide riboside (NR), a form of vitamin B_3, is a precursor to NAD. In fact, your mitochondria prefer NR as an NAD precursor in particular. When taken orally, NR is highly bioavailable and aids in mitochondrial energy production. It exists in high levels in cow's milk.

There is growing evidence that supplementing with NR can promote longevity in life forms ranging from simple worms to mammals like mice. One study showed an average 5 percent increase in the life span of old mice, even though NR supplementation did not begin until the mice were nearing the end of their natural life span (twenty-four months). In people, that would be the equivalent of gaining nearly an additional four years of life, based on today's average life expectancy of about seventy-eight years.

How it works: Nicotinamide riboside has been shown not only to restore NAD+ levels in tissues but also to provide more NAD+ activity than can be obtained from diet alone. NR supplementation is very well tolerated in middle-aged and older adults and can slow cellular aging and improve many age-related metabolic problems, including diabetes and neurodegenerative conditions. In addition, NR has the potential to reduce the declining heart function, high blood pressure, and arterial stiffness that can accompany aging, and it even has beneficial effects on cardiovascular fitness. NR also stimulates a caloric-restriction-mimicking state, which means that it can promote weight loss.

How to do it: Most absorbable, supplemental forms of NR appear under the name Chroma-Dex. Three good NR supplements are Tru Niagen, Elysium Basis, and Thorne ResveraCel, which combines NR with another antiaging compound: resveratrol.

According to the physician who discovered NR, Dr. Charles Brenner, the best way to consume an NR supplement is with one dose in the morning and one in the afternoon, which allows the dosing of the NR to match your body's natural circadian rhythm pulsing of NR. NMN and NAD oral supplements may work similarly, and although research is ongoing regarding the pros and cons of each supplement option, you can think of it this way: at the top of the totem pole in terms of NAD bioavailability and cellular delivery are any mechanisms that bypass digestion or liver metabolism, most notably NAD IVs or patches, or sublingual NMN. The next best option—slightly less potent but more convenient or affordable for many people—is oral NR.

ASTAXANTHIN

Astaxanthin is a carotenoid that's produced by single-celled freshwater algae. When their environment becomes stressful due to excessively salty water, low nitrogen levels, or high temperatures, the algae produce astaxanthin in lipid droplets, which turn the algal cells bright red and allow them to survive the harsh conditions. In humans, astaxanthin performs similar protective functions by promoting cellular survival.

How it works: Astaxanthin protects your mitochondria by acting as both an antioxidant and a free-radical scavenger. As your mitochondria perform normal respiratory functions, they produce free radicals like superoxide radicals, which interact with proteins, fats, and DNA and cause damage to your cells, ultimately contributing to the aging process. Astaxanthin inserts itself into your cell membranes and mitochondrial membranes, where it inhibits free-radical production and helps eliminate the free radicals that are produced. Astaxanthin's antioxidant activity is fourteen times greater than that of vitamin E, fifty-four times greater than beta-carotene, and sixty-five times greater than vitamin C, making it one of the most potent antioxidants.

Astaxanthin also boosts immune system function by promoting anti-inflammatory activity and increasing the activity of natural killer cells. One study examined the effects of astaxanthin on the production of the inflammatory compounds IL-6 and NF-kB following the introduction of lipopolysaccharides, or LPS (remember from chapter 4 that LPS contribute to age-related chronic diseases). The researchers found that astaxanthin suppressed the production of both IL-6 and NF-kB. In another study, researchers found that astaxanthin increased natural killer cell activity and even increased total levels of T and B cells, which both play a role in fighting infection.

How to do it: You can find different brands of astaxanthin online, and Life Extension offers astaxanthin combined with phospholipids to improve absorption. While an effective dose is 12 mg per day, doses up to 40 mg per day can be taken without any negative side effects. If you want to get your astaxanthin more naturally, you can find it in salmon (in fact, it's the compound responsible for the red color in fish and crustaceans). In a kilogram of salmon, you'll get between 26 and 38 mg of astaxanthin.

Astaxanthin is also a fantastic protective treatment for skin radiation from UVA and UVB sunlight rays (almost like edible sunscreen), and I used to dose with 40 mg prior to and after my Ironman triathlons in Hawaii. After these races, I'd experience minimal burning, even with very small amounts of low SPF sunscreen used during the event.

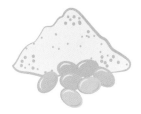

PAU D'ARCO TEA

Derived from the bark of a tropical evergreen tree in the Amazon rainforest, pau d'arco has long been used by people indigenous to Latin America. Dr. Joe Mercola first alerted me to the fact that pau d'arco tea is a simple, highly affordable but little-known way to treat wounds, aches, pains, malaria and other tropical diseases, and inflammation. It also—you guessed it—boosts NAD.

How it works: Pau d'arco contains a compound called beta-lapachone, which acts as a catalyst for NAD. NAD is also a necessary precursor of the sirtuin enzymes discussed earlier in this chapter, which regulate your body's antiaging switches (such as the genes that promote inflammation and control blood sugar management). So by promoting NAD activity, pau d'arco not only promotes mitochondrial health but also helps regulate genetic antiaging processes.

How to do it: You can order pau d'arco tea in bulk online and keep a giant batch of it in the refrigerator for teas, cold drinks, and smoothie bases. Absorption and delivery of the beta-lapochenes in it can be enhanced by blending the prepared tea with a fat source such as coconut oil, coconut milk, sunflower lecithin, fish oil, or any other source of healthy fats. Pau d'arco supplements in capsule form are also available online, but I personally prefer the tea, which has a pleasant nutty flavor.

CURCUMIN

Curcumin is a compound produced by some plants, most notably turmeric (*Curcuma longa*), a member of the ginger family. Technically, curcumin is considered a diarylheptanoid and belongs to the group of curcuminoids, which are natural phenols responsible for turmeric's yellow color.

How it works: Curcumin is a potent antioxidant and free-radical scavenger that protects cellular function from reactive oxygen species such as superoxide radicals, singlet oxygen, nitric oxide, and hydrogen peroxide. It also enhances your body's natural antioxidant capacity by improving the production of antioxidant enzymes like superoxide dismutase, glutathione, and catalase. As a result, curcumin reduces chronic inflammation throughout your body to protect against age-related chronic diseases.

But the effects of curcumin go further. Chronic inflammation is associated with a condition called epigenetic drift. Within your DNA are compounds collectively known as the epigenome, which is responsible for maintaining your DNA's expression and your cells' identity and function. Over time, your ability to keep your epigenome healthy and functioning declines, so as you age, genes that used to be inactive may be expressed, and genes that used to be expressed may go dormant. This drift may cause stem cell production to decline and increase your risk of cancer and cardiovascular diseases. By reducing the inflammatory pathways involved with this downregulation of DNA expression, curcumin can help to prevent epigenetic drift.

How to do it: Curcumin only constitutes about 3 to 5 percent of the turmeric root, so it's more efficient to supplement with curcumin than to simply eat turmeric. Curcumin also has naturally low bioavailability, but this can be increased by combining turmeric with black pepper or piperine (a black pepper extract), exposing it to low heat (such as cooking fish, vegetables, eggs, or curries with turmeric), or combining it with a high-quality fat source, such as butter, ghee, olive oil, coconut oil, or avocado oil. An effective dose is 1,000 mg, but doses as high as 1,500 mg can be absorbed without any negative side effects.

CARNOSINE

Carnosine is a molecule composed of two peptides: beta-alanine and histidine. It is found in high amounts in skeletal muscle, where it can eliminate excess lactic acid and prevent muscular fatigue during exercise—hence its popularity as a performance supplement. But, as you're about to discover, it's also been shown to have potent antiaging effects.

How it works: Carnosine promotes mitochondrial and cellular function by acting as an antioxidant and free-radical scavenger. Not only does it act on its own to inhibit ROS activity, but it has also been observed in rats to promote the endogenous production of antioxidants like glutathione and superoxide dismutase. One in vitro study also showed that carnosine can reduce the rate at which telomeres shorten, which slows aging. It also inhibits the production of advanced glycation end products (AGEs), which contribute to the development of diabetes and other age-related diseases.

How to do it: A standard effective dose is between 500 to 1,000 mg per day. You can purchase carnosine over the counter or online from companies like Life Extension or Thorne. It's important to note that carnosine's effectiveness is cumulative, meaning that its effects become greater the longer you take it and let it accumulate in your body, so be sure to allow ten to twelve weeks to get the full benefits.

ALPHA LIPOIC ACID (ALA)

Alpha lipoic acid (not to be confused with alpha linolenic acid, the other ALA) is a compound derived from sulfur that's involved in mitochondrial aerobic respiration. While the human body can produce very small amounts of ALA, it is obtained primarily from animal dietary sources—particularly cow's liver, although you can also find it in plant sources like spinach, brussels sprouts, yams, and broccoli.

How it works: ALA acts as an antioxidant within mitochondria, has free-radical scavenging capabilities, and upregulates your own antioxidant-producing abilities by recycling "used-up" antioxidants like vitamin C and glutathione. Because of this, ALA is often called the "universal antioxidant." It's both water- and fat-soluble, so it moves through cell membranes and the blood-brain barrier much more easily than most other antioxidants. ALA also helps maintain DNA integrity as you get older by protecting the epigenome, and it also activates telomerase, the enzyme that lengthens your telomeres.

How to do it: In addition to consuming ALA-dense foods, you can supplement with ALA. The recommended dose ranges from 200 to 600 mg per day, but doses up to 2,400 mg per day have been taken with no observed negative effects. It's important to note that ALA supplements should not be taken with food, which can limit absorption. The best time to take ALA supplements is thirty minutes before or two hours after a meal.

APIGENIN

Apigenin is a flavone found in foods such as parsley, onions, and oregano, but it is best known as the primary active compound in chamomile tea, which has been consumed since the time of the ancient Egyptians and has traditionally been used to treat burns, gastrointestinal disorders, infections, and a myriad of other conditions. It also has antiaging effects.

How it works: Apigenin promotes mitochondrial function by inhibiting the breakdown of NAD, a necessary cofactor in mitochondrial redox reactions, which are crucial in the generation of ATP. So apigenin helps maintain mitochondrial energy production, which can decline with age. In addition, apigenin is another epigenome-protecting molecule that preserves DNA integrity.

How to do it: There's sparse research about the ideal dose of apigenin, but the dose in a few cups of chamomile tea or a few servings of fruits and vegetables per day seems to be effective. Supplemental forms usually come in doses of 20 to 50 mg, and higher doses (3 to 10 mg per kg of body weight) are used to treat anxiety.

SULFORAPHANE

As its name suggests, sulforaphane is a sulfur-based molecule found naturally in cruciferous vegetables like broccoli and brussels sprouts. In the early 1990s, it was discovered that sulforaphane had strong anticancer properties, and since then, it's undergone intensive study to discover other potential health effects.

How it works: While researchers are unsure about sulforaphane's ability to act as a free-radical scavenger, research does suggest that it is more effective at activating your body's antioxidant-producing processes than similar compounds such as curcumin and resveratrol, making sulforaphane a strong protector of mitochondrial and cellular health.

It's also an epigenetic modifier that protects the epigenome and prevents DNA deterioration. In addition, sulforaphane induces autophagy (cell death and recycling) and stimulates the production of more mitochondria to enhance the energy output of each individual cell. Finally, one in vitro study showed that a concentrated oral dose of sulforaphane promoted greater stem cell proliferation and protected stem cells from aging.

How to do it: Broccoli sprouts contain extremely high amounts of sulforaphane (up to one hundred times more than broccoli), and you can also supplement with sulforaphane via compounds such as Thorne MediClear or Life Extension Triple Action Cruciferous Vegetable Extract. An effective dose of sulforaphane is about 10 to 35 mg per day for a 150-pound person, 15 to 45 mg for a 200-pound person, and 20 to 60 mg for a 250-pound person.

QUERCETIN

Quercetin is a plant-pigment flavonoid found naturally in red wine, white wine (white wine actually contains more than red wine), gingko biloba, apples, green tea, St. John's wort, and other plants associated with longevity. It occurs in particularly high concentrations in capers, yellow chili peppers, and onions.

How it works: Quercetin is a very powerful antioxidant, and some research indicates it may be one of the most potent flavonoids for combating free radicals in the body. As a word of warning, though low concentrations in the body are highly beneficial, high concentrations can cause quercetin to become an ROS itself. Currently it's unknown what these concentrations equate to in the human body, but for now, just know that more does not equal better when it comes to quercetin.

Quercetin also enhances your own antioxidant-producing abilities, improving the production of glutathione, superoxide dismutase, catalase, and more. It acts as an anti-inflammatory by inhibiting the release of mast cells and histamines, and it may even inhibit the metabolism of resveratrol, making quercetin and resveratrol a potent one-two combo.

How to do it: The typical Western diet provides about 15 to 40 mg per day of quercetin, but recommended doses range from 250 to 1,500 mg, with the average recommended dose falling around 1 g per day. I use quercetin in powder form in a longevity and autophagy tea introduced to me by my friend Dr. Joseph Mercola—you'll find the ingredients on page 325.

This particular blend upregulates both NAD and autophagy pathways and can easily be added to smoothies or consumed in hot or cold water.

EPIGALLOCATECHIN GALLATE (EGCG)

Green tea has been consumed for thousands of years in Asia to promote longevity and improve health. But the primary active compound in green tea, the ester EGCG, can be delivered in higher doses in supplement form.

How it works: Green tea is a strong antioxidant, and EGCG is the primary molecule responsible for this effect. EGCG also acts as a free-radical scavenger and activates endogenous antioxidant production. In fact, research indicates it is more potent than vitamin E and vitamin C, and it does not blunt the hormetic response to exercise as vitamins E and C do.

EGCG is also an epigenetic modifier that protects the epigenome from deterioration. While the exact mechanism of action is unknown, but we do know that the epigenetic effects of EGCG improve skin cancer outcomes. EGCG also promotes cellular autophagy, particularly in the liver and in macrophage and endothelial cells, although it may reduce autophagy in certain eye cells.

EGCG is also known to improve weight loss by increasing fat oxidation (the caffeine in green tea likely enhances this effect). Finally, EGCG easily crosses the blood-brain barrier and is highly neuroprotective, reducing inflammation in the brain. Thus, they help reduce the likelihood of developing age-related neurodegenerative diseases.

How to do it: The ideal dose ranges from 400 to 500 mg per day, and since the average cup of green tea contains up to 90 mg, it may be more strategic to take an EGCG supplement. Higher doses may cause side effects like nausea and heartburn in many individuals.

FENUGREEK

One of the first, most successful, and longest-lasting human civilizations of all time, ancient Egypt, invented many antiaging tricks. One common antiaging food they consumed was fenugreek, an herb found in the Mediterranean region and parts of China and India. The Egyptians processed fenugreek in a lengthy and complicated ritual that involved drying, threshing, winnowing, and boiling to produce an oil that was then applied to the skin to keep it looking soft, bright, and youthful. The famous Egyptian queen Cleopatra smeared this oil it on her face regularly.

How it works: Fenugreek, a semiarid plant most common in South and Central Asia, helps regulate blood sugar levels and prevents the onset of diabetes, or, if you already have diabetes, helps you manage it. But fenugreek's benefits extend far beyond that and deep into your gut, hormone levels, and mitochondria. A powerful antioxidant, fenugreek can mitigate oxidative damage and abate inflammation. Fenugreek has been shown to possess anti-inflammatory capacities that help ease the symptoms of ulcerative colitis, an inflammatory bowel disease. The water-soluble fiber it contains can help relieve constipation. One study concluded that a fenugreek petroleum ether extract containing naturally occurring linolenic and linoleic acids can shut down systemic inflammation and improve arthritis.

Another study found that, in a group of sixty men aged twenty-five to fifty-two with no history of erectile dysfunction, fenugreek significantly increased sexual arousal, energy, and stamina and helped maintain normal testosterone levels. Given the importance of sex in maintaining biological viability, this could be a potent tool for men. Another study has also shown that the active compound of fenugreek, 4-OH-lle, promotes the production of new mitochondria in diabetic patients, who often suffer from low mitochondrial numbers and function. Given the mitochondrial theory of aging, this makes fenugreek a good compound to include in any longevity protocol.

How to do it: Rather than a fenugreek supplement, I prefer organic fenugreek seeds, which are quite tasty and have a delicate maple flavor. You can keep them in a pepper grinder or glass mason jar in your kitchen. Sprinkle or grind them into stir-fries, meat dishes, salads, soups, or anything else for which you desire both the digestion-enhancing and antiaging support of fenugreek seeds. I often combine them with fennel and black pepper for a meat and stir-fry seasoning.

FISH OIL

You'll recall from chapters 4 and 14 that fish oil, whether from supplements or fatty cold-water fish, helps you get the cognitive and physical benefits of the anti-inflammatory omega-3 fatty acids DHA and EPA. It's also important for getting the optimal ratio of omega-6 to omega-3. The anti-inflammatory properties of fish oil make it effective for fighting the signs of aging.

How it works: Both EPA and DHA are precursors of various eicosanoids that are responsible for reducing inflammation. In middle-aged rats, fish oil is known to increase the activities of the antioxidants superoxide dismutase, glutathione peroxidase, and catalase, as well as total antioxidant capacity. It has also been shown to downregulate forty-one genes that are involved in aging and decrease the rate at which telomeres shorten. And because it inhibits inflammatory eicosanoids and cytokines, fish oil has even been shown to be a beneficial replacement for NSAIDs in the treatment of rheumatoid arthritis.

New clinical research studies are now proving fish oil's efficacy for staving off the cardiovascular and metabolic issues, such as diabetes, that can occur with aging, and pharmaceutical companies such as Amarin are now developing drugs based entirely on fish oil. Micronutrients in fish oil such as omega-3 fatty acids and, most notably, vitamin D have also been shown to impact telomere length. Supplemental fish oil at doses of 2.5 g per day has been shown to induce a 32 percent reduction in telomere shortening and also significantly reduce oxidation in blood cells.

How to do it: For my recommended fish oil supplement brands as well as dosages, see chapter 12. You'll also find information on whole-food sources of DHA and EPA in chapter 4.

COENZYME Q10 (COQ10)

Coenzyme Q10 (CoQ10) is a naturally occurring compound found in most aerobic animals, ranging from bacteria to mammals. CoQ10 itself is a powerful tool to have in your antiaging arsenal. Also known as ubiquinone, ubiquinone-Q10, ubidecarenone, vitamin Q10, or coenzyme Q, it is an essential component of the mitochondrial electron transport chain and an antioxidant found in plasma membranes and lipoproteins throughout the body.

Since CoQ10 synthesis can decline as you age, supplementing with it may be extremely beneficial as you get older.

How it works: One study observed the effects of a high CoQ10 intake on old mice with age-related neurodegeneration and found that CoQ10 improves spatial learning and reduced oxidative damage. But these results were not observed in younger mice; they only affected preexisting age-related cognitive decline. It is also known that CoQ10 scavenges free radicals that promote mesenchymal stem cell aging, keeping stem cells younger. Studies have also shown that the antioxidant effect of CoQ10 supplements alleviates cardiovascular disease and inflammation.

How to do it: CoQ10 is found in oily fish like salmon and tuna as well as in organ meats. As a supplement, it's available as capsules, tablets, and oral spray. The ideal dosage ranges from 30 to 90 mg per day divided into several doses, though you can safely take as much as 200 mg per day. As a fat-soluble compound, it is best consumed with a healthy source of fats such as coconut oil or extra-virgin olive oil.

I take CoQ10 in a combination supplement, the Almsbio Glutathione Mito-Therapy+, which contains CoQ10, PQQ, and glutathione (both discussed below), as well as lactoferrin, which is also a good antioxidant. This combination—which you squeeze from a syringe into your mouth, hold for sixty seconds, then swallow—is fantastic for enhancing mitochondrial health. (As a bonus, it tastes like an orange Creamsicle!) Rather than taking separate CoQ10, PQQ, and glutathione supplements, I recommend simply consuming one serving of Almsbio Glutathione Mito-Therapy+ once per day. You'll find a link and discount code on BoundlessBook.com/19.

PYRROLOQUINOLINE QUINONE (PQQ)

Pyrroloquinoline quinone (PQQ) is an antioxidant that's involved in redox reactions, which change the oxidation states of atoms, in living organisms ranging from bacteria to human beings. More than 175 published studies have shown that it has wide-ranging benefits for memory, general cognition, mood, and mental processing power, making it a popular ingredient in many nootropics. PQQ's benefits also include increased mitochondrial density, defense against oxidative stress, improved learning and memory ability, and reduced inflammation.

How it works: In humans, PQQ interacts with cell signaling pathways and mitochondrial functions. It's an ROS scavenger, which protects mitochondria from the damage of oxidative stress. One study even demonstrated that in mice, the antioxidant and DNA-damage-reducing capacities of PQQ played a role in combating osteoporosis. Another study demonstrated that PQQ contributes to the upregulation of certain compounds involved in repairing the microglia and neurons of the cerebral cortex and parts of the hippocampus following traumatic brain injury.

How to do it: PQQ is found naturally in kiwi, celery, papaya, sweet potatoes, green tea, fermented bean products like natto, parsley, and even human breast milk. I don't necessarily recommend that you ask your friends if you can borrow some breast milk from them, but you can certainly consume the other foods or take PQQ in a supplemental form.

Using PQQ in combination with CoQ10 seems to synergistically increase their potency, so I recommend taking a combination supplement that includes both—I prefer the Almsbio Glutathione Mito-Therapy+, mentioned on the previous page. No matter what PQQ source you use, look for a form called BioPQQ. There are countless forms of PQQ on the market today, but BioPQQ is formulated from natural bacterial fermentation, while other varieties contain mostly synthetic forms of PQQ.

GLUTATHIONE

Glutathione is an antioxidant that occurs naturally in your body and primarily consists of the amino acids glutamine, glycine, and cysteine. Glutathione is a true electron trap, placing it high on the list of antioxidants. In fact, it is one of the few antioxidants that is actually produced by your body, rather than being obtained only through food. It is also known to support whole-body detoxification, including most phases of the liver's detoxification pathways, and help cells grow, multiply, and repair themselves.

Because of its wide range of antioxidant activity, glutathione plays a multifactorial role in aging. Overall, there is a decrease in glutathione levels as we age, and this seems to affect the onset of a large number of diseases.

How it works: The depletion of the reduced form of glutathione (often simply referred to as GSH, it's the stable, nonoxidized form of glutathione) has been implicated in many chronic degenerative diseases, including cystic fibrosis, cataracts, macular degeneration, glaucoma, hypertension, asthma, acute respiratory distress syndrome, Alzheimer's, Parkinson's, Huntington's, myocardial infarction, autoimmune conditions, and even the aging process itself. Indeed, GSH levels have been found to parallel the activity of telomerase, the enzyme responsible for maintaining long, strong telomeres. The depletion of GSH has also been found to induce the loss of mitochondrial function due to the accumulation of damage to mitochondrial DNA. Once transferred into the mitochondrial matrix, GSH plays a key role in the defense against ROS and in the detoxification of lipid hydroperoxides (damaged lipids in cell membranes) and electrophiles (which are very similar to free radicals). GSH also critically regulates the release of proteins from the intermembrane space of mitochondria; once released, these proteins engage the machinery of cell death, meaning that GSH is a critical nutrient for the support of mitochondrial health as well as overall cellular activity and health.

How to do it: While we do produce glutathione every day, it is also highly available in supplemental forms as well as in whole-food sources. It is true that some ingested glutathione is broken down and oxidized before being absorbed by your cells, but contrary to popular belief, some does, in fact, get taken up into your mitochondria. Research has indicated that glutathione can cross human intestinal cells intact, and you can take glutathione supplements in forms that protect it from being oxidized before it reaches your bloodstream. Sublingual supplements, for example, are better absorbed than oral glutathione. Glutathione can also be bound within tiny fat droplets called liposomes, which protect the glutathione until the liposomes are taken up by your cells, where they are broken down and the glutathione is released.

The Almsbio Glutathione Mito-Therapy+ supplement mentioned on page 538 contains a form of liposomal glutathione. Jarrow Glutathione is also an excellent supplement and is available online. Whichever supplement you choose, oral glutathione doses should range between 250 and 1,000 mg to increase glutathione levels. Over the course of several months, 500 mg per day can be an effective dose. Pork loin, chicken liver, steak, asparagus, broccoli, potatoes, avocados, zucchini, tomatoes, spinach, parsley, and okra are all excellent sources of glutathione, so a diet to support your mitochondrial health should include these foods.

Here are more ways you can increase your glutathione:

- Consume plenty of vitamin C, which helps maintain your body's supply of glutathione.
- Consume selenium-rich foods like beef, chicken, fish, cottage cheese (if you tolerate dairy well), and brown rice, as selenium is a glutathione cofactor.
- If you don't have allergies or sensitivities, supplement your diet with whey protein, which provides a complete amino acid profile. Glutathione synthesis requires the amino acids glutamine, cysteine, and glycine.
- Consume turmeric: the curcumin it contains can help restore glutathione levels and improve the activity of glutathione enzymes.

MITOQUINONE MESYLATE (MITOQ)

MitoQ is an antioxidant that is attracted to the source of most free radicals: mitochondria. Unlike many other antioxidants, it can accumulate in high concentrations in mitochondria. It delivers CoQ10 directly to mitochondria and is believed to increase mitochondria's ability to produce ATP and simultaneously quench free-radical damage.

While there is not a lot of evidence for MitoQ's efficacy, some studies suggest it may have an effect, particularly for neural dysfunction in humans, and for the sake of thoroughness, I have included it as a potential tactic to improve mitochondrial function and reduce the effects of aging.

How it works: Most of the oxidative stress that mitochondria experience occurs on the matrix side of the inner mitochondrial matrix, which is the space within the inner membrane that contains each mitochondria's DNA, ribosomes, soluble enzymes, and other molecules. MitoQ is believed to reduce the effects of this oxidative stress by supporting a catalase enzyme that removes free radicals from mitochondria. In studies, this can increase rodent life span by 10 percent. MitoQ has also been shown to increase life span and reduce telomere shortening in human cells that have undergone oxidative stress and has extended the life span of transgenic worms with Alzheimer's genes (though it did not do so in normal worms).

But, as I mentioned, there is not much evidence to support the idea that MitoQ has a significant effect on oxidative stress, and one study has actually shown that orally administered MitoQ in healthy mice failed to significantly alter mitochondrial function or gene expression and exerted no overall influence on systemic energy metabolism. Another study demonstrated that MitoQ causes mitochondrial swelling in the cells of kidney proximal tubules, which could lead to renal complications. Finally, MitoQ is so potent at lowering ROS that it may actually interfere with the normal cellular signaling mechanisms that rely on adequate levels of ROS.

How to do it: I'm not yet convinced MitoQ is the ultimate wonder drug, especially since CoQ10's effects are well proven, but should you decide to use it, MitoQ is widely available as an antioxidant supplement. As an antiaging tool, a recommended daily dose of MitoQ is 10 mg. As with many of these compounds, you can monitor the efficacy of your supplementation with oxidative stress tests such as the Oxidative Stress Analysis by Genova Diagnostics.

PTEROSTILBENE

Pterostilbene, one of the bioactive components of blueberries, is a derivative of the antioxidant phenol resveratrol and is structurally very similar, but it appears to be better absorbed than resveratrol and may actually be a more potent antioxidant and anticancer molecule. This is especially useful to know when you consider the recent research published in the *Journal of Food Chemistry* that profiled twenty-one commercial grape seed extract resveratrol products and found that nine of them contained peanut skin extract. The combination of antinutrients, lectins, pesticide contamination, and the prevalence of peanut allergies makes peanut skins a very poor source for resveratrol, so proceed with caution when taking resveratrol supplements. Pterostilbene may be a better bet.

How it works: Doses of pterostilbene as low as 10 mg and as high as 500 mg seem to have significant benefit for reducing cholesterol and glucose in animals. But little is known about exactly how pterostilbene works. Some studies report that it has apoptotic and autophagic effects—in other words, it helps eliminate old and damaged cells, which aids in combating various types of cancer. One study has also shown that pterostilbene exhibits strong anti-inflammatory capacities. In plants, pterostilbene plays a cellular defense role, and it may have the same role in humans. Pterostilbene has been noted to inhibit LPS-induced autoimmune responses and may also inhibit the inducible nitric oxide synthase (iNOS) activity that can cause inflammation. As an NADPH oxidase inhibitor, it may also increase levels of NAD.

How to do it: Low doses of up to 10 mg seem to aid in cognition. Higher doses of pterostilbene, ranging from 250 to 500 mg, aid in reducing cholesterol and glucose levels and improve insulin sensitivity in research animals. Generally, the estimated oral dose range for improving your glucose and lipid metabolism is 20 to 40 mg per kilogram of body weight.

C60

C60, also known as buckminsterfullerene or buckyball, belongs to a unique family of molecules called fullerenes. It is a cage-like fused-ring structure that looks roughly like a soccer ball, contains sixty carbon atoms, and was named after the famous author, designer, inventor, architect, and systems theorist Buckminster "Bucky" Fuller.

How it works: C60 and other fullerenes are produced by passing an electric discharge across the gap between two carbon electrodes in a helium atmosphere. The intriguing fact about C60 is that, because it is not found naturally in living organisms, there is no reason to think that would provide any kind of benefit. However, in 2012, a French laboratory announced that feeding C60 dissolved in olive oil to rats nearly doubled their life spans! The addition of olive oil is critical to the bioactive effects of the buckyballs because pure C60 molecules clump together, clog up cellular metabolism, and appear to be slightly toxic. But when dissolved in olive oil (a process that takes weeks of mixing), the buckyballs provide a host of cellular and mitochondrial benefits.

C60 is a powerful antioxidant that scavenges superoxide, a by-product of mitochondrial energy production that can accumulate and contribute to the development of many age-related chronic diseases. One group of researchers has proposed that C60 has the ability to acquire an overall positive charge by absorbing protons and can thereby penetrate the mitochondria to decrease free-radical production. A carboxyl form of C60 has been proven to prevent nerve cells from dying by dehydration or Alzheimer's-related compounds and allowed mice to live 7 percent longer.

How to do it: C60 is best dissolved in oil—in fact, as noted above, it needs to be dissolved in oil to eliminate toxicity—and this is usually done in a lab with a centrifuge. Most C60 supplements combine C60 with olive oil (although different oils can have different effects—for example, caprylic acid and MCT oil allow C60 to have more activity on brain cells), or you can purchase pure C60 and mix it with extra-virgin olive oil in a blender yourself, although this may be difficult because it can take a lot of blending to get the buckyballs and olive oil to mix. *Always make sure that the buckyballs are dissolved before consuming the concoction.* On BoundlessBook.com/20 you'll find links to several helpful C60 dosing and mixing calculators, DIY oil-dissolving recipes, and other resources. I also highly recommend you go to BenGreenfieldFitness.com/ian to listen to my comprehensive podcast with C60 researcher Ian Mitchell.

MELATONIN

Melatonin is best known as the sleep hormone. It is produced by the pineal gland toward the end of each day to stimulate the sense of being tired so that you will want to go to bed. But melatonin also acts as an antioxidant and mitochondrial protectant.

As you age, melatonin production and deployment can decline, resulting in age-related sleep disorders. Many elderly people—and many health enthusiasts, including myself—take small doses of melatonin to help them sleep. But building evidence suggests that melatonin supplements, especially in larger doses up to 80 mg, can also delay the development of cancers, boost the immune system, and slow the aging process, as well as improve mitochondrial function.

How it works: The interesting thing about mitochondria is that their activity and dynamics exhibit an oscillatory pattern that matches the circadian rhythm–based secretion of melatonin. In fact, melatonin is an antioxidant hormone that is selectively and purposely taken up by mitochondria, where it accumulates in high concentrations. It also acts as a regulator of mitochondrial biogenesis and dynamics, improving the healthy homeostasis of your mitochondria.

In both in vivo and in vitro studies, melatonin has been shown to be effective in preventing the oxidation-induced mitochondrial dysfunction seen in Parkinson's, Alzheimer's, and Huntington's. It is also known to maintain respiratory activity and ATP production in mitochondria.

How to do it: You don't need much melatonin. Many supplement tablets contain 5 mg each, but the truth is that as little as 0.1 to 0.3 mg of melatonin can make a difference, and even that small amount can profoundly increase the quality of your sleep. Many antiaging and cancer physicians prescribe much higher doses, but I'm cautious with high doses because overuse may limit endogenous melatonin production—I only use higher doses if I'm jet-lagged and attempting to reboot my circadian rhythm. I prefer a timed-release version (many brands are available online, but I usually buy Natrol) or the supplement Sleep Remedy, which combines a microdose of melatonin with a few other sleep-supporting compounds, such as vitamin D and omega-3 fatty acids.

SKQS

MitoQ and C60 are SkQs' antiaging cousins. Primarily researched in Russia, SkQs are newly discovered antioxidant compounds that specifically target mitochondria, and they have been studied quite a bit recently to determine if they can slow down the processes associated with aging.

When started late in life, supplementation with SkQ not only prevents age-related decline but also significantly reverses it, acting on pathways for hair loss, low body temperature, body weight loss, and heart, kidney, and liver pathologies, along with stroke, Parkinson's, Alzheimer's, and pancreatic cancer. In doing so, it has been shown to improve mice longevity by about 15 percent. Quite notably, when researchers started giving SkQ to mice in the middle or the end of their lives, it worked to improve quality and quantity of life even at that point, which means it may be an effective antiaging hack for people who spent many decades making poor decisions about their health and lifestyle and then decided to shape up later in life.

In fungi, crustaceans, fruit flies, and mice, SkQ significantly prolongs life span and appears to be especially effective in the early and middle stages of aging. In mammals, SkQs inhibit the development of age-related diseases such as cataracts, retinopathy, glaucoma, balding, osteoporosis, thymus gland degradation, hypothermia, the oxidative damage of lipids and proteins, and a host of other conditions. But that's not all. When eighty-nine animals (dogs, cats, and horses) that had become blind because of retinopathy were given eye drops containing SkQ (now sold under the brand name Visomitin), vision was restored in 75 percent of the animals. The same drops prevented the loss of sight in rabbits and restored vision to animals that had already become blind. So this tiny molecule looks incredibly promising as a therapeutic drug for prolonging youth.

How it works: MitoQ and SkQ both deliver chemical foot soldiers to mitochondria to fight ROS. MitoQ delivers CoQ10, and SkQ delivers plastoquinone. C60 then allows your mitochondria to absorb these compounds via osmosis. So these three molecules—MitoQ, SkQ, and C60—are a mitochondrial stack made in heaven!

SkQ was designed to accumulate inside cells to target free radicals where they do most of their damage: inside mitochondria. Mitochondria pull in SkQ because they are negatively charged and SkQ molecules are positively charged. In research studies, SkQ has been shown to prevent the oxidation of mitochondrial cardiolipin, a crucial component of the inner mitochondrial membrane. Even in very low concentrations, SkQ appears capable of stopping cellular apoptosis that occurs due to DNA damage. At higher concentrations, SkQ prevents the tissue death initiated by ROS.

How to do it: Aside from the relatively inexpensive Visomitin eye drops, SkQ is currently a bit hard to get—and to get the right oral dosage from the eye drops, you'd need to drink nearly an entire bottle at once. As far as dosage is concerned, the approximate midpoint of the range in most mice research, at 5 nm per kg of body weight daily, translates to about 22.4 mcg per kg of body weight in humans, which, for a 70 kg or 154 lb human, would be 1.6 mg per day.

One website selling the raw ingredient used in Visomitin sells 10 mg of SkQ for $225, making this a relatively expensive antiaging supplement for the time being, although several companies are now working on affordable oral solutions. For example, Mitotech SA, a pharmaceutical company founded by Russian researcher Dr. Vladimir Skulachev, is developing SkQ products and drugs that are currently being taken through FDA's regulatory process.

If you want to dive deeper into SkQ science, I encourage you to do some reading of the numerous papers that Dr. Skulachev and his colleagues have published, which are readable and well translated into English. Most of these papers are published in full and are free on the internet, and you'll find links to them on BoundlessBook.com/19.

UROLITHIN A

Urolithin A is produced by the body after you ingest compounds found in particularly high concentration in pomegranates (particularly the bitter components such as the skin and seeds) and can help recycle defective mitochondria. Since it is a metabolite that results from the transformation of the tannins in pomegranate by gut bacteria, it can be classified as a postbiotic.

Some of the earliest research on urolithin A was performed on *C. elegans* worms, which experienced a 45 percent longer life span than worms not given the compound. Rodents given urolithin A experienced markedly improved muscular function and clearance of damaged mitochondria. Compared to a control group, these rodents showed a 57 to 65 percent increase in exercise capacity, 42 percent increase in running endurance, and a 9 percent increase in grip strength—all markers that correlate with longevity.

In addition, researchers have exposed colon cancer stem cells to a mixture containing urolithin A and found it to be effective at inhibiting the number and size of colon cancer stem cells and also in inhibiting the activity of aldehyde dehydrogenase, a marker of resistance to chemotherapy. Urolithin A can also cross the blood-brain barrier to protect against neurotoxicity and amyloid plaque accumulation.

How it works: As you age, ATP production begins to put strain on your mitochondria, and eventually, energy output falls. But when exposed to urolithin A, these failing mitochondria are broken down and eliminated (very similar to taking out the trash!) to make room for new, properly functioning mitochondria to grow.

Ellagitannins and punicalagins are two natural polyphenols found in pomegranates. They have been shown to have anti-inflammatory and anticancer effects, but once metabolized by gut bacteria, they also produce urolithin A in the digestive tract. So supplementation with pomegranate extract, along with specific bacterial species (probiotics) that can help the pomegranate compounds to produce urolithin A, can be an effective approach to maintaining healthy mitochondria.

How to do it: Eating pomegranates, particularly whole pomegranates with skins, seeds, and flesh, can be the first strategy to increase urolithin A. However, concentrated pomegranate extract, particularly when combined with bacterial species called *Gordonibacter urolithinfaciens* and *Gordonibacter pamelaeae*, can allow for significantly higher amounts of urolithin A and the growth of urolithin-producing bacterial strains within the digestive tract.

Very few probiotic formulas actually contain both pomegranate as a prebiotic and the specific bacterial species that have been shown to produce urolithin A, but one company called SEED has produced an impressive formula that contains both. They offer both versions of their probiotic formulas for men and women, and you'll find links to both on BoundlessBook.com/19.

SELECTIVE ANDROGEN RECEPTOR MODULATORS (SARMS)

SARMs are therapeutic compounds that mimic anabolic steroids. The US Anti-Doping Agency points out that the difference between the two is that SARMs have fewer androgenic properties, which permits them to target tissues much more directly and reduces the host of known negative side effects experienced with steroids. Quite simply, SARMs provide the benefit of steroids without many of their dangerous and annoying mental and physical effects. But what many people don't know is that SARMs, in addition to increasing libido, building muscle, and enhancing energy, can stimulate specific pathways that improve mitochondrial health.

How it works: SARMs contain androgen-like compounds that interact with cellular androgen receptors. The androgen receptor then creates a signal that leads to a magnified expression of particular genes, such as those for muscle growth or fat loss. SARMs are a selective receptor modulator, which means that they can either block or activate hormone receptors depending on conditions, so they have the ability—like adaptogenic herbs—to replicate the effects of hormones in one tissue and at the same time reduce the adverse effects of synthetic steroids or hormones in other tissues.

Several SARMs show a ratio of anabolic to androgenic effects of greater than 3:1 and up to as much as 10:1 (for comparison, testosterone has a ratio of 1:1). This means that SARMs produce anabolic to androgenic effects of up ten times that of testosterone but without the sex drive fluctuations, gastrointestinal disturbances, stroke, blood clots, and other health issues associated with anabolic steroids.

One popular, well-researched, and relatively safe SARM is known as Cardarine, or GW501516 (often called "exercise in a bottle"). Technically, it binds to a PPAR (peroxisome proliferator activator receptor), not an androgen receptor as a SARM normally would, but despite this difference, Cardarine offers impressive results because it activates AMPK, which is responsible for stimulating glucose uptake into skeletal muscle tissue and oxidizing fatty acids. In addition to burning fat by stimulating fatty acid oxidation, Cardarine can increase HDL cholesterol by an average of 79 percent while simultaneously decreasing LDL cholesterol. Molecular analyses have revealed that PPAR is involved in exercise-induced reprogramming of muscle fibers and skeletal muscle metabolism by regulating the expression of genes associated with mitochondrial biogenesis and respiration, and since SARMs upregulate PPAR activity, they can be categorized as mitochondrial support.

Cardarine was developed in the 1990s as a way to prevent and cure breast, prostate, and colon cancer. By the early 2000s, it was discovered that it can also help treat metabolic disorders, including diabetes and obesity. When the fitness community caught wind of these benefits, they quickly discovered that it is also a potent endurance-increasing supplement, and indeed, it has been used by athletes for over twenty years with no reported harmful side effects. Cardarine has also been used in research studies in obese, prediabetic men with metabolic syndrome; these studies showed that it reverses metabolic abnormalities and helps control obesity. In laboratory studies on rats and monkeys, it has been shown to burn fat and build muscle, while also eliminating type 2 diabetes, increasing HDL cholesterol, and lowering VLDL cholesterol.

While some early-1990s studies showed that Cardarine can cause cancer and tumor development with long-term, high-dose use, more-recent studies showed that not only is it harmless under normal use, but it also offers many positive health benefits. As a matter of fact, a study published in 2004 by the American Association of Cancer Research stated that PPAR agonists such as Cardarine have been "shown to have no effect on the proliferation of colorectal cancer cells" and that "under normal culture conditions, PPAR activation has no effect on cell growth." Furthermore, in 2008, Cardarine was studied for treatment of breast cancer and colon cancer. These studies concluded that it can inhibit the growth of cancer cells.

Cardarine has also been shown to cause increased endurance, decreased body fat, and decreased recovery time, and it can also protect the brain, benefit the heart, protect the kidneys, protect against liver damage, strengthen the immune system, and heal skin disorders. Sedentary mice treated with it were able to run on a treadmill for 270 minutes before tiring, compared to untreated active mice, which could only run for 160 minutes! So, like MOTS-c, you can consider this to be very much like exercise in a bottle.

How to do it: SARMs can be taken orally rather than via inconvenient injections. The maximum recommended dose of a SARM like Cardarine is 20 mg per day. If your goal is to increase endurance, you'll want to start with about 10 mg per day. If you're looking for greater gains, particularly for fat loss, go with 20 mg per day and, for best results, take it an hour before exercise.

Cardarine has a half-life of sixteen to twenty-four hours, so you can take 10 mg once per day or, if you are taking 20 mg per day, split your dose into two, taking one dose every ten to twelve hours (most SARMs come in liquid bottles, and one dropperful is typically 10 mg).

Of course, Cardarine is just one example of a SARM. On BoundlessBook.com/19, you'll find links to two articles in which I discuss the SARMs LGD-4033 and SR-9009, both of which stack quite well with Cardarine for even more accelerated fat loss or muscle gain.

10. Photobiomodulation

I've talked about using photobiomodulation—basically, exposing your body and brain to certain light wavelengths—in chapter 6 (for cognitive enhancement) and chapter 12 (for improving physical recovery). Turns out, because photobiomodulation (PBM) works on mitochondria, it's also a good antiaging tool.

How it works: Within your mitochondria is an enzyme called cytochrome c-oxidase (CCO), which catalyzes the reduction of oxygen for energy metabolism and ATP production. PBM can increase activity of CCO and also disassociate nitric oxide from CCO, which restores electron transport ATP production by increasing the electrical potential across the mitochondrial membrane. This increased membrane potential is also believed to produce ROS. ROS can exert a mild hormetic effect (similar to heat exposure, cold exposure, or wild plant intake), leading to increased cellular repair, healing, and gene transcription. The low-level oxidative stress that results from these ROS may also cause stem cells to grow and proliferate, and the ROS themselves serve as signaling mechanisms for cell-to-cell conversation.

In addition, stem cell proliferation can occur when light-based stimulation of the mitochondria leads to a switch from anaerobic sugar-burning glycolysis to highly efficient oxidative phosphorylation. This switch increases the amount of oxygen that mitochondria required by the mitochondria, including those in stem cells, and when these stem cells sense this need for more oxygen, they migrate to tissues with low levels of oxygen that may need enhanced repair.

How to do it: Aside from regular, moderate doses of sun exposure, two of the PBM methods I recommend most often are the Vielight and the Joovv. The Vielight is aimed at PBM for your brain, and you'll find more about it in chapter 6. The Joovv is a larger device that's better for full-body treatments, and you'll find more about it in chapter 12.

But as a word of caution, when it comes to PBM, more is not better: the light frequencies produce ROS, and excessive ROS can cause oxidative damage. The recommended use for the Vielight is one twenty-five-minute session every two days, and for the Joovv, ten to twenty minutes per day, but no more. (You'll learn even more about photobiomodulation in the next chapter.)

11. Sulfur Support

One of the most important antiaging pathways in the body is that of the Nrf2 transcription factor, and one of the best ways to support Nrf2 is to eat foods rich in sulfur. I'll get to why in a moment.

Nrf2 is responsible for unzipping and exposing genes that encode for the expression of antioxidant proteins that protect against oxidative damage. Activating Nrf2 switches on a host of antioxidant pathways, increases glutathione production, and can even trigger the expression of an antiaging phenotype. A phenotype is an observable characteristic that results from the interaction of the surrounding environment (including food) with an organism's genes. So the stimulation of an antiaging phenotype results in an increase in the expression of genetic factors that help to combat the effects of aging, such as enhanced detoxification pathways.

Glutathione acts as a powerful antioxidant within the mitochondrial matrix, and other antioxidants that result from Nrf2-induced transcription also benefit mitochondria in a similar manner.

How it works: If you are familiar with sulfur (hydrogen sulfide, or H_2S), you may know it only as a poisonous gas that smells of rotten eggs and flatulence. But H_2S is also a signaling molecule. Brace yourself: we're about to wade through some thick scientific terminology.

H_2S causes the formation of a disulfide bond between two cysteine residues: cys-226 and cys-613. The resulting compound deactivates what are called keap1 ubiquitin ligase substrate adaptors. When these adaptors are activated, they cause a chain of events that suppresses Nrf2. So by deactivating these adaptors, H_2S creates an environment in which Nrf2 can act freely and promote the transcription of powerful antioxidant genes.

How to do it: One of the best ways to increase the activation of Nrf2 factors is to consume a lot of sulfur. So fill your diet with plenty of sulfur-containing foods from the Brassica family, which includes bok choy, broccoli, cabbage, cauliflower, horseradish, kale, kohlrabi, mustard leaves, radishes, turnips, and watercress. (Added bonus: each of these is also high in isothiocyanates, a potent cancer-fighting agent.) These foods, along with sulfurous and stinky eggs, onions, and garlic, contain sulforaphane, an H_2S-containing compound.

Broccoli sprouts, which can be kept in your freezer and added to smoothies, are a quite potent sulforaphane-containing superfood. According to my friend Dr. Rhonda Patrick, freezing and blending broccoli sprouts appears to be an excellent way to increase sulforaphane's bioavailability by up to three and half times!

Another Nrf2 activator is curcumin, which is found in turmeric, the primary spice in Indian curries—I talked about curcumin as a mitochondria-supporting compound earlier in this chapter. Finally, hydrogen-rich water, also discussed earlier in this chapter, is also a good way to activate NrF2 pathways.

12. The Aspirin, Magnesium, and Vitamin D Stack

Aspirin is a nonsteroidal anti-inflammatory drug (NSAID) most commonly used as a pain reliever, to treat fever, and to reduce inflammation. While I am highly skeptical of using NSAIDs to treat pain or inflammation (in chapter 12, I explained the dangers of using NSAIDs), aspirin is one of the most popular and has even been used to decrease the risk of death following a heart attack, as well as to decrease the risk of certain types of cancer. Magnesium, which you have encountered throughout this book, is a mineral with several important physiological properties. Vitamin D, which should also be familiar to you by now, is one of the primary fat-soluble vitamins that the body requires for many important physiological functions.

How it works: An article on the website of the antiaging guru Josh Mitteldorf, who wrote the excellent book *Cracking the Aging Code*, alerted me to two *Science* magazine articles that featured simple and inexpensive basic measures that reduce risks of all major diseases associated with old age. Two strategies were taking baby aspirin daily and increasing your blood levels of vitamin D.

It turns out that daily baby aspirin is associated with a lower risk of heart disease, stroke, dementia, and several kinds of cancer (although, in my opinion, fish oil can work similarly, with fewer potential side effects). High blood levels of vitamin D are associated with a lower incidence of most cancers, heart disease, and dementia; protection against low bone density and autoimmune disease; and a lower incidence of colds, the flu, asthma, diabetes, stroke, multiple sclerosis, and cognitive decline.

Vitamin D's anti-inflammatory properties likely delay telomere shortening. Two different studies on twins have shown that individuals with the lowest levels of vitamin D had shorter telomeres that indicated an additional five years of biological aging compared to their twin. Another randomized controlled trial found that vitamin D supplementation at 2,000 IU per day increased telomerase activity by over 19 percent in the blood cells of people who were deficient in vitamin D. In another study, children whose daily milk was fortified with vitamin D caught half as many colds as children without supplementation, so vitamin D likely has a positive impact on the immune system degradation that can occur with age.

Finally, as you have already learned, glycemic variability and insulin sensitivity are two very important longevity parameters to control. A multitude of studies have documented that higher intake of magnesium helps control blood sugar and retain insulin sensitivity with age.

How to do it: In addition to eating a wide variety of foods rich in vitamin D, fish oils, and magnesium (including fatty fish like tuna, herring, sardines, and salmon for fish oil; cheese, beef liver, egg yolks, and mushrooms for vitamin D; and avocados, almonds, and Brazil nuts for magnesium), take a daily dose of baby aspirin or fish oil with a dose of vitamin D with your first meal of the day. Dosages range from 1 to 20 g for fish oil and 2,000 to 6,000 IU for vitamin D, depending on your activity levels and size. Ideally, combine vitamin D with 50 to 150 mcg of vitamin K_2 to increase its absorption. Then, before bed, take 400 to 600 mg of magnesium. Just remember that more magnesium is not better and can cause loose stools.

13. Rhodiola

Because how it works is not fully understood, rhodiola is in a category of its own. This perennial flowering plant has a rich and almost mythical history of use dating back to at least AD 77, when the Greek physician Dioscorides described it in his medical text *De materia medica*. Vikings consumed it to enhance their strength and endurance, and Central Asians used a tea brewed from it to treat colds and flus. Known as the golden root, the root extract of *Rhodiola rosea* has been shown to be particularly effective in preventing age-related decline.

How it works: A group of geneticists from UC Irvine found that feeding rhodiola root to fruit flies allowed the flies to live 20 percent longer. In another experiment, mice were exposed to a lethal dose of gamma radiation, and 90 percent of the mice given rhodiola thirty minutes before radiation survived just fine, in contrast to a 100 percent death rate in mice not treated at all.

Normally, gamma radiation wreaks havoc in cells and randomly breaks apart a host of molecules. Although scientists aren't sure of the exact mechanism of action, it appears that the body has its own built-in chemical machinery for repairing the damage and that rhodiola upregulates this machinery. There is also some speculation that rhodiola may increase stress resilience in a xenohormetic manner, very similar to the extracts from wild plants. (In fact, many of the strategies in this chapter that extend life span also increase stress resilience in some manner as well, making the phrase "harder to kill" an achievable objective for many people if they simply knew what to do.)

One study found that rhodiola consumption is associated with the regulation of the expression of 1,062 different genes, including 72 cardiovascular genes, 63 metabolic genes, 163 gastrointestinal genes, 95 neurological genes, 60 endocrine genes, 50 behavioral genes, and 62 genes associated with psychological disorders, making it a potent supplement for overall longevity and resilience, particularly if you've been exposed to radiation (as most of us living in a postindustrial era of flying on airplanes have!).

How to do it: Rhodiola can be found in many supplemental forms. You can find it available as a capsule or tablet online. Stephen Buhner, a very good herbalist, recommends an extract form from Woodland Essence, and rhodiola is also a key component of TianChi, one of my favorite

Chinese adaptogenic herb blends. Rhodiola doses as low as 50 mg are effective in preventing fatigue, and acute doses of 300 to 650 mg are helpful in combating fatigue and stress (doses higher than that don't appear to give any additional benefit).

14. Deprenyl

Like rhodiola, deprenyl is in an antiaging category all its own. Also known as selegiline, it was developed to treat Parkinson's disease and Alzheimer's, but as early as the 1980s and 1990s, studies in Europe showed impressive increases in the life spans of animals treated with the drug.

Deprenyl helps prevent the breakdown of dopamine, which naturally increases with age. It's most often used with L-dopa to treat Parkinson's disease, but it may also help prevent the onset of neurodegenerative diseases.

How it works: Production rates and levels of the neurotransmitter dopamine remain fairly stable until about age forty-five. After that, brain levels of dopamine decrease by about 13 percent each decade. When the number of dopamine-producing neurons in the brain deteriorate by about 30 percent, Parkinson's can develop.

Monoamine oxidase B (MAO-B) is the enzyme responsible for breaking down dopamine, among other neurotransmitters, and MAO-B levels increase as you age. Deprenyl is a selective inhibitor of MAO-B. Many rat studies have shown that deprenyl can help prevent the onset of degenerative brain diseases and even treat early stages of Parkinson's.

How to do it: Twice-weekly doses of 5 mg can help you maintain dopamine levels and high amounts of what I can best describe as positive energy. Legally, you need a prescription to obtain it, but you may still have trouble getting your hands on it if you do not have a neurodegenerative condition. It is possible to purchase deprenyl through online pharmacies.

For a less powerful but more affordable solution, many of the smart drugs and nootropics in chapter 5 also support dopamine pathways, and the peptide Semax, also discussed in chapter 5, can give you a feeling of cognitive enhancement very similar to that of deprenyl.

15. Telomerase Activators

As you know by now, telomeres—the caps at the ends of chromosomes—are some of the primary, if not *the* primary, biomarkers for biological age. Your body already possesses the necessary machinery to rebuild telomeres in the form of the telomerase enzyme. The problem is that in adults, the gene responsible for the production of telomerase is almost always turned off, so our cells produce very little of it for most of our lives. However, there are supplements and foods you can consume that may switch on this gene.

How it works: Telomerase is an enzyme that possesses its own RNA molecule and appears especially significantly in stem cells and cancer cells. It copies its RNA molecule and tacks it onto the ends of your chromosomes, thereby elongating your telomeres and keeping them from fraying or becoming excessively shortened.

How to do it: Unfortunately, we can't eat telomerase or administer it intravenously. The molecule doesn't survive digestion and won't migrate from the blood into the cell nucleus, where it performs its work. So the best way to maximize the longevity-enhancing effects of telomerase is to switch on the gene responsible for producing telomerase. There are several supplements and foods you can take that may do this, along with a few lifestyle strategies, all covered below.

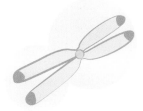

PHARMACEUTICALS

Many pharmaceutical companies are working on preventing aging via telomerase. While some have attempted to create supplements that will deliver telomerase in a form that will reach the cell nuclei, most focus on signaling the cells themselves to turn on the telomerase gene. That way, telomerase will appear right in the cell nucleus where it is needed.

Sierra Sciences, a private drug company based in Reno, Nevada, has screened over 250,000 small-molecule compounds that it believes could lead to an increase in the expression of telomerase. They claim they have found a compound three times more potent than anything previously discovered at increasing the expression of telomerase in cells, and they market it as telomerase activation molecule 818 (TAM-818). When I interviewed Dr. Bill Andrews, the chief scientist of Sierra Sciences and one of the world's leading experts on telomeres, he told me that he personally uses TAM-818, TA-65 (an astragalus extract), a supplement called IsaGenesis, a vitamin D/K blend, vitamin C, fish oil, and flaxseed oil to maximize telomerase activity. (Warning: Aging Care Capsules, the main supplement that contains TAM-818, and TA-65 are currently several hundred dollars per bottle!)

The peptide epithalon is also an effective telomerase activator—for more on that, see page 528.

ASTRAGALUS

Astragalus is an herb that comes from the root of a perennial plant in the northern and eastern parts of China. It may be able to activate telomerase, but it takes a very large amount of astragalus plant to extract an effective dose.

The pharmaceutical company T.A. Sciences has begun to produce an astragalus extract that has been reported to have telomere-lengthening benefits. Their product—quite popular and hotly debated in antiaging circles—is called TA-65. The primary constituent of TA-65 is cycloastragenol, a purified extract of astragalus root. While initial research indicates that cycloastragenol works to activate telomerase, it is still fairly weak: an effective human dosage would be about 1,500 mg per day, but the capsules that are sold currently contain only about 5 to 20 mg and cost several dollars per dose.

Because TA-65 is so expensive and possibly too weak, it may be simpler to use astragalus itself in high doses or use a product such as the adaptogenic herb complex TianChi, which contains high amounts of astragalus in a pure, concentrated extraction. Astragalus has long been used in traditional Chinese medicine—it's considered one of the greatest chi tonics in Chinese herbology—and is often used as an adaptogenic substitute for ginseng. It is said to build upright chi, meaning that when the lungs are strong and the breath is deep, astragalus promotes good posture and holds the organs in place. Traditionally, it is also said to maintain the protective chi that circulates over your skin to ward off seasonal illness.

Even if you don't believe in concepts like protective chi, there is still a lot of research that supports the use of astragalus to enhance your health and longevity. Some, such as my friends at the supplement research website Examine.com, say that astragalus can provide several health benefits but may not actually extend your life. They say that, like resveratrol, astragalus adds life to your years rather than years to your life. But while there are no studies that show an increase in life span, astragalus has been shown to reduce age-related metabolic and physical decline, and it is known particularly for its cardioprotective and anti-inflammatory effects.

One of astragalus's primary effects is protecting mitochondria. Oxidation can damage the lipids that make up mitochondrial membranes, and astragalus inhibits this oxidation. It also been shown to prevent calcium- and oxidant-induced permeation of mitochondrial membranes. Heart mitochondria in particular are protected following astragalus supplementation, which also exerts antioxidant and antitoxin effects on cardiac tissue as well as blood vessels, so the herb can also improve and preserve cardiovascular health.

Because astragalus naturally has poor bioavailability, in traditional Chinese medicine, it is often paired with *Angelicae sinensis* (also known as *dong quai* or female ginseng) to increase the absorption of both. The traditional preparation is a 5:1 ratio—30 g of astragalus and 6 g of *Angelicae sinensis*. Online you can also find supplemental forms of astragaloside IV, the active ingredient of astragalus. The standard dose for astragaloside IV is 5 to 10 mg.

If you prefer shotgun approaches for your supplements, the TianChi Chinese Adaptogenic Herb Complex and the Inner Peace Herb Complex made by my friend and Chinese herbalist Roger Drummer both contain astragalus alongside a host of other supportive compounds, including rhodiola, reishi mushrooms, green tea, and acerola cherry. Links to both can be found on BoundlessBook.com/19.

OTHER SUPPORTIVE STRATEGIES

In addition to astragalus, herbs that can increase telomerase production include ashwagandha, bacopa, boswellia, green tea, horny goat weed, and milk thistle. Other supplements that may stimulate the body to express telomerase include the amino acid carnosine, omega-3 fatty acids from fish oil, curcumin, and resveratrol (found in red wine and grape skin extract).

Several varieties of mushrooms have been studied for their ability to increase telomerase activity, particularly in cancerous cells. These include reishi, cordyceps, oyster, shiitake, and wood ear (often listed on mushroom powder and supplement labels as auricularia or auricula). Green tea, oolong tea, coffee, and even being breastfed as a child can all also increase telomere length and telomerase activity!

Stress management and even meditation have also been shown to measurably increase telomerase activity. And, as you may remember from chapter 9, lifting weights is known to profoundly improve telomere length.

16. Fecal Transplants

Fecal transplantation, also known as fecal bacteriotherapy, is the transplantation of a donor's fecal matter into your colon, either through the rectum or through the mouth (cleverly disguised as a poop pill). The idea behind this fairly extreme longevity tactic is to transplant the healthy gut bacteria in a healthy donor's fecal matter. Extreme measures like this may well be worth the gross-out factor: from 1999 to 2007, deaths from gastrointestinal infections grew from seven thousand to seventeen thousand a year, with 83 percent of these deaths occurring among patients over the age of sixty-five, two-thirds of whom died from *Clostridium difficile* infections.

How it works: Think back to chapter 13's explanation of the brain-gut connection. Your brain can often end up downstream of the good and bad events that occur in your gut, and vice versa. That means that if something goes wrong in your intestines and colon, you could suffer major complications in your nervous system, immune system, and endocrine system.

Older people, particularly those in hospitals and nursing homes, often take antibiotics designed to eliminate infections. *C. difficile* tends to plague this population, especially once other gut bacteria, whether good or bad, have been destroyed. Once settled into your gut, *C. difficile* churns out toxins that can damage the lining of the intestines, leading to symptoms that include diarrhea and potentially severe, life-threatening inflammation of the colon. Fecal transplants have been shown to be effective in shoving *C. difficile* bacteria out of your gut and replacing them with the beneficial bacteria that belong there. Fecal transplants have also been shown to be effective in treating some cases of ulcerative colitis, an autoimmune condition characterized by abdominal pain, bloody diarrhea, ulcers on the colon, and fatigue.

But the effects of a fecal transplant may go beyond simply fixing issues with *C. difficile*. For example, in one study that reminded me quite a bit of the young blood transfusion experiments described earlier in this chapter, transplanting gut bacteria from young fish to old fish extended the mean life span by 41 percent and maximum life span by 30 percent in the old fish. This was due not just to the elimination of *C. difficile* but to a complete overhaul of the entire fish microbiome—or at least that of the colon. This makes sense because one of the primary differences between centenarians and shorter-lived people is that the gut microbiomes of centenarians have specific bacteria that seem to be associated with longevity. So in addition to eating a diet rich in fermented foods, getting dirty by engaging in frequent practices such as being outside, and avoiding antibiotics—all strategies that strengthen the gut microbiome— rebooting our intestinal flora may have a host of benefits.

How to do it: Fecal transplants are best administered by professional medical practitioners in a medical clinic (Dr. Glenn Taylor of the Taymount Clinic is one of the more respected poop-pill practitioners), but they can be performed in your own home using the type of DIY instructions that pop up everywhere from Reddit to Quora. The treatment consists of placing saline-diluted fecal matter into your colon via a nasoduodenal catheter or enema, or consuming encapsulated versions. On BoundlessBook.com/19 you'll find links to websites where you can find clinics that will administer fecal transplants, and you may also want to check out OpenBiome.com, where you can connect with healthy donors for the DIY version.

Should you decide to eschew the fecal transplant, you may be interested in a far more affordable and easy alternative: sunlight exposure. The most recent research seems to indicate that frequent, healthy doses of sun exposure can positively influence the colon's microbiome, if perhaps not as dramatically as a fecal transplant.

Other Strategies

Is what you just read an exhaustive list? By no means! As a matter of fact, I spend plenty of time these days at antiaging conferences, speaking with physicians, poring over studies on PubMed, and reading just about every book I can get my hands on that looks at longevity and life quality. While I tend to slightly favor more natural, ancestral strategies over technological ones, here are just a few of the interesting fields to keep an eye on if you're passionate about antiaging:

- **Cellular reprogramming:** Made popular by longevity researcher Dr. David Sinclair, cellular reprogramming involves, theoretically at a young age such as twenty-five, delivering a genetically engineered virus into your cells. The virus includes Yamanaka factors, which can cause cells to revert to a youthful, stem cell–like state. Then, when aging sets in later in life, an antibiotic is administered that activates the virus, sparking tissue rejuvenation, organ restoration, chronic disease reversal, and even fading of wrinkles and gray hair. Like many new antiaging protocols, the procedure is in research infancy and may carry risks such as cancer and immune system dysfunction, but it's definitely a protocol I plan on paying attention to. Check out Sinclair's book *Lifespan* to learn more.

- **Senolytic medicines:** Senolytics are a class of drugs that selectively induce death of senescent or aging cells, which are thought to be the root cause and driver of many age-related diseases. The company Unity is one that's developing senolytics. So-called senotherapeutic drugs include a class called genoprotectors, which target causes of aging such as damage to the DNA. One particularly intriguing strategy for slowing senescence is combining the pharmaceutical dasatinib with the nutraceutical quercetin, which in mice equivalent to eighty-year-old humans increased survival by 36 percent and in early human clinical trials appears to act similarly for antiaging.

- **CRISPR:** Currently the simplest, most versatile, and most precise method of genetic manipulation, CRISPR is a technology that enables geneticists to edit parts of the genome by removing, adding, or altering sections of the DNA sequence. The company Editas Medicine focuses on translating CRISPR systems into treatments for people with serious diseases. At the time of this writing, they have received FDA approval for a genome-editing trial—although research currently shows that CRISPR is somewhat risky in terms of its potential to wreak havoc on DNA.

- **AI-based drug discovery:** The goal of AI-based drug discovery is to shorten the research, discovery, and preclinical stages, from three to four years to just a few months. This could save time and financial resources in the development stage of antiaging drugs, as well as provide stronger drug candidates for approval. The company Insilico Medicine is working on an AI engine that covers the entire drug discovery process, from hypothesis generation and target identification to real-world evidence collection.

- **mRNA:** Messenger RNA (mRNA) transfers instructions stored in the DNA to make the proteins required for cells. The company Moderna is developing mRNA medicines that teach your own cells to produce proteins that could prevent, treat, or cure diseases.

- **Isotopically fortified organic compounds:** Instead of preventing oxidative stress, isotopically fortified molecules do not get damaged by oxidative stress and can be consumed to replace the natural organic compounds that do, making the body more resilient. The company Retrotope has demonstrated the safety and efficacy of isotopically fortified organic compounds for several pediatric diseases.

- **Machine vision and sensing:** Advances in AI now allow laser-like accuracy in disease detection from easily accessible data like images. For example, Google Brain has developed accurate predictors for multiple diseases using basic retinal scans. Another company, Haut.AI, uses machine vision to monitor skin health and personalize interventions.

- **Wnt pathways:** One of primary signaling pathways that regulate the self-renewal and differentiation of adult stem cells are the Wnt pathways, which play a role in the formation of new tissues as well as repair and regeneration. The company Samumed has identified novel biological targets and developed drugs that that modulate Wnt activity.

- **New organs:** 3-D bioprinting of tissues and organs presents a new way to restore lost tissue structure and function. The company United Therapeutics has developed a range of products to address cardiovascular disease, infectious diseases, and cancer.

To stay up-to-date on these more advanced concepts, subscribe to my free podcast at BenGreenfieldFitness.com and read the books *Juvenescence* by Jim Mellon and *The Kaufmann Protocol* by Dr. Sandra Kaufmann, and follow the work of Peter Diamandis and his A360 organization.

Antiaging Condensed

In case your head is spinning from all the information in this chapter, here's how you can systematize everything you have just read about:

- Don't smoke.
- Minimize your intake of processed and packaged foods.
- Be able to clearly identify and succinctly state your life's purpose.
- Set aside time for friends and family.
- Set aside time to attend to your spiritual disciplines, such as silence and solitude, meditation, gratitude, fasting, or breathwork.
- Have sex regularly.
- Incorporate low-level physical activity throughout your day, and take it outdoors as much as possible.
- Follow a diet low in sugar and vegetable oils and rich in wild plants, dark berries, tannic beverages, herbs, spices, sulfur-rich foods, organ meats, healthy fats, and low-glycemic-index carbohydrates such as legumes and tubers. If you carry genetic factors that predispose you to excess fat storage, an inflammatory response to fats, or difficulty digesting fats, continue to incorporate regular periods of fasting and manage your blood glucose, but shift toward a more Mediterranean approach higher in monounsaturated fats (see chapter 13 for more on this).
- Perform a twelve-to-sixteen-hour intermittent fast every day, a twenty-four-hour dinner-to-dinner fast one to four times per month, and a caloric-restricted or zero-calorie three-to-five-day water fast two to four times a year.
- Drink pure, clean, filtered water and add liquid trace minerals, sea salt, or Celtic salt to it. Also include hydrogen tablets or some other form of hydrogen-rich water at least twice a day, in the morning and evening, if your budget permits.
- Each day, expose your body to a variety of hormetic stressors, most notably cold, heat, sunlight, wild plants, herbs, hyperoxia, and hypoxia (use a hyperbaric chamber or LiveO2 if either fit your budget). Consider supplementing with ketone esters or ketone salts, particularly for long fasting periods, before or after airline travel, or before or during long workouts.
- Prior to any carbohydrate-containing meal, consume insulin-stabilizing compounds such as bitter melon extract, Ceylon cinnamon, apple cider vinegar, berberine, rosemary, turmeric, ginger, fenugreek, *Gymnema sylvestre*, or cayenne.
- If you are up for the task and like the flavor, consume a variety of shellfish and organ meats, including sweetbreads, liver, heart, and kidneys, at least four times a month. If you wind up leaving out the sweetbreads, consider using the peptide epithalon, the peptide thymosin-alpha, or thymus injections.
- If your budget permits, consume a morning or midday smoothie that contains rhodiola, colostrum, chlorella, spirulina, marine phytoplankton, aloe vera, coffeeberry fruit extract, frozen broccoli sprouts, and moringa. You can also include other sirtuin-supporting foods in the smoothie, such as blueberries, cacao powder or cacao nibs, black currant powder, turmeric, quercetin, chamomile, or green tea extract. (See a list of possible ingredients at BenGreenfieldFitness.com/antiagingsmoothie.)
- Increase telomerase activity by consuming one packet of TianChi on an empty stomach at some point in the afternoon, or by supplementing with astragalus or TA-65 and TAM-818.
- If your budget permits, supplement each morning with carnitine, alpha lipoic acid, CoQ10, PQQ, glutathione, pterostilbene, MitoQ, astragalus, vitamin D, fish oil, C60, SkQs, and a good multivitamin/mineral complex, and then supplement each evening with magnesium, melatonin, and, if you are not breast-feeding or having regular sex, oxytocin. Also try to use a daily probiotic that contains pomegranate seed and skin extract (such as the brand SEED).
- The prescription drugs rapamycin, metformin, and deprenyl can also be used but are not, in my opinion, necessary or, in many cases, even recommended.
- If your budget permits, at some point during the day, consume a serving of ketone salts or ketone esters.
- If your budget permits, regularly drink Dr. Mercola's autophagy tea or put the ingredients into one of your smoothies (see page 325 for the recipe).
- If your budget permits, utilize my full peptides protocol from the peptides section of this chapter.
- If your budget permits, purchase and regularly use a Vielight, Joovv light, and a low-EMF infrared sauna.
- If your budget permits, get an NAD IV once a month and sustain levels with daily NR or NMN intake or NAD patches between IVs. Alternatively, and especially for an affordable solution, prepare and drink pau d'arco tea daily.
- If your budget permits, harvest and bank your stem cells and, one to two times per year, have them injected into any ailing joints or into your bloodstream, preferably combined with PRP and exosomes.
- If your budget permits, visit an antiaging or wellness clinic monthly or quarterly for thymus and placental injections, along with a test of your hormones so you can consider bioidentical hormone replacement therapy if needed.

HOW TO QUANTIFY AGING

Of course, the elephant in the room and the million-dollar question is, *How can I actually know whether any of these tactics are even working for me to reverse aging and enhance my health?* So let's finish with a handful of simple techniques as well as more advanced tests that you can use to measure the efficacy of your efforts to increase longevity, reduce the rate at which telomeres shorten, and stave off the aging processes discussed in this chapter.

Resting Heart Rate

In 2018, the body-metric-tracking company Fitbit released over 150 billion hours of heart data. Among a host of interesting conclusions that can be drawn from this data, including the law of diminishing returns with excessive exercise and the extreme importance of regular walking, is the significant suggestion that a high resting heart rate (RHR) is a very strong predictor of early death. If your RHR is 80, for instance, you're twice as likely to die from heart problems than someone whose RHR is below 50, and you're three times more likely to die if your RHR is over 90.

In most cases—outside of extremely overtrained athletes and those with a history of diseases that damage the heart's electrical system, such as coronary artery disease, heart attack, and infections such as endocarditis and myocarditis—the lower the heart rate, the better. On BoundlessBook.com/19 you'll find links to more of this fascinating data, but ultimately, if you begin to track RHR and see it rising over time, that could indicate accelerated aging.

Telomere Testing

Relatively new laboratory technology can measure the rate at which telomeres shorten, along with mitochondrial aging, white blood cell count, cellular damage, and more. At-home testing companies such as TeloYears, SpectraCell, Repeat Diagnostics, and Life Length can use this technology to measure your average telomere length (ATL). ATL is the mean length of all telomeres in a given sample of leukocytes or white blood cells found in a single drop of blood (blood is the standard sample collection method used for telomere measurement because it is typically more reliable than saliva). You can then compare your results to those of other people of your age and gender, and you can even compare your biological age to your chronological age. One caveat is that the accuracy and reliability of most telomere tests appears weak at best. But when I interviewed Dr. Bill Andrews of Sierra Sciences, he recommended Life Length and Repeat Diagnostics because they use a more accurate form of telomere testing referred to as FISH. Another company, SpectraCell, uses a more accurate form of telomere testing referred to as TCR technology.

Another intriguing age-tracking company called Osiris Green works differently: it offers an Epigenetic Age Analysis service that provides you with a biological predictor of age by measuring several different areas of DNA from saliva and then observing what types of changes in the DNA occur over time. According to Osiris Green, over a person's lifetime, DNA undergoes repeated chemical changes, referred to as epigenetic changes, and these epigenetic changes can potentially alter the way genes function, which can have physiological consequences. Many of these epigenetic changes appear random, but some regions of DNA experience consistent and predictable epigenetic changes that progress with age like the ticking of a clock. Their service looks specifically at several of these areas and uses the observed changes to predict your biological age.

White Blood Cell Count

White blood cells are the primary immune system cells that ward off pathogens. But you may be surprised to learn that higher circulating levels of white blood cells are not necessarily indicative of a healthier immune system—quite the opposite, in fact. White blood cell counts on the lower end of normal can predict a better chance of a long life. This seems to be true primarily in healthy individuals, and people who are generally unhealthy or have a compromised immune system should not use low white blood cell counts to predict longevity.

The normal range for white blood cells is 4,000 to 10,000 cells per microliter of blood. You can request a white blood cell count test from your doctor or medical provider, as it is often included in a complete blood count (CBC) test.

Handgrip Strength

Grip strength is known to predict all-cause mortality risk in middle-aged and elderly people even better than blood pressure. Even when controlling for disease status, inflammatory load, inactivity, nutritional status, and depression, grip strength predicts all-cause mortality in older disabled women, and poor grip strength is an independent risk factor for type 2 diabetes.

Aside from mentally tracking whether you can give a firm handshake, the easiest way to test your grip strength is with a simple home device called a digital dynamometer, although you can also track your grip strength with your dead-hang time from a pull-up bar, a farmer's walk for time, or how long you can clutch a weighted barbell or hex bar in your hands.

Walking Speed

People who walk the fastest tend to die later. A study performed in 2013 revealed that out of seven thousand men and thirty-one thousand women who walked recreationally, those with the highest frequent natural walking speed were less likely to die than others. Conversely, a rapid decline in walking speed has been shown to predict death.

To track and test your walking speed, you can use any GPS or wristwatch with speed-measurement capabilities designed for runners, triathletes, or adventure racers. Good brands include Garmin, Suunto, and Timex. I personally find that when I walk, it is best to simply focus on fast foot turnover and to force myself to walk at a slightly faster pace than what I would consider to be a leisurely amble.

Facial Appearance

According to research, the perceived age of your face is likely a better predictor of your risk of mortality than your actual age, cognitive function, or health markers. The obvious way to track this variable is to pay close attention to your "mirror, mirror on the wall." For example, every Wednesday, after administering my clay mask and skin serum, I lean forward to inspect my face for signs of oxidative damage or excessive wrinkling—or the opposite, which I would expect if I, say, added a high dose of astaxanthin or stepped up my sweating protocol in an infrared sauna.

Subjective Evaluation of Your Quality of Life

Chances are, if you are content with your physical and psychological health, social relationships, and immediate environment, you may end up living longer. On the other hand, being discontent or having a poor opinion of your current situation may lead to an early death. A positive subjective opinion of your life is even a better predictor of longevity than objective measurements.

To measure your subjective quality of life, you can take tests or use questionnaires, such as the Quality of Life Scale, to determine how satisfied you are with your current circumstances. On BoundlessBook.com/19 you'll find links to online tests and questionnaires.

Muscle Quantity (with a Caveat) and Quality

Since muscle produces proteins and metabolites that directly regulate your recovery from trauma and injury, lean muscle mass can serve as a metabolic reservoir for healthy aging. Some research suggests that the more muscle you have, at least to a certain extent, the better you can recover from surgeries, burns, falls, breaks, and punctures, and the longer you can stave off sarcopenia (age-related muscle loss). Of course, as you learned in chapter 9, muscle is also directly correlated to longevity because the expression of a longevity-enhancing protein known as kiotho depends on skeletal muscle strength. The only caveat is that the muscle can't be useless, extra body mass that your body has to carry and cool—it must be high-quality, functional, powerful muscle.

So what is the best way to test your muscle quantity and quality? You may be familiar with the body mass index (BMI), which measures your total body mass. But this is not necessarily the best scale to use to determine how much high-quality, functional muscle you have because it measures all of the mass on your whole frame. Instead, the fat-free mass index (FFMI) is an excellent measure of muscularity. Your FFMI is equivalent to your lean body mass in kilograms divided by your height in meters squared. The equation looks like this:

$$\text{FFMI} = (\text{lean body mass in kg}) \div (\text{height in m})^2$$

The average FFMI score for men is about 19 (in between a slight build with low musculature and a normal build with average musculature), and the average score for women is about 15.

Several wearable tracker devices now use noninvasive tendon-force measurement tools to track muscle speed and power during movement, including the M-Power and the Moxy.

Life Purpose

Time and time again, evidence has shown that having a strong life purpose predicts your allostatic load, which is a fancy term for age-related wear and tear, and that people with a stronger life purpose tend to live longer than those who have no clear direction or purpose in life. Make sure that you can express your purpose in one succinct sentence, and if you need help figuring it out, check out Mastin Kipp's book *Claim Your Power*.

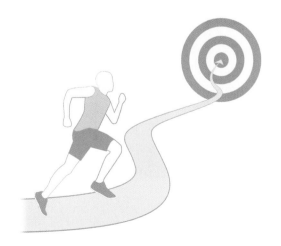

Intelligence

It may not seem very fair, but intelligent people live longer. It has been shown that across all causes of mortality, a higher IQ can protect you. Some have suggested that this is due to the faster reaction times that accompany higher IQs. In other words, if you are smarter and have a quicker brain, you will likely react faster to an incoming car. This may be part of it, but it is not the full picture. Another aspect of intelligence-induced longevity may be that more intelligent people make more intelligent decisions regarding their health, choosing healthy behaviors over self-destructive ones. Basically, the smarter you are, the less likely you are to drink too much, not exercise, overeat fast food, or smoke. Research backs up this theory as well. For example, one recent paper published in the journal *Intelligence* reveals that the more intelligent you are in your late teens and early twenties, the younger you can feel in your seventies!

Although some aspects of intelligence cannot be measured, you can indeed test your IQ. The most reliable, accurate, and accepted results come from tests administered by licensed professionals using validated methods. But it can still be fun to test yourself with apps and online quizzes. The best apps for testing your IQ (and for increasing it via training) are IQ Test Pro Edition, Mensa Brain Training, and IQ Test Free. You'll find links on BoundlessBook.com/19.

Aging Clock Analysis

Finally, researchers are now investigating a new way to quantify aging via a method that looks at your "aging clock." This method analyzes the nucleolus, which is the part of the cell's nucleus where the protein-building ribosomes are located. Part of the nucleolus is occupied by ribosomal DNA (rDNA), which encodes for RNA. There appears to be a direct link between nucleolus aging and markers of accelerated aging in humans, and researchers now hypothesize that measuring the amount of methylation on the rDNA may turn out to be a very accurate way to determine true biological age. But at this point, rDNA measurements aren't widely available or cost effective.

The Bottom Line

If all of that tracking information seemed a little overwhelming on top of everything else I've already covered in this chapter, here is a quick summary and explanation of how you can habitually weave these antiaging measurements into your life:

- Track your resting heart rate daily.
- Get a telomere test, CBC, and mitochondrial profile test annually.
- Get a body fat test quarterly.
- Test your handgrip strength weekly.
- Pay attention to the way your face looks in the mirror weekly.
- Perform a treadmill walking speed test weekly (you can do this as a warm-up or cool-down for any of the workouts from chapter 12).

- If you own a device that tracks muscle speed and power, choose one strength training workout from chapter 12 during which you can measure muscle speed production, or simply keep mental or written track of your strength progressions for specific exercises, and try to track on a monthly basis.

- Take a subjective quality-of-life questionnaire.

- Create a clear, short, succinct, one-sentence purpose-of-life statement, memorize it, and put it into action.

Finally, here's one bonus tip for you. A study entitled "Ability to Sit and Rise from the Floor as a Predictor of All-Cause Mortality" investigated 2002 men and women aged fifty-one to eighty who performed a sitting-standing test to and from the floor, which was scored from 0 to 5: one point was subtracted from 5 for each support used (for example, using both hands and one knee to get up would result in a score of 2, while being able to simply pop up using just one leg would result in a score of 4). The ability to sit down and stand up efficiently and with minimal assistance was directly correlated with a decrease in mortality.

After reading this study, I began making it a goal most days to do a quick two-minute burst of sitting on the floor, extending my legs in front of me, then standing up as many times as I can, using my arms and any other support as little as possible. Try it. It's harder than you may think.

THE LAST WORD

The world's longevity all-stars live longer, but they live better too, with strong connections to family and friends; active lifestyles; clean air, light, and water; a distinct life purpose; an avoidance of smoking; an overwhelmingly plant-based diet that includes fasting; moderate, daily physical activity; and a sprinkling of the other natural practices outlined in this chapter. When asked, centenarians also attribute their long lives to mild amounts of good stress—meaning spartan conditions combined with a life of manual labor, along with a strong sense of community.

In addition, modern biohackers and longevity gurus and scientists are increasingly turning to a host of better-living-through-science tools, technologies, and tactics, with a strong focus on mitochondrial and stem cell support, caloric-restriction and fasting strategies, supplements, IVs, and injections.

ONE THING YOU CAN DO THIS WEEK

One prevailing characteristic of many Blue Zones residents is that their diets include wild and often bitter plants. Our modern produce is fluffy, beautiful, and sugary, far unlike wild nettles growing in the countryside or root shavings collected from a forest floor. But from rosemary to dandelion to clovers, it is not that difficult to either grow or find wild plants and herbs just about anywhere. Your task this week is to use a field guide or an app such as FlowerChecker or PlantSnap to identify one edible wild plant that grows near you and figure out how to harvest it and include it in a recipe.

In addition, most of the longest-lived fit and happy people I know have figured out how to hack their environment to allow them to engage in low-level physical activity all day long, rather than being sedentary and then doing a brutal exercise session at the beginning or end of the day. From keeping a pull-up bar or kettlebell in the office to taking daily walks or using treadmill workstations, the sky's the limit as to how this can be accomplished. This week, choose one way that you can change your environment to allow for more movement, such as only using a chair or a sitting position when you're eating or driving.

For citations for all the research studies mentioned in this chapter and a deeper dive into the topics of this chapter—including links to podcasts, blog posts, recommended tools and supplements, and much more—visit BoundlessBook.com/19.

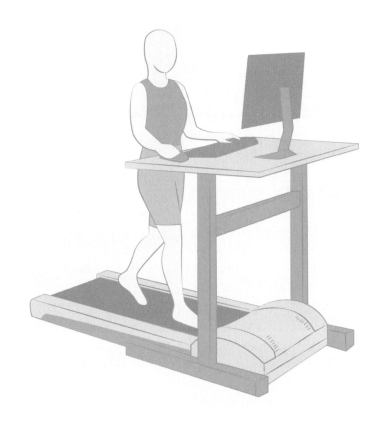

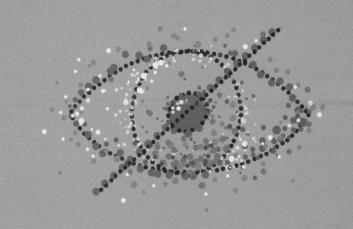

20

INVISIBLE

HIDDEN VARIABLES THAT MAKE OR BREAK YOUR MIND, BODY, AND SPIRIT

I live in a stupid home. That's right: my personal abode deep in the Inland Northwest forest of Washington State is completely stripped of all Bluetooth and wireless signals. There is no WiFi, no microwaves, no fancy internet-connected appliances, no remote-controlled security system, no Alexa, no Google Assistant, no Philips Hue lighting system—just pure, natural power, harnessed from the solar panels on my roof. Save from sleeping in a giant Faraday tent, which my wife has curtly vetoed, I'm about as off-grid as a blogger and podcaster can get.

In addition, the air in my home is pure and clean—inspired by the NASA Clean Air Study, we have abundant air-filtering and toxin-removing plants such as peace lilies, Boston ferns, English ivy, and areca palms, along with the type of multistage space-age HEPA air filters I'll talk more about in this chapter. Essential oil diffusers throughout the house release relaxing and healing scents like lavender, frankincense, and blue spruce, and negative ion generators churn out the same type of ions released by waves crashing into the shore at a beach or tall pines swaying in the wind in a forest.

Then there's the light. The windows, doors, and reflective surfaces are placed to provide natural light throughout the house, and there are no vision-disturbing LED backlit screens, artificial lighting, flickering, or glare. Each room has either full-spectrum incandescent bulbs, which generate extremely low amounts of dirty electricity while providing a spectrum of light similar to that of sunlight, or biological LED, a form of light that can be customized for each room—for example, the gym and office have large amounts of wakefulness-enhancing blue and white light, while the bedrooms and bathrooms have relaxing red light.

Finally, the water is clean, pristine, and thoroughly filtered. After all contaminants and toxins have been filtered from the water, it passes through a structuring unit, which adds natural ionic vibration to the water. The water then goes through a remineralization process that restores minerals, and finally it's exposed to natural UVA, UVB, and infrared rays from the sun to charge the ions and increase the vibration of each individual water molecule.

So why do I place such an emphasis on these invisible, hidden, or frequently ignored environmental factors?

Frankly, even though the modern health and fitness industry places disproportionate value on traditional means of improving one's body—namely movement (exercise) and nutrition (diet)—the reality is that electricity, air, light, and water affect the optimization of the mind, body, and spirit just as much as, if not more than, movement and nutrition. Electricity, air, light, and water can enhance or destroy neural cell activity, muscle recovery, and the strength of the body's key meridians or chakras, through which energy flows.

This chapter will give you all the tools you need to make your environment as pure and health-optimizing as possible. I'll share with you every lifestyle solution and hack possible to make sure the air you breathe is clean, including HEPA air filters, essential oil diffusers, mold testing kits and mold remediation strategies, and more.

When it comes to electricity, I'll show you how to mitigate and minimize the damage from wireless routers, how to introduce negative ion generators and dirty-electricity filters into your home, and how to use natural and safe forms of electricity, such as pulsed electromagnetic field therapy (PEMF) and grounding, to enhance your body. I'll also explain why you should be using air tube headsets for smartphones, antiradiation protective phone cases, and laptop radiation shields.

This chapter will also equip you with everything you need to know to address lighting—especially LED lighting—that may be harming your health. You'll find information about safe lighting alternatives such as red light bulbs for bedroom and areas of rest; blue light bulbs for offices and gyms; blue-light-blocking glasses and blue-light-producing ear and eye devices; software that can reduce screen temperature, flicker, glare, and more; television-based blue-light blockers; and healing and health-enhancing forms of light such as near- and far-infrared therapy and photobiomodulation.

And finally, this chapter will give you the best solutions for optimizing your water, including the best type of water filters, from reverse osmosis to remineralization, and the best glass-bottled waters for travel and home. It will also teach you how to use and create trace minerals and structured water, the optimum way to filter shower and bath water, where to find natural springs, and how to filter water when traveling.

HIDDEN ENVIRONMENTAL STRESSORS

Environmental stressors are ubiquitous in the modern world, whether you're at the gym, the grocery store, or the coffee shop down the street. There's often not much you can do about these toxins, unfortunately, but it's good to know what you may be encountering in public spaces—and it reinforces why it's so important to control these variables where you can, in your own home.

For example, running on the treadmill at the gym can be incredibly stressful to your lungs and hormones if the carpet or flooring in the gym is constantly releasing volatile organic compounds, cleaning chemicals, aldehydes, benzenes, molds, or other toxins. Recent studies have demonstrated that, quite paradoxically, there are concerningly high levels of carcinogens in the average health club, as well as significant amounts of harmful bacteria on the surfaces of fitness equipment such as treadmills and weight-training machines. As a matter of fact, the indoor air quality in some fitness centers can be just as harmful to your health as the pollution in a crowded urban environment (more on all of this later in this chapter).

That same health club, or a basement home gym, or your favorite healthy coffee shop or natural grocery store, can also be chock-full of dirty electricity, also known as electrical pollution or EMF, which is constantly churned out by exercise equipment, appliances, phones, computers, self-quantification devices, and more. Don't get me wrong: I am not opposed to the modern wonders of electricity. But safe, clean electricity has a smooth sine wave that goes up and down sixty times a second, while dirty electricity, a form of electromagnetic pollution that operates in the 4-to-100-kilohertz range, can contaminate both the electrical supply and a human cell's electrically charged membranes. The books *Zapped* by Ann Louise Gittleman and *Dirty Electricity* by Samuel Milham provide a comprehensive treatise on this growing postindustrial health assailant.

Or consider the lighting in a gym, the kitchen of a clean eater, or the average spa or physician's office. Light can have a significant impact on your sleep and your health, and the hidden dangers of light-emitting diode (LED) lighting include the risk of eye issues such as retinal damage and age-related macular degeneration, mitochondrial dysfunction, metabolic disorders, disrupted circadian biology, sleep disruption, increased risk of cancer, and more.

We encounter LED light every day: it's in car headlights, the back of your computer monitor, billboards, traffic signals, camera flashes, mall and airport lighting, and many other locations you encounter, even at night. Large-area LED displays are used as stadium displays, dynamic decorative displays, and dynamic billboards on freeways. Thin, lightweight message displays are used at airports and railway stations and as destination displays for trains, buses, trams, and ferries. LEDs are also used in exit signs, emergency vehicle lighting, ships' navigation lights, brake lights, night vision devices, glow sticks, and more. Unfortunately, these artificial light sources have a host of deleterious health effects in humans.

The average gym or health club and, unfortunately, the average exercise enthusiast's home are also void of clean, pure, electrically charged water. Regular drinking water is often filled with toxic levels of lead, fluoride, glyphosate, chemicals, endocrine disruptors, pharmaceutical drugs, and other contaminants. If the water is filtered, it is often filtered to such an extent that many of the beneficial minerals are removed and the water's natural electrical charge disappears. Between industrial dumping, pesticide runoff, leaky storage tanks, and government mandates, there is a growing issue with water contaminants that may be pouring out of any faucet, including asbestos, chlorine, lead, mercury, volatile organic compounds, arsenic, fluoride, nitrate, and perchlorate.

Environmental stressors may be all around you, but that doesn't mean you're powerless to protect yourself. This chapter will give you the tools to defend your home from pollutants and toxins, and the knowledge to shield yourself as much as possible in public.

ELECTRICITY

There's a reason I keep the wireless router turned off in my home and opt instead to hardwire in via the ethernet, rarely bring my cell phone near my ear, don't use or touch a microwave, and eschew doing any kind of workout with my phone in anything but airplane mode.

It all comes down to a concept called bioelectromagnetics, the interaction between living organisms and electric and magnetic fields, both those produced by organisms and those from other sources. Areas of study in bioelectromagnetics include cell membrane potential and the electric currents that flow in nerves and muscles; the physiological effects of man-made sources of electromagnetic fields such as mobile phones; the ability of living cells, tissues, and organisms to produce electrical fields; and how cells respond to electromagnetic fields.

In the late eighteenth century, the Italian physician and physicist Luigi Galvani was the first to record the phenomenon of bioelectromagnetism while dissecting a frog at the same table where he had been conducting experiments with static electricity. Galvani coined the term *animal electricity* to describe the phenomenon of the frog's muscles twitching. He hypothesized that muscle activation resulted from an electrical fluid or substance in the nerves. It turned out that he was on the right track: short electrical signals called action potentials occur in several types of animal cells, collectively called excitable cells, including neurons, muscle cells, and endocrine cells. These action potentials are crucial to facilitate cellular communication and activate intracellular processes, but they are possible only because of voltage-gated ion channels on the cell, which allow the electrical potential on both sides of a cell membrane to engage in proper signaling.

Bioelectromagnetism is rampant in nature. For example, sharks have bioelectric sensors in their snout that allow them to detect electrical fields produced by other fish, and migratory birds navigate in part by the earth's magnetic field. Another example is the electric eel, which generates a large electric field outside its body for hunting and self-defense.

Like these animals, humans are also big, living batteries—and this is exactly why many of the helpful biohacking devices in this book, such as PEMF, and modern medical imaging such as MRIs actually work. If we were just big skin-covered bags of non-electrically-charged meat, we wouldn't respond to electric or magnetic signals at all. Of course, this also means that our tissues respond to other sources of electromagnetic radiation, including cell phones, cell towers, microwaves, appliances, Bluetooth, WiFi, and beyond.

A number of studies have been conducted on magnetic fields and electric fields to investigate their effects on cell metabolism, cell turnover, cell death, and tumor growth. One of the better summaries of some of the shocking discoveries made in these studies is the book *The Non-tinfoil Guide to EMFs: How to Fix Our Stupid Use of Technology* by Nicolas Pineault, while two of the best books for understanding the voltage potential of the body and the fact that we are all basically giant batteries are *Healing Is Voltage* by Jerry Tennant and *The Body Electric* by Robert Becker.

EMF Is Everywhere

Now that you have a basic understanding of bioelectromagnetism, here's why you should be concerned: the United States alone is wired with half a million miles of high-voltage power lines, and for wireless communication, we depend on over half a million microwave links. We also have tens of millions of broadcasting transmitters flooding our airwaves, use over thirty-five million electromagnetic devices (and that number is increasing at an exponential rate), and plant ourselves in front of hundreds of millions of video and television screens.

Electromagnetic frequency (EMF) radiation is the by-product of this explosion of electronic technology. It's a form of environmental pollution that's emitted by millions of domestic appliances, military installations, industrial machines, computers, broadcast and communications transmitters, and all other electrically powered devices. EMF radiation can cause headaches, vision problems, anxiety, irritability, depression, nausea, fatigue, disturbed sleep, poor physical performance, and loss of motivation.

Even worse, all metallic objects—including electrical circuits, telephone wiring, water and gas pipes, and even the metal objects we carry on our bodies, such as keys, watches, and jewelry—can act as antennae that collect and magnify these energy waves, creating a compounding effect that significantly alters the natural balance of our body's biochemical energy patterns. When you're constantly bombarded in this manner by EMF waves, it can not only distort your internal cellular communications but also entrain your body.

What You Can Do About Radiation

From the Fukushima disaster in Japan to the average airport security line to medical tests that use radioactive compounds, we're constantly bombarded by nuclear, X-ray, and microwave radiation—and it's an unfortunate fact that a nuclear disaster that occurs thousands of miles away can affect you as you sit sipping iced tea in your own backyard.

One problem with radiation is that certain glands and tissues with high amounts of iodine receptors, including thyroid, prostate, and breast tissue, are extremely sensitive to oxidation and cell damage from radiation, especially when these tissues are low in the nutrient iodine. When radioactive iodine (found in most forms of radiation, including all the stuff that gets blown into the atmosphere after a disaster such as Fukushima) gets into areas of your body that have numerous iodine receptors, if these receptors are lacking iodine, then the radioactive iodine latches on and begins ionizing, oxidizing, and harming these tissues. As you can imagine, if the receptors have had adequate dietary exposure to iodine, then they are already filled with normal iodine and do not readily grab the radioactive version of iodine.

The other issue with radiation, as I alluded to above, is that it is highly capable of causing oxidation—just as eating a lot of heated vegetable oil or sugar can cause free-radical damage, but to a much greater extent. Radiation exposure is the equivalent of a bunch of tiny bullets passing through your tissues.

Contrary to popular belief, you simply cannot stop ionizing radiation from entering or passing through your body by taking some special nutritional supplement or drug. To get complete protection from radiation, you'd have to shelter in an underground bunker and get lead or concrete walls between you and the source of the radiation. Good luck with that.

So rather than running from radiation, I recommend you speed your body's ability to repair damaged tissues and organs, and equip yourself with high amounts of the proper nutrients to counteract the effects of ionizing, oxidizing radiation, including these:

- Oral magnesium in supplemental form (around 400 to 600 mg per day, or until you get loose stool). Magnesium offers strong protective effects against small daily doses of radiation.

- Algae, which can naturally protect against radiation. In addition to organic chlorella and spirulina tablets, which you can eat, swallow, or sprinkle into smoothies, you can liberally include sea vegetables in your diet.

- A full spectrum of antioxidants from a diet rich in wild plants, herbs, and spices, along with the antioxidants in chapter 19

- Additional antioxidants from a supplement that contains high-quality omega-3, vitamin D/K, and vitamin A. I recommend Living Fuel SuperEssentials Omega combined with a good multivitamin like Thorne's.

If acute radiation exposure occurs or you're frequently traveling to irradiated areas, also include:

- 6 mg of nascent iodine per day in a glass of water

- One or two servings of edible clay each day. Clay can draw out stored radioactive compounds from your body, and, yes, it literally tastes like eating dirt. I recommend food-grade bentonite clay, which can easily be ordered from Amazon or found at many health-food stores.

Finally, to learn more about naturally protecting yourself from radiation and the huge problem with radiation exposure in our modern era, I highly recommend you read Dr. Mark Sircus's book *Nuclear Toxicity Syndrome*.

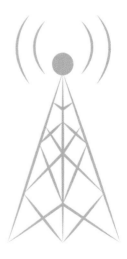

Entrainment, also known as "sympathetic resonance," is the tendency of an object to vibrate at the same frequency as an external stimulus. It's why grounding (which I talked about in chapter 7) works so well. But while the frequencies used in grounding take advantage of the natural frequency of the earth, when you become entrained to any disruptive external frequency—such as the frequency emitted by your wireless router—you can lose the integrity of your intrinsic frequencies (like the natural vibration of your cells), which can degrade physical and mental performance and create huge potential for some serious downstream health issues.

Years ago, in my book *Beyond Training*, I admitted that a direct cause-and-effect relationship between electromagnetic radiation and illness or cellular damage has been difficult to prove, but since then, the number of studies on the link between EMF and human biological damage has exploded. In addition to the books mentioned earlier, to understand the seriousness of this issue and get the nitty-gritty details on protecting your home and body against the ravages of EMF, I recommend you read the books *Zapped: Why Your Cell Phone Shouldn't Be Your Alarm Clock and 1,268 Ways to Outsmart the Hazards of Electronic Pollution* by Ann Louise Gittleman and *Disconnect: Truth About Cell Phone Radiation, What the Industry Has Done to Hide It, and How to Protect Your Family* by Devra Davis.

In Pineault's book *The Non-tinfoil Guide to EMFs* and a host of studies at EMF-Protection.us, I discovered several shocking facts, including these:

- In the last one hundred years, the microwave radiation we're exposed to has increased a quintillion times (yes, that's a real number), and it's still steadily increasing!

- EMF exposure triggers oxidative stress in your cells after just five seconds.

- In 2017, the Phonegate Alert report, devoted to exposing phone misinformation and scandals, found that 90 percent of all cell phones in the world exceed acceptable radiation standards.

- One study gave thirty healthy volunteers a simple memory test without any exposure to WiFi radiation, then gave them the test again while they were exposed to a 2.4 GHz WiFi. Half the participants experienced noticeable decrease in memory accompanied by a change in brain activity and a drop in brain frequency levels related to alertness.

- Children generally absorb twice the amount of radiation as adults (and their bone marrow alone absorbs up to ten times more!). Exposure to radio frequency radiation from WiFi and cellular phones can disrupt normal cellular development, especially in babies and children. Several studies have linked radiation exposure to delayed kidney development; the disruption of protein synthesis is so severe that the authors of one study noted, "This cell property is especially pronounced in growing tissues, that is, in children and youth. Consequently, these population groups would be more susceptible than average to the described effects."

- A 2007 study investigated the impact of low-frequency cell phone signals on sleep. Participants were exposed to the signals from real phones or a placebo signal from fake phones. Those exposed to the real signals had a significantly more difficult time falling asleep and experienced changes in brain wave patterns deleterious to sleep.

- Finally, in a now-classic study, a group of Danish high schoolers placed one group of plants in a room that was shielded from wireless radiation, and they placed another group in a room with two WiFi routers, which together emitted the same amount of radiation as a cell phone. The plants in the room with the radiation didn't grow nearly as well as those in the other room, and the closer a plant was to a router, the sicklier it was. In photos, they appear to be colorless and shrunken.

The emerging and increasingly popular 5G technology is particularly problematic. 5G uses bandwidths of extremely high-frequency millimeter waves (MMW), between 30 GHz and 300 GHz, in addition to some lower and midrange frequencies. But high-frequency MMWs travel a short distance, don't travel well through buildings, and tend to be absorbed by rain and plants, leading to signal interference. This means 5G infrastructure will require a host of cell towers situated closer together, with more input and output ports than there are on 4G towers. This will result in wireless antennas every few feet, on every lamppost and utility pole in your neighborhood (just scan the telephone poles as you drive and you can already see 5G boxes popping up nearly everywhere). In addition to posing a serious environmental threat to plant and insect health, this new 5G signal may have these effects:

- DNA single- and double-strand breaks
- Excess oxidative damage that leads to tissue deterioration and premature aging
- Disruption of cell metabolism due to cell membrane damage
- Increased permeability of the blood-brain barrier (see chapter 2)
- Melatonin reduction (leading to insomnia and, because melatonin has an antioxidant effect, increasing cancer risks and further oxidative damage)
- Disruption of brain glucose metabolism

What You Can Do

Are you convinced yet that you may need to be thinking about this problem? Here's a quick, practical guide to jump-start your EMF radiation protection.

READ MY BOOK *HOW TO BIOHACK THE ULTIMATE HEALTHY HOME.*

It's available at BenGreenfieldFitness.com/healthyhome and includes a detailed interview with a building biologist named Bryan Hoyer, whom I hired to analyze my entire home with dirty electricity meters. The most interesting findings of my building biology analysis? The simple act of switching off the WiFi router and installing dirty-electricity filters in each outlet of my house had a profound impact on lowering EMF, although my home is still blasted with signals from cell phone towers as far as two miles away. (I politely declined Bryan's recommendation to spend $15,000 on a Faraday paint job for every room and Faraday curtains for every window in my home, but I must admit that I thought seriously about it after seeing the number of cell tower signals bouncing through my stupid home in the forest.)

In addition, both he and Dr. Joseph Mercola recommended that I get an Acoustimeter, a simple, affordable device that allows me to test microwave, dirty electricity, and radio frequency (RF) of any of my own devices, technology, appliances, along with any hotel room I stay in. A reading of more than 3.0 µW/m2 on the meter is considered dangerous to cellular biology, and, most concerningly, my own body spikes to that level when I'm merely holding my iPhone if it isn't in airplane mode. Scary, eh?

USE DIRTY-ELECTRICITY FILTERS IN ALL THE MAIN ROOMS OF THE HOUSE.

I personally use and recommend Shielded Healing, Greenwave, and Stetzer filters. If you want to take out your pocketbook and just install a whole-house dirty-electricity filter, Shielded Healing makes a model called the Power Perfect Box. Shielded Healing also has a dirty-electricity filter that can be installed in just one outlet in each room of the house (whereas you need multiple Greenwave or Stetzer filters in each room); they also have a solar power panel dirty-electricity-filtering option that limits the amount of electrical pollution during DC to AC conversion.

CONSIDER PURCHASING A NEGATIVE ION GENERATOR.

A negative ion generator, as you might expect, releases negative ions. These charged particles are abundant in nature, from the beach to the mountains to the forest. HEPA air filters (which I'll talk about more later in the chapter) often come with a built-in negative ion generator. Himalayan rock salt lamps also naturally produce high amounts of negative ions.

LIMIT ELECTRICAL POLLUTION IN YOUR WORKSPACE.

On BoundlessBook.com/20 you'll find a link to a video in which I explain seven ways to limit electrical pollution in your office. In addition to installing dirty-electricity filters and plugging a negative ion generator into the wall outlet, some of these simple steps include buying a grounding cable for any laptops that don't have a three-prong charging cable, hardwiring your computer into the router or wall via an ethernet cable, and placing a Schumann resonance generator or any other 7.8 Hz frequency generator, such as a PEMF device, in or near your working space.

WHEN YOU'RE NOT USING YOUR WIRELESS ROUTER, UNPLUG IT OR SWITCH IT OFF WIRELESS MODE.

You can even purchase a digital wall timer that will automatically turn off your WiFi between, say, 10 p.m. and 6 a.m. In addition, place your router in the garage, a corner of the basement, or as far away from living spaces as you can. If you are building a home, you can do as I did and hard-wire the entire home with metal-shielded Cat 6 ethernet cable so no WiFi is necessary. (I actually recommend running all electrical wiring in a new building through metal conduits to reduce EMF.)

LIMIT ARTIFICIAL LIGHT RADIATION, FLICKERING, AND EMF FROM LIGHTING.

I'll cover all this and more later in this chapter.

DITCH THE BLUETOOTH.

Instead of Bluetooth, use a wired headset or, better yet, an air tube headset for your phone, which allows sound to travel through tubes rather than wires, so you are not exposed to any radiation from wires—I recommend the headsets by Aircom, DefenderShield, and A3. And when you have to talk on your phone, use the speaker setting. I realize this is inconvenience in an era of fancy earbuds that allow you to tune in to your devices without being wired down, but think of it this way: you only have one brain, and it's smart to protect it however you can.

MAINTAIN SOME DISTANCE BETWEEN YOU AND ELECTRONIC SIGNALS.

Keep your cell phone or laptop several inches away from your skin whenever possible, and put your cell phone on airplane mode if you need to put it in your pocket or near your head while sleeping or exercising. If you keep your cell phone in your pocket, consider purchasing a DefenderShield case or an inexpensive Faraday pouch to put it in.

If you need to place an electronic device such as a laptop in your lap, use an EMF-blocking pad such as a DefenderShield pad or Harapad to protect your precious crotch.

AVOID USING YOUR CELL PHONE WHEN THE SIGNAL IS WEAK.

A weak signal amplifies EMF—including that single bar you desperately try to connect to as the airplane is about to land (you know who you are!). You can also turn off the Enable LTE or 4G option on the Settings/Cellular page on your iPhone. This reduces radiation by 84 percent!

SLEEP IN A FARADAY CAGE OR BLANKET.

If you're absolutely surrounded by WiFi signals and you're very concerned about dirty electricity in your home or surroundings, you can purchase a Faraday cage or Faraday sleeping blanket so that you are protected for the approximate third of your life that you are in bed. LessEMF.com sells these and many different forms of shielding fabrics and clothing.

TRAVEL WITH EMF PROTECTION.

For travel or the office, when you're often exposed to WiFi and other EMF that you can't turn off, consider purchasing a personal protection device called the Blushield. It was designed by a team of engineers in New Zealand who pioneered a completely new way of creating an electrical field using crystal photonics (light) rather than magnetic fields or RF (old-school ways of creating interference with EMF or high voltage). It's based on the idea that cells use biophotons (light) to communicate with the internal environment of the human body as well as with the external environment. Mitochondria have evolved to sense and adapt to changes in the external environment (temperature, light, and so on). A crystal photonic scalar signal is built into a Blushield, which produces an efficient and clean way to signal these frequencies around the body for long-term protection, specifically by affecting the subatomic space between atoms.

The Blushield microprocessor generates multiple waveforms similar to what you would find in the millions of frequencies you experience in nature, rather than the repetitive frequency you find in EMF-generating devices such as cell phones or WiFi devices. The company that makes Blushield has shown that blood cells become less "sticky" in response to EMF exposure when using the device, likely because it limits damage to calcium channels, which results in less clumping of cells and has a positive effect on cell membrane strength.

Resources for Learning More

If you do everything listed above, you'll be well on your way to protecting yourself and your home from electrical pollution, but if you really want to geek out on EMFs, perform a thorough test of EMF levels in your home, or upgrade your home with low-EMF technology, then visit the website LessEMF.com, where you'll find a host of content on EMF-proofing your home, along with the equipment you'll need to do so.

Another excellent resource, in addition to the books already listed in this chapter, is EMFCenter.com, which is chock-full of free videos and e-courses. It also offers on-site professional consulting and EMF-proofing for your home or office. Finally, Nicolas Pineault, whom I mentioned earlier, has a fantastic EMF-mitigating course called ElectrosmogRx, which you can access through BoundlessBook.com/20.

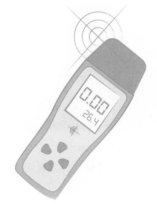

LIGHT

Most of us think of light as just a wave of energy that signifies the absence of darkness, but the fact is, light has a profound impact on human biology, for better or worse. Chapter 7 explained the effects of artificial light on circadian rhythms and sleep, and other sections of this book described biohacks that use light, such as photobiomodulation, near-infrared, far-infrared, UVA, and UVB.

But the effects of light go far beyond its potential for positively hacking sleep or enhancing recovery, especially when it comes to the potential for artificial light to damage your overall wellness. The negative health impact of artificial light sources includes the risk of cataracts, blindness, age-related macular degeneration, mitochondrial dysfunction, metabolic disorders, heart disease, and more. Multiple recent studies have also reported that exposure to artificial light can cause breast cancer, circadian phase disruption, and sleep disorders. One 2015 meta-analysis reviewed eighty-five scientific articles and showed that outdoor artificial lights, such as street lamps and outdoor porch lights, are a risk factor for breast cancer and that more-intense indoor artificial light elevates this risk. This study also showed that exposure to artificial bright light at night suppresses melatonin secretion, increases sleep onset latency, and increases alertness, and that the circadian misalignment caused by artificial light exposure can have significant negative effects on psychological, cardiovascular, and metabolic functions.

The Dangers of LEDs

One perfect example of the hazards of modern light is LEDs (light-emitting diodes), which are rapidly replacing compact fluorescent (CFL) bulbs, primarily because LEDs, unlike CFLs, do not contain mercury, and they're far more energy efficient. LED lighting is used in aviation lighting, car headlights, emergency vehicle lighting, advertising, traffic signals, camera flashes, and general lighting. Large-area LED displays are also used in stadium signage, dynamic decorative displays, and dynamic billboards on freeways. But LEDs pose significant environmental risks and toxicity hazards because they contain high amounts of arsenic, copper, nickel, lead, iron, and silver.

LEDs can also cause irreversible retinal damage to the photoreceptors in your eye and have been shown to induce necrosis in eye tissue. The American Medical Association even put out an official statement warning of the health and safety issues associated with white LED street lamps. Things get even worse once dimming and color-changing features are introduced into LED lighting, which is a common feature in smart homes.

The problem is that, unlike incandescent and halogen lights, LED lamps are a form of digital lighting. In a color-changing system that allows you to dim or adjust the color of the lights, there are typically three LED sources: red, green, and blue. The intensity of these sources has to be changed to achieve different colors, and this means the LEDs rapidly alternate between on at full intensity and completely off over and over again, resulting in a lighting phenomenon called *flicker*. Even though it appears to your naked eye that the LEDs really aren't changing color or intensity that much, your retina perceives this flicker, and you can often observe this phenomenon if you use an older camera or a device called a flicker detector to record an LED light in your house or an LED backlit computer monitor. This trick doesn't work with newer cameras and smartphones, which have a built-in algorithm that detects the flicker frequency and automatically changes the shutter speed accordingly, but I've found that by switching my iPhone to slow-motion video recording, I can often detect flicker in a monitor or light. Although this flicker is present in all LED systems, it's the worse in LEDs that can change color or have intensity-dimming functions.

Research has shown that this flicker can irreparably damage the photoreceptor cells in the retina, resulting in headaches, poor eyesight, brain fog, lack of focus, increased risk of cataracts, and sleep disruptions. Unfortunately, energy-saving lamps such as compact fluorescent lamps (CFLs) can also cause similar issues, along with endocrine and hormonal damage, and they can also induce oxidative stress damage that affects not only the eyes but also sensitive photoreceptors on many other areas of the skin.

The Benefits of Natural Light (and Dark)

But light can be good for you, too, and in fact, the therapeutic use of full-spectrum light—also known as photobiology—offers many surprising health benefits. In the 1700s, scientist and inventor Andreas Gärtner built the first phototherapeutic device, which was a foldable hollow mirror he used to concentrate sunlight onto the aching joints of his patients. A gold leaf on the mirror absorbed UV radiation from sunlight and then transformed this light into near-infrared and red wavelengths, which can penetrate deeply into the tissue. Similarly, many people today use infrared saunas to manage joint pain.

In the 1800s, General Augustus Pleasonton published the book *Influence of the Blue Ray of the Sunlight*, in which he described the "Blue Ray of Sunlight and Blue Colour of the Sky" as instrumental in "Restoring Health from Acute and Chronic Disorders to Humans and Domestic Animals." In the late 1870s, Dr. Edwin Dwight Babbitt published his book *Principles of Light and Color*, in which he reported on his own research on the therapeutic effects of using colored lights on different parts of the body. In 1897, Indian physician Dinshah Ghadiali used chromotherapy in the form of indigo-colored light as a treatment for gastric inflammation and colitis, and in the late nineteenth century Niels Ryberg Finsen of Denmark, who was awarded the Nobel Prize for Physiology in 1903, used red light to treat smallpox and other light spectrums to address chronic diseases such as tuberculosis. In the decades following, Finsen phototherapy developed into a cutting-edge therapeutic intervention, explained in the groundbreaking book *Light Therapeutics* by Dr. John Harvey Kellogg and in work by Dr. Oscar Bernhard, a Swiss surgeon who used heliotherapy (sun therapy) during surgeries.

Light can drastically affect metabolism too. mTOR, the master fuel sensor in our cells, facilitates protein synthesis and growth while inhibiting the recycling of damaged cells, and more natural light can activate mTOR. This is one reason plants and humans grow more in the summertime—not only is there more food abundance, but there's more natural light, too. But your body also needs darkness, and winter. The master fuel sensor in the winter and in darkness, including at night, is AMP-0-activated protein kinase (AMPK), which optimizes energy efficiency and stimulates the recycling of cellular materials.

Now, consider what happens if you are constantly exposed to light: your hormones and metabolism shift toward constant mTOR activation growth and anabolism, which, in excess, is generally associated with cancer and shortened life span. On the flip side, when you experience periods of darkness (along with, ideally, fasting), you strike a balance between constant anabolism with no cellular cleanup and smart catabolism with adequate time for natural cell turnover.

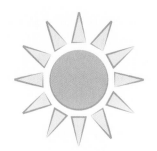

11 Ways to Biohack Light to Optimize Your Body and Brain.

So how can you mitigate the damage done by the wrong kind of light and maximize the benefits of the right kind of light and a balance between light and darkness? You're about to learn my top eleven tips.

1. CHOOSE YOUR LIGHTING CAREFULLY.

One way to ensure you are purchasing a healthier light bulb is to look at a value on the label or box called the color rendering index (CRI). CRI is a quantitative measure of the ability of a light source to reveal the colors of various objects accurately. For example, sunlight, incandescent light bulbs, and candles all have a CRI of 100. When purchasing an LED, look for an R9 (full red spectrum) with a CRI of close to 97, which is the highest you are likely to find and gets you as close as possible to natural light. You also need to look at the color temperature of the light, which is expressed in Kelvin (K). For example, the sun has a physical color temperature of 5,500 K and a correlated color temperature—how the light source appears to the human eye—of about 2,700 K. Many LEDs have a color temperature of up to 6,500 K, but an ideal choice would be an LED with a color temperature as close as possible to 2,700 K. (Most incandescent lamps have a maximum color temperature of 3,000 K because the light filament would melt at a higher temperature.)

You can also consider using a biological LED. The company Lighting Science produces a line of biological bulbs that give off light meant to complement the circadian rhythm, not disrupt it. The light that emanates from Lighting Science's Sleepy Baby bulb, for example, does not interfere with melatonin production and is designed to be as close to candlelight as possible. In contrast, their GoodDay bulb, inspired by morning sunlight, is engineered to provide a rich white illumination with high color rendering to support alertness, mood, and performance—all from light energy largely missing from conventional LED, fluorescent, and incandescent sources. Unfortunately, while these light bulbs are a decent option for customizing areas in your home where you're active (like your office, gym, and garage) and areas where you want light that won't disturb your sleep (like your bedroom and master bathroom), my own testing and the testing of the building biologist I hired to audit my home both showed that they still produce a significant amount of flicker.

For the ultimate solution, although it can be more expensive and far less energy efficient, I recommend switching as many light bulbs in your home and office as possible to the old-school clear incandescent bulbs or a candlelight-style organic light-emitting diode (OLED), which is a human-friendly type of lighting because it is blue-hazard-free and has a low correlated color temperature illumination. This means the candlelight style is deprived of high-energy blue radiation, and it can be used for a much longer duration than normal LEDs without causing retinal damage.

If you decide to go with incandescent, keep in mind that many incandescents are coated with white to make them more aesthetically pleasing. Steer clear of these: the coating changes the beneficial wavelengths. Instead, choose a 2,700 K incandescent light bulb or a low-voltage halogen lamp.

The one benefit of low-voltage halogen lights is that they are more energy-efficient than standard incandescent lamps. But most halogens operate on an alternating current (AC), which generates a large amount of dirty electricity, so you must use a direct current (DC) transformer with them. The problem is that to do this, you need an inverter-switching power supply to convert AC to DC, and this can cause high voltage transients (dirty electricity) and relatively high electrical fields, both of which were measured by my friend Dr. Mercola when he tried to pull this off. So the only way to make a halogen lighting solution work is to go off-grid and switch your entire house to all DC power, or to use solar panels with no AC inverter installed and use the solar power battery to run the halogens. I suspect this is too much trouble for most folks, and because of that, the best option seems to be limited use of biological LED along with either low-temperature incandescent bulbs or blue-hazard-free candlelight OLED lighting.

2. GET MORNING SUN.

Unless you're trying to shift your circadian rhythm forward by sending your body a message that it isn't morning yet (review chapter 7 for information on timing your sun exposure, circadian rhythm, and sleep), you should expose yourself to as much natural sunlight as possible first thing in the morning. In fact, the more sun you get in the morning, the more melatonin you make at night. A fasted morning walk in the sunshine is one of the best ways to optimize your overall health, and the full spectrum of UVA, UVB, near-infrared, and far-infrared rays from sunlight can also mitigate some of the damage done by artificial light the rest of the day. You can also purchase a UVB-generator light, such as the SolRx 1000-Series full-body light panel.

Interestingly, research by my friend Chris Masterjohn shows that if you are deficient in the fat-soluble vitamins A and D, your photoreceptors become less sensitive and the strategy of getting adequate sunlight becomes less effective—so be sure to implement everything that enables sunlight to charge your internal battery, including a diet rich in healthy fats and minerals, clean, pure water, and frequent skin contact with the earth.

This is also yet another reason I am a fan of the Living Fuel SuperEssentials Omega supplement. Not only does it have high amounts of vitamins A and D from purified fish liver oil, but it also contains a full milligram of astaxanthin, which can protect photoreceptors from oxidative damage generated by artificial light. As a matter of fact, I used to use 10 mg of astaxanthin when racing Ironman Hawaii to protect myself during ten hours of intense UVA and UVB radiation on the island of Kona. Other compounds similarly supportive for skin damage from excess sun radiation include collagen or amino acids and vitamin C.

3. USE BLUE-LIGHT BLOCKERS.

Seven years ago, in an attempt to minimize the slight headache and eye discomfort I often experienced after working on my computer for long stretches, I purchased my first pair of biohacked glasses from a company called Gunnar. While these glasses significantly reduced my exposure to monitor flicker and even allowed me to wander through malls and grocery stores without being bothered by the harsh artificial lighting, blue-light-blocking technology has come a long way since then.

Many companies, such as Ambr, Felix Gray, and Swannies, now produce untinted antiglare glasses that can block the higher range of the blue light spectrum, and other brands, such as Spektrum, produce slightly tinted glasses that reduce even more of the blue light spectrum. Gunnar and Swannies now make yellow-tinted glasses that block most blue light, and Ra Optics, Uvex, and TrueDark make orange- and red-tinted glasses that block all blue light. I personally wear clear or yellow lenses for daytime computer work, nighttime dinners out, and driving at night, and I switch to the more effective but far less attractive orange or red lenses for evenings at home. If you want to specifically block the most harmful wavelengths of light, make sure the glasses block the spectrum of 400 to 485 nm (the Ra Optics glasses are an example of lenses that block that specific spectrum).

4. AVOID ARTIFICIAL LIGHT NOT ONLY AT NIGHT BUT IN THE MORNING TOO.

You'll often hear that you should be careful with isolated and concentrated sources of blue light at night, but this rule applies in the morning too. Especially until you've gotten out into the sunlight, you should avoid artificial light as much as possible in the morning, particularly by limiting harsh, concentrated sources of blue light such as artificial home and office lighting or bright screens, and instead open curtains to allow as much natural light into your home and office as possible. In addition, you'll often find me wearing blue-light-blocking glasses for the first couple hours of the morning, and I avoid turning on the kitchen lights and bedroom lights unless absolutely necessary (trust me, making a big cup of hot coffee in the dark isn't a good idea).

5. USE RED LIGHT IN THE EVENING.

For the bedroom, consider red incandescent bulbs, particularly in the light fixtures near the bed. Candles are also an excellent option for both the bedroom and the dinner table, although you must choose fragrance-free candles because many scented candles are riddled with paraffin, soy, toxic dyes, and of course artificial fragrances. If your phone or e-reader has the option, always turn on night shift mode or, better yet, red-light mode in the evening (on BoundlessBook.com/20 you'll find a handy hidden trick to easily switch your phone to red-light mode).

6. INSTALL IRIS SOFTWARE ON ALL MONITORS.

I first became aware of Iris when I interviewed a brilliant young Bulgarian computer programmer named Daniel Georgiev on my podcast. Daniel invented a special piece of software that goes far beyond the blue-light-blocking computer software called f.lux, which many people are already familiar with. Iris controls the brightness of the monitor with the help of your computer's video card, allows you to have adequate brightness without monitor flicker, reduces the color temperature of your monitor, optimizes screen pulsations to reduce eye strain, adjusts the brightness of your screen according to the light around you, and even automatically adjusts your computer monitor's settings based on the sun's position wherever you happen to be in the world. It has settings for pre-sleep, reading, programming, movies, and many others, and even allows you to receive pop-up reminders for activities such as eye exercises and stretching. There's a link to Iris-Tech and my podcast with Daniel on BoundlessBook.com/20.

7. USE AN ANTIGLARE COMPUTER MONITOR.

Fancy, modern LCD monitors are not flicker-free, even though many people think they are because they don't look as harsh as older monitors. These LCD monitors originally started out by using cold cathode fluorescent lamps as a backlight source for the monitor, but in recent years manufacturers have shifted to using LEDs. If you have a thin monitor or a laptop, then you probably have an LCD monitor with LED, and if you are unsure, you can find the model number on the back of the monitor and google it. Due to the way brightness is controlled on LED backlights, it produces the same LED light flicker you've already learned about.

The monitor I use is an Eizo FlexScan EV series, which regulates brightness and makes flicker unperceivable, without any drawbacks such as compromised color stability. It allows you to lower the typical factory preset color temperature setting of 6,500 K down to the more natural 2,700 K, and it also has a Paper Mode feature, which produces long reddish wavelengths and reduces the amount of blue light from the monitor. The Eizo monitors also have antiglare screens, which reduce eye fatigue by dissipating reflective light that otherwise makes the screen difficult to see.

8. USE LIGHT-BLOCKING TAPE OR STICKERS.

Even if you are blocking light from reaching your eyes at night by using blue-light-blocking glasses, a sleep mask, and blackout curtains, you still need to be cognizant of items in your bedroom that have LED lights, such as televisions, clocks, power strips, or computer chargers. This is because even if your eyes are covered, your skin has photoreceptors that can detect all these sources of light.

Even if you have mitigated all light sources in your own bedroom, walking into any hotel room at night presents you with a veritable Christmas tree–like lighting experience.

Fortunately, you can easily purchase simple and affordable light-blocking pieces of tape, such as Lightdims, which act like blackout shades for LED lights on electronics. They can dim or completely cover unwanted LED glare or flare in any room. You simply peel off a sticker and apply it to your electronics, keeping them functional while dimming annoying LEDs to a comfortable or completely unnoticeable level. If you ever feel like you are being bombarded with LEDs or external sources of light in any room—even when you've shut off everything you can—these stickers work perfectly.

9. USE A DRIFTTV FOR YOUR TV.

A driftTV is a small box that you plug into your TV. It removes a percentage of blue light from the content you watch and allows you to view the TV screen at night with far less artificial-light exposure. You can set how much blue you want to take out—for example, you can set it to remove 50 percent of all blue light over a period of one hour (that way, the transition is seamless and virtually unnoticeable if you're watching a movie at night).

10. DON'T OVERUSE SUNGLASSES.

Unless I'm trying to avoid snow blindness from a day of snowboarding on a glaring bright white slope or I'm at a windy beach getting sand blown in my face, you'll rarely find me sporting sunglasses. Why? Our bodies are perfectly designed to cope with sunlight. The retina in your eyes registers how bright your environment is and then secretes hormones to keep you safe from the sun.

Specifically, sunlight stimulates your pituitary glands via the optic nerve to produce a hormone that triggers the melanocytes in your skin to produce more melanin, which allows you to tan and offers some protection from excess UV radiation. When you wear sunglasses, less sunlight reaches the optic nerve, and thus less protective melanin is made and the higher your risk of a carcinogenic and uncomfortable sunburn.

However, if you don't happen to have a set of blue-light-blocking glasses handy, there can be an advantage to wearing sunglasses at night, especially while driving: car headlights are notorious sources of concentrated blue light from LED!

11. USE PHOTOBIOMODULATION DAILY.

Photobiomodulation therapy involves using light of all wavelengths, including visible light, ultraviolet light, and near-, mid-, and far-infrared wavelengths to combat the effects of artificial light and to also elicit some surprising research-proven health benefits for the entire body. For example, blue light therapy has been shown to be good at relieving joint pain, although it can be harsh on the eyes and the circadian rhythm if you overdo it. Red light has a host of research proving its efficacy for relieving inflammation, balancing blood sugar, reducing body fat, improving macular degeneration, assisting with melatonin production, increasing blood flow to the brain, building

Your Skin Is an Eye

Okay, I'm going to stop for a second and go down a rabbit hole here. You may be wondering why on earth you should limit the amount of light that your skin is exposed to. In brief, it's because your skin is an eye.

In the animal kingdom, light-sensing photoreceptors that go far beyond the eyes are quite prevalent. Most of these photoreceptors are located in the brain or the nerves (or, in insects, on the antennae). But a number of different photoreceptors have been found on animals' skin, particularly in color-changing cells or skin organs called chromatophores. You likely know these as the black, brown, or brightly colored spots on fish, crabs, frogs, octopuses, and squid. Many animals can control these chromatophores, matching the color and pattern of a background for camouflage or producing colorful marks to signal aggression or to attract a mate.

It appears that in addition to those vital roles, chromatophores help to maintain a normal circadian rhythm, even without precise knowledge of a light source's location in space or time (such as the location of the sun overhead). These circadian rhythms include the timing of daily cycles of alertness, sleep and wake, mood, appetite, hormone regulation, and body temperature. In some animals, chromatophores have a quite different task: magnetoreception, which is the ability to detect the earth's magnetic field for the purposes of finding direction, an underlying mechanism for orientation in birds, bees, and cockroaches.

It turns out that people have nonvisual photoreceptors too. With the discovery of light-sensitive retinal cells that convert light into signals that can stimulate biological processes, it became obvious that humans must use some sort of nonvisual pathway for some behaviors and functions. For example, pupil size and circadian rhythms vary with changing light even in blind people who have lost all rods and cones due to genetic disorders. Research on rodents at Johns Hopkins University suggests that these nonvisual pathways can regulate mood and learning ability.

Just like in animals, photoreceptors in humans go far beyond the eyes: they are found in our skin, subcutaneous fat, central nervous system, and other areas in the body. Because our skin is exposed to a wide range of light wavelengths, one study investigated whether opsins, the light-activated photoreceptors in the eye, are expressed in the skin to potentially serve as photosensors. The study showed that four major opsins are indeed expressed in two major human skin cell types—melanocytes and keratinocytes—and that these opsins are capable of initiating light-induced signaling pathways to the rest of the body.

Another study discovered melanopsin, another photoreceptor used in retinal nonvisual photoreception, inside blood vessels. The researchers found that this light-sensitive protein can regulate blood vessel contraction and relaxation, and can be damaged by exposure to blue light. Interestingly, melanopsin tends to be much weaker and more susceptible to this damage when levels of vitamins A and D are low.

Another finding backs up the fact that it is not only the light that falls on our eyes that determines our circadian rhythms. In this study, it was shown that shining a bright light on the skin (in this case, behind the knees) has the same effect as shining light on the retina when it comes to regulating our twenty-four-hour circadian clock. Scientists suggest that one reason that people have circadian rhythm photoreceptors on their skin is that when light falls on blood vessels near the skin, it increases the concentration of nitric oxide in the blood, which can significantly shift the circadian clock. This should be especially important to you when you learn this: blue light can penetrate skin as deep as blood vessels, which means that artificial light on your skin can directly affect your circadian rhythm.

Then there's a photoreceptor protein called neuropsin, which is primarily found in the retina but is also located in the skin and helps run the body's master clock. Neuropsin responds to UVA and violet light, while melanopsin seems more sensitive to blue and red light. This may partially explain why going out into the sun during the day (which activates neuropsin) may work so well for regulating your circadian rhythm.

Finally, it seems that these photoreceptors strongly interact with hormone production and fat burning. In one study, researchers put some fat cells under lamps that simulated the sun for four hours and kept other samples in the dark. After two weeks, the cells under the lamps had fewer lipid droplets (the organelles that store fat) than the cells that didn't get any light. This means that exposure to adequate sunlight (on both the skin and the eyes) could cause your cells to store less fat—and based on a number of compelling studies, artificial light (especially blue light) may have the complete opposite effect!

If you want to take a deep dive into how profoundly light can interact with the skin, you should check out the work of my former podcast guest Dr. Jack Kruse, who talks about how light exposure affects carbohydrate sensitivity, thyroid activity, hormone production, and much more. You'll find a few helpful links to sections of Jack's website on BoundlessBook.com/20.

stem cells in bone marrow, and enhancing kidney and thyroid function. Perhaps most surprisingly, Olympic athletes are now using red light therapy to increase time to exhaustion.

One of the most commonly used wavelengths of light in photobiomodulation is near-infrared, which begins at about 750 nm and goes all the way into 1,200 nm. In the lower range, near-infrared penetrates beneath the skin, and at the high range it penetrates deep into the body, resulting in a significant release of nitric oxide and stimulation of mitochondrial pathways that assist with ATP production. Far-infrared is another spectrum frequently used in photobiomodulation, especially in the form of heat lamps or infrared saunas. It is absorbed by the water in your body, which is why it cannot penetrate as deeply as near-infrared, but it also has significant healing effects, especially if you are well hydrated on some form of structured water while using it (read Gerald Pollack's book The Fourth Phase of Water for more on this).

As a word of warning, there appears to be a Goldilocks effect when it comes to photobiomodulation. Most photobiomodulation devices use a power density between 10 and 20 mW/cm^2. That is the equivalent light dose of 1 joule per 100 seconds, and since approximately 10 joules is considered to be a therapeutic dose of light, you really don't need to use photobiomodulation for much more than twenty minutes per day (depending on the power of the device you use and your distance from the device). In addition, all light emits a frequency, and it appears that the ideal frequency is 10 to 40 Hz, with higher frequencies potentially causing a negative biological effect. As mentioned in earlier chapters, I personally use a photobiomodulation panel of clinical-grade red and near-infrared light called a Joovv (placed near the stand-up desk in my office) for twenty minutes per day, along with a head-worn device called a Vielight for twenty-five minutes every other day, and, finally, a far-infrared sauna for thirty minutes three times per week.

AIR

Every day, we inhale an average of fifteen thousand liters of air, and any toxins present in that air pass through our lungs and are circulated to the heart, liver, kidneys, brain, and other organs. According to the World Health Organization, long-term exposure to air pollution leads to a marked reduction in life expectancy, primarily due to an increased risk of death from cardiopulmonary and lung cancer, and according to recent research from MIT, air pollution causes about two hundred thousand early deaths a year in the US alone. When pregnant women are exposed to air pollution, it can cause preterm births and is associated with asthma, autism, lower IQ, and worse performance on standardized tests in their children. In 2018, CNN reported on a major study showing that the same air pollution that results in cognitive decline now affects 95 percent of humans worldwide!

Indoor air pollution is caused by particles like pollen, dust, pet dander, mold spores, and smoke combined with ozone, gases, and volatile organic compounds emitted by building materials, furniture, carpeting, paint, household cleaners, and personal care products. The most common sources of outdoor air pollution are motor vehicles and solid fuel–burning industry and factories, but other sources include smoke from bushfires, herbicides, pesticides, windblown dust, and even pollen and mold spores released by vegetation.

One of the key ways air pollution causes damage is by causing inflammation, along with sabotaging cellular methylation processes (which impact just about every aspect of physiology) and impairing immune system T cell function. Air pollution has been shown to cause inflammation that hardens the arteries, and free radicals from gasoline, diesel, and jet fuel incite a host of oxidative stress on the body. New studies suggest that exposure to high pollution levels can increase the risk of autism and dementia, accelerate the rate of calcium deposits in the arteries, increase the risk of heart attack and stroke, and affect pancreatic function. (Research has now found that air pollution caused 150,000 cases of diabetes in America in 2016 alone!)

Frustratingly, air pollution is hard to avoid, unless you can somehow manage to live upwind from the industrial section of the city or settle in the countryside. Even then, factories pop up in new areas, new highways get added to accommodate increasing traffic, and airplanes and crop dusters fly overhead—not to mention your neighbor's daily lawn-spraying ritual, muffler-free vintage truck, or loud gasoline lawn mower.

But in your home or other areas where you can control your environment, such as your office, there are indeed strategies you can implement to enhance air quality and combat the threat posed by various places you visit throughout the day.

Exercise and Air Pollution

Studies have shown that there are concerningly high levels of carcinogens in the air of the average fitness center, as well as significant amounts of harmful bacteria on the surfaces of fitness equipment such as treadmills and weight training machines.

I'll address the problem with air pollution in gyms in a moment, but I want to address the elephant in the room first: compared to skipping exercise altogether, it's still better to exercise even if you're exercising in a polluted environment. But at the same time, the CDC, the EPA, and plenty of medical journals have found that exposure to air pollutants in urban areas is linked to higher rates of asthma and abnormal heart rhythms and increases your risk of death from cardiovascular disease, respiratory diseases, and all causes, and recent data shows that the indoor air quality in some fitness centers may be just as harmful to health as the air pollutants in urban areas. What this means is that if you have the choice between, say, exercising in your backyard or a nearby park or forest and exercising in the gym, you'd be far better off with the former.

WHAT YOU'RE BREATHING AT THE GYM

The idea that the air quality in some gyms is as bad as outdoor air pollution in cities may seem surprising, but it's backed up by the data. For example, one study in the journal Building and Environment found unacceptably high levels of carbon dioxide, formaldehyde, and other volatile organic compounds (VOCs) as well as particle pollution in multiple indoor fitness centers.

Let's look first at carbon dioxide (CO_2). Since expiration (the primary mechanism by which we lose fat) releases CO_2, its levels significantly rise when there are lots of people huffing and puffing in a room, especially if that room is poorly ventilated. So the more folks you cram into an indoor space who are running on treadmills, rowing, riding bikes, lifting weights, and jumping around, the worse the air quality in that space. This is why I'm a bigger fan of home gyms than commercial gyms, and I'm also a fan of getting in and out of a gym quickly by utilizing a strategy such as high-intensity interval training.

Another study showed the highest levels of CO_2 within a fitness center were in an interior room used for indoor cycling spin classes. I'm not saying that these CO_2 levels are toxic and going to kill you, but they're not completely harmless either. This is all the more concerning when you consider that most building owners (gyms often lease from building owners) save money by recycling used air instead of heating or cooling fresh air from outside.

And then there's mold. On the website SurvivingMold.com, you can learn plenty more about hidden sources of environmental mold that deleteriously affect the health of more than a hundred million people worldwide. Indoor mold can be even more damaging than well-known pollutants such as asbestos and lead, and, unfortunately, mold is common in gyms, locker rooms, swimming pool areas, and saunas because these areas are full of bacteria and moist air. Inhaling mold toxins can be just as harmful as eating mold on a piece of old food.

I've worked at plenty of gyms and health clubs and know for a fact that the cleaning procedures at many, many facilities are less than stellar, and that mold is often ignored or left to hang out for long periods of time. (A good test for the cleanliness of your gym is to leave a small piece of chewed gum in a corner, ledge, crack, or space and see how many days it takes to disappear. You'd be shocked at how long it can take!) So if your gym or the locker room area in your health club is somewhat humid, smells like sweaty socks, or has frequent puddles or pools of water throughout the day, it likely has mold and fungus issues.

Next, there's the problem of particulate matter in indoor spaces such as gyms. Particulate matter is a mixture of solid and liquid droplets such as nitrates, sulfates, organic chemicals, metals, and soil or dust. It can come from rubber mats, metal plates, and dumbbells banging together, and even has pieces of dead skin from other people working out (ew!). The problem is that these particles are small enough to pass through your nasal cavities and enter your lungs, especially when you're breathing hard in an indoor environment.

Unfortunately, over a quarter of the gyms in the study in *Building and Environment* exceed the indoor limit for these kinds of particles. It is true that HEPA air filters and a good cleaning protocol can help out quite a bit in this situation—unless the cleaners are made of toxic chemicals, which can then enter the air and get recirculated. Even school gymnasiums have been found to contain significant levels of particulate matter, such as dust, soil, and bacteria, all of which can trigger immune, asthmatic, and allergic responses in susceptible children.

Next is the issue of volatile organic compounds (VOCs). Exposure to high levels of VOCs can cause skin irritation, neurotoxicity, and hepatotoxicity (toxicity of the liver). The scary fact is that over 80 percent of the gyms that have been studied exceed the acceptable level of unsafe VOCs, which include compounds such as formaldehyde, fire retardants, acetone, and other substances that off-gas from carpeting, furniture, cleaners, and paint. Levels of VOCs tend to be higher in gyms with newer equipment and in spaces that have been recently cleaned (because of the cleaning chemicals used).

Finally, there are all those synthetic fragrances, colognes, and deodorants that your fellow gym-goers have plastered all over their bodies and that are filling the air around you. I address these types of hormonal and endocrine disruptors in my podcast episode on estrogen dominance, which is linked to on BoundlessBook.com/20, but the bottom line is that these are a serious issue that, frustratingly, can be out of your control unless you have the courage to ask the woman running on the treadmill next to you to slather on a bit less perfume next time.

WHY YOU SHOULD EXERCISE OUTDOORS

Now, let's compare all this to outdoor exercise. In one podcast episode (linked to on BoundlessBook.com/20), my guest Evan Brand and I discussed research that shows that something as simple as spending time among trees, walking in forests, exercising on nature trails, and hiking outdoors exposes you to tiny particles and phytochemicals that plants release, and these particles and phytochemicals help decrease cortisol, depression, and anger.

In addition, stepping outside the constant comfort of air-conditioning and heaters and instead getting frequent exposure to temperature fluctuations and weather—cold air, snow, rain, sun, heat, and other environmental variables—can increase stress resilience, burn more calories, increase cardiovascular performance, and get you more fit quickly.

An article in the *Journal of Physiological Anthropology*, "Natural Environments, Ancestral Diets, and Microbial Ecology: Is There a Modern 'Paleo-Deficit Disorder'?," highlighted research from as early as the 1960s showing that early-life experience with microbiota and other bacteria found in outdoor situations, along with environmental stress, can positively influence longevity and health. The authors recognized the coevolutionary relationship between microbiota and the human host and pointed out that there is worse health, more anxiety and depression, and higher incidence of immune-related diseases in developed nations that have become too sanitized—where people aren't outside around dirt, trees, animals, and other natural areas of microbial ecology (which, by the way, is far different than man-made bacteria and synthetic toxins and chemicals in gyms).

In a Japanese study of *shinrin-yoku* (defined as "taking in the forest atmosphere" or "forest bathing"), researchers found that elements of the environment, such as the smell of wood, the sound of running streams, and the scenery of the forest, can promote relaxation and reduce stress, and those taking part in the study experienced lower levels of cortisol, slower heart rates, and lower blood pressure.

This should all really come as no surprise. Scientists have long known that sunlight can lower depression, especially depression from seasonal affective disorder (SAD). One study from the University of Essex found that something as simple as a walk in the countryside reduced depression in 71 percent of participants. These same researchers found that nature therapy, also known as ecotherapy, and spending as little as five minutes in a natural setting, whether walking in a park or gardening in the backyard, improved mood, self-esteem, and motivation.

Health-care professionals are also finding that being in a natural environment has numerous benefits for kids and can combat obesity, anxiety, depression, and other health issues. In an article on WebMD, nurse Stacy Bosch of the Clark County School District in Nevada noted that more often than not, students who are overweight or have type 2 diabetes spend little time outside. To get the kids and their parents away from the TV or computer and increase their physical activity, which can help control weight and blood sugar, Bosch writes a prescription for the entire family to go into natural areas and simply take a walk.

HOW TO GET STARTED GETTING OUTSIDE

So now that you know that constantly being indoors in a gym may not be the best thing for your health and that being outdoors in nature provides you with a myriad of benefits, what are some ways you can start exercising outdoors? The following are five quick-and-dirty tips.

1. Commute with your body.

It always surprises me when folks drive just a few miles (or less!) to the gym so they can move when it would have been just as easy to bike or walk to the gym. Say you have a concurrent strength-endurance workout that involves running and lifting. Why not run to the gym, do your lifting, and run back? Too far? Allow me to introduce you to a novel machine called a bicycle, available for rent or purchase anywhere in the world. It's rare these days that I use my truck at home for anything except hauling alfalfa for the goats or transporting a paddleboard, and it's also rare for me rent a car or use public transport when I travel. If I can engage in low-level physical activity all day long, including commuting with my body, I can spend less time in the cardio section of the gym. Of course, you can always step up your commuting a notch with a weighted vest or weighted backpack.

2. Find a park.

Anytime I'm traveling, I use the "find nearby" option on Google Maps to find the nearest park where I can do dips and push-ups on park benches, pull-ups from bars or tree branches, mini workouts at the children's play area (if it doesn't creep out the parents too much), a jog or run on the park trails, yoga in a quiet grassy area, or skips, hops, bounds, and sprints on a wide-open section of grass. One of my standby workouts? Run the circumference of the park, choose three exercises (such as push-ups, burpees, and lunge jumps), do a high-rep set of all three, then run again.

3. Use nature as a gym.

In my article "Strongman Workouts for Fat Loss, Muscle Gain, and Performance" (there's a link on BoundlessBook.com/20), I give you plenty of backyard and outdoor gym ideas, including these:

- Make a sandbag: I made my sandbag in about thirty minutes by purchasing a couple of military duffel bags online, putting pea gravel into plastic contractor bags, and putting the gravel-filled plastic bags in the duffel bags. You'll find other good sandbag instructions on BoundlessBook.com/20.

- Get a tire: I pulled into my local tire store and asked them if they had any old heavy tires they didn't need anymore. They gave me four of them for free and even offered to help toss them into the back of the pickup truck for me! Afterward, I realized that a true strongman competitor probably would have put the tires into the truck himself.

- Hunt down a tree: Whenever I go on a hike, I make it a goal to find at least one log and carry it for a little while, either overhead, clutched in my arms, or on my shoulders. The past couple of times, I've taken the heavy logs home so that I have them in my backyard for easy access.

- Find a rock: My nearby river has some nice big rocks that I transported to my yard in my pickup. These decently large river rocks are smooth and don't give you as many scrapes and cuts as some of the rougher varieties.

- Push a vehicle: Have a manual car or truck, and a driveway or access to a big empty parking lot? Simply put your vehicle into neutral and get ready for the workout of your life.

Want even more? Check out my friend Zach Even-Esh's excellent book *The Encyclopedia of Underground Strength and Conditioning* and consider approaching outdoor exercise sessions as if you're trying to mimic a nineteenth-century farmer who's pushing, pulling, lifting, hoisting, bending, twisting, and moving all day long. While you may not have a farm or want to build a giant wooden barn or till a field, you can still inject a little extra fitness in your daily routine with activities such as these:

- Go to your local hardware store, buy a rope, attach it to a tire or cinder block, and practice dragging it in your driveway or backyard.

- Plant a small patio garden and go outside (moving!) to water, pick, plant, and care for your plants.

- Go to a park that has a safe and sturdy wooden fence and climb over and under it, or even balance on top of it.

- Find a heavy river rock and carry it up or down a hill, or (more practically) build a wall or firepit in your backyard with large rocks.

You get the idea.

4. Hike.

Hiking solo is one of my favorite ways to recharge and reboot my body, but hiking is also a great activity to do with friends or family because it allows you to socialize, forage for plants, and get nature therapy while you're exercising. With a little research on your local area, you can often find short hikes that offer good scenery that aren't too difficult and don't require special equipment.

Contrary to popular belief, hiking doesn't need to be a passive, easy walk. More-difficult hikes with weight packs, boulder scaling, and even stops to carry heavy rocks or logs can provide you with an extreme fitness challenge that's just as tough as any hard class you might take at a gym. My go-to app for hunting down hikes just about anywhere is AllTrails.

5. Find water.

From swimming to kayaking and canoeing to paddleboarding, getting out on rivers, lakes, or the ocean gives you the benefits of cold thermogenesis, a non-weight-bearing form of exercise, and exposure to even more elements of nature—without all the chlorine and mold issues of fitness center pools. Beach workouts that involve sprints, burpees, push-ups, mountain climbers, lunges, and squats can easily be combined with forays into the water for freestyle and underwater swimming. (For these type of workouts, a good underwater mp3 player can spice things up a bit.)

WHAT ABOUT OUTDOOR AIR POLLUTION?

Of course, no consideration of exercise and air pollution would be complete without addressing air pollution outdoors, which in some major metropolitan areas can be just as concerning as indoor air pollution. In 2013, the American Lung Association published a report on the latest measurements of soot particles and ozone in the air for almost one thousand countries and cities in the United States.

The results come as no surprise, especially for major cities like Los Angeles. In fact, LA is one of the most polluted cities in the US, and not too far behind are the highly urbanized cities of Houston, Washington, New York, Cincinnati, and Philadelphia. On the other hand, cities in North and South Dakota, as well as Palm Beach, Florida, are considered the cleanest.

Whether you live in a polluted city or not, you've surely had to make do with working out along busy, polluted roads at some point in your life. Whether you're a serious athlete or a recreational cyclist or runner, it's prudent to educate yourself on whether working out in polluted areas causes damage to your lungs and your brain.

According to an Australian review of pollution studies worldwide, during exercise, even a minimal concentration of air pollutants can damage the lungs. This damage is as severe during minimal exposure during exercise as it is during exposure to high concentrations of soot and air pollutants when not working out! The researchers concluded that individuals who work out outdoors, especially in highly polluted areas, should be worried about their health.

Harmful particles in the air can get past the nasal hairs, the body's first line of defense, and end up in the lungs, where they cause inflammation and irritation. Sometimes they end up in the bloodstream as well, and when this occurs, the risk for heart attack and stroke increases. Because working out means taking deeper breaths, more of these particle pollutants get past your nasal filtering.

Yet another study, this one from the *New England Journal of Medicine*, concluded that women who live in areas with high amounts of soot in the air are more likely to die from a heart attack than women who live in cleaner air. Said researchers concluded that soot particles are especially harmful to athletes who take in higher concentrations during exercise.

In a similar study at the University of Edinburgh, healthy subjects were made to exercise for thirty minutes on stationary bikes inside a laboratory that piped in diesel exhaust fumes at levels similar to that of a busy highway during rush hour. Researchers found that their blood vessels were less able to distribute blood and oxygen to the muscles, and their levels of tissue plasminogen activators, which are naturally occurring proteins that dissolve clots in the blood, significantly decreased. Because of these findings, the researchers concluded that working out along polluted roads may possibly set in motion the preliminary stages of a heart attack or stroke.

But new research offers some glimmer of hope to athletes and exercise enthusiasts who have no choice but to exercise in polluted urban areas. In a study in the journal *Medicine and Science in Sports and Exercise*, an extended timeline was utilized to study the effects of air pollution during exercise. It's crucial to note that this study was quite unlike previous ones that took measurements immediately after exercise—this one looked at the effects over time. Two groups of mice were subjected to regular doses of diesel exhaust fumes for five weeks. The first group did not exercise, while the second did. In the mice that did not exercise, there was an alarming spike in lung inflammation and free radicals at the end of the five weeks. Astonishingly, the mice that were made to exercise while exposed to diesel exhaust fumes seemed to undergo changes that allowed their bodies to combat the harmful effects of the pollution.

These findings led researchers to conclude that long-term aerobic exercise may protect against the effects of pollution, potentially because of the body's ability to naturally produce antioxidants. Granted, the study was conducted on mice. So what about the effects of pollution during exercise on humans?

It's no secret that the more polluted the air is in a particular area, the more hospital admissions there are for cardiovascular and respiratory issues. But on the other hand, the health benefits of exercise seem to more than balance the harmful effects of air pollution. A 2010 study in the Netherlands utilized epidemiological data and estimated that short daily trips using a bicycle in polluted cities would take away between 0.8 to 40 days from a person's average life span. But the researchers also found that the additional exercise would lengthen an individual's life span by three to fourteen months. It appears, therefore, that exercising outdoors is indeed better than not working out at all, even in an urbanized and polluted area.

Yet another study was conducted at the University of British Columbia's Environmental Physiology Lab. The research utilized two groups of individuals for seven straight weeks. The first group was made to cycle at various intensities while exposed to diesel engine exhaust. The second group, meanwhile, performed a similar activity in an environment with filtered air. The subjects who cycled in polluted air appear to have adapted and showed signs of combating the harmful effects of pollution the way that the mice in the earlier study did.

Of course, additional studies have to be conducted to truly establish as fact the anti-inflammatory effects of exercise against pollution. But even the limited studies available right now may help allay your concerns—they all suggest that going outdoors to exercise is better than not exercising at all even in a polluted area.

But while your body may have a built-in mechanism to protect itself from the harmful effects of air pollution, it's still prudent to take additional steps to lessen the damage. So consider the tips below if you exercise outdoors near polluted roads—or indoors in polluted gyms.

1. Know when to exercise.

As you probably already know, air quality is most compromised when temperatures are highest. Sunlight and heat essentially charge up the air along with all the chemical compounds that are present in the atmosphere. This concoction then combines with the nitrogen oxide in the air to create smog, which is a harmful combination of smoke, soot, and chemical fumes. So it's a good idea to schedule your workouts for the cooler mornings or early evenings.

2. Avoid working out along roads.

Steer clear of roads, particularly busy streets, as these areas tend to have a higher concentration of airborne pollutants. Simply choosing to run, walk, or cycle a few meters from the road can do wonders. Of course, altogether avoiding busy roads is by far the best choice if you truly want to minimize your exposure to airborne pollutants.

3. Educate yourself about your community's air pollution levels.

Before a major run or bike session, check AirNow.gov, where you will find the latest EPA air-quality forecasts for all the major cities in the US. That way, you can schedule your workouts for the least-polluted hours of the day.

4. Don a mask.

Wearing a filtration mask is a smart move as well. Athletes who wear filtration masks during their workouts in polluted urban areas tend to have fewer incidences of pollution nausea than those who don't wear masks. Sure, you may look like a bird flu hypochondriac, but if you're going to be running alongside traffic, it's a small price to pay to avoid the adverse effects of air pollution.

5. Take antioxidants regularly.

Though your body produces its own antioxidants, they may not be enough to combat the daily stress that pollutants subject your body to. To help your body fight harmful free radicals, boost your intake of antioxidant-rich fruits like cherries, pomegranates, and blueberries, as well as dark green vegetables like kale, bok choy, Swiss chard, and purple cabbage; bitter herbs and spices such as rosemary, turmeric, and curry powder; and foods high in sulfur such as garlic, onions, broccoli, and cauliflower.

So that's it. Don't stop exercising—even in gyms and polluted areas. Just do as much as you can to mitigate the damage, and if you ever have the option to exercise outdoors in fresh, clean air, do that instead.

Protecting Yourself from Air Pollution and Toxins

So aside from exercising outdoors whenever possible and taking the steps above to protect yourself during exercise, what can you do to minimize the effects of air pollution? Here are my top eight suggestions.

1. BREATHE THROUGH YOUR NOSE WHENEVER POSSIBLE.

The air we breathe is first processed through the nose, which is lined with tiny hairs called cilia that filter, humidify, and warm or cool the air before it enters the lungs. It is estimated that these cilia protect us from over twenty billion particles of foreign matter every day.

And there are many other benefits to nasal breathing. For example, breathing in and out through the nose helps you to take fuller, deeper breaths, which stimulates the lower lungs to distribute greater amounts of oxygen throughout the body. The lower lungs are rich with the parasympathetic nerve receptors associated with calming the body and mind, whereas the upper lungs, which are used in chest and mouth breathing, are associated with hyperventilation and trigger sympathetic nerve receptors, which are involved in fight-or-flight reactions.

Here's another benefit: the lungs actually extract oxygen from the air during both exhalation and inhalation, and because the nostrils are smaller than the mouth, air exhaled through the nose creates a backflow of oxygenated air into the lungs. Plus, because we tend to exhale more slowly through the nose than we do through the mouth, the lungs have more time to extract oxygen from the air we've already taken in.

Proper nose breathing also reduces hypertension and stress and keeps you from overexerting yourself during a workout. Finally, your sinuses produce nitric oxide, which, when carried into the body through the breath, can open blood vessels and combat harmful bacteria and viruses.

2. BRING THE OUTDOORS INSIDE.

As with light, the simplest place to start cleaning the air is to get as much help from nature as possible. Opening windows and doors to circulate air regularly is key (install screens if necessary). Of course, if you're living in a relatively polluted area, this means that you need to pay close attention to the next two strategies.

3. GET PLANTS.

To ensure that the air circulating in your home is pure, clean, and filtered, have air-cleaning plants in as many rooms as possible. NASA actually did a clean air study and found that plants such as peace lilies, Boston ferns, English ivy, areca palms, and other easy-to-grow indoor plants can absorb toxic chemicals through their leaves, roots, and even the soil that they rest in, removing many of the compounds that may be lurking in our environment, including benzene, formaldehyde, and trichloroethylene. Of course, added benefits of plants are that they help us de-stress and emit beneficial aromatic polyphenols, similar to an essential oil diffuser (more on that later).

4. INSTALL A HEPA AIR FILTER IN YOUR HOME.

A good HEPA (high-efficiency particulate arrestance) filter removes not just particles but also volatile organic chemicals and gases. For a stand-alone unit, I recommend at least one but preferably several AirDoctor HEPA filters placed throughout your home. The filter it contains can capture 99.99 percent of ultrafine particles, along with VOCs like formaldehyde. It also has a negative ion generator, which I recommended earlier in this chapter.

If you want to spend more money, you can upgrade to another stand-alone unit, a Molekule, which contains nanotechnology that destroys pollutants at the molecular level. Many harmful pollutants such as viruses and some smaller VOCs are smaller than 0.3 microns, and even AirDoctor HEPA filters can't remove all of them. Molekule's technology, called photoelectrochemical oxidation (PECO), works at the molecular level to eliminate all indoor air pollution and is able to destroy pollutants one thousand times smaller than HEPA filters.

Finally, if you don't want AirDoctors or Molekules spread all over your house, you can do as I did and install a HEPA filter with an ozonator and negative ion generator in the central air duct of your home. Look for one that traps particles smaller than 2.5 microns and is approved by the California Air Resources Board, which is one of the most strict regulatory bodies for air quality. I use a whole-house brand called AllerAir.

5. USE ESSENTIAL OIL DIFFUSERS.

Saturate the air throughout your house with strategically placed essential oil diffusers, which can release a variety of different scents and help purify the air due to the antifungal, antiviral, and antibacterial properties of many essential oils, most notably lemon, thieves, oregano, peppermint, rosemary, and lavender.

6. USE NATURAL HOUSEHOLD CLEANERS.

From toilet bowl cleaners to laundry detergent, synthetic, chemical-based cleaners are an enormous source of health issues and environmental pollution. For example:

- Tide laundry detergent has high levels of 1,4-Dioxane, a carcinogenic contaminant. (In people who are sensitive to molds and mycotoxins, Tide is a major trigger for chemical sensitivity reactions.)
- Most fabric softeners contain synthetic fragrances that can cause respiratory irritation, headaches, and autoimmune reactions.
- All-purpose cleaners contain the sudsing agents diethanolamine (DEA) and triethanolamine (TEA). When these substances come into contact with nitrites in the environment or your body and mouth, they react to form nitrosamines carcinogens.

In contrast, if you peek into the cleaning cabinet of the Greenfield home, you'll see three basic ingredients: lemons, baking soda, and white vinegar. These three ingredients form the basis of our household cleaning solutions, from disinfectants to window cleaners. Sure, occasionally we'll throw in essential oils such as tea tree, oregano, thieves (a blend of cloves, lemon, cinnamon, eucalyptus, and rosemary—I talked about it at length in chapter 15), or lemon, but even then, you'll find no strange chemicals.

Fact is, there are many inexpensive, easy-to-use natural alternatives that can safely be used in place of commercial household products. You'll find a list of the best natural household cleaning ingredients and recipes for cleaning solutions on pages 588 to 589. There are also plenty of additional helpful recipes on BoundlessBook.com/20.

7. CHOOSE THE RIGHT FURNISHINGS.

Your new carpet or cabinet could be slowly poisoning you with chemicals such as benzene, ethylene glycol, or formaldehyde via a process called off-gassing. In one test of furniture for a baby's nursery, a rocker put off seven times more formaldehyde than the State of California considers safe, the paint for the nursery contained five times the amount of chemical gases as the recommended limit, and more than one hundred chemicals wafted from the crib mattress, including alcohols and industrial solvents.

The good news is that many furniture items emit low or no levels of hazardous chemicals, especially those with a Greenguard certification. Stem Furniture is one company that produces furniture with absolutely zero VOCs. When it comes to engineered wood, such as flooring or cabinets, look for an indoor-air-quality low-emission certification, such as one from Greenguard or SCS Global Services. In addition, look for non-VOC paint, and as an alternative to vinyl flooring, consider natural linoleum.

8. BE HIGHLY COGNIZANT OF MOLD AND MYCOTOXINS.

Mycotoxins, as you may recall from chapter 4, are toxic compounds produced by various species of mold. Among a variety of other health issues, they can cause mitochondrial dysfunction, asthma and other breathing issues, cancer, cardiovascular disease, altered kidney and liver function, disrupted sleep, stunted muscle recovery, miscarriage, and a bad case of fuzzy brain. There are a host of mycotoxins and molds in foods that are commonly perceived to be healthy, and the website SurvivingMold.com is a fantastic tool for discovering whether a food you frequently eat may be tainted with dead organic matter that is deleteriously affecting your health and performance.

In a nutshell, unless you completely trust the source or the amount of time it's been around, I'd seriously reconsider the blue cheese at the salad bar and other potentially moldy foods, including sour cream, buttermilk, and sour milk; cured, pickled, and smoked meats and fish; prepackaged meats, like lunch meats, salami, smoked fish, and some sardines; commercial, store-bought pickles, olives, capers, salad dressing, or ketchup; vinegar and soy sauce; and the average hotel room coffee. I'm not saying you have to live your life completely abstaining from these foods, but you should go out of your way to avoid them if you don't know how they were packaged or how long they have been open to the environment.

But mycotoxins aren't just found in food. By getting a test such an ERMI (environmental relative moldiness index) from a licensed contractor (I don't recommend this as a DIY project), you may find that your house has toxic mold that produces bacteria that can often be more deadly than what you find in food. When an area of moisture forms in your house, within twenty-four to forty-eight hours mold can form, chomp down, and multiply on just about any part of your home that mold considers a food source, including dust, wood, paint, paper, cotton, oil, and modern building materials like drywall.

To avoid mold formation and exposure, I recommend you do the following:

- Keep house dust to a minimum. Mop all floors and dust all surfaces at least once a week. Use a vacuum cleaner with a HEPA filter (I use a brand called Rainbow). HEPA-filter vacuums capture the widest range of particles and potential allergens.

- Use a dehumidifier in mold-prone rooms such as basement bathrooms.

- Use an oscillating fan in the bathroom after showering and fix any leaks as soon as possible.

- Regularly clean surfaces where mold usually grows—around showers and tubs and beneath sinks.

- Be conscious of toxins in carpeting, especially in products made from synthetic materials. Buy natural-fiber wool and cotton rugs. If you really want to take things to the next level, replace your wall-to-wall carpeting with hardwood floors, all-natural linoleum, or ceramic tiles, and use nontoxic glues, adhesives, stains, or sealers for installation.

- Seal or replace particle board walls, floors, and cabinets, which often contain formaldehyde, which emits unhealthy fumes. Avoid any synthetic, strong-smelling plywood, fiberglass, fiberboard, and paneling.

- Consider adding a WaterCop to your house around every drain, sink, and bathtub. This device will shut the water off to the house at the first sign of a leak. Most models are wireless, but there are wired options too.

If you want to know if you have been exposed to mold, there are a few options. In the US, you can get mold exposure tests that you'll learn about momentarily, or you can simply pay attention to symptoms. If you suddenly begin to experience allergy-like symptoms such as asthma, congestion, frequent sickness, headaches, joint pain, or brain fog, and you've recently moved into a new house or apartment or haven't changed anything in your diet, you should suspect mold.

Chapter 4 explained how to get tested for mold exposure and some exercises you can do if you have been exposed. I also recommend revisiting chapter 13 and following the detoxification instructions there. Two especially potent supplements in the case of mold exposure are liposomal glutathione and oil of oregano. But to really get to the best resources on symptoms, treatment, and remediation, I'd visit the website SurvivingMold.com.

Finally, if the laundry list of potentially mold-containing foods above makes you extremely nervous or stressed about your diet, I recommend you do a simple Coca pulse test after you eat a meal that is a frequent staple in your diet and you suspect may be causing symptoms. This basically involves using a phone app (I use one called NatureBeat) and a connected chest strap heart

The Best Natural Household Cleaners

The natural cleaning ingredients below can all be used alone or combined to create nontoxic cleaning solutions for many applications. At right are recipes for some of my favorites, and you can find many more thorough instructions for anything you'd ever need at Eartheasy.com, which is an organic-living website owned by my friend Aran Seaman.

Of course, if you don't have time, you don't have to create your own cleaning supplies. There are a growing number of commercial nontoxic home-cleaning products, and you can find these and other organic, natural products, from kitty litter to diapers, on websites such as ThriveMarket.com or OrganicConsumers.org. On BoundlessBook.com/20, you'll find links to some of the products I recommend most.

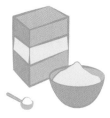

Baking soda cleans and deodorizes.

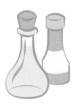

White vinegar cuts grease and removes mildew, odors, some stains, and wax buildup.

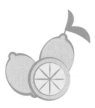

Lemon is a natural acid that is effective against most household bacteria.

Rubbing alcohol is good for cleaning floors, especially tile.

Washing soda, also known as SAL soda, is sodium carbonate decahydrate, a natural mineral. It cuts grease, removes stains, softens water, and cleans walls, tile, sinks, and tubs.

Cornstarch can be used to clean windows, polish furniture, and clean carpets and rugs.

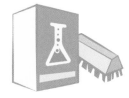

Borax, despite its scary name, is simply sodium borate. It cleans, deodorizes, disinfects, softens water, and cleans wallpaper, painted walls, and floors. It is also good for killing mold.

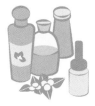

There are dozens of **essential oils**, but we stick to three when we need to kill bacteria or clean our bodies or kitchen counters: oregano, thieves, and lemon.

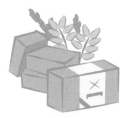

Unscented natural **soap**, such as castile soap, goat's milk soap, and coconut oil soap, comes as a liquid, flakes, powders, or bars. It's biodegradable and will clean just about anything, and you can make it at home yourself. We get most of our soap-making goods from Mountain Rose Herbs.

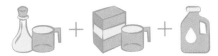

All-purpose cleaner: Mix ½ cup vinegar and ¼ cup baking soda into ½ gallon of water. You can also use natural fiber cloths, which remove dirt, grease, and dust on their own, without any cleaning solution, because they are formulated to penetrate and trap dirt. You'll find a number of brands listed on BoundlessBook.com/20.

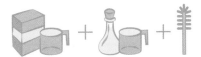

Toilet bowl cleaner: Mix ¼ cup baking soda and 1 cup vinegar, pour it into the toilet bowl, and let it sit for a few minutes. Scrub with a brush and rinse. A mixture of two parts borax and one part lemon juice will also work.

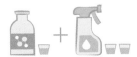

Mold remover: Mix one part hydrogen peroxide (3 percent) with two parts water in a spray bottle and spray on areas with mold. Wait at least one hour before rinsing or using the shower.

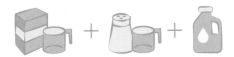

Oven cleaner: Mix ¾ cup baking soda, ¼ cup salt, and ¼ cup water to make a thick paste, and spread it throughout the oven. Let sit overnight, remove with a spatula, and wipe clean.

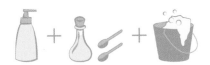

Dishwashing soap: Use any nontoxic liquid soap, such as Dr. Bronner's. For tough jobs, add 2 or 3 tablespoons of vinegar to the warm, soapy water

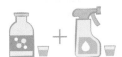

Stain remover: For stains on clothes, you can use a 1:1 solution of water and 3 percent grade hydrogen peroxide to soak out grass, underarm, and many food stains.

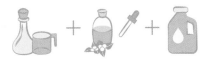

Floor cleaner and polish: For vinyl and linoleum, mix 1 cup vinegar and a few drops of olive oil in 1 gallon of warm water. For wood, use a solution of ¼ cup vinegar and ½ gallon of warm water. For polishing wood, apply a thin coat of equal parts vegetable oil and vinegar and rub in well.

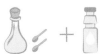

Window cleaner: Mix 2 teaspoons of white vinegar with 1 quart of warm water. Spray it on windows and glass and wipe it off with crumpled black-and-white newspaper or a cotton cloth. Alternatively, you can buy Citra Clean natural window and glass cleaner.

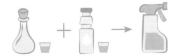

Carpet cleaner: Mix equal parts white vinegar and water in a spray bottle. Spray directly on the stain, let it sit for several minutes, and then clean with a brush or sponge using warm soapy water. For fresh grease spots on the carpet, you can sprinkle cornstarch onto the stain and then wait 15 to 30 minutes before vacuuming. For a heavy-duty carpet cleaner, mix ¼ cup each of salt, borax, and vinegar, rub the paste into the carpet, and leave it for a few hours before vacuuming.

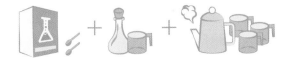

Disinfectant: Mix 2 teaspoons borax, ¼ cup vinegar, and 3 cups hot water.

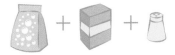

Dishwasher soap: Mix equal parts washing soda, baking soda, and salt.

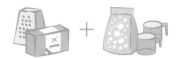

Laundry detergent: Grate one 5-ounce bar of castile soap and mix it with 2 cups of washing soda. You can also try Eco Nuts, an effective laundry detergent made from the dried fruit of the soapberry tree.

rate monitor to track your heart rate before, during, and after eating. If your heart rate increases by five or more beats after eating, you may have an allergy to the food, or there may be mycotoxins in it. In plain terms, the change in your heart rate indicates that your body is going into fight-or-flight mode after eating—which is not a good sign!

Need more resources? Two good books for discovering how to de-mold your house are *My House Is Killing Me!* and *The Mold Survival Guide*, both by Jeffrey C. May.

WATER

In my hometown of Spokane, Washington, they don't fluoridate the water, and boy, am I glad.

Fluoride is certainly a crucial compound—in pesticides, that is. That's right: sodium fluoride is a registered insecticide and rodenticide that is used in rat and roach poisons. It is a toxic waste by-product of the manufacturing of phosphate fertilizers and the aluminum-refining industry, which means it also has a lot of lead as well as other toxic substances in it. But it's cheaper to simply dump fluoride into our water supply than to pay toxic waste disposal fees. Unfortunately, this can cause cancer, hip fracture, dental fluorosis, stained teeth, neurological impairment, lower IQ in children, and learning disorders.

Sure, fluoride certainly has a good antidecay effect when you apply it directly to the tooth itself—but you don't have to swallow the stuff, and frankly, when it comes to tooth decay, there is little to no difference between countries with fluoridated water and countries with nonfluoridated water. If you really want to dig into the issue with fluoride, listen to a podcast that I recorded with Paul Connett, coauthor of the eye-opening book *The Case Against Fluoride* (the podcast is linked to on BoundlessBook.com/20), or read the book *The Fluoride Deception* by Christopher Bryson.

Of course, fluoride isn't the only issue with water. Since 2004, testing by water utilities has consistently found thousands of pollutants in the tap water we drink on a daily basis. More than half of the chemicals detected are not subject to health or safety regulations and can legally be present in any amount. Unfortunately, at least in America, the federal government has not set a single new drinking-water standard since 2012—and water utilities spend nineteen times more on water-treatment chemicals every year than the federal government invests in protecting lakes and rivers from water pollution in the first place.

Chlorine is probably one of the more common chemicals that many health enthusiasts encounter in the gym or in drinking water. Particularly in swimming pools that are not naturally cleaned, we soak up chlorine through our skin while simultaneously breathing in chloramines, the toxic by-products that form when chlorine reacts with organic matter such as dead skin cells.

If you're a swimmer or triathlete or someone who hits the pool or hot tub often, you're likely getting exposed to plenty more chlorine than you're drinking in your municipal water supply or from a glass of tap water at a restaurant. And even if you're not a swimmer, you're still getting significant skin exposure to chlorine simply from showering or bathing in your city's water (if you're not using the filtration methods I'll describe shortly). This chlorine exposure can cause both cell wall damage and internal soft tissue damage, along with autoimmune, asthma, and allergy issues. If you're not filtering your water, chlorine can even vaporize from toilet bowls and into the air as you wash your clothes or dishes!

But perhaps you're already aware that chemicals in water are an issue. Perhaps you're also aware of the importance of drinking enough water, and that your body consists mostly of water, which is needed for just about every physiological process and biochemical reaction that exists, including blood circulation, metabolism, body temperature regulation, and detoxification.

But did you know there are different types of water that go far beyond regular H_2O?

EZ Water and DDW

In his TEDx Talk "Water, Cells, and Life" and his books *The Fourth Phase of Water* and *Cells, Gels, and the Engines of Life*, Gerald Pollack explained the role of water in the functioning of cells and the importance of negatively charged structured water, also known as exclusion zone (EZ) water. This water can both hold and deliver electrical energy, much like a battery. Typical tap water is simply H_2O, but EZ water is actually H_3O_2, which is more viscous and alkaline than regular water and has a refractive index about 10 percent higher, allowing it to more readily respond to light photons from sources such as an infrared sauna, photobiomodulation light panels, and sunlight.

It is also the same kind of negatively charged water that your cells and extracellular tissue naturally contain. This is important because cell membranes are hydrophilic (water-loving) surfaces with a net negative charge, and EZ water can accumulate next to these hydrophilic surfaces. As negatively charged particles from the water and the cell membranes repel each other, energy is created. This is because a key factor that allows positive charges to migrate into a cell is the water surrounding the cell. The electrical conductivity of water acts like a battery that drives the cellular machinery by inducing a charge separation that is able to shuttle positive protons along the cellular cytoskeleton while leaving negatively charged electrons in the water. If you always thought this was achieved by a sodium-potassium pump, as most biology textbooks still teach, then you should look up the work of Gilbert Ling on PubMed, where you'll find research articles that thoroughly debunk the notion of a sodium-potassium pump.

My friend Dr. Thomas Cowan wrote in his books *Human Heart, Cosmic Heart* and *Cancer and the New Biology of Water* about how this negative charge allows blood, which consists largely of water, to more easily navigate through the chambers of the heart, reducing cardiovascular strain and increasing overall heart health. In addition, my former podcast guest Dr. Stephanie Seneff has an excellent TEDx Talk about how negatively charged ions in EZ water help to generate sulfate, which enhances cell fluidity and reduces any tendency for cells to clump, particularly when sunlight is present. EZ water may even upregulate p53, a transcription factor that acts as a potent tumor suppressor and modulator of DNA damage, making it potentially useful for cancer therapy.

Then there's deuterium-depleted water (DDW). DDW—which can be purchased in bottles or created by a DDW generator—is also known as "light water" and contains a very low concentration of deuterium. Deuterium is a hydrogen isotope that has roughly double the mass of a hydrogen atom. This means that high amounts of deuterium in the body—which are often found in people who have been exposed to pesticides, herbicides, municipal water, a high-sugar or acidic diet, or many other unhealthy scenarios—can displace hydrogen and deleteriously impact cell function. Reducing levels of deuterium can restore proper cell function and health. I strongly suspect that hydrogen-enriched water (which I talked about in chapter 12), structured water, and DDW are three forms of water that are going to receive plenty of attention in the wellness world over the next decade as people come to realize that not all water is created equal.

According to Pollack, you can build EZ water naturally in your cells by not only drinking pure and preferably structured water (pay attention to the water filtration strategies in this section), but also by chilling your water, exposing your water to sunlight or infrared light, drinking fresh vegetable juice, drinking coconut water blended with turmeric, exposing your bare skin to sunlight, using an infrared sauna, and walking barefoot outside, which allows you to absorb negatively charged ions from the surface of the earth. According to Robert Slovak, whom I interviewed in a podcast (linked to at BoundlessBook.com/20), the same can be said for DDW: by lowering your carbohydrate intake and increasing your healthy fat intake, you can cause your body, through the process of beta-oxidation, to produce its own DDW!

Who knew water was so much more complex than just H_2O?

How to Manage Exposure to Metals

I step into my basement infrared sauna at least once a week, and usually far more often than that, because saunas have been shown to be an excellent way to release metals through the skin, and because I know that everything from brake dust on the road to metals in airports and airplanes to the occasional sushi binge exposes me to my fair share of metals. If it's not cleaned up in and removed from the body, this type of chronic metal exposure can cause chronic fatigue, poor mood, disrupted sleep, headaches, poor immune system function, low hormones levels, and brain fog.

The biggest culprit for metal exposure is modern dentistry. Even though about 50 percent of dentists in the US are now mercury-free, only an estimated 10 percent of dentists fully understand the health risks associated with amalgam fillings—which contain toxic mercury, despite what the term *silver filling* might lead you to believe.

If you decide you want to pull the metal out of your mouth, then you should know that the process of removing and replacing amalgam fillings comes with the risk of acute toxicity from the mercury released during the removal process, and this can cause serious damage to organs such as your liver and kidney.

Because of this, and because other metals can get absorbed into your mouth when you're at the dentist, my family and I only go to a holistic dentist (also known as a "biological dentist"). These dentists make a special effort to limit your exposure to toxins and chemicals. When they're removing amalgam fillings, they use a cold-water spray to minimize mercury vapors, put a dental dam in your mouth so you don't swallow or inhale any toxins, use a high-volume evacuator near the tooth at all times to evacuate the mercury vapor, wash out your mouth out immediately after the fillings have been removed, and use powerful air purifiers in each room. They also take precautions during regular cleanings, such as using natural products to ensure you are not exposed to chemicals and toxins.

The following organizations can help you to find a holistic dentist:

- Consumers for Dental Choice
- International Academy of Biological Dentistry & Medicine (IABDM)
- Dental Amalgam Mercury Solutions (DAMS)
- Huggins Applied Healing
- Holistic Dental Association
- International Association of Mercury Safe Dentists

Unfortunately, you can get heavy-metal exposure from all sorts of sources that go way beyond metal in your mouth. These sources include:

- Smog
- Car keys
- Toys made in China
- Secondhand cigarette smoke
- Pesticides and herbicides
- Protein powders and dietary supplements
- "Pristine" water (like my local Lake Coeur d'Alene) that in fact has high amounts of mining runoff
- Food stored in metal containers
- Big fish like tuna and dolphin
- Nuclear fallout from the Fukushima disaster in Japan

You can get tested for heavy metals through a company like DirectLabs or Cyrex, but if you've been exposed to any of the above, you can assume you'd benefit from pulling metals out of your body. Binding heavy metals and pulling them out of your body is called chelation, and many substances can do this. The metals generally exit your body in stool, urine, hair, breath, and sweat. Some forms of chelation are accomplished with drugs such as DMPS, but the website DMPSBackfire.com shows you some of the serious problems that can be caused by conventional chelating drugs.

Chelators bind by way of ionic bonds, which are the attractions between the positive charge of a heavy metal and the negative charge of the chelating molecule. Because of this, chelation can extract precious minerals from your body, but it can also spread metals throughout your body, so that they wind up deposited elsewhere. So to get heavy metals out of your body, I do not recommend chelation drugs or natural chelation. Instead, I recommend you use natural compounds that can gently draw heavy metals out of your body.

As with most detoxification programs, you can't simply pop a supplement or chug a giant bottle of activated charcoal water and walk away. Instead, to ensure that metals and other toxins are actually removed and don't travel throughout the body, you need to follow a specific, systematized detox protocol. For metals, the two programs I recommend highest are Dan Pompa's True Cellular Detox program and Dr. Chris Shade's Detox Qube. Review chapter 13 for more information on proper detoxification.

Best Practices for Pure Water

You're no doubt aware that we live in a modern postindustrial era in which our water is filled with chemical contaminants from bleach, salts, pesticides, metals, toxins, and drugs, along with biological or microbial contaminants that include bacteria, viruses, protozoans, and parasites, and even radiological contaminants such as cesium, plutonium, and uranium.

So what can you do to ensure you're protecting yourself from contaminants and chemicals in your drinking water, bathwater, and cooking water, while at the same time consuming water that is in the most natural, ancestral, mitochondria-supporting state possible? Here are my top six tips.

1. FILTER YOUR WATER.

When it comes to filtering your water, the gold-standard method is to install a whole-house reverse osmosis (RO) system. RO removes chlorine, inorganic and organic contaminants, about 80 percent of fluoride, and most water disinfectant by-products. For a whole-house system, a tankless RO system (which won't accumulate bacteria) with a compressor is the best option; the companies iSpring, Hydrologic, and Purify Guru all make this system.

Unfortunately, when you use a reverse osmosis system, the good minerals such as calcium, magnesium, and potassium are filtered out along with the bad minerals like fluoride. In addition to depleting your body of precious electrolytes, demineralized water is also more acidic. So to make your water healthy with good minerals once again, and to increase its alkalinity, you can remineralize it with trace liquid mineral drops, use sea salt liberally, make Hunza water (structured water rich in hydrogen and minerals that also has a naturally high pH—you can find instructions for making it on BoundlessBook.com/20), or take a daily shot of a trace liquid minerals supplement.

To transform your RO water into EZ water, you may want to install a whole-house structured water system along with your RO system. The website GreenfieldNaturals.com, owned by my father, Gary Greenfield, has a variety of both whole-house and portable structured-water filters that easily allow you to create your own EZ water (the Hunza water mentioned above is also naturally high in EZ water). A relatively new option for whole-house water filtration called the Hydro Energiser was designed by my father and combines activated carbon with minerals in a highly porous block filter. This unique adsorbent can soak up a variety of organic and inorganic substances, including chlorine and chloramine, which is more difficult to remove. It provides the highest-quality drinking water possible from a carbon block filter and simultaneously structures the water, which enhances both absorption and hydration. You get the best of both worlds—filtration from the carbon and structuring from the minerals all at once.

2. USE FILTERS ON ALL FAUCETS.

If you forgo a whole-house RO system, then at least purchase a countertop RO system and showerhead and faucet filters. In a conversation I had with renowned water expert Robert Slovak, he told me about a reverse osmosis purifier that presents none of the bacteria issues of a standard tank-based RO system, is incredibly affordable, and can be placed on any countertop. Called an AquaTru, it uses a miniaturized version of the same reverse osmosis technology used by all the major bottled-water brands.

I highly recommend you also install a KDF showerhead and faucet or Fixt showerhead filter in your bathroom (after all, if you're filtering the water that goes into your mouth but not the water that comes in through your skin, it's a bit of a wasted effort). You'll find links and discount codes on BoundlessBook.com/20.

3. USE GLASS INSTEAD OF PLASTIC BOTTLES.

This is a no-brainer: just don't use plastic. If you must travel with a plastic bottle or drink from a plastic bottle while exercising, use a BPA-free brand that will also filter your water, such as Berkey, LifeStraw, Fixt, or LifeDefender. This will save you plenty of money on bottled water like Pellegrino and Gerolsteiner, especially while traveling through airports. I also highly recommend stainless steel bottles from a company such as Yeti.

Finally, don't get stuck in a hotel with the average hotel plastic bottled water, and definitely don't pay $8.75 for the glass bottle in the minibar. Instead, do as I do and make your first stop anywhere you go a grocery store where you can grab filtered water in glass bottles.

4. FIND A LOCAL NATURAL SPRING.

If you want to get as close to a natural source of water as possible, visit FindASpring.com to browse through a user-created database of natural springs around the world. You'd be surprised at how much free, mineral-rich, clean spring water flows in an area that's often just a few minutes from your front door. Armed with a glass carboy, you can legally and inexpensively harvest it for drinking or bathing!

5. MAKE SURE YOU GET THE RIGHT MINERALS AND VITAMINS.

Sulfate, cholesterols, and minerals are incredibly important for adequate water absorption. Get sufficient amounts of cobalamin (vitamin B12), glutathione, iron (preferably from grass-fed animal sources), sulfur (from cauliflower, broccoli, garlic, onions, and liver), zinc (shellfish and black ant extract are quite good sources), fresh air, grounding or earthing, and sunlight. Avoid exposure to glyphosate and heavy metals.

6. MANAGE CHLORINE EXPOSURE.

To mitigate the damages of chlorine, especially on days that you're in a chlorinated pool or hot tub, fight the oxidation by getting the following into your body:

- 2 to 5 g of vitamin C
- 2,000 to 4,000 IU of vitamin D
- 10 to 20 IU of a natural source of vitamin E that includes tocotrienols and mixed tocopherols, mixed with omega-3 fatty acids (I recommend Living Fuel SuperEssentials Omega)
- Lots of wild plants, herbs, and spices

Unfortunately, most soaps and shampoos that are designed to strip chlorine from your skin and hair are laden with many endocrine disruptors and dangerous personal care product chemicals. There is one product, SwimSpray, that's a natural, vitamin C–based spray that will remove chlorine odor, but it's not going to stop chlorine from getting absorbed into your body. So the best thing you can do is equip yourself internally to handle the ravages of chlorine. If you need to test your antioxidant levels to see how well equipped your body is to fight chlorine damage, I recommend the Ion Panel with 40 Amino Acids from Genova.

Finally, if you have the luxury of a home pool or a hot tub, treat it with a healthy alternative to chlorine. Several companies make natural minerals and enzymes that can clean water without the use of chlorine. Other options include saline water, filters that include ozonator generators to kill bacteria, non-chlorine shock, and bromine. Many of these options still require trace amounts of chlorine. For example, for my own hot tub, I use an ozone generator and small amounts of non-chlorine shock, but it still needs about 2 tablespoons of chlorine each week to keep it sparkling clean.

I'll admit it: I don't eat organic, completely pesticide-free produce all the time. Sometimes I end up with conventionally grown, pesticide-laden produce. Usually that happens when I'm at a backyard barbecue or a friend's home for dinner, and that spinach salad or handful of cherries just looks so appealing.

But the majority of the time, I buy organic produce (and when I don't, I use a simple vinegar-based cleaning trick I'll tell you about shortly). Many people seem to feel just fine when they eat pesticide-laden produce. This is because you won't necessarily feel the effects immediately after pesticide exposure. In fact, the biggest danger from pesticides is the harm that comes from repeated low-dose exposure.

Recent data collected by the EPA reports that in the US alone, approximately five billion pounds of active pesticide ingredients are applied to our foods annually. That's a tremendous amount of poison entering our bodies, and, sure enough, a 2002 University of Washington study found that 109 out of 110 urban and suburban children had pesticides in their urine samples, which is even scarier when you consider how prevalent pesticide exposure has become since then.

Food grown on certified-organic farms contains significantly less pesticide residue than food grown with synthetic pesticides. That may seem obvious, but the evidence for this fact has only been available since 2002, when research proved that children fed organic food have lower residues of certain pesticides in their bodies than children fed conventionally grown food.

So buy certified-organic produce. And if you really want to make an educated decision and fill your body with the most nourishing and least damaging produce, I recommend you check out the book *Rich Food, Poor Food*. Mira and Jayson Calton have an excellent list of the produce items that tend to be most laden with, not only harmful pesticides, but also GMOs, chemical fertilizers, various synthetic substances, sewage, and irradiation. Following their advice allows you to reduce your pesticide exposure by 80 percent and avoid genetically modified produce 100 percent of the time.

And for that simple vinegar trick I mentioned to remove the pesticides and herbicides from nonorganic produce? Simply mix a solution of ½ cup vinegar and 5 cups water as a bath in your kitchen sink and then briefly place your nonorganic vegetables or fruit in the solution, swish them around, and rinse thoroughly in plain water.

But solving the produce problem doesn't address the entire scenario: you also need to watch out for the pesticides and herbicides in your yard. After all, the average suburban lawn soaks up ten times as much chemical pesticide per acre than conventional farmland, with over seventy million tons of fertilizers and pesticides applied to residential lawns and gardens annually!

I'll admit, I'm not a huge fan of lawns. My wife and I prefer to dig up most of the trimmed, neat grass or sod in the yard and replace it with fruit trees and a big, dirty vegetable garden. But if you do want that pristine expanse of green grass, the only way to reduce your dependence on chemical lawn fertilizers is to develop a healthy lawn that is naturally resistant to weeds, insects, and disease, using the following steps:

1. **Improve the soil.** You can get a lawn pH tester for a few bucks. When you test, it should read between 6.5 and 7.0, which is slightly acidic. Soil that is too acidic needs a sprinkling of lime, and soil that is not acidic enough needs a sprinkling of sulfur.

2. **Choose native grass.** Grasses vary in preferred climate, required water and nutrients, shade tolerance, and the degree of wear they can withstand. Ask your local garden center to recommend grass that is well adapted to your area.

3. **Mow often, but don't trim the grass too short.** Giving your lawn a marine cut is not the best idea because surface roots become exposed, the soil dries out faster, and surface aeration is reduced. Don't cut off more than one-third of the grass at any one time, and shoot for grass that's about 2.5 to 3.5 inches high. When your lawn is finished growing for the season, cut it a bit shorter, to about 2 inches. This will minimize the risk of mold buildup during the winter.

4. **Water deeply, but not too often.** Regular watering encourages your lawn to develop deep root systems, which make the lawn hardier and more drought-resistant. But be sure you let the lawn dry out before rewatering. Most healthy lawns require only 1 inch of water per week, which is about fifteen to twenty minutes' worth of sprinkling once per day. It's best to water in the early morning, when less water will be lost to evaporation.

5. **Use natural lawn fertilizer.** I recommend the Ringer brand, which is a mix of certified-organic minerals.

An excellent resource for more chemical-free yard recommendations is *The Organic Lawn Care Manual* by Paul Tukey. I also highly recommend you flip back to chapter 13 to read about glyphosate and the proper supplements to protect your gut.

THE LAST WORD

Ultimately, you can't do much about invisible assailants like the diesel exhaust getting piped out of the trucks that drive on the roads you run or bicycle on, the chemical-laden disinfectants that gets sprayed on the treadmills and the exercise equipment at the gym, the pesticides and herbicides that litter the grass at a public park, your neighbor's WiFi signals, or street lights and bright headlights of oncoming cars.

But there is plenty that you *can* control, and now you're equipped with what you need to know to maximize your protection against modern invisible assailants and ensure that electricity, air, light, and water are fully optimized in your environment, without having to go completely off-grid or to move to a pristine Himalayan mountaintop.

Perhaps your head is spinning with all your newfound knowledge about the dizzying array of steps you can take. But don't let that stress you out. Start with the small steps, like these:

- Install Greenwave or Stetzer dirty-electricity filters in every room of your house.
- Buy an air tube headset and DefenderShield case for your phone, and keep it in airplane mode when you don't need to have it on.
- Turn off your WiFi router when you aren't using it, or hardwire in with an ethernet cable.
- Replace your regular water bottles with glass jars or BPA-free plastic bottles.
- Begin to glance at the labels of your personal care products and household cleaners and understand what you're smearing on your body, your desk, or your countertop.
- If you need a fast air and water solution, buy an AirDoctor HEPA filter and an AquaTru water purifier, and if you want a more permanent solution, install a whole-house reverse osmosis filter and central HEPA air filter in your home.
- Purchase and use a set of blue-light-blocking glasses and switch your phone to red light at night.

ONE THING YOU CAN DO THIS WEEK

This week, do an experiment to see how little you can use artificial light. Sunlight? Fine. Candles? Check. Have a fireplace in your living room? Great. A real paper book at night instead of the phone or Kindle? Perfect. Forgoing switching on the kitchen lights in the morning and instead making coffee in the dim morning light? That counts too. Grow accustomed to less light and see what happens to your sleep cycles. I suspect you'll be pleasantly surprised.

> For citations for all the research studies mentioned in this chapter and a deeper dive into the topics of this chapter—including links to podcasts, blog posts, recommended tools and supplements, and much more—visit BoundlessBook.com/20.

ROUTINES AND RITUALS

A PLAN FOR YOUR PERFECT DAY

I stared out the window at the doe gently padding its way from the tree line of the forest and across my driveway. It stopped and glanced in my direction. Could it possibly hear the loud buzzing emanating from the modified car buffer I was massaging my head with as I stood barefoot in the kitchen, staring off into the wilderness behind my home? As the doe crossed the driveway and entered the trees on the other side, I moved the car buffer from the right side of my skull to the left, the rapid vibrations gently digging into the tight craniosacral muscles at the back of my head.

Why such a strange morning habit? It improves the blood flow to my skull, provides a bit of a wake-me-up buzz for my head, and lowers my blood pressure and stress for the entire remainder of the day by relaxing my neck and trapezius muscles. But my morning routine is not limited to applying a car buffer to my head. Indeed, my entire day spanning into the afternoon and evening is rife with elaborate routine.

Why? Consider just a few brief snippets of the daily routines of a handful of successful pop culture, historical, and political icons, all from the book *Daily Rituals: How Artists Work*:

Secretary of state and president John Quincy Adams skinny-dipped in the Potomac River in the morning, always trying to see how long he could swim without touching the bottom (he got up to 80 minutes before his wife told him to stop).

After putting his kids to bed, President Obama goes over briefing papers and does paperwork, and then reads a book for pleasure for a half hour before turning in.

Stephen King writes every day of the year without exception, beginning work between 8:00 and 8:30 a.m. He has a glass of water or cup of tea and takes a vitamin pill each day, ensuring he is in the same seat and his papers and desk are arranged in the same way every single day. King has a daily writing quota of two thousand words and rarely allows himself to quit until he's reached his goal.

The 31-year-old Harvard dropout and founder of Facebook, Mark Zuckerberg, is well known for almost always wearing a plain gray T-shirt, saying in a 2014 interview that wearing the same shirt helps allow him to make as few decisions as possible.

I don't know any successful people who do not have some kind of structured and occasionally elaborate daily routine. The book quoted above, *Daily Rituals*, notes that novelist Franz Kafka, frustrated with his living quarters and day job, wrote in a letter to his fiancée Felice Bauer in 1912, "Time is short, my strength is limited, the office is a horror, the apartment is noisy, and if a pleasant, straightforward life is not possible then one must try to wriggle through by subtle maneuvers."

Kafka is just one of the 161 great minds profiled in the book. These novelists, poets, playwrights, painters, philosophers, scientists, and mathematicians all had daily rituals (often automated and slightly subconscious), such as waking early or staying up late; self-medicating with a morning doughnut or a hot bath; drinking vast quantities of coffee (it is said the philosopher Voltaire consumed forty to fifty cups per day); or taking long daily walks. Novelist Thomas Wolfe, for instance, wrote standing up in the kitchen, the top of the refrigerator as his desk, dreamily fondling his male configurations (and you thought my infrared-light-on-the-balls trick was strange!). Philosopher Jean-Paul Sartre ingested ten times the recommended dose of corydrane (a mix of amphetamine and aspirin) each day. Philosopher René Descartes preferred to linger in bed, his mind wandering in sleep through woods, gardens, and enchanted palaces where he experienced every pleasure imaginable. British author Anthony Trollope made himself write three thousand words each morning (precisely 250 words every fifteen minutes for three hours) before going off to his job at the postal service, which he kept for thirty-three years, during which he wrote more than two dozen books. Choreographer George Balanchine did most of his work while ironing, and composer and pianist George Gershwin worked for twelve hours a day from late morning to midnight, composing at the piano in pajamas, a bathrobe, and slippers.

While I don't necessarily endorse beginning each morning with a doughnut or spending the entirety of your waking hours lingering in bed for enhanced productivity, I do know this for a fact: not only does a daily routine give structure and efficiency to each day, but it also gives you something to fall back on and depend on in times of stress. Routine serves as a fantastic source of comfort, peace, and relaxation when life gets moving fast or becomes difficult.

In this book, I've presented countless ways to optimize your mind, body, and spirit, with tools, supplements, dietary hacks, exercises, regular practices, and much more. I cannot recommend highly enough that you pick the suggestions that work best for you and systematize them into daily, weekly, monthly, and yearly routines. You'll find my routines, as well as more advice for creating your own, on BoundlessBook.com, and in the rest of this chapter I'll provide done-for-you exercise, diet, and supplement programs that you can use or adapt as you like.

THE BOUNDLESS WEEKLY PROGRAMS

These programs for exercise, diet, and supplements weave a host of the principles, habits, and guidelines in this book into a single week of living, moving, and eating. While they don't necessarily include every single boundless biohack, supplement, trick, tool, and tactic, they will allow you to easily develop a rock-solid foundation that you can build upon with additional strategies if you see fit.

Each program includes beginner, intermediate, and advanced options so that you can take as deep a dive into a boundless life as you'd like. Enjoy!

BOUNDLESS EXERCISE PROGRAM

In chapter 10, I gave you a glimpse into an ideal exercise program that targets all vital components of your fitness. In this section, you'll discover how those same concepts can be adjusted and customized to your specific time availability and fitness goals.

The beginner program below will give you maximum results with the absolute minimum effective dose of exercise. The intermediate program includes elements that further enhance sports performance, mobility, fat loss, and muscle maintenance or muscle gain. The advanced program is designed to give you the best body possible and can be used by athletes and hard-charging high achievers who are preparing for a more intense event, such a triathlon, marathon, obstacle race, or other serious sporting endeavor.

If you don't know how to do an exercise, then look it up on YouTube. Most of these exercises are quite common and can be found there.

Daily Habits

15 MINUTES OF MORNING MOVEMENT

Beginner: Walk for 15 minutes, preferably in the sunshine.

Intermediate: Perform one or a combination of the following exercises for a total of 15 minutes.

- Yoga: Warrior poses and Sun Salutations (there's a good routine on BoundlessBook.com/21)
- ELDOA stretches (see chapter 17)
- Foam rolling and deep tissue work on any sore or tight areas (see chapter 17)
- Sunshine walk with deep nasal breathing and box breathing (see chapter 3)
- Mini-trampoline rebounding or time on a vibration platform (see chapters 11 and 12)
- Foundation Training (see chapter 17). You're going to need the excellent book *True to Form* by Dr. Eric Goodman to do this properly (or the Foundation Training app for your phone).

Try to avoid music, podcasts, or audiobooks during this time and instead focus on silence, breathing, and meditation.

Advanced: Choose from any of the intermediate routines. On as many days as possible, either later in the morning or immediately after this routine, if time permits, perform 20–30 minutes of fasted, aerobic cardio, such as an easy walk in the sunshine, a yoga routine, sauna, hot-cold contrast, a swim, or a bike ride. Preferably finish with a 2-to-5-minute cold shower. If time does not permit for this in the morning, instead do a 20-to-30-minute evening pre- or post-dinner walk.

Tabata Set

Warm up for 2–5 minutes, then complete 8 sets of 20 seconds of a single exercise (burpees, jumping jacks, mountain climbers, kettlebell swings, squats, treadmill, bike, rowing machine—you choose), with 10 seconds of rest after each 20-second effort. Go at your all-out, maximum-intensity pace for every 20-second effort. Cool down for 5–10 minutes after 8 sets.

LOW-LEVEL PHYSICAL ACTIVITY THROUGHOUT THE DAY

Beginner: If you work indoors, use a standing or treadmill workstation. Walk and use the stairs as much as possible everywhere you go.

Intermediate: Adopt the beginner protocol, but stop every hour for 100 jumping jacks.

Advanced: Continue the beginner and intermediate protocols, but throughout the entire day, every 30–60 minutes, take quick stops or Pomodoro-esque breaks for burpees, kettlebell swings, jumping jacks, high-knees running, stairs, mountain-climbers, mini-trampoline jumping, vibration platform work, or 1-to-2-minute bursts of any other quick, explosive activity. In addition, on any three days of the week, slip away and perform a single Tabata set (see the box at left).

Finally, during any of the day's activities, try to practice hypoxia. For example, during the rebounding session, you could hold your breath for the first 15 seconds of every minute. Or during the sauna or yoga, you could hold your breath during certain movements. You can even practice breath-holds during the last few reps of a weight-training exercise. In addition, during every activity you do in this program, unless absolutely necessary (for instance, you are gasping for breath or getting light-headed), attempt to only breathe through your nose using abdominal belly breathing.

Monday

SUPER-SLOW STRENGTH

This routine is ideally performed in the late afternoon or early evening, at least three hours prior to bedtime.

Beginner: Warm up with 5–10 minutes of aerobic exercise. Complete each of the following exercises very slowly, with an 8-to-10-second count up and an 8-to-10-second count down. Focus on keeping your muscles tight and tense for each rep, and do not rest between reps but instead maintain constant muscle tension. Complete a single round of the entire circuit. Each exercise should be completed as one single set to complete failure.

Each exercise should take you a minimum of 90 seconds and ideally 2 to 2½ minutes to complete:

- Machine chest press (or dumbbell chest press, push-up, or other horizontal pushing variation)
- Machine pull-down (or pull-up, assisted pull-up, or other vertical pulling variation)
- Machine shoulder press (or dumbbell shoulder press, handstand push-up, or other vertical pushing variation)

- Machine seated row (or cable row, bent-over dumbbell row, or other horizontal pulling variation)
- Leg press (or squat, goblet squat, dumbbell squat, or other squatting or lunging variation)

Intermediate: Warm up with one or two sets of 3–6 fast, explosive reps for each exercise in the beginner routine, and finish each of the super-slow sets with as many fast, explosive, partial-range reps as you can complete.

Advanced: Warm up for 5–10 minutes, preferably with a gymnastics routine, Animal Flow, a Foundation Training routine, or anything else that dynamically prepares the body for movement and elevates the heart rate. Next, from the list of Strength exercises on page 602, choose one upper-body push, one lower-body push, one upper-body pull, one lower-body pull, and one full-body move. Pair that exercise with one exercise from the Core & Mobility list on the same page.

Gradually adding weight and decreasing repetitions or maintaining repetitions with each strength set (as long as you keep good form), complete 3–8 repetitions of the upper-body push exercise in a slow, controlled fashion. Next, complete 10–20 repetitions of a Core & Mobility movement of your choice (for active recovery), preferably one that does not exhaust or work the same muscles that you used during your strength set.

Then return to the Strength set, do another set of the same exercise, and follow it up with the same Core & Mobility exercise. Repeat until you have completed 3–5 sets of both the Strength move and the Core & Mobility move, and then move on to the lower-body push. Continue this pattern until you have finished all movement categories: upper-body push, lower-body push, upper-body pull, lower-body pull, and full-body move.

Cool down with deep breathing, box breathing, sauna, walking, or any of the easier movements programmed for the day.

HOT AND COLD

Beginner: Take a hot-cold contrast shower in the morning and/or evening, alternating 20 seconds of cold water and 10 seconds of hot water. Ensure the water touches all parts of your body during the shower, particularly the armpits, insides of the thighs, face, head, and other areas of high blood flow.

Intermediate: Take a hot-cold contrast shower and do the following routine if time permits:

- Spend 15–30 minutes in a dry sauna or infrared sauna. Stay in at least long enough to begin sweating, and ideally long enough that you begin to get uncomfortably hot.
- Take a 2–5 minute cold shower, cold soak, or easy cold-water swim (55 degrees Fahrenheit or less).

Advanced: Exercise in the sauna if possible. It is okay to kill two birds with one stone and do any of the day's sessions in the sauna (such as Foundation Training, mobility, or meditation) or to do yoga or detox strategies such as dry skin brushing in the sauna. You can also simply read, breathe, and relax. Just stay away from phones, WiFi, Bluetooth, and other forms of EMF.

Other techniques that are good for the sauna or pool (just be careful and responsible!) are resisted breathwork, restricted breathwork, breathing exercises, and breath-holds. Optionally, either in the sauna or after your shower, complete a full-body dry skin brush (this should take 2–5 minutes).

Finally, consider using Cool Fat Burner or Cool Gut Buster cold thermogenesis gear for 20–60 minutes at some point during the day. Or, if you have more time, you can lie on your back in the sauna and do the full 60-minute holotropic breathwork routine found in week 3 of Niraj Naik's SOMA breath routine (there's a link on BoundlessBook.com/21).

Strength Exercises

You can substitute kegs, logs, rocks, kettlebells, and sandbags for most of these Strength moves if you'd rather train outdoors or strongman-style (see Zach Even-Esh's *The Encyclopedia of Underground Strength and Conditioning* for good examples).

UPPER-BODY PUSH

- Machine chest press
- Barbell or dumbbell bench press
- Incline barbell or dumbbell bench press
- Standing overhead press
- Standing cable press
- Loaded push-up with weighted vest, or super-slow push-up with body weight

UPPER-BODY PULL

- Machine pull-down
- Bent barbell or dumbbell row
- Weighted or super-slow pull-up
- Weighted or super-slow horizontal pull-up
- Fast single-arm cable or dumbbell row
- Lat pull-downs
- Seated row

FULL-BODY MOVES*

- Man Maker
- Turkish get-up
- Bear complex (power clean, front squat, push press, back squat, and second push press)
- Dead lift to overhead press
- Overhead squat

* Get more excellent full-body complexes at BenGreenfieldFitness.com/complexes.

LOWER-BODY PUSH

- Leg press
- Barbell squat
- Goblet squat
- Front squat
- Single-leg squat
- Front lunge
- Reverse lunge
- Barbell or dumbbell step-ups

LOWER-BODY PULL

- Back extension machine
- Dead lift
- Suitcase dead lift
- Romanian dead lift
- Hexbar dead lift

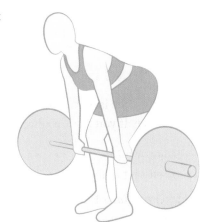

Core & Mobility Moves

- Torso twists
- Cat/cow
- Birddogs (opposite arm-leg extensions)
- Yoga Sun Salutation series
- Banded side-to-side walks

- Mountain climbers
- Foam rolling
- Bridging
- Banded side-walks
- Lunging mobility exercises

For more excellent ideas, see BoundlessBook.com/21.

Tuesday

FUNCTIONAL FITNESS

This routine is ideally performed late afternoon or early evening, at least three hours prior to bedtime. If you don't have time to do it on Tuesday, do it on Thursday instead.

Beginner: Perform the 7-minute workout from chapter 12. If time permits, attempt to do 2–3 rounds. Use good form on every exercise and move as quickly and explosively as possible!

Intermediate: Perform 2–3 rounds of the 7-minute workout. If possible, use blood-flow restriction or Kaatsu bands on both arms and legs. Start or finish this routine with a mitochondrial training set of 4 rounds of 30–60 seconds of all-out effort followed by 4 minutes of active recovery using any bodyweight or cardio movement, such as bicycle, treadmill, elliptical, or rowing (you can also perform this at a different time of day).

Advanced: Perform the intermediate routine above, or, along with the mitochondrial training set above, perform the full-body kettlebell training routine at right.

Wednesday

MORNING DETOX SESSION

This routine is ideally performed late afternoon or early evening, at least three hours prior to bedtime. If you don't have time to do it on Tuesday, do it on Thursday instead.

Beginner: Do 5–15 minutes of tai chi shaking (google it!), rebounding on a mini trampoline, or vibration platform work.

Intermediate: Do a clay mask (see chapter 17). While the mask dries, do 5–15 minutes of rebounding on a mini trampoline or standing on a vibration platform. Rinse off the mask, then move to the sauna for 20–30 minutes. While in the sauna, do full-body dry skin brushing and any yoga movements or other stretching movements that feel good. Finish with a 2-to-5-minute cold shower or cold soak. Dry off, then apply topical magnesium to all joints and any sore spots, or take a warm magnesium salt bath later in the day.

Advanced: Do a clay mask (see chapter 17). While the mask dries, do 5–15 minutes of rebounding on a mini trampoline or standing on a vibration platform. Next, perform a coffee enema (a link to instructions is on BoundlessBook.com/21). Rinse off the mask, then move to the sauna for 20–30 minutes. While in the sauna, do full-body dry skin brushing and any yoga movements or other stretching movements that feel good. Finish with a 2-to-5-minute cold shower or cold soak. Dry off, then apply topical magnesium to all joints and any sore spots, or take a warm magnesium salt bath later in the day.

Full-Body Kettlebell Training

Do 3–5 rounds of the following:

- 5 Turkish get-ups per side
- 30 swings, split into 3 sets of 10 with 10 seconds' rest between each set
- 5 goblet squats
- 30 snatches per side, split into 3 sets of 10 with 10 seconds' rest between each set
- 5 bottoms-up presses per side
- 60 seconds of walking with two kettlebells "racked" on your chest or held farmer's carry–style at your side

Ideally, use hypoxia during the 30-to-60-second hard cardio mitochondrial efforts, such as a Training Mask or LiveO2.

CROSS-TRAIN! ACTIVITY OF CHOICE

Beginner, Intermediate, and Advanced: Today is your free day to engage in a hobby of your choice and a chance to challenge both your brain and body at the same time. If you're sore or beat up, try something like an easy paddleboarding session, a new yoga class, hiking on a new trail, frisbee golf, or regular golf. For more of a challenge, try tennis, basketball, ultimate frisbee, soccer, kickboxing, or jujitsu.

Just don't beat yourself up too much: Thursday and Friday are both relatively physically intense. If you do want to perform a more structured workout, do the Functional Movement / Animal Flow routine at the bottom of this page.

BRAIN TRAINING

Beginner, Intermediate, and Advanced: At any time of day, choose any new skill or hobby, or an existing skill or hobby for which you are learning a new technique—for example, you could cook a new recipe, play a new board or card game, play the guitar, ukulele, harmonica, piano, or any other musical instrument, or create a watercolor or oil painting. Anything on your bucket list for learning counts. You can also use any of the tools, biohacks, or brain aerobics exercises discussed in chapter 6.

Thursday

HOT AND COLD

Beginner, Intermediate, and Advanced: Spend 10–30 minutes in a dry sauna, steam sauna, or (preferably) an infrared sauna. Stay in at least long enough to begin sweating, and preferably long enough that you begin to get uncomfortably hot.

It is okay to kill two birds with one stone and do any of the day's sessions in the sauna, such as Foundation, mobility, or meditation, or to do yoga or a brief workout. You can also simply read, breathe, and relax. Just stay away from phones, WiFi, Bluetooth, and other forms of EMF.

Finish this sauna session with a 2-to-5-minute cold shower, soak in a cold bath or cold pool, or any other cold thermogenesis activity.

Functional Movement / Animal Flow

This workout is flexible but needs to be primarily bodyweight and functional and should include elements such as crawling, carrying, lunging, hanging, traversing, and swimming. Total workout time is 30–60 minutes. Examples of workouts include these:

1. Riding your bike to a river or lake to go for a swim

2. Completing a bodyweight or functional CrossFit WOD like "Fat Amy"

3. Walking briskly on a nature trail and stopping at park benches or other areas for dips, push-ups, squats, hanging from tree branches, pull-ups, etc.

4. Doing a circuit like the following:

   - Farmer walk—20 meters
   - Bear crawl—10 meters
   - 60-second asymmetrical carry (like carrying two heavy objects of different weights farmer's carry-style); swap sides at the 30-second mark
   - Frogger—10 meters
   - Overhead walk—single hand, swapping hands at the 10-meter mark
   - Duck—10 meters

   Repeat for five total rounds.

You get the idea! This is your chance to mix things up and try new moves. The only rules: don't lift heavy, and make it fun and functional.

Warm up for 5–10 minutes, preferably with a gymnastics routine, Animal Flow, a Foundation routine, or anything else that dynamically prepares the body for movement and elevates the heart rate.

Next, from the Strength list on page 602, choose one upper-body push, one lower-body push, one upper-body pull, and one lower-body pull, and choose one core/carry/move exercise from the list on page 606. Pair each exercise with one exercise from the Power list on page 607 that falls into that same movement category.

Gradually adding weight and decreasing repetitions or maintaining repetitions with each strength set (as long as you keep good form), complete 3–8 repetitions of the upper-body push exercise in a slow, controlled fashion. Next, complete 3–8 repetitions of the corresponding upper-body push Power movement as quickly and explosively as possible. If the Power move is a carry (like a fast farmer's carry), then rather than completing a certain number of repetitions, complete 20–30 seconds as quickly and explosively as possible.

Then recover for 2–3 minutes. During your recovery period, you can walk, do more mobility exercises, do foam rolling, dance, or do anything else you want that doesn't exhaust those same muscle groups. Then repeat the Strength exercise and the subsequent Power exercise. Continue this scenario until you have completed 3–5 sets of both the Strength move and the Power move, and then move on to the next movement category. Continue this pattern until you have finished all movement categories.

Cool down with deep breathing, box breathing, time in a sauna, walking, or any of the easier movements programmed for the day.

VO$_2$ MAX TRAINING

Beginner: Complete 4 rounds of 4 minutes of intense intervals (the maximum sustainable pace that you can maintain without your form suffering) with 4 minutes of easy aerobic active-recovery sessions between each round. The mode of exercise is your choice and can include a bike, treadmill, rowing machine, swimming, elliptical trainer, or running outdoors.

Intermediate: Do the beginner workout, but for the first 2 rounds, wear a Training Mask during the work efforts, and for the next 2 rounds, wear a Training Mask during the recovery efforts.

Advanced: Do the intermediate workout, or use a LiveO2 trainer set at hyperoxia for the first 2 rounds of work efforts and hypoxia for recovery efforts, and set at hypoxia for the next 2 rounds of work efforts and hyperoxia for recovery efforts.

Friday

SUPER-SLOW STRENGTH

Beginner and Intermediate: Repeat Monday's routine.

Advanced: Repeat Monday's routine. Alternatively, perform the complex sets routine at the top of this page.

Strength Core/Carry/Move Exercises

- Walking dumbbell lunge
- Walking overhead dumbbell lunge
- Farmer's walk
- Incline sit-up
- Incline sit-up with rotation
- Any version of a knee-up, V-up, or get-up
- Any version of a hanging bent- or straight-leg raise
- Reverse hyperextension
- Slow torso twists
- Turkish get-ups

Saturday

FOAM ROLLER OR MASSAGE

Beginner: Get a 30-to-90-minute full-body massage.

Intermediate: Get a 30-to-90-minute full-body massage, if possible while lying on some type of PEMF or earthing device (such as a Biomat, BodyBalance PEMF mat, or Pulse Center's Pulse XL Pro table) and while listening to Michael Tyrell's sound healing tracks.

Advanced: Get the same intermediate massage or do the full-body foam-roller workout described in chapter 12. I highly recommend the RumbleRoller and Training Mask for this routine to spice things up a bit more. Bonus points for doing this in a dry or infrared sauna.

ADVENTURE OF CHOICE

Beginner, Intermediate, and Advanced: Choose your own adventure, preferably outdoors. It can be, for example, hiking, skiing, snowboarding, road cycling, mountain biking, or playing on an obstacle course. Don't make this too epic in terms of physical intensity but instead use it as an opportunity for nature therapy, challenging your brain, and doing something novel. This can last anywhere from 45 minutes to 3 hours. For an added fat-burning effect, perform this workout in a fasted state.

Sunday

SOCIAL SPORT

Beginner, Intermediate, and Advanced: Choose any sport or activity that allows you to be with other people, such as badminton, volleyball, tennis, frisbee golf, golf, or a group exercise class. Use Meetup.com if you find it helpful.

BRAIN TRAINING

Beginner, Intermediate, and Advanced: At any time of day, choose any new skill or hobby, or an existing skill or hobby for which you are learning a new technique—for example, you could cook a new recipe, play a new board or card game, play the guitar, ukulele, harmonica, piano, or any other musical instrument, or create a watercolor or oil painting. Anything on your bucket list for learning counts. You can also use any of the tools, biohacks, or brain aerobics exercises discussed in chapter 6.

Power Exercises

UPPER-BODY PUSH

- Overhead push press
- Explosive or clap push-up
- Medicine ball chest throw or overhead throw
- Snatch
- Burpees

UPPER-BODY PULL

- Jumping pull-up
- Explosive horizontal pull-up
- Battle rope
- Fast single-arm cable or dumbbell row
- Muscle-ups

LOWER-BODY PUSH

- Jump squat
- Lunge jumps
- Explosive step-ups

LOWER-BODY PULL

- Power clean
- Hang clean
- Clean and jerk
- Kettlebell swing
- Medicine ball slam

CORE/CARRY/MOVE

- Lunge jumps
- Box jumps
- Fast farmer's walk
- Sled push
- Explosive stair climbs
- Explosive torso twists
- Medicine ball side throw
- Rowing machine
- Bicycle
- Treadmill or another sprint
- Banded side-to-side walks
- Mountain climbers
- Burpees
- Muscle-ups

HOT AND COLD

Beginner: Take a hot-cold contrast shower in the morning and evening, alternating between 20 seconds of cold water and 10 seconds of hot water. Try to ensure the water touches all parts of your body during the shower, particularly the armpits, inside of thighs, face, head, and other areas of high blood flow.

Intermediate: Take a hot-cold contrast shower and do the following routine if time permits:

- Spend 15–30 minutes in a dry sauna or infrared sauna. Stay in at least long enough to begin sweating, and preferably long enough that you begin to get uncomfortably hot.
- Take a 2-to-5-minute cold shower, cold soak, or easy cold-water swim (55 degrees Fahrenheit or less).

Advanced: Exercise in the sauna if possible. It is okay to kill two birds with one stone and do any of the day's sessions in the sauna (such as Foundation Training, mobility, or meditation) or to do yoga in the sauna. You can also simply read, breathe, and relax. Just stay away from phones, WiFi, Bluetooth, and other forms of EMF.

Other techniques that are good for the sauna or pool (just be careful and responsible!) are resisted breathwork, restricted breathwork, breathing exercises, and breath-holds. Optionally, either in the sauna or after your shower, complete a full-body dry skin brush (this should take 2–5 minutes).

Finally, consider using Cool Fat Burner or Cool Gut Buster cold thermogenesis gear for 20–60 minutes at some point during the day. Or, if you have more time, you can lie on your back in the sauna and do the full 60-minute holotropic breathwork routine found in week 3 of Niraj Naik's SOMA breath routine (there's a link on BoundlessBook.com/21).

A Note for Athletes

While the program described above will develop excellent athletic, full-body functional fitness, if you are a serious athlete who is looking for a program specifically designed for sports performance, I highly recommend you read my book *Beyond Training: Mastering Endurance, Health & Life* (BeyondTrainingBook.com), which includes several programs specifically tailored to athletes.

THE BOUNDLESS DIET

There are a host of diets out there that are designed to optimize health, and which works best for you depends entirely on your biochemical individuality. Here, I've compiled the best of the best of these diets and grouped them into beginner, intermediate, and advanced categories based on a trajectory from a very clean and somewhat restrictive reset diet to a more liberal eating plan with a larger selection of foods, and finally to a widely varied diet that's easy to sustain for life. In other words, unlike in the exercise program, the beginner, intermediate, and advanced categories have nothing to do with how difficult a diet is; it's all about taking you from a standard American diet to a more ancestral, health-optimizing, widely varied way of eating.

For each diet, I've listed test results and symptoms that may make the diet the right one for you, and I've provided a sample week of meals for each. If you've read chapters 13 and 14 and done much of the self-quantification from chapter 16, you are already equipped with most of the information you need to customize your diet, but if you're looking for something "done-for-you," the protocols below will give you plenty to work with.

No matter which diet you decide to pursue, make sure you adhere to the following principles:

- Incorporate regular intermittent fasts or longer fasting periods.
- Ruthlessly eliminate inflammatory foods and control glycemic variability.
- Rather than engaging in long-term calorie and carbohydrate restriction, occasionally refeed your body with adequate calories and carbohydrates.
- Occasionally engage in periods of more intense detoxification.
- Whenever given the option between real food and packaged or processed food, choose the former.
- Eat a very wide variety of multicolored plants, herbs, and spices.
- Whenever possible, choose clean, organic, wild, non-GMO foods and ingredients.
- Whenever possible, eat locally grown in-season foods.
- Review the longevity tips in chapter 19 and incorporate those principles into your diet as often as possible.

Beginner

The diets in this section are extremely clean eating protocols designed to reboot and reset your entire body, especially the gut. These are somewhat restrictive plans that I do not necessarily recommend following for life, unless you have a serious condition such as celiac or Crohn's disease or severe food allergies.

If you've been eating a diet or living a lifestyle that has caused gut damage, inflammation, sugar dependency, or similar gut problems, I recommend that you follow any of the diets in this section for a minimum of four to eight weeks prior to progressing to an intermediate plan. If you have more serious gut issues, autoimmune symptoms, or a condition like dysbiosis, stick to this type of diet until symptoms subside, which can take three to six months (in the case of the GAPS diet, it is recommended that you follow it for up to two years to fully heal a leaky gut). If you need to detox or cleanse at any point throughout the year, you can return to these diets—for example, you can perform a one-to-two-week liver cleanse in the spring and winter or follow an Elemental Diet for the first thirty days of each year.

Rather than simply recommending one single diet—which you know from chapter 14 is a flawed approach—I'm instead equipping you with a number of diets that you can use to heal your gut, ease digestion, detox your body, and prepare your digestive system for more variety.

AUTOIMMUNE PALEO DIET (AIP)

Also known as the Paleo autoimmune protocol, the AIP diet is a much stricter version of the Paleo diet (which is based on meat, fish, vegetables, nuts, and seeds). It eliminates dairy, grains, eggs, nightshades, legumes, and other foods that may cause inflammation in people with a leaky gut. As explained in chapter 13, leaky gut can lead to an autoimmune response in which your own immune system tags your tissues, such as your eyes or your nervous system, with certain types of antibodies, including those listed in the table on page 610. This falsely signals to your immune system that those tissues are foreign invaders, and your immune system then attacks those tissues. Each autoimmune disease also has markers specific to that condition, and BoundlessBook.com/21 includes more information on which antibodies are specific to which diseases. By focusing on nutrient-rich foods and avoiding inflammatory ones, the AIP diet aims to heal inflammation and any holes in the gut.

People who follow the AIP diet should typically follow it strictly for four to eight weeks and then slowly reintroduce foods that they have been avoiding. I recommend following this plan if you've completed any food allergy panels such as Cyrex's and discovered that you have sensitivities to wheat, soy, gluten, dairy, or eggs, or if you've tested your gut and know you have inflammation. It's a good choice if you have any of the indicators of autoimmunity listed in the table. The best book to accompany this diet is *The Autoimmune Paleo Cookbook* by Mickey Trescott. After you've spent at least four to eight weeks on one of the diets in this section, the Wahls Protocol (outlined in the intermediate section later in this section) is also an excellent diet for managing autoimmunity.

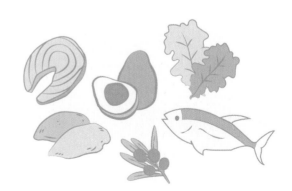

You may want to follow this diet if you have...

	MARKERS	TESTS
Blood	• Sm/RNP antibodies (Smith/ribonucleoprotein) • SS-A and SS-B antibodies (Sjogren's-syndrome-related antigens A and B) • Scl-70 antibodies (scleroderma-70) • Jo-1 antibodies (John P.-1) • centromere B antibodies • ribosomal P antibodies • high aluminum	You can order autoimmune blood tests online through Quest Diagnostics, such as their Inflammatory Bowel Disease Differentiation Panel, ANCA Screen, and Lactoferrin Quantitative Immunoassay.
Urine	• proteinuria (high protein levels in urine) • hematuria (blood in urine, which may or may not be visibly detectable) • active sediment (red or white blood cell casts in urine)	You can ask your doctor or medical provider to perform a urinalysis that includes these markers, or order the Urinalysis, Complete with Microscopic Examination online through DirectLabs. An Intestinal Permeability (Leaky Gut) Kit by Genova can indicate whether you have a leaky gut.
Stool	• calprotectin (a protein released by neutrophils that can indicate inflammation) • imbalances in gut microbiota (research suggests that commensal bacteria can play a role in the pathology of autoimmune diseases)	You can request a calprotectin stool test from your doctor or medical provider as well as a comprehensive stool analysis to analyze gut levels of commensal bacteria. You can also order a comprehensive stool analysis through labs such as the Great Plains Laboratory and Genova Diagnostics.
Genes	There are over 1,000 gene variants associated with susceptibility to autoimmunity, but important ones to look at or ask your medical practitioner about are these: • AIRE • FOXP3 • FAS • PI3K • CTLA4 • CD25 deficiency • STAT3 and STAT1 gain-of-function • IL-10 deficiency • STING gain-of-function • PLCG2 gain-of-function	You can order a genetic test through 23andMe, then upload your raw data into a genetic analysis tool like StrateGene, Genetic Genie, FoundMyFitness, or MyHeritage. You can also get a more comprehensive analysis through services such as Bob Miller's TreeOfLife, The DNA Company, or Health Nucleus.
Symptoms	• inflammation • fatigue • muscle aches • difficulty concentrating • hair loss • rashes	

A Sample Day of the AIP Diet

For detailed recipes, instructions, and layout of the meal plan, visit BoundlessBook.com/21.

BREAKFAST	LUNCH	DINNER	SNACK
Go Greenfields Mint Smoothie Bowl	Tuscan Pesto Chicken Skillet	Black Sesame Seared Tuna with Wasabi Citrus Aioli	Blueberry Pie Energy Balls

SPECIFIC CARBOHYDRATE DIET (SCD)

The specific carbohydrate diet (SCD) was first described by Sidney V. Haas in 1924 as a way to treat celiac disease and was further refined in the 1951 medical textbook *The Management of Celiac Disease*. It was later repopularized in 1987 by Elaine Gottschall, the mother of one of Haas's patients.

The SCD is a gluten-free and grain-free diet and was a popular treatment for celiac disease decades before gluten was even discovered. I recommend you follow this plan if you have IBD, IBS, bloating, gas, or gut inflammation, particularly if these issues are brought on by gluten or grain consumption. It's a good choice if you have any of the indicators of inflammation and celiac disease listed in the table. The best book to accompany the SCD program is *Breaking the Vicious Cycle* by Elaine Gottschall.

You may want to follow this diet if you have...

	MARKERS		TESTS
Blood	• autoantibodies • tissue transglutaminase antibodies • total serum IgA (immunoglobulin A)		You can order a blood test that checks for these markers through your physician. If you prefer to order them yourself online, DirectLabs offers tests for tissue transglutaminase and IgA, and Quest Diagnostics offers tests for tissue transglutaminase and total IgA.
Urine	• red urine • proteinuria • hematuria		The Urinalysis, Complete with Microscopic Examination from DirectLabs can determine proteinuria and hematuria, and you can typically determine whether your urine is red just by looking at it. Red urine is frequently caused by hematuria. An Intestinal Permeability (Leaky Gut) Kit by Genova can indicate whether you have a leaky gut.
Stool	• foul-smelling stool • fatty stool • diarrhea		These markers are pretty obvious (fatty stool is indicated by excess bulk and a pale, oily appearance, and often coincides with a particularly awful odor), but you can also order a stool test through labs like Great Plains Laboratory and Genova Diagnostics.
Genes	• HLA-DQ2 • HLA-DQ8		You can order a genetic test through 23andMe, then upload your raw data into a genetic analysis tool like StrateGene, Genetic Genie, FoundMyFitness, or MyHeritage. You can also get a more comprehensive analysis through services such as Bob Miller's TreeOfLife, The DNA Company, or Health Nucleus.
Symptoms	• abdominal discomfort • bloating • gas • gastritis • skin rashes	• nausea • vomiting • nerve damage (manifesting as nerve tingling) • fluid retention • fatigue	

A Sample Day of the SCD

For detailed recipes, instructions, and layout of the meal plan, visit BoundlessBook.com/21.

BREAKFAST	LUNCH	DINNER	SNACK
Asparagus, Tomato & Fontina Frittata	Slammin' Salmon Burgers	Ginger-Spiced Chicken Skewers	Paleo Pumpkin Chia Pudding

GUT AND PSYCHOLOGY SYNDROME (GAPS) DIET

Dr. Natasha Campbell-McBride, a neurologist and nutritionist, developed the GAPS diet based on the SCD; like the SCD, it removes potentially problematic foods, particularly grains and gluten-containing foods, but it also focuses on adding healing, nutrient-dense foods.

If you have cognitive issues, irritation, brain fog, or nervous system–based problems affected by the gut, such as ADD/ADHD, this is a good diet to follow. It's a good choice if you have any of the indicators of leaky gut or ADD/ADHD listed in the table. The best book to accompany the GAPS diet is *Gut and Psychology Syndrome* by Dr. Campbell-McBride.

You may want to follow this diet if you have...

	MARKERS	TESTS
Blood	• antibodies associated with large proteins from foods like dairy, grains, shellfish, and nuts, and the proteins themselves (a Cyrex lab test can identify these) • high levels of zonulin (the compound that controls intestinal permeability) • high LPS (lipopolysaccharides)	There is a new blood test based on blood cell membrane potential that may indicate ADHD by testing your MPR ratio. You can order this blood test through your physician. A Cyrex food allergy panel (especially Array 10C) is excellent for identifying antibody reactions to specific food proteins.
Urine	• proteinuria	The urine albumin-to-creatinine ratio indicates if you have proteinuria. You can also order a urine test for proteinuria through your doctor or online through DirectLabs. An Intestinal Permeability (Leaky Gut) Kit by Genova can indicate whether you have a leaky gut.
Stool	• zonulin • alpha-1-antitrypsin • increased levels of colonic gram-negative *Enterobacteriales* • reduced levels of *Lactobacillus and Bifidobacterium* (although some recent evidence suggests that excessive levels of *Bifidobacterium* may contribute to ADHD)	You can order a stool test through your doctor or purchase a Microbiology Analysis online through Genova Diagnostics.
Genes	• the NOD2/CARD15 genetic mutation 3020insC (leaky gut, ADD/ADHD) • the ATG16L1 (autophagy-related 16 like 1) polymorphism rs2241880 (leaky gut, ADD/ADHD) • the IRGM (immunity-related GTPase M) polymorphisms rs13361189 and rs4958847 (leaky gut, ADD/ADHD) • the 7-repeat allele of the 48-base pair of the VNTR section of the DRD4 gene (ADD/ADHD) • the rs27072 polymorphism of the SLC6A3 gene (ADD/ADHD) • the rs1611115 polymorphism of the DBH gene (ADD/ADHD)	You can order a genetic test through 23andMe, then upload your raw data into a genetic analysis tool like StrateGene, Genetic Genie, FoundMyFitness, or MyHeritage. You can also get a more comprehensive analysis through services such as Bob Miller's TreeOfLife, The DNA Company, or Health Nucleus.
Symptoms	• irritable bowel syndrome • gastric ulcers • food allergies • small intestine bacterial overgrowth • infectious diarrhea • Crohn's disease • ulcerative colitis • other autoimmune diseases • a propensity to gain weight • lack of focus • low motivation • difficulty with organization • avoidance of activities that require sustained attention • forgetfulness	

A Sample Day of the GAPS Diet

For detailed recipes, instructions, and layout of the meal plan, visit BoundlessBook.com/21.

BREAKFAST	LUNCH	DINNER	SNACK
Sweet Potato Toast	Tomato Soup with Coconut and Curry	Keto Meatloaf	Cheesy Turmeric & Garlic Kale Chips

SWISS DETOX DIET / COLORADO CLEANSE

Both the Swiss Detox Diet, developed by Dr. Thomas Rau, and the Colorado Cleanse, developed by Dr. John Douillard, are comprehensive approaches to healing and detoxifying the gut, liver, and gallbladder. Both these programs are simple and consist of foods such as kitchari, olive oil, and celery juice.

If you need a liver or gallbladder cleanse, these protocols work well, and they can also be used as seven-to-fourteen-day jump-starts for any of the other diets in the beginner, intermediate, and advanced sections. They're good choices if you have any of the indicators of liver or gallbladder issues listed in the table. The best books to read to better understand the protocols and get more recipes are Dr. Thomas Rau's *The Swiss Secret to Optimal Health* and Dr. John Douillard's *Colorado Cleanse, Eat Wheat,* and *Body, Mind, and Sport.*

I am a big fan of using either of these protocols as a cleanse one or two times each year, especially when I am not traveling and can give my body a little extra rest and recovery. I also highly recommend a visit to the Swiss Mountain Clinic in the Swiss Alps for a done-for-you retreat that incorporates the Swiss Detox Diet; you can learn more about it at BenGreenfieldFitness.com/swissclinic. I've personally attended a complete colon and liver detox at this facility, which combines European biological medicine practices with a detox diet for treatment of excessive toxins and also Lyme, Parkinson's, mold and mycotoxin overload, cancer, and beyond.

You may want to follow this diet if you have...

	MARKERS	TESTS
Blood	• low or high levels of alanine transaminase • low or high levels of aspartate transaminase • low or high levels of alkaline phosphatase • low or high levels of bilirubin • low or high levels of albumin • low or high levels of gamma-glutamyl transferase • high white blood cell count • abnormal liver enzyme counts	Abnormal liver enzyme levels can indicate gallbladder inflammation resulting from gallstones. You can get a blood test that analyzes these markers through your doctor or order a Liver Profile, Complete from DirectLabs or a White Blood Cell (WBC) Count from LabCorp.
Urine	• dark urine • bilirubin • urobilinogen • abnormal levels of the enzymes amylase and lipase	You can order a urinary test through your doctor or use urine test strips easily available online to test for liver damage markers such as bilirubin and urobilinogen.
Stool	• pale or clay-colored stool (indicating low liver bile production or blocked liver bile ducts) • bloody or tar-colored stool (indicating potential liver failure) • yellow stool (indicating excessive bilirubin production) • higher levels of proteobacteria than *Firmicutes* (types of gut bacteria that can indicate nonalcoholic fatty liver disease) • fatty stool • bile acid diarrhea (may indicate liver or gallbladder dysfunction)	Some of these issues are detectable just by examining your stool's color, but to test for imbalanced gut bacteria and excess bile, you can also order the Genova Diagnostics Comprehensive Digestive Stool Analysis from your doctor or online from DirectLabs.
Genes	• the rs58542926 variant of the TM6SF2 gene • the rs2228603 variant of the NCAN gene for increased risk of NAFLD • the rs1799945 variant of the HFE gene for hereditary hemochromatosis (excessive iron absorption) and subsequent liver cirrhosis or liver failure • the rs20417 variant of the PTGS2 gene for increased risk of gallbladder cancer	You can order a genetic test through 23andMe, then upload your raw data into a genetic analysis tool like StrateGene, Genetic Genie, FoundMyFitness, or MyHeritage. You can also get a more comprehensive analysis through services such as Bob Miller's TreeOfLife, The DNA Company, or Health Nucleus.
Symptoms	• jaundice (yellowing of the skin and eyes) • abdominal pain, especially in the mid and upper-right section of the abdomen • swelling of the abdomen, legs, and ankles • vomiting • itchiness • loss of appetite • fever • chills • nausea • chronic fatigue	

A Sample Day of the Swiss Detox / Colorado Cleanse

For detailed recipes, instructions, and layout of the meal plan, visit BoundlessBook.com/21.

BREAKFAST	LUNCH	DINNER	SNACK
Chia Yogurt Custard	Rosemary, Squash & Pear Soup	Quinoa-Stuffed Eggplant	Maple Baked Apples

THE ELEMENTAL DIET

Should you need to pull out all the stops to manage gut inflammation, small intestinal bacterial overgrowth (SIBO), candida, yeast, fungus constipation, FODMAP sensitivities, or leaky gut, or if you simply want to push the reset button on digestion altogether, you can spend two to four weeks on an elemental diet. It's a good choice if you have the indicators of SIBO or FODMAP sensitivities listed in the table on page 616. Both SIBO and FODMAP sensitivities are discussed in detail in chapter 13.

The elemental diet is the simplest and, admittedly, most boring of all the beginner diet options. It involves consuming only a meal replacement powder for breakfast, lunch, and dinner, along with a few extra oils, fats, and amino acids for added nutrients. For your meal replacement drink, I recommend one or two servings of Thorne's Mediclear SGS. For each shake, I recommend that you add 10–20 g essential amino acids, along with a teaspoon or tablespoon of extra-virgin olive oil and MCT or coconut oil.

Most of my clients who follow this diet have had the best success blending the meal replacement powder with organic bone broth. I personally prefer this approach, and I add ice and vanilla-flavored liquid stevia so that each meal is like a giant bowl of ice cream. Should you want more variety, you can include soups, broths, and steamed vegetables in your evening meal. To learn more about the elemental diet, I recommend Dr. Allison Siebecker's website, SIBOInfo.com.

A note on testing for SIBO and FODMAPs sensitivity: SIBO on its own won't necessarily show up in a blood test. Instead, one of the most common tests for SIBO is a breath test, which measures the amount of gas produced by the bacteria. You can order this test online through QuinTron Breath Testing and perform it in the comfort of your own home. This test also evaluates your sensitivity to lactose and fructose, both of which are common FODMAPs. Two other relatively accurate SIBO tests are the Organix Dysbiosis test, which tests urine for signs of yeast and bacteria in the small intestine, and a stool analysis such as the Genova GI Effects panel, which can show elevated levels of all bacteria, a result that can be indicative of SIBO.

While looking at symptoms is important, constipation and diarrhea are symptoms of both FODMAP sensitivity and a host of other gastrointestinal problems, so when considered by themselves, these may not indicate FODMAPs sensitivity. It's more effective to look at the results of multiple types of tests, such as a breath test, as noted above, and a stool test and urine test (these are discussed in the table on page 616). Or, in the case of FODMAPs, you can simply eliminate the major triggers from your diet and observe how you feel—chapter 13 has a list of high-FODMAP foods to avoid.

You may want to follow this diet if you have...

	MARKERS		TESTS
Blood	• anti-CdtB antibody (indicator of IBS, which can be linked to FODMAPs) • anti-vinculin antibody (indicator of IBS, which can be linked to FODMAPs)		A food-sensitivity test and blood panel test for food particles could together indicate SIBO. Cyrex Labs offers food-sensitivity blood panels, such as the Array 10, Array 10-90, and Array 10-90x, as well as the Array 2 Intestinal Antigenic Permeability Screen. Just note that if you test positive for one of these panels, it doesn't necessarily mean that you have SIBO, especially if you lack other markers and symptoms. You can order the IBSchek Blood Test for Irritable Bowel Syndrome, which can indicate FODMAPs sensitivity, through Commonwealth Diagnostics International.
Urine	**SIBO (but may point to other GI problems as well)** • indican • high concentration of drug metabolites • conjugated para-aminobenzoic acid	**FODMAP sensitivity** • histamines (however, there aren't established levels that indicate sensitivity) • p-hydroxybenzoic acid • azelaic acid	Currently, there are no comprehensive urine panels that test for all the metabolites listed above, but the Organix Dysbiosis profile by Genova Diagnostics will test for many and can be quite useful for getting an overall snapshot of gut health.
Stool	• nasty, horrible-smelling, pale, and oily stools • fecal Reg 1β • fecal calprotectin		You can order a quantitative Fecal Fat test through LabCorp.
Genes	• There are no well-known genetic markers that predict or contribute to SIBO or FODMAP problems, but research suggests genotypes that contribute to underproduction of interleukin-1 receptor antagonist (IL1RN) may be associated with IBS-related SIBO.		A full microbiome analysis through Viome or Onegevity can tell you if you possess genes linked to high levels of methane-producing bacteria, which often go hand in hand with SIBO.
Symptoms	**SIBO** • abdominal bloating • gas • abdominal pain • food allergies or intolerances • brain fog • constipation • diarrhea	**FODMAP sensitivity** • gas • cramping • depression • fatigue • headaches • brain fog • constipation • diarrhea	

A Sample Day of the Elemental Diet

For detailed recipes, instructions, and layout of the meal plan, visit BoundlessBook.com/21.

BREAKFAST	LUNCH	DINNER	SNACK
Morning Smoothie	Steamed Broccoli	Mind, Body & Soul Vegetable Soup	Organic Applesauce

Intermediate

After following any of the beginner diets for eight to twelve weeks, your gut will be ready for a wider variety of foods. In this section, I'll introduce you to my favorite diets that are clean and easy to digest, primarily consist of real, whole foods, and are appropriate for most people.

Many of the diets below are low-carbohydrate or ketogenic. This is not because a ketogenic diet is perfect for everyone but because eating carbohydrates throughout the day can lead to blood sugar fluctuations and inflammation, and a low-carbohydrate or ketogenic approach is an excellent way to avoid this.

For athletes, extremely active individuals, and folks with the AMY1 gene variant (which allows them to consume more carbohydrates), I typically add a nightly or weekly carbohydrate refeed to the diets in this section. In a nightly refeed scenario, you eat 50–200 g (depending on your size and activity levels) of safe starches in the form of sweet potatoes, yams, taro, other tubers, parsnips, carrots, beets, rice, or properly prepared (either soaked, sprouted, or fermented) grains. In a weekly refeed scenario, you eat carbs ad libitum (without limit) one day a week, and on that day, carbs typically make up about 40 percent of your daily caloric intake.

THE WAHLS PROTOCOL (LOW-CARB VERSION)

After she was diagnosed with MS, Dr. Terry Wahls began studying food and vitamins and created a nutrient-rich, Paleo-esque diet. Within a year of changing her way of eating, she was out of her wheelchair and biking miles at a time.

On the Wahls Protocol, you eat lots of meat and fish, vegetables (especially green, leafy ones), brightly colored fruit like berries, and fat from animal and plant sources (especially omega-3 fatty acids), and you avoid dairy, eggs, grain, legumes, nightshades, and sugar. The low-carb version of the Wahls Protocol is especially good for managing autoimmune conditions while introducing a bit more variety than AIP. This diet can also work quite well for those with mast cell issues aggravated by mold and mycotoxins or Lyme, and for those with mitochondrial dysfunction or poor nervous system health overall. It's a good choice if you have any of the indicators of mast cell/histamine issues or Lyme, mold, or mycotoxin issues listed in the table. The best book to accompany this meal plan is *The Wahls Protocol* by Dr. Wahls.

You may want to follow this diet if you have...

	MARKERS		TESTS
Blood	• elevated levels of serum tryptase		Your physician can order a tryptase blood panel online through LabCorp. Lyme disease is tested for via a blood test that detects antibodies that fight the disease, and your physician can also order a Lyme disease antibodies test through LabCorp. For information on testing for mold exposure, revisit chapter 4.
Urine	• N-methylhistamine (the major metabolite of histamine and a sign of both mast cell/histamine and Lyme/mold/mycotoxin issues)		A 24-hour N-methylhistamine test is available online through LabCorp. To test for Lyme disease, you can order the Ceres Lyme Antigen test. For information on testing for mold exposure, revisit chapter 4.
Stool	There are no well-established stool markers for mast-cell-induced histamine problems, Lyme disease, or mold and mycotoxin exposure.		
Genes	• -1112C/T polymorphism of the interleukin-13 (IL13) promoter gene (associated with systemic mastocytosis, in which mast cells accumulate in high numbers) • CYP1A2 and CYP3A4 variations in the cytochrome P450 (CYP450) genes (indicate greater susceptibility to poisoning via mycotoxin exposure)		You can order a genetic test through 23andMe, then upload your raw data into a genetic analysis tool like StrateGene, Genetic Genie, FoundMyFitness, or MyHeritage. You can also get a more comprehensive analysis through services such as Bob Miller's TreeOfLife, The DNA Company, or Health Nucleus.

	Lyme disease	**Mold exposure**	**Mast cell/histamine issues**
Symptoms	• severe headaches • bull's-eye rash • neck stiffness • severe arthritis or joint swelling and pain • irregular heartbeat • loss of muscle tone	• brain fog • impaired memory, balance, and concentration • insomnia • anxiety • shortness of breath/asthma • eye irritation • headache • fatigue • skin irritation	• flushing • urticaria • diarrhea • wheezing • low blood pressure • shortness of breath • weight loss • enlarged lymph nodes

A Sample Day of the Wahls Protocol

For detailed recipes, instructions, and layout of the meal plan, visit BoundlessBook.com/21.

BREAKFAST	LUNCH	DINNER	SNACK
Spinach, Onion & Goat Cheese Omelet	Avocado, Apple & Chicken Salad	Balsamic Dijon–Glazed Beef Tenderloin with Chimichurri	Keto Deviled Eggs

THE PLANT PARADOX DIET

The Plant Paradox diet, developed by Dr. Stephen Gundry, eliminates lectins (a natural plant-based defensive protein that can cause gastric distress in many people and is found in foods such as green beans, lentils, and edamame) and limits sugar and polyunsaturated omega-6 fats. It also limits phytates, which are a source of energy for sprouting seeds; when people eat them in plants (as phytic acid), they bind to nutrients like manganese, iron, and zinc, making them indigestible and increasing your risk of being deficient in those minerals.

The Plant Paradox diet usually starts with a three-day cleanse, wherein you repopulate your gut bacteria with leafy greens, cruciferous vegetables, clean protein, and good fats, and then has a second phase in which you eat only from the list of approved foods for at least six weeks. Here, I've simplified the diet to skip the two phases and still give you a lectin-free protocol; this version also uses a ketogenic strategy to control blood sugar.

I recommend this diet if you want to eat a rich variety of vegetables but have difficulty digesting them and are sensitive to lectins, phytates, oxalates, and other built-in plant defense mechanisms—it lets you consume a diverse array of plants that are prepared in a manner that makes them easier to digest. It's a good choice if you have any of the indicators of plant-, legume-, or grain-digesting issues listed in the table. The best book to accompany this diet is Dr. Stephen Gundry's *The Plant Paradox*.

You may want to follow this diet if you have...

	MARKERS	TESTS
Blood	• blood TNF-alpha levels over 3 pg/mL • adiponectin levels over 16 mcg/mL • elevated interleukin-6 levels (the ideal range is 2 to 6 pg/mL) • fasting insulin below 2.5 uIU/mL (the lectin wheat germ agglutinin reduces insulin levels by increasing insulin binding) • white blood cell count below 5 K/uL • ferritin under 70 ng/mL for men and under 50 ng/mL for women • adiponectin levels over 16 ug/mL • free T3 under 3 nmol/L	Through LabCorp online, your physician can order TNF-alpha, white blood cell (WBC) count, and ferritin tests. Through DirectLabs, you can order adiponectin, interleukin-6 (IL-6), insulin, and free T3 (FT3) tests. Gluten sensitivities can be tested with the Cyrex Array 3X, which tests for a host of blood markers, including a variety of agglutinin- and gliadin-related antibodies. Through LabCorp, you or your physician can order tests for iron, zinc, and manganese—all of which may be low if you're consuming too many phytates, which prevent them from being absorbed. In addition, Cyrex has a host of panels that are highly accurate for food protein sensitivities, particularly their arrays 3, 4, 5, 6, 7, 8, 10, 11, and 12.
Urine	There are no well-established urinary markers or tests for lectin sensitivities, although research suggests that IgA nephropathy may be correlated with lectins found in wheat (but that requires a kidney biopsy to investigate!). There are also no urinary tests for gluten sensitivity, but the Gluten Detective test (available online) can determine whether you have consumed gluten within the previous 24 hours that's not being properly digested. If you eat gluten and some of it doesn't get digested, metabolites of it will eventually end up in your urine, so this test is helpful for determining compliance with a gluten-free diet and an inability to properly digest gluten. There are no publicly available urinary tests that determine if you are consuming high levels of phytic acid.	

	MARKERS	TESTS
Stool	• diarrhea • creatinine, lactulose, and mannitol levels (may indicate increased intestinal permeability)	While there are no well-established stool tests for lectin sensitivity, there are stool tests for IBS and IBD, and if you have these, a lectin-elimination diet may improve symptoms. Genova Diagnostics offers an Intestinal Permeability Assessment. LabCorp offers a Calprotectin, Fecal test that screens for Crohn's disease, and DirectLabs offers IBStatus, a comprehensive look at the overall health of your gastrointestinal tract. Celiac disease can be tested by measuring the levels of fat in your stool. Your doctor can order this test, or you can get LabCorp's Fecal Fat, Quantitative test. There are no well-established stool tests for excess phytic acid consumption.
Genes	• the rs1049353 variant of the CNR1 gene • the rs1801133 and rs1801131 variants of the MTHFR gene • the rs4680 variant of the COMT V158M gene • all variants of the SOD2 gene • the rs9891119 variant of the STAT3 gene • the rs10758669 variant of the JAK2 gene • the rs2395185, rs10484554, rs3135388, and rs3135391 variants of the MHC gene	You can order a genetic test through 23andMe, then upload your raw data into a genetic analysis tool like StrateGene, Genetic Genie, FoundMyFitness, or MyHeritage. You can also get a more comprehensive analysis through services such as Bob Miller's TreeOfLife, The DNA Company, or Health Nucleus.
Symptoms	**General concerns** • irritable bowel syndrome • Crohn's disease • colitis **Problems digesting lectins** • brain fog • systemic inflammation • abdominal pain or discomfort • nausea **Problems digesting gluten** • bloating • abdominal pain or discomfort • headaches • fatigue • diarrhea • constipation • skin rashes **Mineral deficiencies due to phytates** • paleness (iron deficiency) • dizziness (iron deficiency) • dry hair and skin (iron deficiency) • restless legs (iron deficiency) • anxiety (iron deficiency)	• headaches (iron deficiency) • fatigue (iron deficiency) • diarrhea (zinc deficiency) • hair loss (zinc deficiency) • poor immune function (zinc deficiency) • loss of appetite (zinc deficiency) • impaired glucose tolerance (manganese deficiency) • low fertility (manganese deficiency)

A Sample Day of the Plant Paradox Diet

For detailed recipes, instructions, and layout of the meal plan, visit BoundlessBook.com/21.

BREAKFAST	LUNCH	DINNER	SNACK
Homemade Maple Coconut Yogurt	Cilantro Lime Sardine Salad	Lemon Garlic Chicken Drumsticks	Parmesan Daikon Radish Fries

THE MEDITERRANEAN DIET (LOW-CARB VERSION)

The Mediterranean diet is a plant- and omega-3-rich diet that is prevalent in many longevity hot spots and Blue Zones (although it is possible that the diet's positive health effects may also be caused by lifestyle factors such as fasting, seasonal eating, social meals, high intake of tannin-rich beverages and wild plants, and limited meat consumption).

The ketogenic diet, which is described in chapter 13, is also prevalent in many hunter-gatherer and healthy ancestral populations and has been shown not only to induce effective weight loss but also to improve several cardiovascular risk parameters.

A ketogenic Mediterranean diet merges the well-known beneficial effects of the Mediterranean diet with the positive metabolic effects of a ketogenic diet. This approach can be particularly effective for managing cardiovascular conditions and improving heart health, along with overall health and longevity. It's a good choice if you have any of the indicators of cardiovascular issues listed in the table. An excellent book to accompany this plan is *The Ketogenic Mediterranean Diet* by Robert Santos-Prowse.

In addition to those outlined in the table, helpful tests for cardiovascular issues include a resting and exercise ECG, an echocardiogram, an MRI or CT scan, and a calcium scan score.

You may want to follow this diet if you have...

	MARKERS	TESTS
Blood	• abnormally high levels of cardiac troponins (indicates damage to the heart muscle) • high levels of hs-CRP (indicates inflammation and an increased risk of cardiac events) • high levels of B-type natriuretic peptide (BNP) and N-terminal-pro-BNP (indicates probable congestive heart failure) • elevated levels of lipoprotein phospholipase A2 (known to promote atherosclerosis)	Your physician can order tests for all these markers online through LabCorp.
Urine	• high levels of urinary protein and blood (indicates kidney damage, which, in turn, often causes high blood pressure)	Through LabCorp you can order a urinary Protein Total Quantitative test and Urinalysis, Routine with Microscopic Examination on Positives.
Stool	There are no well-established stool tests for determining cardiovascular disease or predicting cardiovascular events.	

	MARKERS	TESTS
Genes	• the rs429358 and rs7412 variants of the APOE gene (predict hyperlipoproteinemia, the accumulation of excess lipids and cholesterol in the blood) • the rs2200733 variant of the PITX2 gene (predicts atrial fibrillation, irregular heartbeat) • the rs8055236 variant of the CDH13 gene (predicts coronary artery disease, the blockage of coronary arteries) • the rs1746048 variant of the CXCL12 gene (predicts heart attacks) • the rs1051730 variant of the CHRNA3 gene (predicts peripheral arterial disease, the blockage of arteries to your limbs) • the rs1801133 variant of the MTHFR gene (predicts venous thrombosis, blood clotting) • the rs7961152 variant of the BCAT1 gene (predicts hypertension)	You can order a genetic test through 23andMe, then upload your raw data into a genetic analysis tool like StrateGene, MyHeritage, or Genetic Genie to determine if you carry any of these variants.
Symptoms	• chest pain, pressure, or tightness • shortness of breath • nausea • fatigue • faintness • cold sweats	• pain in the back, left shoulder, jaw, elbows, or arms • fluttering in the chest • racing heartbeat • pale gray or blue skin • swelling in the abdomen, legs, hands, ankles, feet, and around the eyes

A Sample Day of the Mediterranean Diet (Low-Carb)

For detailed recipes, instructions, and layout of the meal plan, visit BoundlessBook.com/21.

BREAKFAST	LUNCH	DINNER	SNACK
Jalapeño Bacon & Cheese Cauliflower Muffins	Salmon Arugula Salad with Creamy Balsamic Dressing	Macadamia-Encrusted Mahi Mahi with Cucumber Avocado Salsa	Keto Bacon Burger Bombs

Advanced

Although any of the intermediate meal plans can be followed indefinitely as a diet for life, I am a big fan of a more widely varied diet, especially if your gut is healthy and weight loss isn't your primary goal. If your blood glucose and inflammation are under control; your other labs, blood, and biomarkers look good; your body weight is where you want it to be; you've achieved full-body wellness and want to enjoy and experiment with as many foods as possible and even try eating according to your ancestry, any of the strategies from this section will work for you.

THE PALEO DIET

The Paleo diet is flexible and can be adapted for your specific needs, but it essentially cuts out modern agricultural foods that can cause an inflammatory reaction in many people and focuses on foods that our Paleolithic ancestors would likely have eaten, depending on seasonal availability.

One of the fundamental concepts behind Paleo is that humans were hunter-gatherers far longer than they've been farmers and cultivators. As a result, our genes evolved to favor the nutrient-dense plants and meats of those hunter-gatherers, not the high-sugar, high-dairy, high-refined-carb modern Western diet.

The standard Paleo diet includes meat (especially organ meats like liver and kidneys, bone broth, and marrow); high-quality animal fats; seafood; eggs (ideally pasture-raised); nonstarchy vegetables; low-glycemic-index fruits like berries, citrus, and stone fruits; coconut oil, olive oil, and avocado oil; nuts and seeds; and herbs and spices. The inflammatory foods excluded from the Paleo diet include grains like wheat, barley, oats, corn, and rice; dairy; refined sugar; processed foods; and vegetable oils (such as soybean, peanut, corn, and canola oils). Foods that are eaten in moderate amounts (if they are well-tolerated) include legumes like lentils and chickpeas and nightshades such as tomatoes, white potatoes, red potatoes, and peppers.

This diet would be very appropriate for someone sensitive to grains, legumes, and dairy who wants to expand their diet beyond AIP. Some research even suggests that type 2 diabetes may improve with a Paleo diet. This is because insulin resistance may be caused by inflammation, and the Paleo diet eliminates common inflammatory foods. It's a good choice if you have any of the indicators of dairy sensitivities, autoimmune disorders, or gut inflammation listed in the table. An excellent book on the Paleo diet is *The Paleo Solution* by Robb Wolf.

A note on dairy: You can consume dairy on a Paleo diet if you tolerate it well and it comes from grass-fed cows, which produce milk that is higher in anti-inflammatory omega-3 fatty acids and lower in inflammatory omega-6s. Grain-fed cows absorb gut-irritating lectins from their feed that are then concentrated in their milk, which can contribute to inflammation in people who consume that milk. Ideally, any milk consumed on a Paleo diet (or, in my opinion, any other diet) should be A2 milk, which has more A2 than A1 casein—A1 casein can produce significant gut inflammation in many individuals. The casein concentrations vary among different breeds of cows, with some breeds—such as Guernsey and Jersey cows—having very little to no A1 casein. You can find more details at A2Milk.com.

You may want to follow this diet if you have...

	MARKERS	TESTS
Blood	• lactose- or dairy-related antibodies (indicates dairy or lactose sensitivities) • markers for autoimmune diseases • bacterial cytotoxins and cytoskeletal proteins (associated with gut inflammation)	Cyrex offers the Array 10, Array 10-90, and Array 10-90X, which test for sensitivities to different forms of dairy, like goat's milk, hard and soft cheeses, and yogurt. LabCorp offers the Allergen Profile, Milk, IgE with Component Reflexes, which tests for sensitivity to cow's milk. Cyrex has five panels that screen for autoimmune disorders: the Array 5, 6, 7, 7X, and 8. For gut inflammation, Cyrex also offers an irritable bowel/SIBO screen that tests for bacterial cytotoxins and cytoskeletal proteins.

	MARKERS		TESTS
Urine	• proteinuria (may indicate an autoimmune disorder) • hematuria (may indicate an autoimmune disorder) • active sediment (may indicate an autoimmune disorder)		There are no well-established urine tests for dairy sensitivities, specific autoimmune disorders, or gut inflammation. However, DirectLabs offers a Urinalysis, Complete with Microscopic Examination, which measures the general markers for autoimmune disorders.
Stool	• lactic acid in stool (a sign of undigested, unabsorbed lactose in the gut) • fecal calprotectin (indicates gut inflammation, which may indicate an autoimmune disorder) • lactoferrin (indicates gut inflammation, which may indicate an autoimmune disorder)		LabCorp offers a pH, Stool test that screens for acidity in stool. DirectLabs offers a Calprotectin, Stool test that may indicate an autoimmune disorder such as Crohn's, celiac, lupus, or ulcerative colitis. LabCorp offers a Lactoferrin, Fecal, Quantitative test for gut inflammation.
Genes	If you lack these gene variants, it's likely you're genetically predisposed to be lactose intolerant: • the rs4988235 and rs182549 variants of the MCM6 gene in those of European ancestry • the rs1459469881 variant of the MCM6 gene in those of sub-Saharan African ancestry • the rs41380347 and rs41525747 variants of the MCM6 gene (regardless of ancestry)	For the long list of genes that predict autoimmune diseases and gut inflammation, see BoundlessBook.com/21. A sample, all for genes related to ulcerative colitis: • the rs76418789 variant in the IL23R gene • the rs4728142 variant in the IRF5 gene • the rs1830610 variant near the JAK2 gene • the rs1555791 variant near TNFRSF14 • rs6478108 in TNFSF15	You can order a genetic test through 23andMe, then upload your raw data into a genetic analysis tool like StrateGene, Genetic Genie, FoundMyFitness, or MyHeritage. You can also get a more comprehensive analysis through services such as Bob Miller's TreeOfLife, The DNA Company, or Health Nucleus.
Symptoms	**Dairy sensitivity** • diarrhea • nausea • vomiting • gas • bloating • abdominal pain • fatigue • psoriasis • rashes • headaches	**Autoimmunity** • diarrhea • nausea • vomiting • gas • weight fluctuations • bloating • abdominal pain • fatigue • headaches • rashes • lack of focus and concentration • swelling and redness • muscle aches • hair loss	**Gut inflammation** • diarrhea • gas • bloating • abdominal pain • new food intolerances and allergies • chronic fatigue • poor sleep • weight fluctuations • heartburn

* In addition to the markers in the table above, look for the grain and legume markers listed for the Plant Paradox diet on pages 619 to 620.

A Sample Day of the Paleo Diet

For detailed recipes, instructions, and layout of the meal plan, visit BoundlessBook.com/21.

BREAKFAST	LUNCH	DINNER	SNACK
Sweet Potato & Poblano Hash	Chopped Broccoli Salad with Balsamic, Walnuts & Cranberries	Beef Taco Stuffed Avocados	Basil & Peach Sherbert

THE WESTON A. PRICE DIET

In chapter 17, I talked about the Weston A. Price diet as the ultimate diet for increasing beauty and symmetry and ensuring you eat a full spectrum of fat-soluble vitamins. This diet is the closest representation of the way that my family and I eat, although we vary our selections widely based on what is in season, what I have hunted, what is available at the local farmers market, and where our travels take us. The best book to read to learn more about this diet is *Nourishing Traditions* by Sally Fallon. Follow this diet if you simply like to eat just about everything on God's green earth, and you're willing to take the time to prepare it using ancestral methods, including soaking, sprouting, and fermenting.

A Sample Day of the Weston A. Price Diet

For detailed recipes, instructions, and layout of the meal plan, visit BoundlessBook.com/21.

BREAKFAST	LUNCH	DINNER	SNACK
Tex-Mex Eggs Benedict with Grilled Potato Slabs & Avocado Lime Hollandaise	Avocado & Greek Yogurt Chicken Salad	Chili with Beef, Beans & Chicken Livers	Salt & Vinegar Sweet Potato Chips

THE ANCESTRAL DIET

There are a variety of ways in which you can customize the Weston A. Price diet to be specific to your ancestry—a concept explored in chapter 19. In the book *The Jungle Effect*, Dr. Daphne Miller explained the dietary wisdom of traditional cultures whose diets are specific to their genes and ancestry. In her research for the book (you can listen to my podcast with her, linked to on BoundlessBook.com/21), Miller traveled to locations around the world that she identified as "cold spots"— the opposite of hot spots!—that had a remarkably low incidence of diseases such as diabetes, heart disease, depression, colon cancer, breast cancer, and prostate cancer. It turned out that many of the traditional cultures in these areas ate whole-foods, Weston A. Price–like diets that were specific to their traditions, ancestry, and local environment. Many cold-spot inhabitants who relocate and switch to a modern Western diet develop the very diseases for which their traditional environments are cold spots!

The following are examples of cold spots and foods frequently eaten in their ancestral diets:

- Copper Canyon, Mexico (diabetes cold spot): corn, beans, squash, peppers, nopal cactus, onions, cilantro, tomatoes, jicama, nuts, avocados

- Crete (heart disease cold spot): olive oil, chickpeas, lentils, whole-grain pasta, potatoes, Swiss chard, kale, arugula, fish, red wine, figs, walnuts
- Iceland (depression cold spot): fish, walnuts, purslane, flaxseed oil, barley, rye, black tea, beans, split peas, potatoes, organic dairy products, omega-3-enriched eggs, wild game, cabbage, bilberries
- Cameroon, West Africa (colon cancer cold spot): millet, teff, collard greens, mustard greens, spinach, okra, plantains, beans, nuts, fish, wild poultry and game, onions, tomatoes, bananas, yogurt, kefir, fermented vegetables
- Okinawa, Japan (breast and prostate cancers cold spot): tofu, tempeh, miso, fish, cabbage, bok choy, broccoli, kale, cauliflower, brown rice, green tea, sea vegetables, sweet potatoes, mushrooms, tomatoes, watermelons, grapefruit

For more information, read Dr. Miller's book. Two other very good titles on ancestral eating are Dr. Michael Smith's *Returning to an Ancestral Diet* and Stephen Le's *100 Million Years of Food*. Follow this eating plan if you know your genetics and family history, and you simply want to eat more like your ancestors!

In my opinion, a whole-foods diet that adheres to Weston A. Price principles and incorporates the traditional foods your ancestors ate is ideal for health, cognition, performance, fertility, and longevity—and this is how I eat when I'm home and have ample time for meal prep and cooking.

THE ULTIMATE BIOHACKED DIET

When I have an especially busy day that demands more of me both cognitively and physically, I often fall into what I call the "Ultimate Biohacked Diet." It blends ancestral foods with modern science, skips lunch, and incorporates a neural-enhancing, nutrient-dense, relatively simple dietary approach consisting of the following groups:

- **Meals:** primarily meat, wild-caught fish, bone broth, bitter greens, and wild plants— some of the most nutrient-dense foods you can find
- **Beverages:** black and green tea, red wine, and coffee—all chock-full of antioxidants and longevity-enhancing compounds
- **Supplements:** exogenous ketones, fish oil, creatine, essential amino acids
- **Nootropics:** a microdose of psilocybin blended with lion's mane mushrooms and niacin (a mind-bending, productivity-enhancing, brain-spinning stack made popular by mushroom expert and mycology researcher Paul Stamets)

Here's how a sample day looks on this diet:

- **Morning supplements:** creatine, fish oil, mushroom stack
- **Breakfast:** Salmon and dandelion greens with green tea; or sardines or anchovies over mixed greens with green tea; or a green smoothie; or a fatty coffee blended with mushrooms
- **Snack:** 1 cup of bone broth; or exogenous ketones and essential amino acids mixed into water
- **Lunch:** fasting—black coffee only
- **Preworkout:** 1 cup of bone broth, exogenous ketones, and essential amino acids, or a Kion clean energy bar

- **Dinner:** Celebration of a day of hard work with a bone-in, grass-fed, grass-finished rib-eye steak accompanied by red wine and nettle leaves or other wild plants; or, alternatively, salmon on a bed of roasted vegetables. If I worked out, I usually include a serving of a safe starch, such as sweet potatoes, yams, beets, taro, parsnip, or white rice. I'll often also include hefty doses of Dr. Thomas Cowan's vegetable powders because they are a fast way to get nutrient-dense plant extracts without much chopping or food prep.

I've found this approach to work quite well on cognitively demanding days when I'm at home, when my wife and children are gone, and when I need to buckle down and tackle a good twelve to sixteen hours of deep work, which I occasionally do.

Finally, I'm often asked about what I personally eat. Though I often travel and immerse myself in the local cuisine wherever I happen to be, at home my diet tends to be a mash-up of the bio-hacked diet above when busy and a Weston A. Price approach when I can—along with one or two yearly cleanses or detoxification protocols, a daily twelve-to-sixteen-hour intermittent fast, and a weekly twenty-four-hour fast. That's it.

THE BOUNDLESS SUPPLEMENT PROGRAM

Due to the inherent complexity of the human body, this section was difficult for me to write. In an ideal world, you would be able to fully customize every supplement you take to your unique physiology rather than following a cookie-cutter program. But in my coaching, consulting, research, and experimentation, I've developed supplementation protocols that paint with a relatively broad brush and cover most bases for beginner, intermediate, and advanced goals, as you'll see below.

Beginner

This is for you if you are on a budget, want the lowest-hanging fruit to give you 80 percent of the results with 20 percent of the expense and effort, or need the minimum effective dose of supplementation to look, feel, and perform as good as possible each day. Include:

- A multivitamin-multimineral complex, such as the Thorne Multi
- A good fish oil, such as Living Fuel SuperEssentials or Thorne—2–3 g per day with a meal
- Creatine—5 g per day, taken with a meal or smoothie or another beverage, split into two 2.5 g servings (one in the morning, one in the evening). The brand is not important as long as there are no added sweeteners or fillers. I prefer Thorne Creapure.
- If you are traveling or unable to eat a wide range of plants, greens powder such as Athletic Greens, Organifi Greens, or Living Fuel SuperGreens
- If you are injured, a natural anti-inflammatory such as Kion Flex or Thorne Meriva (see chapter 12)
- If you have difficulty sleeping, 200–500 mg magnesium, 50–100 mg CBD, or 1–2 packets of Sleep Remedy in the evening before bed (see chapter 7)
- If you have gut issues or are unable to eat a wide variety of fermented foods, a good probiotic and gut support blend, such as Seed Probiotic or Thorne Bio-Gest (see chapter 13)

Intermediate

This is for you if you have a slightly higher budget and want to add supplements that can further enhance performance, longevity, and mental function without necessarily breaking the bank. Follow the beginner protocol and add the following:

- 10–20 g of essential amino acids (EAAs) per day—preferably pre- or postworkout without a meal

- Prior to your largest meal or largest carb-containing meal of the day, insulin-stabilizing foods or supplements like bitter melon extract, Ceylon cinnamon, apple cider vinegar, berberine, rosemary, turmeric, ginger, fenugreek, *Gymnema sylvestre*, or cayenne

- On more cognitively demanding days, caffeine or green tea blended with stabilizing compounds such as L-theanine, tulsi, or astragalus (see chapter 5)

- Once or twice a year, use any of the detoxification systems from Dr. Pompa, Dr. Shade, or Dr. Walsh described toward the end of chapter 13.

Advanced

This is for you if you are willing to invest in better living through science so you can live as long as possible and perform at a high level, and you desire to incorporate a full-blown boundless supplements protocol. Follow the intermediate protocol and add the following:

- Qualia, TianChi, nicotine, or another nootropic stack or adaptogenic herb blend on more cognitively demanding days (see chapter 5)

- Immune support via mushroom blends in your morning coffee or tea and oregano oil in your morning or evening water (see chapter 15)

- Ketone salts or ketone esters for longer workouts or longer periods of fasting, especially on more-active days

- Occasional microdoses of psilocybin, LSD, or other psychedelics (see chapter 5)

- Hydrogen-rich water (whether you dissolve tablets in water, purchase canned hydrogen-rich water, or use a hydrogen water–generating machine)

- Several times per week in a morning or midday smoothie: rhodiola, colostrum, chlorella, marine phytoplankton, aloe vera, coffeeberry fruit extract, frozen broccoli sprouts, and moringa. You can also include other sirtuin-supporting foods from chapter 19 in the smoothie, such as blueberries, cacao powder or cacao nibs, black currant powder, turmeric, or green tea extract.

- Daily supplementation with longevity-supporting compounds, including CoQ10, PQQ, glutathione, rapamycin or metformin, pterostilbene, MitoQ, astragalus, C60, nicotinamide riboside (NR), and SkQs (see chapter 19)

Finally, at my company, Kion, I am currently developing a suite of flagship formulations that will allow you to get all the supplements above in a minimum number of products. Over the next three years, you will see appearing at Kion complete, done-for-you formulas for the following seven needs: gut and digestion, longevity and mitochondria, joints and recovery, weight management and blood sugar control, hormone balance, sleep, and immunity. Once each of these supplement formulas is fully developed, you will no longer need to venture to the four corners of the planet to hunt down everything you need for supplementation. I highly recommend you subscribe to the newsletter at GetKion.com to receive an instant alert each time I release a new formulation.

CONCLUSION

Congratulations. You are now fully equipped to be boundless.

We began this book asking important questions about how to truly get the most out of life and live a life as fulfilling, adventurous, and joyful as possible, imagining what would be possible if you and I could leap out of bed each morning and tackle the day with the extreme ferocity of an electrified tiger; envisioning what we would be capable of if not just our bodies but also our minds and our spirits were fully optimized and firing on all cylinders; conceiving the possibility of walking around with the body of a finely tuned superhero, the mind of a professional poker player, and the spirit of an enlightened monk—able to speed-read, memorize cards, remember the names of everyone at the cocktail party, wear any jeans we want, step onto a beach with our chests out and abs in, age gracefully without Botox and liposuction, and have an intense feelings of peace, love, joy, happiness, and true satisfaction, purpose, and meaning in life.

The ability to look, feel, and perform at the human body's full capacity isn't the stuff of lore—it's all completely attainable. You really can have it all: total optimization and holistic balance of body, mind, and spirit. And now you know exactly how to get there.

Come back and visit this book regularly. Consider it your cookbook for looking good naked, performing at peak capacity, upgrading your brain, living a long time, and discovering—using the perfect blend of ancestral wisdom and modern science—true purpose, happiness, and the boundless energy that flows through all of us.

Connect with that boundless energy, nourish it, feel it, taste it, and experience it for the rest of your long and fulfilled life, and share this message and the strategies you've discovered with as many people as you can (feel free to use #beboundless if you'd like!).

Finally, let's face it: the world is constantly changing—new scientific breakthroughs occur, new secrets of our ancestors are unearthed, and knowledge we once accepted as orthodox and established is replaced by even better research and more up-to-date ideas. To help you keep your finger on the pulse of everything that it takes to continue your boundless journey, here are a few resources for you.

BoundlessBook.com

All resources, links, blogs, podcast, articles, studies, downloads, books, and (literally) hundreds of pages of additional content and science are all available on this official *Boundless* website.

Facebook.com/ BGFitness

Each week, I publish photos, short articles, giveaways, caption contests, controversial stories and other items guaranteed to make you a smarter, more productive, healthier human.

GetKion.com

My company for products, coaching, and solutions that empower you to live a more adventurous, joyful, and fulfilling life. Anytime I create a new supplement—including flagship formulations for longevity, digestion, brain, sleep, recovery, hormones, weight management, and beyond—you will find it here. I also have a mentoring program called KionU, where personal trainers, physicians, nutritionists, and other health professionals can become certified in all my advanced coaching methods (you can apply to join at GetKion.com/become-a-kion-coach).

BeyondTrainingBook.com

This is the website for my *New York Times* bestselling book on striking the ideal balance between performance, health, and longevity. You can also visit my Amazon author page to see all the other books I've written on subjects from triathlon training to low-carb diets to raising superhuman kids.

YouTube.com/ BenGreenfieldFitness

On YouTube, you can find videos on subjects such as ice-cold showers, ways to boost testosterone, and cognitive enhancement, along with product reviews, free conference talks, and much more.

Twitter.com/ BenGreenfield

On a daily basis, I use this platform to tweet science, research, articles, and any other fascinating snippets I find.

Instagram.com/ BenGreenfieldFitness

Entertaining and inspirational photos and videos, along with behind-the-scenes stories from my family and me. This is where you'll find raw, live footage of everything from feeding goats to cooking new recipes to brewing coffee enemas.

BenGreenfieldFitness.com

Once a week, I publish a new long-form article similar to the chapters in this book, and twice a week I post a podcast in which I answer listener questions and interview the world's leading experts in biohacking, nutrition, fitness, self-improvement, longevity, and beyond.

As you already know if you've read all of *Boundless*, my clear and distinct purpose is to empower people just like you to live a more adventurous, joyful, and fulfilling life—to discover and unlock their boundless energy. I trust that this book has done just that for you.

Now go forth and be boundless!

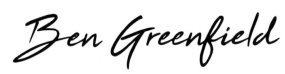

ACKNOWLEDGMENTS

I first conceived of the idea for *Boundless* four years ago, and I admit: I initially thought that writing an all-encompassing book on mind, body, and spirit optimization would be a far easier task than it turned out to be. Heck, if you're reading this, you know that it's a bit of a monster, this book. It's big. It's comprehensive. It's steeped in science. As a result, its writing spanned over three years, and even after it was complete there were plenty of additions and edits that I'm certain wound up driving my editing team and publisher absolutely batshit crazy.

But I made—no, *we* made it. I never would have finished this book had it not been for an amazing team of supportive individuals who provided me with advice, direction, and plenty of heavy lifting throughout the entire process.

First, I'm thankful to my wife, Jessa, and our boys, River and Terran—the former for graciously smiling and putting up with me when I'd whip out my laptop on family vacations and slip away to the basement on early mornings to work on the book, and the latter for inspiring me to become boundless so that I'm able to chase them, play with them, see them grow up, and meet their children and perhaps, if I practice everything within the book, their children's children.

I'm also grateful for Alex, my go-to handyman for research and editing throughout the entire book project, as well as dear Marge and Jojo for their support and hard work on research and website.

Penny, James, and Kristina were integral throughout the launch of the book, planning out all the nitty-gritty details that would have driven me insane—from promotions to marketing and beyond.

This book would also have never happened without the encouragement, direction, and inspiration of my entire team at Kion, most notably my friend and CEO Angelo, but also the phenomenal team of Jillian, Kelsey, James, Hayden, Kirk, Jordan, Kim, Mike, and Brandon.

The team at Victory Belt, including Erich, Erin, Lance, and Susan, was a dream to work with on my book *Beyond Training* and continued their pattern of success and support throughout the creation of *Boundless*. And yes, not only am I grateful for you, but I'm sorry for all those emails, questions, and demands, including the last-minute edits whenever I'd find yet another tip or fact I wanted to add to the book!

My thanks to Kate, for teaching me so much about the book publishing industry and providing so much support along the way. My thanks to JJ Virgin, for conceptualizing the concept of boundless energy and inspiring the title *Boundless*. And my thanks to all those brilliant minds I learn so much from: Dr. Cook, Dr. Koniver, Dr. Mercola, Dr. Pompa, Dr. Shah, and so many others.

To my dear dad and mom, thank you for making me read, write, and type so damn much when I was a kid. Even though I hated that little red pen you always used, it turns out that it has molded me into a bit of an author, and for that, I'm eternally grateful.

Finally, I thank God, for breathing the boundless breath of life into me, and I thank you, my reader, for taking the daring plunge into becoming boundless yourself. May your journey be blessed.

INDEX

hordenine HCL, 96

hormetic stress, antiaging and, 502–509

hormone regulation
  fat burning and imbalances in, 178
  insulin and, 169

hormone testing, 402–403

household cleaners, 586, 588–589

HPA axis
  fixing, 47
  stress and, 43–47

HRV (heart rate variability), 170–171

hs-CRP (high-sensitivity C-reactive protein), 393–394

huperzine, in brain-boosting stacks, 106

hydration
  immune system and, 352
  sex and, 465
  sleep and, 131, 157

hydrogen-rich water, antiaging and, 504–505

hygiene hypothesis, 371

hyperbaric oxygen therapy (HBOT)
  antiaging and, 503
  for recovery, 250

hyperthermia therapy, antiaging and, 507–508

hypothyroidism, fat burning and, 181

I

ibogaine, 110

ibuprofen, 262–263

IGF-1 (insulin-like growth factor 1), 399

immune responses, insulin and, 169

immune system
  about, 344–350
  aging and, 487
  building, 351–386
  mind, 375–386
  sex and, 456
  sleep and, 131

incline treadmill, 232–233

inflammation
  aging and, 485
  fat burning and, 164–166
  leaky brain and, 37–38
  reducing, 55

infrared sauna
  about, 237–238
  for recovery, 253–254

injections, for antiaging, 524–529

inositol, 36

insulin
  benefits of, 169
  self-quantification and, 399
  insulin-like growth factor 1 (IGF-1), 399

intelligence, 558

inversion, for recovery, 256

inversion table, 230

iodine
  children and, 338
  plant-based diet and, 329

Iris software, 574

iron
  absorption of, 329
  children and, 339
  self-quantification and, 401–402

isotopically fortified organic compounds, 553

J

jump rope, 221

K

kale, as brain food, 83

Kaolin clay, 451

keg, 229

kelp powder, 451

ketamine, 110–111

keto flu, 320

ketogenic diet, 315–326

ketone esters, antiaging and, 511, 514

ketones
  about, 28
  testing, 410–411

ketosis, 10, 75–76

kettlebell, 221

Kundalini energy, 49–50

L

lard, 59

L-ascorbic acid, 451

L-deprenyl (Selegiline), 89

leaky brain
  fixing, 34–40
  symptoms of, 33–34

LEDs, 570–571

legumes
  longevity and, 492
  plant-based diet and, 329

life purpose, longevity and, 496, 557

light
  about, 570
  biohacks for, 572–577
  LEDs, 570–571
  natural, 571

light-blocking tape/stickers, 575

lighting
  choosing, 572–573
  radiation from, 568

lion's mane, in brain-boosting stacks, 105–106

lipopolysaccharides (LPS), 70–71

lithium orotate, 101

LiveO2, 236–237

longevity
  about, 477–479
  advanced biohacks and strategies for, 499–554
  habits for enhancing, 487–499
  how we age, 480–487
  muscle building and, 184–187
  quantifying aging, 555–559

LPS (lipopolysaccharides), 70–71

LSD, 109

L-theanine
  about, 98
  in brain-boosting stacks, 105
  sleep and, 150–151

lymph flow, 351–354

M

maca, 459

macadamia nut oil, 59

machine vision/sensing, 553

macronutrients, sex and, 464–465

magnesium
  for antiaging, 547–548
  ketogenic diet and, 321
  leaky brain and, 37
  for recovery, 264–265, 266
  sex and, 461
  sleep and, 150
  sources of, 81

magnesium threonate, 101

magnets, for recovery, 249–250

manosphere, 473–474

manual treadmill, 434

MAO (monoamine oxidase), 13

MAOA gene, 25, 26

MAOB gene, 26

marine phytoplankton, for antiaging, 521–522

massage, immune system and, 353

mat, 434

mattresses, for sleep, 446–447

maximum mitochondrial density, 209, 211

maximum muscular endurance, 207

MCT oil
  about, 28
  ketogenic diet and, 321–322

Medical Doctor (MD), 416

medicine ball, 223

Mediterranean diet, 621–622

melatonin
  about, 146–147
  for antiaging, 542
  sleep and, 150, 156–157

memory, creatine and, 24

menstrual periods, sex and, 457

mesenchymal stem cells (MSCs), 243–246

metabolic acidosis, 202

testosterone, 397–399, 462–463

testosterone optimization therapy, 474–475

thiamine
about, 27
plant-based diet and, 329

thieves oil, 354–356

3-D bioprinting, of tissues/organs, 553

thymus, antiaging and, 527–528

thyroid function, insulin and, 169

TianChi, in brain-boosting stacks, 107

tire, 229

toxins
about, 19–20
fat burning and, 179

traditional Chinese nootropics, 91

traditional global nootropics, 94

training, two-week plan, 214–217

training mask, 224

trans fats, 67

travel
with EMF protection, 569
sleep and, 155–158

triglycerides, 394–396

triglyceride-to-HDL ratio, 394–395

TrueForm treadmill, 233

tryptophan, 149

tulsi, in brain-boosting stacks, 105

turmeric, as brain food, 84

U

Ultimate Biohacked Diet, 626–627

UltraMind Solution Companion Guide, 17

umbilical stem cells, for antiaging, 518–519

undermethylation, 486

underwater audio player, 228

uridine monophosphate, 95

urinary system, aging and, 482

urine testing
about, 74, 334
for autoimmune Paleo diet (AIP), 609–610
for elemental diet, 616
for Gut and Psychology Syndrome (GAPS) Diet, 612
for Mediterranean diet, 621
for Paleo diet, 624
for the Plant Paradox diet, 619
for Specific Carbohydrate Diet (SCD), 611
for Swiss Detox Diet and Colorado Cleanse, 614
for the Wahls Protocol, 618

urolithin A, for antiaging, 544

UVA/UVB radiation, antiaging and, 508–509

V

vagus nerve, leaky brain and, 37

vanillin, 91

vaporizer, 93

Vasper, 234–235

vegetables, cruciferous, 178

VersaClimber, 232

vibration therapy, 248, 351

vibration trainer, 234

vinpocetine, 96

visualization, 380–381

vitamin A
about, 72
body symmetry and, 424
children and, 339

vitamin B supplements, 22, 23, 36

vitamin B_1, 99

vitamin B_3, 99

vitamin B_5, 99

vitamin B_6, 22, 23, 36, 100

vitamin B_{12}
about, 22, 23, 36, 100
children and, 339
plant-based diet and, 330

vitamin C, 72, 100
children and, 340
immune system and, 366–367
for recovery, 258–259

vitamin D
for antiaging, 547–548
body symmetry and, 424–425
children and, 340
plant-based diet and, 330
sex and, 461
sleep and, 145, 151

vitamin D_3, 100

vitamin E, 425

vitamin K, 461

vitamin K_2
body symmetry and, 424
children and, 340

vitamins, water and, 594

VO_2 max, 210

W

Wahls Protocol, 617–618

walking speed, 556

walnut oil, 59

walnuts, as brain food, 83

water
about, 590
best practices, 593–594
deuterium-depleted water (DDW), 591
exclusion zone (EZ), 591
filtering, 178

water filters, 593

weight training
about, 188–189
for genitals, 462

weighted backpack, 222

weighted vest, 222

Weston A. Price diet, 423–426, 625

white blood cell count, 556

Wim Hof breathing, 53–54

wireless router, 568

Wnt pathways, 553

women
sex and, 459
testosterone and, 462–463

workplace, body symmetry and, 433–439

X

X3 bar, 231–232

Y

yeast, 290–292

yoga, 381

yoga trapeze, 229–230

yogurt, 364–365

yohimbine, 460

Z

zinc
children and, 339
immune system and, 358–359
sex and, 461
sleep and, 150
sources of, 81

zinc picolinate, 101